GERIATRIC NUTRITION

CLINICAL GUIDANCE FOR NUTRITIONAL NEEDS AND INTERVENTIONS

José Adán Amaya Duarte and
Kareling Alexandra López Sandoval

ALLIED HEALTH PRESS

Geriatric Nutrition: Clinical Guidance for Nutritional Needs and Interventions

Authors: **José Adán Amaya Duarte and Kareling Alexandra López Sandoval**

Allied Health Press
4164 Lakeshore Road
Burlington ON L7L 1A4
Canada
www.alliedhealthpress.com
Email: orders@arclereducation.com

ISBN: 978-1-77956-834-2

Allied Health Press publishes wide variety of books and eBooks. For more information about Allied Health Press and its products, visit our website at www.alliedhealthpress.com

ABOUT THE AUTHORS

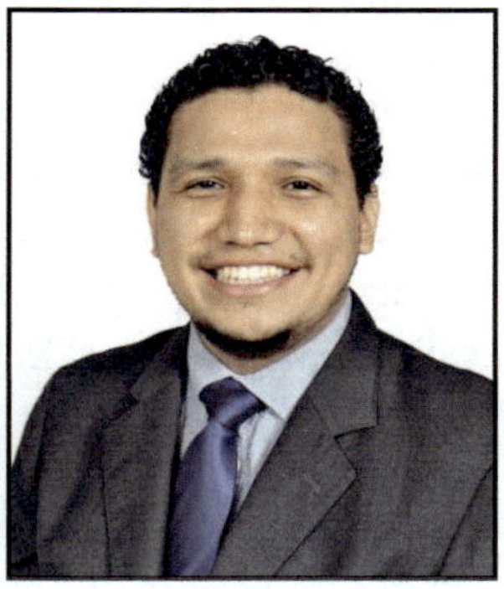

José Adán Amaya Duarte is a medical doctor, academic consultant, and entrepreneur with extensive experience in the industrial, educational, and public health sectors. He currently serves as General Manager (CEO) and co-founder of INVALA S.A., a manufacturing company in Nicaragua, where he has led operational and financial development since 2019.

With a medical degree from UNAN-León, where he also worked as a university professor and research assistant, his profile combines scientific rigor with advanced managerial skills. He also has worked as a medical academic content consultant on global platforms such as Upwork and as a technical advisor and instructional designer for the Pan American Health Organization (PAHO/WHO), participating in multiple virtual training projects, course design, and the updating of pedagogical health content.

In the academic field, he has served as an online tutor, academic coordinator, and designer of educational materials, including audiovisual media, for the Virtual Campus of Public Health. He has also conducted workshops and collaborated in international seminars on topics such as Biofabrication, anatomy, environmental toxicology, educational innovation, and human resource management.

Adán is fluent in English (advanced level) and has basic knowledge of German. In addition, he possesses strong skills in digital tools, ERP/CRM systems, data analysis (SPSS), audiovisual editing, and basic programming (AS3, Swift, Java). His multidisciplinary approach and leadership capacity position him as an influential figure at the intersection of medicine, virtual education, and business management.

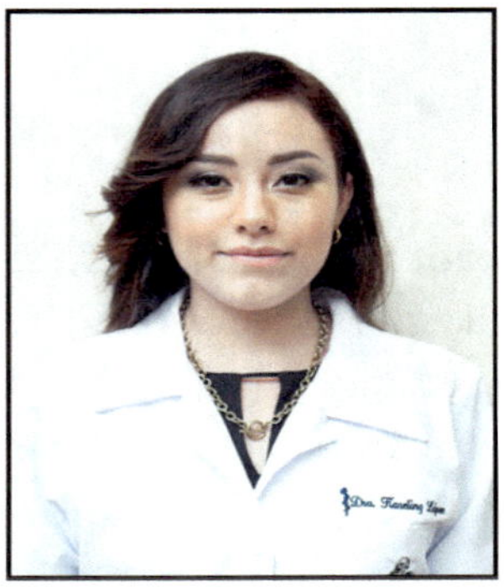

Kareling Alexandra López Sandoval is a medical doctor with experience in clinical care, healthcare operations supervision, and medical translation. She currently serves as Clinical Operations Supervisor at Oclinicals/GI Alliance, coordinating remote teams and maintaining direct communication with clinics in the United States to ensure high standards of patient care.

Graduated as a Doctor of Medicine and Surgery from the National Autonomous University of Nicaragua (UNAN-León), Kareling has worked across various medical areas, developing solid skills in patient assessment, diagnosis, and education. Her career includes roles in both hospital and remote settings, allowing her to adapt to diverse healthcare environments.

In the academic and scientific communication field, she has worked as a medical content reviewer for academic texts, medical article writer based on scientific evidence, and translator of medical documents (Spanish English) with technical accuracy. Her C2-level English proficiency has enabled her to collaborate on international projects, ensuring terminological precision and effective communication with global healthcare teams.

With a combination of clinical training, operational expertise, and medical communication skills, Kareling stands out for her commitment to quality, self-discipline, and continuous improvement in the healthcare sector.

Brief Table of Contents

Detailed Table of Contents

CHAPTER 3

Carbohydrate, Fat, and Fluid Requirements in Older Adults 63

CHAPTER 4

Vitamin Nutrition in Older Adults 87

CHAPTER 7

Smell, Taste, and Oral Somatosensation: Age-Related Changes and Nutritional Implications 179

CHAPTER 8

Aging Gut 211

CHAPTER 11

Dietary Guidelines for the Elderly 307

CHAPTER 12

Supplement Use and Nutrient Interactions in Geriatric Nutrition 333

CHAPTER 13

Screening for Geriatric Nutritional Risk 363

CHAPTER 14

Geriatric Sarcopenia and Nutrition in the Case of Cachexia before Exitus 393

CHAPTER 15

Geriatric Nutrition in the Prevention and Treatment of Disease 427

LIST OF FIGURES

PREFACE

Aging is followed by numerous alterations in the composition of the body, its energy needs, and its economy with which nutrients are used. Lean tissue declines and fat mass increases with age, thus altering the load placed upon diet and lifestyle. The capacity to absorb, transport, and utilize vitamins, minerals, proteins, and other nutrients in the diet alters over time. These alterations are a result of changes in the synthesis of digestive enzymes, transit time of the gut, and organ function. Apart from the physical alterations, the hormonal alterations influence appetite, sensitivity of taste, and the body's signals of thirst and satiety. All these alterations combined serve to generate unique challenges in meeting nutritional needs later in life.

Increased than simply increasing caloric intake or supplements are required to maintain health during the latter part of life. Dietary programs must be formulated from a sense of the effects of aging on metabolism, immune function, and tissue-repair machinery, holding tissue integrity. The senses governing food selection, taste, smell, oral sensitivity, can become less sensitive, reducing foods' appeal that tasted appealing before. Digestive tract function can become slower, resulting in inadequate absorption of necessary nutrients. Fluid balance is also less secure when the sense of thirst is diminished, and the kidneys' water-retaining ability is lost. A complete dietary regimen must then consider quality as well as quantity, in terms of the ratio of proteins, carbohydrates, fats, vitamins, minerals, and water which will be used to maintain day-to-day function, as well as long-term health.

This text, *Geriatric Nutrition: Clinical Guidance for Nutritional Needs and Interventions*, synthesizes the latest information on how aging alters the body's regulation of nutrients. It gives simple guidance on dietary intake in older individuals, explains how nutritional risk is measured, and distills interventions that can prevent or delay age-related disease. Physicians, nutritionists, and home care workers will learn how to plan meals, choose supplements, and track status in a way that optimizes strength, cognition, and general health throughout the aging process.

- Chapter 1 lays a comprehensive foundation by setting the framework of geriatric nutrition. Body composition changes, energy expenditure, and macronutrient and micronutrient functions are addressed. The influence of aging on the gastrointestinal tract, endocrine activity, and muscle protein turnover is specifically addressed. The reader will gain an understanding of why nutritional needs shift and how they can be assessed using anthropometry, biochemical markers, and functional tests.
- Chapter 2 focuses on older protein metabolism and requirements. It explains how synthesis rates in muscles, amino acid oxidation, and protein turnover vary with age. The chapter

compiles evidence for increased protein requirement to maintain lean body mass, discusses optimal phasing and timing of protein intake, and discusses the benefit of multiple sources of protein, including plant, dairy, and fortified foods.

- Chapter 3 addresses the needs of carbohydrate, fat, and fluid. It explains the changes in glucose tolerance, lipid control, and insulin sensitivity with time, and formulates recommendations on the use of complex carbohydrates to maintain stable blood sugar levels. The chapter also addresses the role of the essential fatty acids in heart and brain function and addresses the necessity of maintaining fluid consumption in order to maintain renal function and prevent dehydration.
- Chapter 4 covers vitamin nutriture, including the ways that absorption and tissue levels of fat-soluble and water-soluble vitamins can decline. Each vitamin is covered in terms of function, status indicators, food sources, and dangers of insufficiency. Special focus is given to vitamins D and B12, which are too frequently less than ideal in older adults, and to the realities of options for foods and fortification.
- Chapter 5 considers mineral requirements, from phosphorus and calcium to build healthy bones, through to sodium and potassium to control blood pressure. It discusses how changes in renal function and hormonal regulation that come with aging may influence mineral equilibrium. Chapter 5 provides guidance on how to achieve adequate mineral supply via diet and, where necessary, supplements.
- Chapter 6 covers trace metals—iron, zinc, selenium, copper—and their roles in antioxidant protection, immune defense, and enzymatic function. It discusses how absorption efficacy can differ, the impact of chronic illness on trace metal status, and the risks of deficiency and excess. The chapter offers recommendations for achieving balance through diet selection and monitoring.
- Chapter 7 explains changes in smell, taste, and oral somatosensation. Impairments in olfactory and gustatory function with age and tactile sensitivity of the mouth can reduce hunger and affect food choice. The chapter explains mechanisms for sensory loss, its nutritional effect, and ways to alter flavor and texture to promote adequate intake.
- Chapter 8 covers the ageing gut, ranging from alterations in the microbiome population to changes in the gut barrier function and motility. The chapter reviews how these factors impact nutrient absorption, immune signaling, and systemic inflammation. It also covers mechanisms for enhancing gut health with dietary fiber, probiotics, and other functional foods.
- Chapter 9 integrates macronutrient and micronutrient needs into an analysis of common deficiencies among the elderly. It identifies risk factors, prevalence rates, and clinical signs of nutrient deficiency. The chapter also includes materials and intervention strategies to treat imbalances before contributing to disease.
- Chapter 10 discusses hydration and fluid balance. It explains the physiological changes—reduced renal concentrating ability, impaired sensation of thirst—that make older adults extremely vulnerable to dehydration. The chapter includes guidelines for measuring fluid status, fluid intake targets by day, and safe methods for increasing intake.
- Chapter 11 sets forth dietary guidelines specifically tailored to the older adult, translating nutrition requirements into meal planning data. It covers portion size, number of meals, food group items, and cultural adaptation. The chapter identifies functional guidance for food shopping, food preparation, and food serving that delivers enough nutrition and yet remains acceptable.

- Chapter 12 covers the application of supplements and nutrient-nutrient interactions. It reviews the evidence regarding vitamin and mineral supplements in elderly individuals, examines common over-the-counter products, and describes how certain nutrients may interfere with or enhance the absorption of others. Chapter 12 offers decision-making aids to healthcare practitioners and patients considering supplementation.
- Chapter 13 outlines screening approaches to nutritional risk, such as evidence-based tools, the Mini Nutritional Assessment and the Malnutrition Universal Screening Tool. It outlines results interpretation, how to integrate into practice, and how to return for a full assessment when risk is identified.
- Chapter 14 covers geriatric sarcopenia and cachexia nutrition before the end of life. The chapter covers the pathophysiology of muscle loss, accelerators of tissue wasting, and targeted nutritional and exercise interventions to preserve function. Ethical and quality-of-life considerations in feeding support in advanced illness are also covered.
- Chapter 15 covers the way nutrition can be used to prevent and treat leading diseases of aging—cardiovascular disease, osteoporosis, diabetes, dementia, and cancer. It encapsulates eating patterns shown to lower disease risk, dietary modifications that support treatment objectives, and interdisciplinary approaches between dietitians and other healthcare professionals.

This text is directed to registered dietitians, doctors, nurses, pharmacists, occupational and physical therapists, caregivers, and health science students. It will be a resource for older adults and their families as a source of reliable information on food choice, meal planning, and working with healthcare teams to maintain strength, vitality, and independence in the latter part of life.

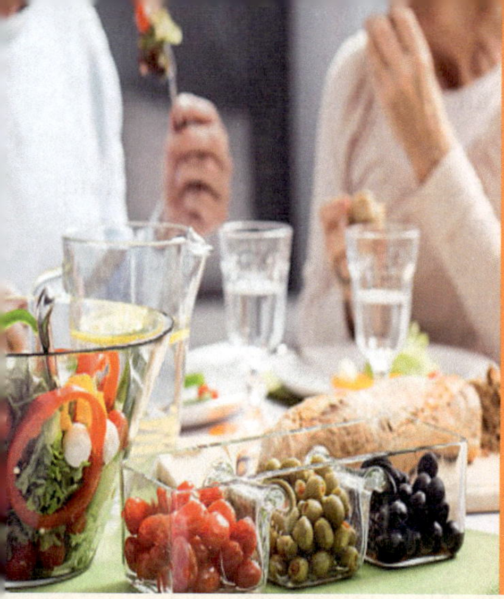

Chapter 1

INTRODUCTION TO GERIATRIC NUTRITION

Contents

Introduction

Geriatric nutrition requires a complete understanding, as it plays a very important role in the health and quality of life of the aged. An older population generally goes through several physiological and psychological changes that may affect their nutritional needs and food intake. For instance, illnesses like decreased appetite, altered taste sensation, and chronic disorders may render nutrient absorption challenging. It is critical for healthcare providers to determine these factors so they can create effective nutritional interventions that address the particular needs of older adults. Perhaps most importantly, ensuring sufficient protein intake is critical in the prevention of frailty and muscle atrophy, two age syndromes common in older adults. Moreover, ongoing education regarding nutrition and diet may allow older adults to make positive choices about their own well-being, which can result in a higher quality of life. It is understanding the psychosocial and social determinants affecting meal patterns in elderly individuals. Social isolation, a common state among the elderly, can lead to severe food intake reduction and loss of desire to prepare meals. This complicates the need to consider nutrition and psychosocial factors because interventions that only address calories and nutrient content may prove to be inadequate. Interventions to promote social interaction, such as shared meal programs and communal dining spaces, can foster a more facilitative environment for older individuals. In addition, the literature indicates that there is a need for healthcare professionals to provide holistic assessments that include not only physical well-being but also social connections and mental health in older nutrition planning (Lampugnane et al., 2017). Lastly, the effective management of geriatric nutrition requires an interdisciplinary approach to providing personalized nutritional care to elderly patients. Interprofessional teamwork among medical professionals like geriatricians, nurses, dietitians, and social workers can facilitate holistic understanding of a senior's food needs and tastes. The establishment of specialized education programs for healthcare professionals can maximize their ability for comprehensive geriatric assessment, unambiguously establishing the specific needs of older patients (Nolan et al., 1997). Besides, such collaboration fosters comprehensive care that transcends the prescription of medical care, understanding the importance of nutrition in sustaining optimal health and preventing disease among older individuals. Finally, with the growing population of elderly individuals, a rigorous focus on geriatric nutrition will be vital to enhancing the health of the elderly and mitigating their complex health needs (Figure 1.1).

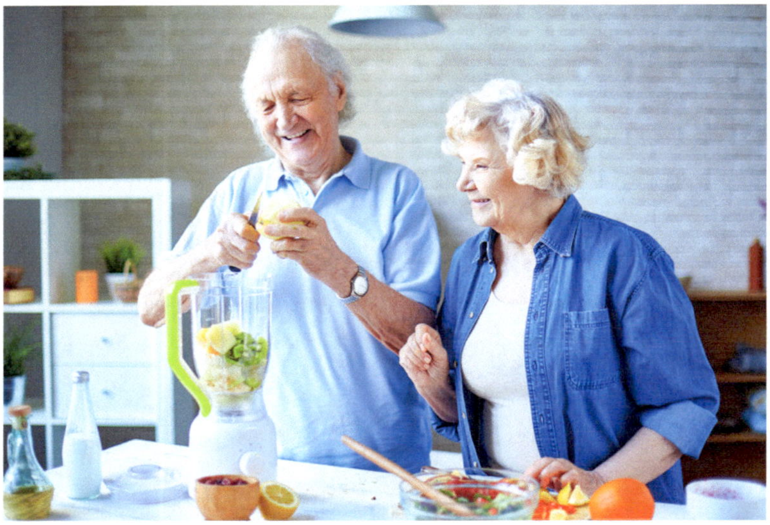

Figure 1.1. Geriatric nutrition.

Source: http://biodietz.com/wp-content/uploads/2018/03/GeriatricNutrition.jpg.

Definition of Geriatric Nutrition

The definition geriatric nutrition establishes a distinct practice in the delivery of dietary needs and nutritional intervention unique to older adults. As the population ages, it is increasingly important to understand the unique nutritional concerns of this patient population. Geriatric nutrition not only addresses the physiological changes that are part of aging, such as the shift in metabolism and muscle wasting, but it also addresses the multifaceted interaction between comorbidities and medications that characteristically define the older patient. As many elderly people suffer from symptoms such as decreased appetite, oral illness, or decreased cognitive functioning, a thorough nutritional evaluation is essential in designing individually tailored dietetic regimens that ensure maximal health. Incorporation of effective approaches in geriatric nutrition has the potential to significantly enhance the quality of life, functional status, and the prevention of frailty and sarcopenia, thereby emphasizing the multiple roles of nutrition in geriatric care. Moreover, the application of geriatric nutrition is not just the provision of adequate caloric intake, but also significant factors related to nutrient density and variety, thereby bridging the very specific inadequacies common among the aging population. For instance, vitamins B12 and D and calcium and protein are crucial in maintaining bone integrity and muscle function, both of which play key roles in the prevention of age-conditioned diseases such as osteoporosis and sarcopenia. This condition, which is characterized by muscle mass and strength loss, is a significant challenge among the elderly, with a high risk of falls and dependency on care for activities of daily living. Under such circumstances, monitoring and understanding of factors such as age-related metabolic alterations and nutrient utilization are essential. Interventions to optimize nutrition through dietary and supplement means become the underpinnings of excellent geriatric care, ultimately providing enhanced health and life satisfaction for older adults (Ji et al., 2024). With awareness of the complexity of geriatric nutrition, interdisciplinary practice is clearly required. Nutritionists, physicians, and caregivers must collaborate to develop comprehensive plans of care that are congruent with the older adult's preferences and values. This interactive process involves assessment of functional capacity, cognitive function, and anything that could interfere with optimal nutrition, such as social isolation or financial stress. The effect of frailty, deficiency in nutrients, and cognitive decline cannot be overemphasized as it plays a significant role in the nutritional status of the elderly. In addition, the perioperative period is a time in which nutritional optimization is of the utmost importance because surgical interventions have the tendency to place further stress on a compromised physiological state. Adequate feeding not only facilitates recovery but also minimizes complications during and after surgery. Consistently, multidisciplinary approaches that target geriatric care effectively provide a holistic model of treatment based on the complexities of the ageing population (Zabolotskikh et al., 2022).

Relevance of Nutrition in Elderly Individuals

Nutrition plays a pivotal role in an ageing population not just in promoting physical wellbeing but also in enhancing the ageing person's quality of life. As individuals age, their metabolic processes and nutritional requirements are altered, and this necessitates reconsideration of diet. A balanced intake of basic nutrients like proteins, vitamins, and minerals is crucial to provide muscle tone, mental clarity, and overall energy levels. Adequate nutrition prevents the untoward effects of aging, such as compromised immune function and increased susceptibility to chronic disease. Therefore, the use of dietary strategies uniquely addressing the special needs of the elderly represents a topmost agenda in geriatric nutrition. Attainment of these nutritional needs can significantly reduce the prevalence of malnutrition and lead to better health status and richer life experience. In addition, the characteristics of gastrointestinal aging have extensive influences on nutritional absorption and overall health of the elderly. Along with progressive aging, there are various physiological alterations in the gastrointestinal tract like reduced motility, reduced secretion of digestive enzymes, and impaired nutrient absorption, which can hinder appropriate nutrient consumption. These changes can cause malnutrition, and consequently, increase the risk of developing a multitude of health issues, including cardiovascular diseases, impaired immunity, and muscle weakness. Studies stress the significance of information concerning the interaction between gastrointestinal physiology and nutritional requirements of the elderly. By identifying the effect these changes in physiology have on eating habits, healthcare professionals can more effectively develop successful nutritional interventions that are specifically designed for the unique requirements of older adults, ultimately contributing to healthier aging and improved wellness results (Rémond et al., 2015). It is also important to understand that nutritional interventions need to be complemented with systemic caregiving and policy systems to facilitate the well-being of the elderly in a successful way. Evidence-based policy must prioritize comprehensive interventions that encompass nutrition education, enhancing supportive community services, and healthy food access. Alignment of these elements is crucial, especially in the context of socio-economic factors that hinder older individuals' nutritional status.

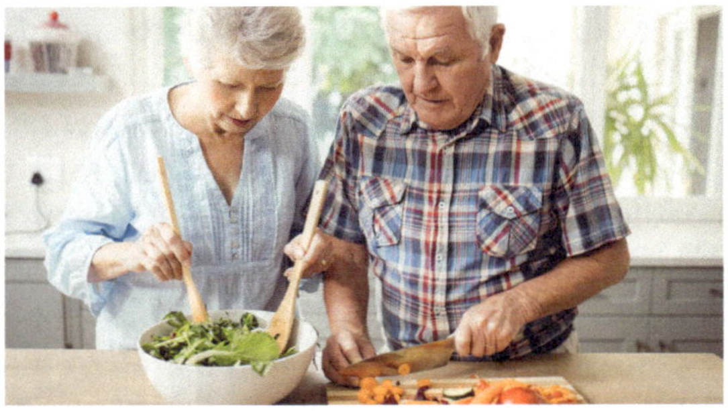

Figure 1.2. Nutrition in older adults.

Source: https://cdn.shopify.com/s/files/1/0038/0878/8544/articles/FeaturedImage_NutritionOlderAdults.png?v=1601919556.

For instance, intensified care coordination models can potentially advance patient self-management, thus encouraging enhanced nutritional practice among the elderly. As emphasized by research, current policies have a tendency of overlooking the significant role of nutrition to the health and well-being of older individuals, making a call for policy transformation at its core (The Stern Center for Evidence-Based Policy, 2015). As we seek to enhance the dietetics among older individuals, understanding the interactions between nutrition, policy, and health will be critical in establishing an inclusive framework that caters to aging populations (Figure 1.2).

Special Nutritional Needs of the Elderly

At one age, his or her physiological changes require specific nutritional adjustments in order to remain healthy and maintain a good quality of life. One of the imperative requirements for the elderly populations is their intake of required nutrients, primarily proteins, vitamins, and minerals. With increasing age, disorders such as loss of appetite, masticatory dysfunction, and metabolic changes can lead to deficiencies of nutrients. It is vital that these problems are recognized by healthcare providers and dietary suggestions tailored accordingly. For instance, protein supplementation to maintain muscle and calcium and vitamin D supplementation to combat osteoporosis are necessary. Water intake also cannot be overlooked because dehydration is a common problem in the elderly population and carries severe health consequences. Resolution of these issues through individualized meal planning will enhance the nutrient status and general well-being of the elderly, making geriatric nutritional management crucial. In addition to the physical challenges of aging, mental well-being also influences elderly food consumption patterns. Depression, particularly in individuals with chronic disease, can significantly influence appetite and intake of nutrients. Studies imply that higher rates of unrecognized depression in the elderly could lead to substantial lowering of retention of nutritional information and adherence to dietary recommendations. For instance, one study isolated the relationship between higher scores on the Geriatric Depression Scale and lower nutrition quiz scores in older adults as a problem with good practice in screening. This exchange emphasizes that the treatment of mental health is as important as nutrition education in promoting healthy eating among older adults. Addressing mental health problems along with nutritional deficiencies can have improved health outcomes and higher nutritional compliance among the elderly population, which is important because of population aging. Furthermore, social and environmental aspects of geriatric nutrition cannot be overlooked. The majority of elderly people face unique barriers like social isolation, lack of access to healthy food options, and financial constraints, all of which have the potential to disrupt their ability to maintain a balanced diet. These conditions normally create an increased reliance on convenience foods that tend to have limited nutritious value. In addition, caregivers and families can also play a vital role in supporting the nutritional needs of elderly individuals because their intervention can lead to increased planning and preparation for meals. Community-based interventions, such as nutrition education and food delivery, can also encourage increased healthy food consumption among older adults. By addressing these social determinants of health, the nutritional requirements of the elderly can be addressed more effectively, not just for proper nutrition but also for support for a meaningful lifestyle.

1.1. Common Nutritional Challenges in the Elderly

The elderly population suffers from various nutritional problems that can significantly impact their overall health and quality of life. One of the most critical problems is the widespread occurrence of unintentional weight loss, in most developed countries caused by a mix of some or all of the factors mentioned above, like reduced appetite, changes in taste and smell, and physical impairment that makes food preparation difficult. The problems can cause malnutrition, which worsens frailty and is responsible for decreased functional status. The majority of older adults also have diseases that affect their intake of nutrients, such as dementia or chronic obstructive pulmonary disease, further making it challenging for dietary adherence. One cannot overstate the importance of addressing these nutritional complications because proper nutrition is critical in maintaining cognitive function, immune function, and overall health in aging individuals, making specific nutritional interventions for this age group imperative (Lampugnale, 2017). Moreover, mental status is closely related to the diet of older adults, and depression is a primary concern. A significant majority of older adults have unrecognized depression, which generally leads to low motivation for self-care as well as inappropriate dietary intake. It has been reported that an inability to concentrate, a primary symptom of depression, can significantly undermine the capacity to retain essential healthcare education, including knowledge about nutrition (Wynn-Grundy, 2016). This connection demonstrates a cyclical system whereby poor mental health leads to poor nutrition habits, in turn exacerbating physical health conditions. Hence, treatment for mental health goes hand in hand with nutritional education so that elderly patients can make sound decisions regarding their dietary habits. Through the treatment of both sections, healthcare experts are in a position to improve the state of health and enhance the well-being of older people. In addition to psychological factors, socio-economic determinants also play an integral role in the nutritional problems of the elderly. Many elderly people live on fixed incomes that may limit exposure to nutrient-dense food. The availability of supermarkets and the price and accessibility of fresh, lower-cost fruits and vegetables also vary significantly from one location to another, contributing to nutritional disparities within this population. Social isolation among older people is also a common occurrence that leads to irregular eating habits and consumption of convenience foods that are lacking in essential nutrients. Overcoming such socio-economic constraints requires a mix of strategies that involve community support schemes, funds for purchasing healthy food, and social interaction-improving programs with food sharing or communal eating programs. These measures are vital to enhancing eating habits and preventing elderly people from lacking the diet that promotes their health and well-being (Figure 1.3).

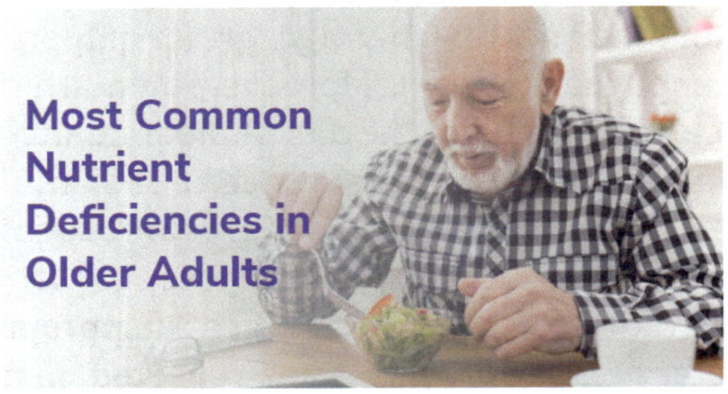

Figure 1.3. Common nutrient deficiency in older adults.

Source: https://www.reanfoundation.org/wp-content/uploads/2021/09/most-commom-nutrient-defencies-in-olderAdult-blog-image.jpg.

1.1.1. Physiological and Metabolic Changes with Aging

Aging is associated with a sequence of gradual physiological changes that significantly impact the body systems, particularly the gastrointestinal tract (GIT). With progressive age, alterations in the mechanical and chemical processes of digestion become evident. Reduced gastrointestinal motility and altered gastric acid secretion may compromise the efficacy of nutrient absorption. In addition, the structure of the intestinal wall may be altered, weakening its ability to transport essential nutrients into the blood. Such alterations not only compromise nutrient uptake but also predispose elderly individuals to malnutrition, a condition that can further exacerbate pre-existing disorders such as cardiovascular disease and immunocompromised dysfunction.

The older adult also exhibits significant changes in metabolism and digestion, which influence his or her nutritional status. The degradation of basal metabolic rate (BMR), which is quite common due to loss of muscle tissue, results in decreased energy expenditure. This decrease has the potential to cause weight gain unless calorie consumption decreases, something that is particularly unsafe given the fact that obesity and associated diseases are prevalent among older individuals.

Aging also alters the hormonal regulation of hunger and fullness, e.g., through changes in levels of leptin and ghrelin, with effects on satiety and hunger cues that help lower appetite. Again, as indicated elsewhere, these changes in metabolism necessitate a reappraisal of carbohydrate, fat, and fluid requirements particular to older people for optimizing health and preventing obesity- and metabolic disorder-related disease. Research has indicated that changes in taste and olfactory senses, common among the elderly, lead to decreased caloric intake and poor nutrition. As stated above, older adults tend to eat calorie-dense, nutrient-lean foods that consist mainly of saturated fats and sugar. This feeding behavior not only exacerbates metabolic impairment but also increases the risk for cardiometabolic diseases.

The influence of aging on metabolism goes beyond macronutrient requirements to include micronutrient needs as well. Based on studies, some micronutrient deficiencies have been determined to be caused by physiological changes due to aging, e.g., reductions in absorption capacity and eating habits. Deficiency in these essential micronutrients, such as vitamins B12, D, and C, as well as minerals zinc and iron, has been linked to many age-related illnesses, including cognitive impairment and increased risk of chronic diseases. For instance, oxidative stress and neurodegenerative conditions such as Alzheimer's disease have meaningful implications for the function of antioxidant micronutrients in the diet (Staehelin, 2017).

As the population ages and undergoes such physiological alterations, the comprehension of the dynamic interaction between such gastrointestinal alterations and their impact on nutrient consumption becomes critically important. The inability of the gastrointestinal system to effectively absorb and utilize essential nutrients can also add to frailty and chronic disease, calling for specific dietary therapy. Moreover, aging metabolism is also characterized by increasing loss of muscle mass, a condition referred to as sarcopenia, with decreased energy expenditure and altered nutrient utilization. Sarcopenia not only weakens physical strength but also threatens older adults with greater morbidity and impaired mobility. Regular aerobic and resistance exercise can correct many of these characteristics of the disorder, citing the role physical exercise has in addition to proper nutrition (Deutz et al., 2014). Proper nutrition, including protein, is particularly relevant because it helps to sustain muscles and functional capacity. As the body's metabolism slows down, proper intake of protein is required in order to combat age-related muscle loss and recover, ultimately optimizing metabolic health in older adults. The effects of these metabolic and gastrointestinal changes cascade far beyond individual health, into population-based public health measures as well. Malnutrition, fueled by the challenges of metabolic economy and nutrient utilization, represents a major threat for older individuals, leading to various health problems that are not only bodily but also psychological and affect quality of life (Rémond et al., 2015). For dietary advice to be properly personalized to respond to such challenges, however, it must be reinforced by a detailed review of the aging body's needs. Tailored food products and nutrition therapies that optimize nutrient access and supplement the unique functional capacities of the aging GI tract are key to preventing malnutrition. Continued research and intervention development will be important to educating healthcare professionals about the best nutritional interventions for the elderly patient population in an effort to maximize health outcomes and add to longevity.

1.1.2. Impact of Chronic Diseases on Nutrition

Chronic disease has a substantial impact on the nutrition of older people, seriously threatening their health and well-being. With a growing population of older people facing a number of chronic diseases, such as diabetes, cardiovascular diseases, and arthritis, such diseases tend to result in modifications in dietary needs and preferences. For instance, individuals with diabetes will require control of carbohydrate intake, whereas individuals with cardiovascular diseases might require restriction in sodium. The complexity of these nutritional requirements can exacerbate already prevailing nutritional problems in the absence of appropriate assistance and resources towards nutritional education and meal planning. Hence, it is extremely important to understand these chronic conditions to formulate effective nutritional strategies that can address the unique needs of elderly patients. The physiological and mechanical changes of the aging gastrointestinal tract are a significant contributor to nutritional concerns among the elderly. As outlined in the latest studies, the old gut has diminished motility, impaired digestion, and decreased absorptive capacity, leading to poor nutrient intake and malnutrition (Rémond et al., 2015). These physiological changes do not happen randomly; they may have a cascading effect on health status, influencing the intensity of chronic diseases, in addition to increasing comorbidity risk. For example, poor protein absorption can jeopardize muscle mass and strength, which could worsen diseases like sarcopenia, which is prevalent among older adults. Hence, satisfying these gut-related factors is crucial for creating balanced nutritional interventions that could potentially enhance the health and well-being of older adults with chronic diseases. Besides, the link between chronic disease and diet extends beyond individual food needs to influence broader system-based issues within the health care policy landscape. Evidence-based policy actions are required to facilitate improved geriatric nutrition management through prevention, care coordination, and patient self-management (The Stern Center for Evidence-Based Policy, 2015). As indicated by the evidence, there is a substantial gap between strong evidence for effective nutrition interventions and their implementation. This imbalance must be addressed through policy that encourages nutritional education, access to healthy food, and support for caregiving families, the nutritional health of the aged can collectively be addressed. By creating an integrated approach for both medical and nutritional care, we can mitigate the impact of chronic disease on nutrition and promote healthier aging among the geriatric population (Figure 1.4).

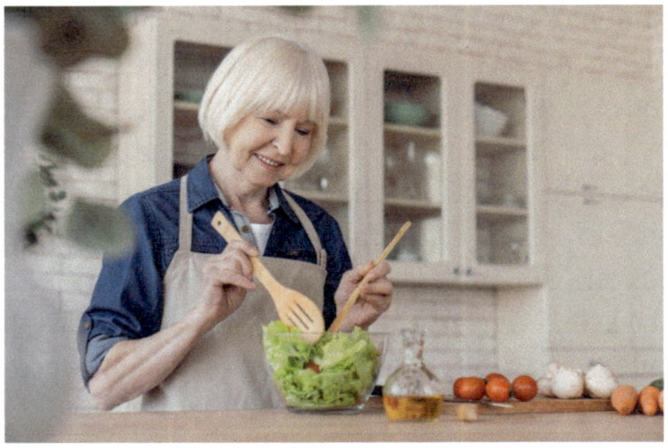

Figure 1.4. Prevent common chronic diseases in older adults.

Source: https://continuing.mcmaster.ca/app/uploads/2024/09/elderly-person-rcm-article-scaled.jpg.

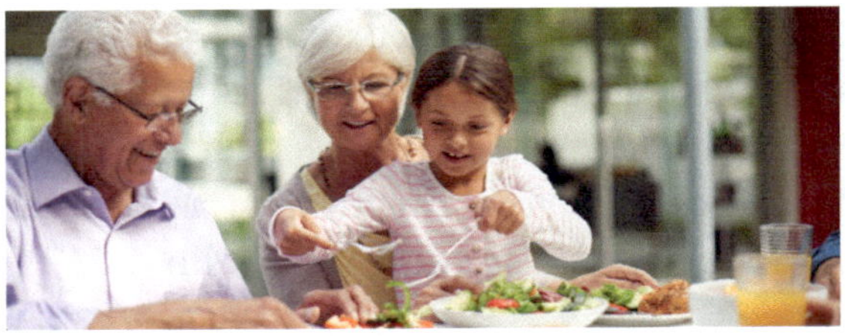

Figure 1.5. Food & healthy eating.

Source: https://external-content.duckduckgo.com/iu/?u=http%3A%2F%2Ftimiskamingh u.com%2Fwebsites%2Ftimiskaminghu.com %2Fimages%2Fphotos%2FFood%2520and %2520Healthy%2520Eating%2520section_ older%2520adults%2520icon.jpg&f=1&nofb= 1&ipt=3d094928c3efa01ba355e475d47cc13b 551d217c6169def330ccddae594ae5d9.

1.2. Nutritional Requirements for Older Adults

It is necessary to realize the nutritional requirements of older adults since the age population is increasing, and the requirement is continuously on the rise. Older adults mostly undergo physiological changes like decreased metabolism and altered organ function, which can influence their nutritional requirements. For instance, the number of calories to be ingested in order to remain healthy and weigh the same can be fewer with age, but the requirement of nutrients like vitamins and minerals remains the same or even greater. This paradox can lead to malnutrition unless appropriate dietary modification is undertaken. Studies indicate that improper intake of nutrients can exacerbate chronic diseases, forming a cycle of negative health effects, which can lower the quality of life in the elderly, making targeted nutrition intervention for this group important. Malnutrition frequently presents as a principal problem in geriatric populations, particularly in residential aged care facilities. Evidence suggests that approximately half of all residents suffer from some level of malnutrition, most frequently resulting from factors of reduced appetite, dietary restrictions, and problems with gastrointestinal absorption. Malnutrition is severe with implications of high morbidity and mortality rates as well as increased risks of infection, falls, and readmission. Specifically, elderly patients with conditions like hip fractures are more likely to have compromised outcomes of recovery in cases of malnutrition, validating the necessity of comprehensive nutritional evaluation and treatment as part of geriatric management. Nutritional management developed in a multidisciplinary approach in such settings can significantly enhance physical recovery, as well as general health. Efficient nutritional intervention presents an urgency in addressing the targeted nutritional needs of the elderly. Evidence supports the value of ongoing nutrition screening and assessment on admission to residential care so that individual dietary requirements are recognized and met. Interventions can include individualized meal plans emphasizing nutrient-dense foods, with accommodations for residents' choice to enhance compliance and satisfaction. The positive impact of such interventions has been confirmed in various studies, with enhanced nutritional status and functional recovery in aging adults who are treated with proper care. As noted, early and sustained focus on nutritional issues in paved protocols can potentially prevent, to a great extent, the complications of malnutrition, ultimately resulting in a healthier and more robust elderly population (Agarwal et al., 2016; Malafarina et al., 2017) (Figure 1.6).

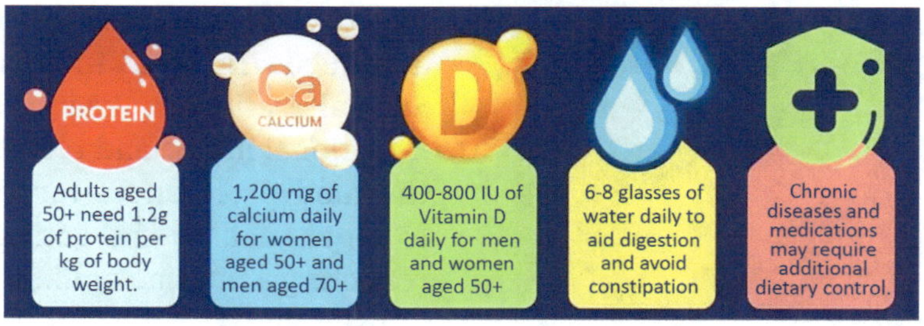

Figure 1.6. Nutritional requirements for older adults.

Source: https://ninkatec.b-cdn.net/wp-content/uploads/2024/01/Ninkatec-Infographic_Nutritional-Needs-of-the-Elderly.jpg.

1.2.1. Essential Nutrients for Aging Populations

As age progresses, nutritional demands become more complex due to physiological changes affecting digestion, absorption, and metabolism of the major nutrients. One of the main concerns is the elderly GIT, which progressively undergoes mechanical and functional impairments. These alterations can potentially develop barriers to nutrient acquisition and bioavailability. A detailed investigation of the impact of aging on the GIT is necessary to provide appropriate dietary counseling. With the rising incidence of malnutrition among older adults, it is essential to develop dietary interventions that have been tailored for these changes in GIT functions. This will not only avoid malnutrition risks but also enhance the overall health status of elderly adults (Rémond et al., 2015). Essential nutrients such as protein, vitamins, and minerals are essential in maintaining health while growing older. Adequate consumption of protein is required to preserve muscle mass, immunity, and recovery from illness or injury. It has been established that there is a need for higher protein intake among older populations to counteract sarcopenia, which is the loss of muscle mass with age. Similarly, vitamins B12 and D contribute to the preservation of mental acuity and bone density, respectively. Calcium and magnesium also ensure the maintenance of bone density and heart health. According to these nutritional dynamics, certain dietary advice that considers the unique demands of aging populations is of significant concern. Policymakers are required to prioritize actions that bridge such nutritional gaps and ensure that old people adhere to healthy diets (The Stern Center for Evidence-Based Policy, 2015). In addition to highlighting the focus on single nutrients, it is also essential to be aware of the broader context of nutrition and aging for older adults. Economic constraints, sensory changes, and comorbidity effects can further complicate food decisions in older adults. It is essential to incorporate these factors in framing nutritional interventions and policies.

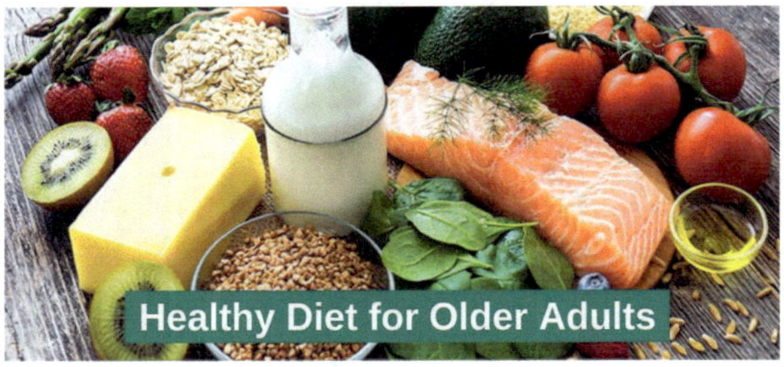

Figure 1.7. Proper nutrition can ensure healthy aging.

Source: https://external-content.duckduckgo.com/iu/?u=https%3A%2F%2Fukcareguide.co.uk%2Fmedia%2FHealthy-Diet-for-Older-Adults-min.jpg&f=1&nofb=1&ipt=b16d3f4e5c9551d75b5578cab0c13242c7d4494aee8ffd06c1eae6828e732c85.

For instance, programs that are local and help make available nutrient-dense foods can significantly improve the eating habits of the elderly. Furthermore, self-management education can empower older individuals to make better dietary choices without any support. Addressing such compound issues requires an all-encompassing approach that welcomes cooperation among healthcare professionals, policymakers, and societies toward enhancing the nutritional well-being of older individuals (The Stern Center for Evidence-Based Policy, 2015).

1.3. Dietary Patterns and Food Choices

Knowledge of food and eating patterns is essential in geriatric nutrition, as they can greatly influence health outcomes among older people. As people grow older, their taste for specific food groups tends to shift as a result of physiological changes, lifestyle changes, and cultural factors. For instance, there is research that has found older people are likely to have a taste for less firm foods with a reduced interest in more complex flavors. Such alterations make it difficult to have proper nutritional intake and result in imbalances. Also, the food preferences for this group are likely to be shaped by the eating habits of the past, reflecting a lifetime of liking and disliking foods. Consequently, a careful examination of these food preferences is important in order to make effective nutritional interventions for health and well-being improvement in the elderly so that practitioners can provide individualized dietary recommendations in accordance with both personal taste and nutritional needs. Additionally, research on gender-specific food preferences reveals notable variations affecting the consumption of food in the elderly population. For instance, research identifies males as typically preferring processed and red meat, while females show a preference for prepared fruits and vegetables. Such identification suggests variations in indigenous nutrition habits and patterns typical among genders at old age (Lombardo et al., 2024). These findings are critical in the development of gender-sensitive nutrition programs because these food preferences significantly influence dietary intake and total health. Additionally, identifying these gender dynamics can help in developing more effective educational materials that speak more effectively to older adults, ensuring they make healthier food choices. Thus, resolving these differences in food preferences can result in more effective engagement strategies in geriatric nutrition interventions. Lastly, recent initiatives aimed at introducing healthier dietary practices highlight the importance of traditional diets, such as the Mediterranean diet, in promoting longevity and health over old age. Displacement of such diets poses individual health as well as environmental sustainability risks (Grosso et al., 2024). Projects like the DELICIOUS project underscore the importance of educational approaches that sensitize children and adolescents to the nutritional and environmental benefits of adhering to conventional dietary patterns. The interventions must, however, be conceptualized in the context of elderly people as well and keeping in view their individual nutritional constraints, preferences, and life realities. Teaching and equipping the older generation with functional skills in meal planning and nutrition can set the stage for a reversal of better eating habits, ultimately resulting in a general enhancement of their health and quality of life towards the end years of their lives (Figure 1.8).

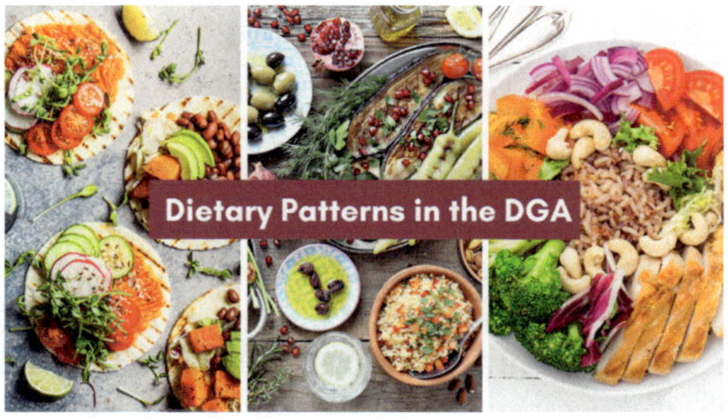

Figure 1.8. Healthy dietary patterns.

Source: https://foodinsight.org/wp-content/uploads/2021/02/dga-diets-.png.

1.3.1. Overview of Healthy Dietary Patterns

Healthy dietary patterns are an important area to consider in geriatric nutrition in order to foster overall health among elderly populations. With advancing age and associated physiological changes, the body may change nutrient absorption and metabolic rate, making it essential to address nutrition in a specifically individualized way. Studies have shown that a well-balanced diet containing plenty of fruits, vegetables, whole grains, and lean proteins can effectively enhance the quality of life among the elderly. Despite this, the majority of older people are malnourished, and this could be due to a combination of sociological, physiological, and economic causes. A comprehensive review of food behaviors among this population reveals that a high percentage of older people are suffering from inadequate nutrient intake, which often accompanies inadequate knowledge of diet and nutrition (Agbozo et al., 2018). This highlights the importance of intervention at school to bring about a greater awareness of diet and eating healthy foods. Furthermore, research yields correlations between health status and the quality of diet in elderly groups. For instance, a proper diet has been established to decrease the risks of chronic diseases like hypertension and diabetes, both prevalent in this age group. The incorporation of required nutrients—such as vitamins, minerals, and fiber—into daily meals can possibly improve age-related conditions. Some nutritional elements, such as zinc, have also been known to influence cognitive processes among the elderly, validating the possibility of dietary changes improving not only physiological but also cognitive functioning (Maylor et al., 2006). Therefore, setting age-specific dietary standards within accessibility is critical in the management of nutritional problems among the elderly. Setting healthy dietary lifestyles requires a poly-categorical approach that addresses the individual preferences, cultural, and socioeconomic lifestyles. Involving community programs with nutrient education and health food availability is paramount in convincing older adults to lead healthy eating habits. Evidence exists to demonstrate that if older individuals are motivated to improve eating habits, significant gains in nutritional status can be made (Agbozo et al., 2018). Social interaction, such as sharing a meal and a cooking class, can also increase motivation and adherence to improved eating habits. Finally, there is an integrated strategy involving education, access, and social support mechanisms that can facilitate older adults' adoption of healthier diets, enhance their independence, and improve their well-being as they age.

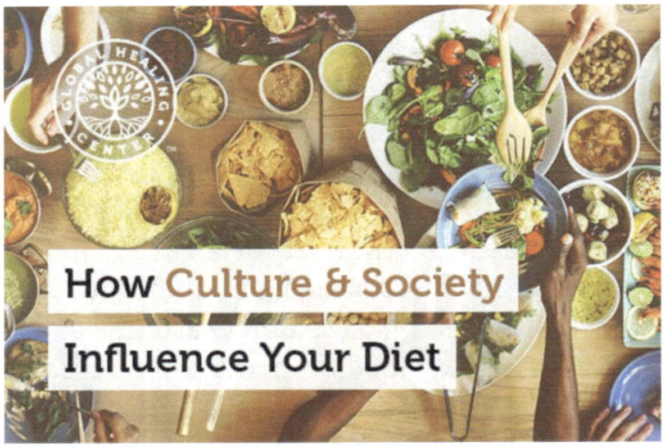

Figure 1.9. Culture influences health food habits.

Source: https://cdn.shopify.com/s/files/1/0675/8635/9598/files/healthy-eating.jpg.

1.3.2. Role of Supplements in Geriatric Nutrition

Provision of adequate nutrition in the elderly is a multifaceted problem that sometimes requires supplementation. With the process of aging affecting the gastrointestinal tract, nutrient absorption and digestion are greatly reduced, and deficiencies are likely to arise and aggravate existing health conditions (Malafarina et al., 2017). The majority of the elderly are denied food due to underlying health problems, mobility issues, or economic constraints, which contribute to further diminishing the consumption of essential nutrients. Nutritional supplements therefore, become essential in plugging in the gaps. Supplementation with major nutrients, i.e., vitamin D, calcium, and B12, has the potential to lower malnutrition risk and enhance all-around well-being. Not only does supplementation maintain physiological functioning, but it also facilitates the elderly in leading a good quality of life through enhancing their energy levels and mental functioning. Moreover, the impact of malnutrition on the recovery after health episodes, like hip fractures, is very clear amongst the elderly population. Prevalence of malnutrition has been recognized as high in geriatric patients admitted due to hip fracture, with nearly 18.7% of the patients found to be malnourished (Malafarina et al., 2017). Such inadequacies in consumption can lead to increased hospital complications and disrupt the process of functional recovery after fracture. Nutritional supplementation has been found to improve recovery outcomes, along with decreasing mortality in these patients. By addressing deficiencies, healthcare providers can improve nutritional status, thereby enhancing rehabilitation. As the incidence of malnutrition in older adults is very high, supplements also play a critical role in improving recovery and preserving independence with increasing age. Considering these barriers, medical practitioners and caregivers need to advocate for comprehensive nutritional screening among older individuals. Identifying seniors at risk of malnutrition needs to be an interconnected strategy for consideration of eating habits, individual health status, and social settings. Integration of supplements into daily nutrition programs needs to be designed in line with specific nutritional deficiencies and health conditions. Educational programs are also important to motivate older adults to make intelligent dietary decisions with effective supplementation. By focusing on the unique needs of the geriatric population, practitioners are in a position to make certain that nutritional advice reflects the intricate nature of aging and puts emphasis on the functional impairments it brings (Rémond et al., 2015). The personalized approach to geriatric nutrition will ultimately result in maximized health benefits, maximized quality of life, and longevity among the aging population.

1.4. The Role of Caregivers and Healthcare Professionals

The reliance of caregivers on healthcare professionals provides a fundamental foundation for the profession of geriatric nutrition. Caregivers, such as family and friends in most instances, provide needed care to the elderly, particularly those who have difficulties associated with illness or disability. The caregivers play a critical role in ensuring proper nutrition by assisting in the preparation of meals, monitoring food likes and dislikes and recognizing changes in appetite and nutritional status. Their daily active involvement can go a long way to promote the welfare of the elderly, particularly in terms of facilitating complex nutritional needs arising from disease conditions. Harmonization with medical practitioners further commercializes this relationship by offering exposure to nutritional services, adjusting diet regimes based on evolving health statuses, and providing learning on nutritional issues. This partnership is intended to optimize dietary outcomes with a focus on the basic interdependence between care and wellbeing among the elderly. Healthcare professionals possess advanced knowledge that complements the support caregivers provide to ensure an integrated approach for geriatric nutrition. They are capable of performing nutritional risk assessments, particularly for vulnerable groups of individuals with dementia. Evidence supports the fact that nutritional deficiencies have the potential to increase the symptoms of dementia, therefore decreasing the quality of life of patients and their caregivers. Continuous assessment and immediate intervention from doctors can be employed to prevent such risks, validating the essence of multidisciplinary team working. For example, evidence supports the fact that an early identification of nutritional risk and personalized interventions are critical in caring for individuals with dementia living in the community.

These interventions are not only limited to nutrition education but are even broader support systems integrating emotional aspects of caregiving, optimizing the effectiveness of nutrition care and reducing family caregivers' stress (Mole et al., 2018). The organizational framework of nutrition care needs to continue checking and refining itself to meet changing challenges facing caregivers and healthcare professionals. Current evidence sheds light on the variations between nutritional interventions, particularly in community-living older adults. Home care workers and healthcare providers' duty is interwoven with nutrition policy, addressing the complexities of the aging population. As identified by studies, a large proportion of elderly individuals are susceptible to malnutrition, and a successful policy framework can aid in the application of evidence-based interventions and promote health education programs targeted at this age group. This is particularly significant because caregivers often have no training in planning dietary needs and navigating the healthcare system effectively. Therefore, the reinforcement of support and education for caregivers along with healthcare workers becomes a number one priority in advocating geriatric nutrition and quality of life outcomes (The Stern Center for Evidence-Based Policy, 2015) (Figure 1.10).

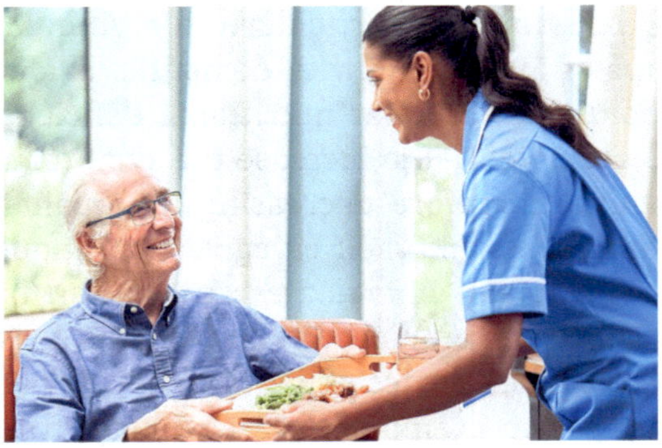

Figure 1.10. Role of caregivers and healthcare professionals in geriatric nutrition.

Source: https://edyncaregiverservices.com/wp-content/uploads/2023/05/Elderly-Nutrition.jpg.

1.4.1. Importance of Nutrition Education for Caregivers

Of paramount concern in the case of geriatric nutrition is the caregiver's role, as they have a direct bearing on the eating patterns and health of the elderly. Nutrition education equips caregivers to be confident and competent about the unique dietary requirements of the elderly, which can help improve their health and well-being. With an older population comes issues like increased susceptibility to chronic diseases, and caregivers must be given the answers to such issues through informed dietary choices. Basic nutrition knowledge provides caregivers with the skills to implement sensible meal planning, look for nutrient gaps, and drive healthier eating habits among older adults to ensure that this susceptible group is given the best diet care necessary for complete well-being. Also, caregivers who undergo nutritional education are in a better position to detect and respond to a wide range of health issues likely caused by poor nutrition, such as frailty or malnutrition. The integration of nutritional assessments, as indicated by geriatric studies, reflects the utmost significance of caregivers advocating for individualized nutritional interventions. Training initiatives focusing on the relationship between health outcomes and diet expose caregivers to the impact of diet choice in the context of chronic illnesses present among elderly patients. In-depth understanding of the Mini-Nutritional Assessment will equip caregivers with the recognition of the at-risk individual who is malnourished, allowing intervention for improvement in physical and mental well-being, thus fostering better health outcomes among the elderly under their care (Lampugnane et al., 2017). In addition, nutritional education provides caregivers with the ability to handle cultural food sensitivities and food preferences around food, which is essential in providing an environment that supports compatible healthy eating. By acquiring the skill of respecting and incorporating cultural food preferences when planning meals, caregivers not only make meals more acceptable but also ensure psychological health and identity for older adults. Apart from this, the significance of preventative nutrition interventions is actualized through the training of the caregivers since they can effectively implement health promotion and disease prevention programs. Meal coordination and interacting with dietary limitations are vital means in a caregiver's toolkit, ultimately contributing to improved health outcomes and a higher quality of life for the elderly population (The Stern Center for Evidence-Based Policy, 2015).

1.4.2. Strategies for Supporting Nutritional Needs

It takes an interdisciplinary approach to meet the nutritional needs of the geriatric population by considering their unique physiological changes and nutritional requirements. With age, individuals are predisposed to experiencing altered metabolism, loss of appetite, and susceptibility to medical conditions that could complicate nutrition. Interventions for enhanced nutrition supplementation must include systematic evaluations of individual needs, particularly through the use of the Mini-

Nutritional Assessment—a well-established method of identifying risk for malnutrition in older persons. Lastly, initiatives to raise awareness among healthcare providers on the importance of personalized nutrition plans can significantly strengthen geriatric patients' nutrition status and ultimately enhance their health outcomes and quality of life. Adding these evaluations to routine practice will be able to provide targeted intervention to address the unique nutritional requirements of this population (Lampugnale, 2017). Health literacy is part of educating and empowering the patient and caregiver in the holistic approach towards nutrition among the elderly. How much one can make informed food choices, particularly with regard to high-level conditions, relies on health literacy. Educational programs, such as family workshops or one-to-one counseling, may increase nutrition awareness and enhance healthier eating practices. Further, the incorporation of caregivers and family members into nutrition planning can contribute to compliance with dietary recommendations and create a support network for older adults. Through a focus on self-management and the provision of practical support, health professionals are able to empower older people to take an active role in their own nutritional health, such as food preparation and portion control. This is essential to maintaining independent living and a decrease in institutionalized dependency (The Stern Center for Evidence-Based Policy, 2015). Moreover, collaboration among healthcare professionals like physicians, dietitians, and social workers is also needed in creating an equitable system of nutrition care for the elderly. Collaboration is important to ensure that every factor of a patient's condition, including mental condition and social support system, is included in his or her nutritional treatment program. Providing access to multidisciplinary teams can encourage providers to develop individualized nutrition plans that are tailored not only to dietary preference but to preferences based on medical conditions and physical limitations. With the routine administration of geriatric assessments that evaluate the social determinants of health, such as food and transportation availability, providers will have an opportunity to recognize barriers to optimal nutrition. Breaking down these barriers collectively with evidence-based policies and community resources will lead to improved health among the elderly and ultimately their overall well-being (The Stern Center for Evidence-Based Policy, 2015; Lampugnale, 2017) (Figure 1.11).

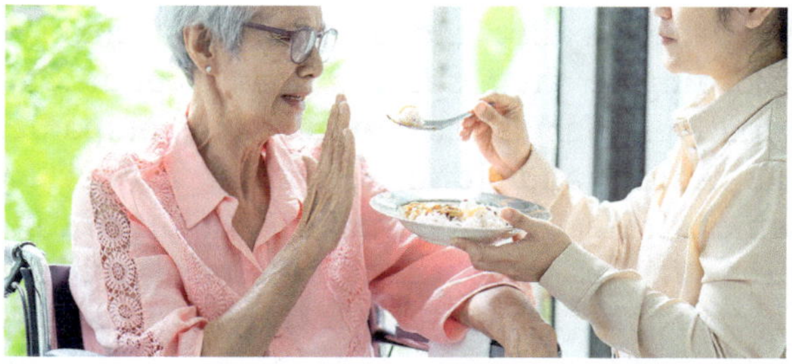

Figure 1.11. Ways to improve nutrition in the elderly.

Source: https://www.samvednacare.com/blog/wp-content/uploads/2020/01/5-Ways-to-Improve-Nutrition-in-the-Elderly.jpg.

1.4.3. Collaboration Between Healthcare Providers and Nutritionists

Co-operation between health care professionals and nutritionists is key in addressing the specific nutritional needs of older people. As the geriatric population increases, health care systems must adapt to provide holistic and comprehensive care. Nutritionists introduce valuable knowledge in designing dietary plans for the prevention and management of age-related diseases such as obesity, diabetes, and malnutrition. By working closely with the medical team, including doctors and nurses, nutritionists can ensure that food interventions are not only appropriate for the medical conditions of the patients but also acceptable in terms of individual tastes and eating cultures. Such an interdisciplinary approach is beneficial to ensure better health outcomes and optimal quality of life for the elderly, which substantiates that cooperation is essential for good geriatric care. In the management of complex care, the collaboration among nutritionists and medical practitioners can lead to more effective interventions. Older patients, who often have many chronic diseases, can have their nutritional interventions included in their global care plan, which affects their treatment efficiency as well as the recovery pattern. For instance, the nutritionist can assess the patient's diet and propose food changes according to their specific health conditions. Initiatives such as those in place in companies like Aetna and Johns Hopkins University demonstrate the advantage of incorporating nutrition into more comprehensive systems of care management, which can enable a team-based care approach among different professionals dedicated to patient care with a common purpose of achieving shared health goals. These interprofessional teams not only promote improved communication among team members but also ensure that all aspects of a patient's health are addressed, leading to improved outcomes at reduced costs. Furthermore, the utilization of ordered communication channels between nutritionists and healthcare professionals is imperative in ensuring successful cooperation. Intermittent interdisciplinary consultations and shared electronic health records can facilitate information exchange on dietary adherence and patient outcomes. This helps in the early detection of potential setbacks and timely intervention. Given the increasing complexity of older persons' needs in geriatric nutrition, well-established guidelines on inter-professional collaboration can enhance care deficiencies and patient engagement. A multidisciplinary approach is critical in the provision of quality services among the elderly, according to the key requirements of quality care (Allum et al., 2018). Lastly, creating effective partnerships among healthcare professionals and nutritionists is key in creating a responsive care atmosphere focused on the nutritional health of the older adult population (Figure 1.12).

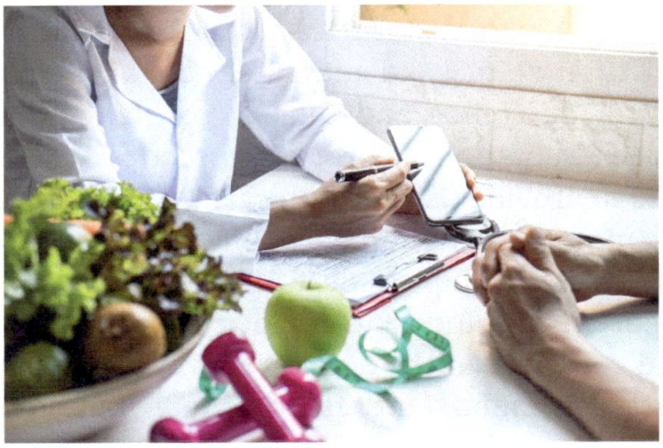

Figure 1.12. Collaboration between healthcare providers and nutritionists plays a pivotal role in addressing the unique nutritional needs of older adults.

Source: https://www.oncozine.com/wp-content/uploads/2019/08/Fotolia_274813027_Subscription_Monthly_M.jpg.

1.5. Addressing Malnutrition in Older Adults

Management of malnutrition among the elderly demands an in-depth understanding of the intricate factors surrounding the condition. Aging affects the gastrointestinal tract (GIT) in a way that affects the mechanics of food digestion and absorption. The generated changes in the form of malfunctioning gastrointestinal motility and impaired nutrient bioavailability greatly hinder the ability of the older groups to meet their nutritional needs. As the function of the GIT becomes impaired, there is an increased risk of malnutrition, with a direct effect on health outcomes. This impairment not only diminishes physical health but also compounds chronic conditions, creating a vicious circle that tends to lead to greater morbidity and mortality among the older population. Thus, interventions for enhancing dietary and nutritional status should consider the aging gastrointestinal system's complexity and its impact on overall nutritional status (Rémond et al., 2015). In addition, the treatment of malnutrition is vital in reducing the onset of comorbid diseases present in older individuals. Research indicates that malnutrition increases susceptibility to a range of pathologies in critical organ systems such as the nervous system, musculoskeletal system, and cardiovascular system. Such is the situation that proactive nutritional strategies have become part and parcel of the delivery of geriatric care. Such strategies may include personalized dietary programs aimed at the unique physiological changes experienced by the older individuals, e.g., decreased appetite and depressed taste. The healthcare providers also need to emphasize the importance of social support and psychological treatment because depression and isolation can aggravate the complications of malnutrition. By creating an interdisciplinary system that integrates nutritional and psychosocial requirements, practitioners can maximize the quality of life for older adults (Rémond et al., 2015). To ensure effective intervention implementation, there must be coordination across healthcare providers, caregivers, and the community. Education is central to this process, and medical providers need to become educated in how to conduct comprehensive nutritional assessments that detect malnutrition risk factors. Incorporating training in the predictive domains of geriatric evaluation, like the Mini-Nutritional Assessment, into medical school curricula can yield physicians with a greater ability to detect and treat malnutrition in older persons. Moreover, interventions that facilitate community engagement, such as nutrition workshops and meal planning classes, can give empowerment to older adults through the skills to choose healthy foods. Collectively, a concerted effort towards optimization in nutrition in older adults can yield beneficial health impacts and healthier aging (Lampugnale, 2017) (Figure 1.13).

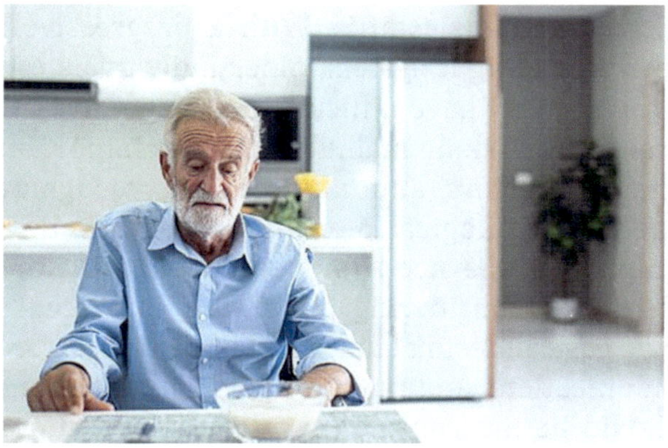

Figure 1.13. Malnutrition in older adults.

Source: https://domf5oio6qrcr.cloudfront.net/medialibrary/16144/conversions/gettyimages-1403932695-thumb.jpg.

1.5.1. Identifying Signs of Malnutrition

It is crucial to identify the signs of malnutrition in elderly individuals to ensure their good health and well-being. With the world's population aging, it is more necessary than ever before to recognize what specific signs characterize malnutrition. The most common signs are apparent weight loss, fatigue, and weakness, which are often overlooked by caregivers. Another sign of nutritional deficiency is loss of appetite, e.g., no interest in food or difficulty chewing and swallowing. Not only do these signs point to deficiency, but they can also promote a decline in the state of overall health. Ongoing assessment and screening can detect these changes early on and allow for intervention at this point that can interrupt the cycle of malnutrition. It is therefore imperative in geriatric nutrition to institute an active approach to monitoring these signs to maintain quality of life and improve outcomes in older adults. The aging gut undergoes several alterations that significantly affect nutrient intake, digestion, and absorption. Some of these alterations include decreased gastrointestinal motility, changes in saliva secretion, and alteration of the gut's microbiome, all of which can potentially alter nutritional status. With a progressively less efficient gut system, older individuals can progressively have difficulty drawing nutrients from food, risking malnutrition. It is important that caregivers and nutritionists recognize these physiological alterations because they emphasize the need for personalized dietary therapies, considering the elderly individual's own gastrointestinal functions. Both food texture modifications and nutrient-dense food options should be incorporated in these interventions to improve digestion and bioavailability of nutrients. Recognition of these physiological barriers is an integral part of the diagnosis of malnutrition in older adults, allowing for selective application of nutritional interventions to address deficiencies and enhance overall health. The nexus between malnutrition and medical complexity is most pronounced in older individuals, with severe consequences for their quality of life. Malnutrition is not only associated with weight loss and muscle atrophy but is also associated with increased risks of chronic diseases such as cardiovascular disease and autoimmune conditions. Malnutrition can also compromise recovery from illness and susceptibility to infection. The widespread impact of malnutrition necessitates a combined approach through the detection of biomarkers of nutrient deficiency and the establishment of particular dietary guidelines according to the unique requirements of the elderly. Implementing these regulations would decrease malnutrition-related risks, ensuring better health outcomes. It requires cooperation between caregivers, patients, and healthcare providers to make known the importance of awareness and guarantee that elderly people reach suitable nutritional levels throughout the aging process, which eventually leads to increased longevity and quality of life.

1.5.2. Interventions to Prevent Malnutrition

Aging has the tendency to expose one to malnutrition due to varied physiological, social, and environmental factors. Preventive measures against malnutrition in geriatric populations have become increasingly important, particularly in health care settings. A comprehensive nutritional assessment is key to the detection of high-risk individuals and facilitating early interventions for their specific requirements. Tools like the Geriatric Nutritional Risk Index can effectively detect complications of nutrition and guide management.

Moreover, the application of goal-directed nutritional support, including oral nutritional supplements with protein and carbohydrates, has been shown to avert weight loss and facilitate improved functional outcomes after surgery. The active engagement of healthcare consumers in co-designing interventions also enhances acceptability and efficacy, predisposing the holistic treatment of elderly nutrition (Gumuskaya et al., 2024). Hospital food quality is also a key variable influencing geriatric malnutrition. Patients often complain about meals served during hospital stay, to the exclusion of nutritional uptake and general recovery. Literature shows that satisfaction in foodservice translates directly into dietary consumption and a number of barriers that make meals unattainable. For instance, a study assessing the Malaysian Geriatric Patients' Hospital Foodservice Protocol showed that while there was overall reasonable satisfaction among most patients, a significant number still had barriers affecting their ability to eat adequate meals. In fixing these barriers and in streamlined foodservice delivery, hospitals can provide an environment conducive to better nutritional success, hence alleviating malnutrition among the elderly (Omar et al., 2022). Effective multimodal intervention is now recognized to be more effective than single-modality intervention in preventing geriatric malnutrition. Such intervention encompasses combining preoperative care through optimization of nutrition, hydration protocols, and cooperative programs for various health conditions, such as smoking cessation and management of chronic diseases.

These strategies are also most advantageous for elderly frail patients, as they not only increase nutritional intake but also surgical outcomes and quality of life. There is evidence for the belief that preoperative hydration decreases surgical stress and enhances recovery, and this topic will likely need to be further researched to allow for a thorough understanding and incorporation. By integrating the various dimensions of care—nutritional, medical, and psychological—healthcare providers can make a dramatic difference in the health outcomes for the elderly at risk of malnutrition (Gumuskaya et al., 2024) (Figure 1.14).

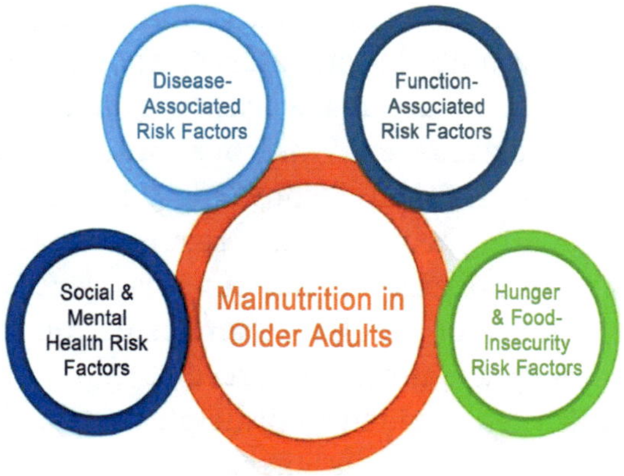

Figure 1.14. Aging often predisposes individuals to malnutrition due to various physiological, social, and environmental factors.

Source: https://slideplayer.com/slide/14442779/90/images/9/Contributing+Factors+of+Malnutrition+among+Older+Adults+Illustrate+the+Need+for+a+Coordinated%2C+Comprehensive+Solution.jpg.

1.5.3. Community Resources and Support Systems

Effective geriatric nutrition is as much about tailored food interventions as it is about robust community resources and support systems that are crafted to cater to the needs of older adults. In an increasingly aging population, it is as important as ever to develop support infrastructures to enhance nutritional well-being. Among the community resources are neighborhood food pantries, meal delivery programs, and senior centers that together work to combat food insecurity in the elderly. Through the provision of access to nutritious food and health education regarding the consumption of well, these facilities are essential to the improvement of the health outcomes of the elderly. Prevention policies and care coordination, as noted by The Stern Center for Evidence-Based Policy (2015), play a crucial role in ensuring that elderly people have an efficient means of accessing these facilities and receiving complete nutritional care in their communities. Older adult support networks are multifaceted, incorporating both formal and informal family and friend support and formal services. Social support should not be discounted; emotional, practical, and informational support can exert strong influences on health behaviors, such as food choices. The integration of social networks and access to community resources can assist in improving the effectiveness of nutritional interventions. For instance, when family caregivers are provided with nutrition education as suggested by Lampugnane (2017), they are better placed to advocate and offer better sources of food to elderly family members. The boosting of community support systems can thus lead to improved nutrition and overall health status among geriatric populations with a call for systemic intervention in the management of special dietary needs of older individuals. Besides, the problems of geriatric nutrition become increasingly complex, necessitating an efficient, well-coordinated effort involving healthcare professionals, community organizations, and families caring for older adults. Healthcare interventions must navigate through barriers such as mobility impairments and transportation availability that may limit older persons' access to nutritional food. Comprehensive assessments like geriatric assessments are necessary to ascertain every individual's requirements and tailor nutrition appropriately. By encouraging collaboration between health professionals and community resources, as defined in The Stern Center for Evidence-Based Policy (2015) and Lampugnale (2017), we can encourage environments that not only cater to the nutritional needs of older adults but also the overall health concerns. More and more, building up these community resources and support systems will contribute to healthier eating and improved quality of life in older adults.

1.6. Innovations in Geriatric Nutrition

Geriatric nutrition has made significant strides in recent years to meet the specific nutritional needs of the elderly. Elderly individuals have a common set of special problems in terms of altered taste, impaired mastication or swallowing function, and vulnerability to chronic disease, making it difficult to obtain sufficient nutrition. Technologies such as texture-modified foods and nutritionally enriched meal options now enable elderly people to enjoy palatable foods without any loss of health. Further, food fortification processes have been enhanced to allow the addition or enrichment of foods by producers with vitamins and minerals specifically tailored for the elderly to provide optimal nutritional content. These nutrition boosts not only simplify dietary compliance but also improve the general health of older individuals, highlighting the focal role that tailored nutrition plays in impacting quality of life. Application of technology in geriatric food is another revolutionary innovation that is transforming how older adults eat. Smart kitchen appliances and meal planning programs enable senior citizens to monitor their nutritional needs independently, making it possible for them to enjoy nutritious diets despite physical limitations.

Telehealth programs are also a chance for nutritionists to conduct remote consultations, thereby bridging the gap between health professionals and older adults with dietary issues. These technologies allow for individualized nutrition programs sensitive to individuals' health status and personal preferences, as well as increasing the sense of control over health in older adults. Adoption of these new technologies reflects a shift toward patient-centered approaches to geriatric nutrition consistent with the general goals of improving health outcomes and healthy aging. Furthermore, community activities and programs designed to promote geriatric nutrition have become important aids to regulating the eating needs of older populations. Findings suggest that community-based interventions such as neighborhood dietary workshops and group cooking classes can improve older adults' nutritional skills and knowledge. In addition to providing educational resources, these programs facilitate social support, reversing the feelings of loneliness and isolation that the elderly are normally forced to experience. Organizations, guided by principles established by task forces for intergenerational health care, aim to promote physical and social health among older individuals through enhanced nutrition. The impact of such community programs can be observed since they cause older citizens to form healthier patterns of eating, contributing their fair share toward overall strategy in order to guarantee greater longevity and reduced health care costs associated with nutrient imbalance (Fretwell & Feeney, 1993) (Figure 1.15).

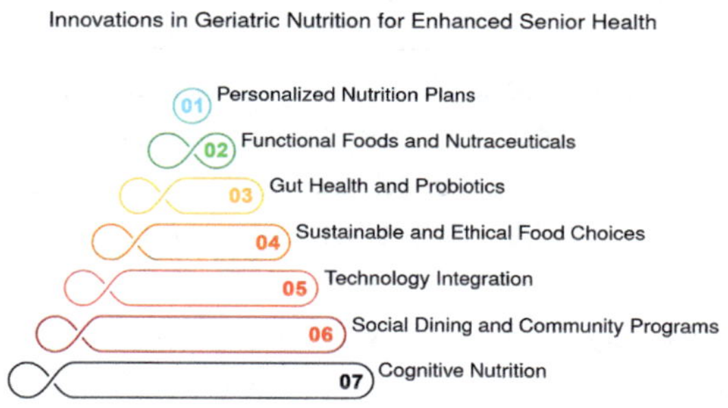

Figure 1.15. Innovations in geriatric nutrition.

Source: https://fastercapital.co/i/Geriatric-Nutrition-Service-Silver-Spoon-Startups--Nourishing-Geriatric-Nutrition-Services--Innovations-in-Geriatric-Nutrition-for-Enhanced-Senior-Health.webp.

1.6.1. Advances in Nutritional Science

Nutritional science has made significant advances, particularly in the nutritional needs of older people. With the world facing the dilemma of an ever-growing geriatric population, there has been an increased emphasis on how nutrition influences the health of older people. Malnutrition, dietary restrictions, and food choice are some of the issues that need to be understood in perspective to aging physiology. As a notable example, evidence has shown that targeted nutritional treatments can improve the functional status and quality of life of older adults, marking an important intersection of advances in geriatric care and nutritional science. Moreover, as presented by recent research, the range of food patterns and their associated health benefits is essential for developing impactful nutritional recommendations for older adults in a manner that there can be a more effective intervention in geriatric nutrition and, therefore, enhanced health equity in the risk group (Burholt & Dobbs, 2012). Through the application of frontier research methodology, the science of nutritional sciences has further advanced. Through bibliometric analysis, scholars have graphed trends in literature on the dietary needs of older adults, and it has turned out that there is growing recognition of the contribution of nutrition to the aging process. Bibliometric analysis has not only identified growth in publications about food innovation created for the elderly but has also signaled research gaps that need to be examined. By grouping keywords within thematic areas, researchers are in a position to effectively pinpoint major subjects such as the quality of diet, food security, and nutritional status that are pivotal to addressing the unique issues of the aged. Recent evidence underlines the necessity of interdisciplinarity in tackling these urgent issues and directs attention to the importance of evidence-based advice on nutrition tailored specifically to the older population (Puteri & Febriansyah, 2024). The evolution of nutritional science also encompasses examining the global concerns in rural ageing and how these affect food security. The United Nations' decade-long change of research interest suggests a growing awareness of how geographical and socioeconomic factors converge with older people's nutritional needs, especially in rural communities. As evolving agricultural practices and weather conditions influence food supply, the nexus of rural ageing and nutrition has become critical. Researchers posit that comprehension of these dynamics is central to informing public health programs that can respond to food security issues in these populations. Consequently, consideration of advances in nutritional science should be prioritized within the convergence of social, economic, and technological factors to formulate far-reaching strategies that contribute to the improvement of the nutritional status of older people living in different settings (Burholt & Dobbs, 2012).

1.6.2. Technology and Nutrition Monitoring

Technology incorporation into nutrition monitoring represents a promising innovation in geriatric medicine, with the ongoing increase in the number of elderly people. This has resulted in the creation of advanced tools and software aimed at monitoring food intake, determining nutritional requirements, and providing tailored meal planning. Technology can significantly contribute to the prevention of malnutrition, a major problem among residents in care homes for older people, where research indicates that, on average, half of all residents are malnourished. By implementing the use of digital platforms, caregivers can perform routine nutrition screenings and assessments that enable nutritional approaches to be directed towards each person's individual health requirements. Not only does this innovation make data collection more effective, but interventions can also be made more effectively, which can mitigate the adverse effects of poor nutrition in elderly populations. Including technology in monitoring nutrition also enables a timelier effort in the treatment of conditions most apt to strike older individuals. With real-time data in hand, health care providers are able to identify and treat nutritional deficiencies and imbalances promptly. This capability is essential because aging itself is a multi-factorial process where individual interventions cannot suffice. Current evidence indicates the increase in protein-energy malnutrition incidence is linked to growing multi-morbidities among aged care residents, increasing the need for effective nutritional strategies. Technology tools can be employed to track such trends so that interventions remain timely and appropriate. They can also accelerate communication among multidisciplinary teams, thereby improving coordination of efforts crucial to integrated patient care planning and delivering effective nutrition programs. Besides, the utilization of technology can also be a key factor for the active involvement of families as caregivers in the nutritional care of older individuals. By the provision of user-friendly applications and platforms, family members are able to engage with nutritional monitoring systems to improve their understanding of the dietary requirements of the elderly, thereby establishing an enabling environment for optimal nutrition. This engagement can promote improved compliance with dietary regulations and more empowered decisions on diet. The focus of the Stern Centers on prevention and care coordination reflects the potential that technology has to bridge practice and policy gaps in geriatric nutrition. With the progress of discipline, it is increasingly important that novel technological strategies are complemented with evidence-based interventions so that the elderly population receives the best possible health, delivering what they need and maintaining nutritionally (The Stern Center for Evidence-Based Policy, 2015; Agarwal et al., 2016) (Figure 1.16).

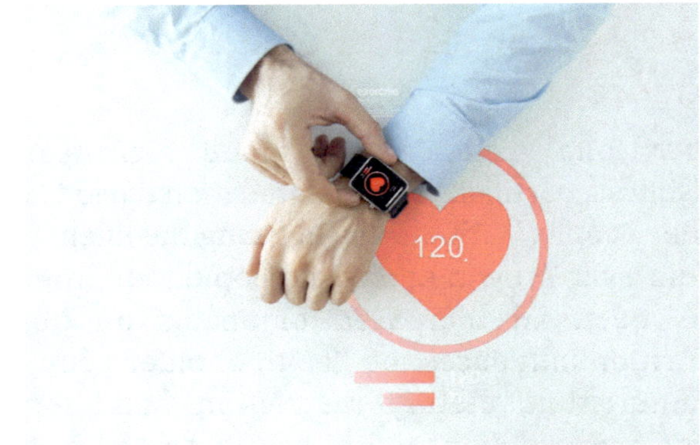

Figure 1.16. Digital technologies for effective geriatric care.

Source: https://www.news-medical.net/images/news/ImageForNews_754284_16899272689454231.jpg.

1.6.3. Future Trends in Geriatric Dietary Practices

As the number of older individuals increases, so too are dietary habits of the elderly modified to meet their bespoke nutritional needs. New trends will involve a shift to more personalized nutritional treatments based on the health, diet, and ethnicity of the individual. With new technologies such as wearables and mobile health applications, caregivers will be better placed to monitor the consumption of diets. Such tailoring will not only enhance meal satisfaction but also improve health outcomes by addressing specific dietary deficiencies often prevalent among ageing populations. Moreover, dietary education programs specifically geared towards caregivers and elderly individuals will become essential, emphasizing the importance of acquiring an understanding of the contribution of nutrition in managing chronic disease as well as promoting overall well-being. With the identification that nutrition is a part of the overall quality of life among the elderly, food technology and meal preparation innovations are likely to be pivotal. For example, the creation of nutrient-rich, convenient meal choices can reduce frustration in aspects like chewing or swallowing difficulties, which many seniors experience. Furthermore, convenience foods that align with dietary recommendations but are low in added sugars and sodium will most probably feature more prominently in the future. Adoption of the Wellspring model, which has pledged some success in improving the quality of care in nursing homes, means that a systematic process for meal planning will be key in the future. This strategy can enhance dietary quality and satisfaction among residents, leading to better health status (Bowers et al., 2002). Further, increased awareness of the social aspect of eating will be set to transform geriatric meal patterns in the future. Future interventions may involve social dining occasions, thereby facilitating socialization among residents and preventing loneliness, a frequent issue among most elderly. Promoting palliative care and self-management strategies, as outlined in studies highlighting evidence-based policy, implies a move towards more holistic approaches to care (The Stern Center for Evidence-Based Policy, 2015). These models of care not only target meal planning but also consider the psychological and social dimensions of eating. By integrating these trends into geriatric nutrition, practitioners are able to create a more affirming and stimulating environment that recognizes the importance of food in the body and soul care.

SUMMARY

Geriatric nutrition is increasingly recognized as being important in fulfilling the special needs of the elderly. The nutritional requirements of individuals change with age due to physiological alterations and the greater prevalence of chronic health disorders. Understanding the changes is essential for clinicians to develop useful diet plans. The diet plans not only have to enhance nutritional intake but also to take care of the specific health problems that are encountered in older people, like malnutrition and its multiple effects on health. Implementation of geriatric assessment into daily clinical practice is essential so that clinicians can identify nutritional deficits and develop individualized interventions to foster well-being. This alludes to the growing significance of geriatric nutrition in maintaining health and quality of life in the older population, ultimately maximizing the efficacy of medical treatment as the aging of the population continues to rise. Further, more recent data have established the alarming prevalence of malnutrition in elderly patients, compounded further by its acceleration with age due to decreased gastrointestinal function. The aging gut is subject to mechanical and chemical changes that affect nutrient uptake, hence predisposing the elderly to malnutrition (Rémond et al., 2015). Intervention against these risks demands that one understands how such changes can impact food consumption and health (Rémond et al., 2015). There is a demand for healthcare systems to implement approaches that effectively diagnose the elderly's nutritional status in time for intervention. By educating clinicians regarding the interaction between nutrition and aging, we can facilitate an active response to the management of geriatric conditions that develop due to malnutrition, thereby improving long-term health outcomes in this group. Basically, as geriatric nutrition becomes more advanced, there is little doubt that interdisciplinary cooperation among geriatricians, nutritionists, and allied healthcare workers is necessary. Such teamwork would make that holistic assessment, as suggested by recent literature, part of mainstream older patient care (Lampugnale, 2017). By multidisciplinary teamwork and a focus on geriatric training for future healthcare staff, we can equip them better to deal with the issues caused by an aging population. The proposed educational interventions will, apart from enhancing knowledge of the primary areas of geriatric assessment, trigger a systems approach to managing oncogeriatric patients. Overall stress on nutrition and health will end up leading to improved surgery outcomes and an improved quality of life for aging populations, highlighting the significant impact of geriatric nutrition on the delivery of care in this population.

Geriatric nutrition is a field that encompasses a number of important considerations that have a direct impact on both the physical and mental well-being of older adults. As the population shifts and the number of individuals over the age of 65 continues to rise, particularly with an estimated 20% of the United States population being this age by 2029 (Wynn-Grundy, 2016), it is increasingly important that their nutritional needs are acknowledged. Nutritional deficiencies have the impact of aggravating already existing health issues as well as inducing a loss of functional capacity. The fundamental understanding of tailoring nutritional interventions to address the unique physiological requirements of older individuals is essential for all medical caregivers working with this group. With the body undergoing so many changes, the inclusion of adequate nutrition education is of paramount importance in enhancing longevity and quality of life. Moreover, the interplay between mental health and nutrition among aged populations must be stringently examined. Depression in older populations that remains undiagnosed has been labelled as a significant problem, with some estimates suggesting that up to 40% of older populations with chronic disease remain undiagnosed for depression (Wynn-Grundy, 2016). This has significant implications for cognitive function because symptoms such as an inability to focus undermine the storage of essential healthcare education, including nutritional information. The relationship between mental health and knowledge of diet emphasizes the necessity for comprehensive measures that not only address physical health but also account for psychological considerations. Mental illness screening is crucial in making sure elderly people can fully utilize and comprehend dietary advice particular to their case. Lastly, as the field of nutrition evolves, it also contains data discovered in other animals, such as dogs and cats, which sheds light on underlying principles applicable to human aging. Aging in companion animals parallels human geriatric aging, and improved veterinary care, diet, and lifestyle contribute to increased lifespan. Such analogies can augment geriatric nutritional knowledge by alluding to the benefit of diet-specific accommodations made for aging physiologies. Through the transfer of knowledge acquired in both veterinary and geriatric nutrition, healthcare providers can better manage the complex interaction between diet, disease, and health in older adults. As we move on to look at these interacting dimensions in greater detail, we see that international nutrition strategies come into play in securing improved health in the aging population.

A CLOSER LOOK

NUTRITIONAL NEEDS OF OLDER PERSONS

Nutritional needs of older persons highlight that with aging come physiological, psychological, and social alterations whose immediate effect is on dietary requirements and food intake. With advancing age, metabolism slows down, and there is a lower energy requirement, but nutrient-dense food is required to maintain health, immunity, and strength. Protein is necessary to prevent wasting of muscles (sarcopenia) and to heal wounds and maintain immunity. The elderly should take high-quality protein foods such as lean meat, milk, legumes, eggs, and fish. Calcium and vitamin D are critical to maintain bone density and prevent osteoporosis, while vitamin B12 absorption decreases with advancing age, putting more people at risk of deficiency, affecting cognition and red blood cell production. Iron, zinc, and folate are important for energy, immunity, and cell function (Figure 1.17).

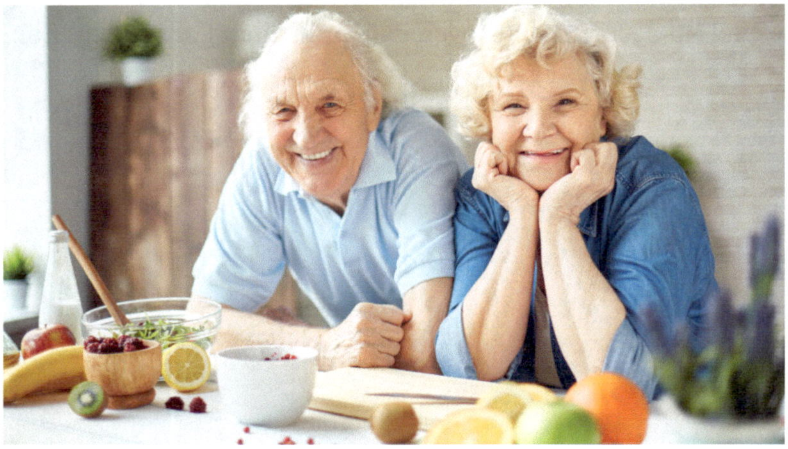

Figure 1.17. Nutritional needs of older people.

Source: https://extension.usu.edu/nutrition/images/older-nutrition.png.

Hydration is also a common issue among the aging due to the compromised sense of thirst, and therefore, encouraging proper fluid intake—especially water—is important. Foods with fiber, like fruits, vegetables, and whole grains, enhance digestion and prevent constipation, which is a common issue among aging populations as well. Decreasing the consumption of salt, saturated fat, and added sugar also reduces the risk of chronic disease development, like hypertension, diabetes, and cardiovascular disease. Social determinants such as loneliness, mobility impairment, reduced income, and oral disease may also affect food consumption and meal frequency, so interventions in the form of community meal services, counseling, and low-cost cooking education are useful. Overall, a balanced, multicolored, and individualized diet helps in sustaining health, independence, and quality of life in old age.

REFERENCES

1. Mole, L., Kent, B., Abbott, R., Wood, C., & Hickson, M. (2018). The nutritional care of people living with dementia at home: A scoping review. *Health & social care in the community, 26*(4), e485–e496. https://doi.org/10.1111/hsc.12540(accessed on 12th July 2025).
2. Agarwal, E., Isenring, E., Marshall, S., et al. (2016). Optimizing nutrition in residential aged care: A narrative review. https://core.ac.uk/download/196601588.pdf (accessed on 12th July 2025).
3. Agbozo, F., Amardi-Mfoafo, J., Dwase, H., et al. (2018). Nutrition knowledge, dietary patterns and anthropometric indices of older persons in four peri-urban communities in Ga West municipality, Ghana. https://core.ac.uk/download/478290013.pdf (accessed on 12th July 2025).
4. Allum, W., Alsina, M., Andritsch, E., et al. (2018). ECCO essential requirements for quality cancer care: Oesophageal and gastric cancer. https://core.ac.uk/download/157587654.pdf (accessed on 12th July 2025).
5. Maylor, E. A., Simpson, E. E., Secker, D. L., Meunier, N., Andriollo-Sanchez, M., Polito, A., Stewart-Knox, B., McConville, C., O'Connor, J. M., & Coudray, C. (2006). Effects of zinc supplementation on cognitive function in healthy middle-aged and older adults: the ZENITH study. *The British journal of nutrition, 96*(4), 752–760.(accessed on 12th July 2025).
6. Ash, S., Harvey, K., & Vivanti, A. (2010). Developing a quick and practical screen to improve the identification of poor hydration in geriatric and rehabilitative care. https://core.ac.uk/download/10895888.pdf (accessed on 12th July 2025).
7. Deutz, N. E., Bauer, J. M., Barazzoni, R., Biolo, G., Boirie, Y., Bosy-Westphal, A., Cederholm, T., Cruz-Jentoft, A., Krznariç, Z., Nair, K. S., Singer, P., Teta, D., Tipton, K., & Calder, P. C. (2014). Protein intake and exercise for optimal muscle function with aging: recommendations from the ESPEN Expert Group. *Clinical nutrition (Edinburgh, Scotland), 33*(6), 929–936. https://doi.org/10.1016/j.clnu.2014.04.007(accessed on 12th July 2025).
8. Volkert, D., Beck, A. M., Cederholm, T., Cruz-Jentoft, A., Goisser, S., Hooper, L., Kiesswetter, E., Maggio, M., Raynaud-Simon, A., Sieber, C. C., Sobotka, L., van Asselt, D., Wirth, R., & Bischoff, S. C. (2019). ESPEN guideline on clinical nutrition and hydration in geriatrics. *Clinical nutrition (Edinburgh, Scotland), 38*(1), 10–47. https://doi.org/10.1016/j.clnu.2018.05.024(accessed on 12th July 2025).
9. Rémond, D., Shahar, D. R., Gille, D., Pinto, P., Kachal, J., Peyron, M. A., Dos Santos, C. N., Walther, B., Bordoni, A., Dupont, D., Tomás-Cobos, L., & Vergères, G. (2015). Understanding the gastrointestinal tract of the elderly to develop dietary solutions that prevent malnutrition. *Oncotarget, 6*(16), 13858–13898. https://doi.org/10.18632/oncotarget.4030(accessed on 12th July 2025).
10. Bowers, B., Hawes, C., Phillips, C. D., Zimmerman, D., Fielding, J. A., Jacobson, N., Stone, R. I., et al. (2002). Evaluation of the Wellspring Model for Improving Nursing Home Quality. https://core.ac.uk/download/71351187.pdf (accessed on 12th July 2025).
11. Burholt, V. and Dobbs, C. (2012) Research on Rural Ageing: Where Have We Got to and Where Are We Going in Europe? Journal of Rural Studies, 28, 432-446. https://doi.org/10.1016/j.jrurstud.2012.01.009 (accessed on 12th July 2025).
12. Donini, L. M., Lenzi, A., Perna, S., Poggiogalle, E., Rondanelli, M., & Spadaccini, D. (2018). Are

the therapeutic strategies in anorexia of ageing effective on nutritional status? A systematic review with meta-analysis. https://core.ac.uk/download/188830393.pdf (accessed on 12th July 2025).

13. Puteri, N. E., & Febriansyah, M. I. (2024). Scientific Mapping of Elderly Food Studies: A Bibliometric Approach. Journal of Nutrition Science, 5(1), 20–28. https://doi.org/10.35308/jns.v5i1.9560 (accessed on 12th July 2025).

14. Marsha D. Fretwell, M.D. Aging 2000, SJS Inc. Marian S. Feeney University of Rhode Island (1993). Alternatives and consequences of health care prototypes and developing a public policy education program. https://core.ac.uk/download/pdf/7052050.pdf (accessed on 12th July 2025).

15. Grosso, G., Busó, P., Mata, A., Abdelkarim, O., Aly, M., Pinilla, J., Fernandez, A., et al. (2024). UnDErstanding consumer food choices & promotion of healthy and sustainable Mediterranean diet and LIfestyle in children and adolescents through behavioral change actionS: The DELICIOUS project. *The European Journal of Public Health, 34.* https://www.semanticscholar.org/paper/f2b263188a28ad561becdb5f8bb1df54ba8429aa (accessed on 12th July 2025).

16. Gumuskaya, O., Skendri, S., Birkenhead, K., & Sarkies, M. N. (2024). Perioperative nutrition in older patients: What are the priorities? *Current Opinion in Clinical Nutrition and Metabolic Care, 28,* 6–13. https://www.semanticscholar.org/paper/c91a91bd2cdff72332c93b0e17aefca148b3cda3 (accessed on 12th July 2025).

17. Ji, S., Jung, H., Baek, J., Jang, I. Y., & Lee, E. (2024). Sarcopenia as the mobility phenotype of aging: Clinical implications. *Journal of Bone Metabolism, 31,* 1–12. https://www.semanticscholar.org/paper/9a5294441bfba7a4d15514f72a1ed93eae64f67f (accessed on 12th July 2025).

18. Lampugnale, C. A. (2017). Surgical assessment of the geriatric oncology patient. https://open.bu.edu/bitstream/2144/26707/5/Lampugnale_bu_0017N_13146.pdf (accessed on 12th July 2025).

19. Lombardo, M., Feraco, A., Armani, A., Camajani, E., Gorini, S., Strollo, R., Padua, E., et al. (2024). Gender differences in body composition, dietary patterns, and physical activity: Insights from a cross-sectional study. *Frontiers in Nutrition, 11.* https://www.semanticscholar.org/paper/41e1ec705b373b6bd0c09bc24a5fd295dd343c08 (accessed on 12th July 2025).

20. Malafarina, V., Reginster, J. Y., Cabrerizo, S., et al. (2017). Nutritional status and nutritional treatment are related to outcomes and mortality in older adults with hip fracture. https://core.ac.uk/download/pdf/212756692.pdf (accessed on 12th July 2025).

21. Matringe, C. H. (2007). Nutrition and eating behavior in older adulthood. https://core.ac.uk/download/41538217.pdf (accessed on 12th July 2025).

22. The Stern Center for Evidence-Based Policy (2015). The Stern Center for Evidence-Based Policy, 2015. The Stern Center for Evidence-Based Policy ("Stern Center"), University of Pittsburgh's Health Policy Institute. https://core.ac.uk/download/75783019.pdf (accessed on 12th July 2025).

23. Nolan, M. (1997). Gerontological nursing: Professional priority or eternal Cinderella? https://core.ac.uk/download/56526.pdf (accessed on 12th July 2025).

24. Omar, N., Shafiee, S. I., Nor'hisham, S. H., Ibrahim, Z., Jamaluddin, R., Rahamat, S., Mohd Yusof, B. N., et al. (2022). A logical framework (MYGERYFS) for hospital foodservice to prevent

malnutrition among geriatric patients in hospitals, Malaysia: Protocol for a feasibility study. *JMIR Research Protocols, 12*. https://www.semanticscholar.org/paper/2329c4ad9798988cbe02d098788e8ba36c9a0427 (accessed on 12th July 2025).

25. Presley, R. G. (2014). Food intake of hospitalized older adults after exposure to volunteer feeding program. https://core.ac.uk/download/72840102.pdf (accessed on 12th July 2025).

26. Wynn-Grundy, N. J. (2016). Undiagnosed depression in the elderly and healthcare education. https://core.ac.uk/download/70426926.pdf (accessed on 12th July 2025).

27. Zabolotskikh, I., Gorobets, E., Grigoryev, E., Kotovskaya, Y., Lebedinskii, K. M., Musaeva, T., Mkhitaryan, E. A., et al. (2022). Perioperative management of elderly and senile patients. Recommendations. *Annals of Critical Care*. https://www.semanticscholar.org/paper/e01ca676503024b8e474fbd8834e6dce9bf576ee (accessed on 12th July 2025).

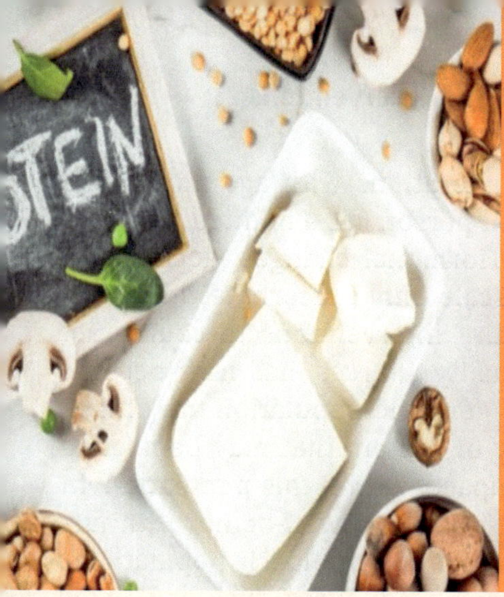

Chapter 2

PROTEIN METABOLISM AND REQUIREMENTS

Contents

Introduction

Gaining an understanding of the intricacies of protein metabolism when addressing the dietary needs of elderly individuals is essential. The physiological processes of the body change very dramatically with age, and such changes include alterations in muscle mass, metabolic rate, and nutrient absorption. This population is particularly vulnerable to disorders such as sarcopenia, a syndrome of loss of muscle mass and strength, which can lead to impairment of mobility and increased morbidity. Current studies have suggested that inadequate protein intake is a significant factor in these age-related declines and warrant a closer examination of the dietary protein requirements unique to geriatric populations." This chapter aims to analyze the biochemical pathways of protein metabolism and how the pathways can be optimized for greater health benefits among the elderly, thereby increasing their quality of life and independence. Protein is not only a fundamental macronutrient; it plays a crucial role in various functions of the body, including tissue repair, muscle development, and disease resistance. With geriatric nutrition, there is a focus on how the alterations with age impact the utilization and digestion of protein. Evidence highlights that the aged person has a blunted response to protein in the diet, which is inhibitory for muscle synthesis. Hormonal changes, decrease in physical function, and prevalence of chronic diseases on a large scale only exacerbate this issue. The challenge therefore, still lies in identifying appropriate dietary interventions to counteract these deficits. A higher protein intake, particularly from good-quality sources, has now become an essential recommendation; however, specific guidelines in the geriatric population are still in progress. This calls for critical research into not only the quantity of protein that may be needed but also the timing and type of protein that may have beneficial impacts within this population. In addition, the effects of poor protein consumption are not limited to muscle well-being, with far-reaching implications on overall metabolic function and health outcomes among elderly populations. Untreated protein-energy malnutrition will result in serious health consequences, such as greater susceptibility to infections, slow healing of wounds, and eventually increased mortality. It is important for healthcare professionals, nutritionists, and caregivers assisting elderly populations to understand these implications. New evidence highlights the necessity for thorough nutritional evaluations to customize dietary interventions for effectiveness. Interventional strategies can be through the inclusion of protein supplements or fortified foods to address the nutritional deficit in affected individuals due to low protein consumption. With an understanding of the complexities of protein metabolism and specific needs of the geriatric age group, it is now possible to formulate specific dietary guidance that not only addresses their short-term nutritional need but also facilitates long-term healthy and active lifestyles, thus ensuring a robust quality of life at older age (Figure 2.1).

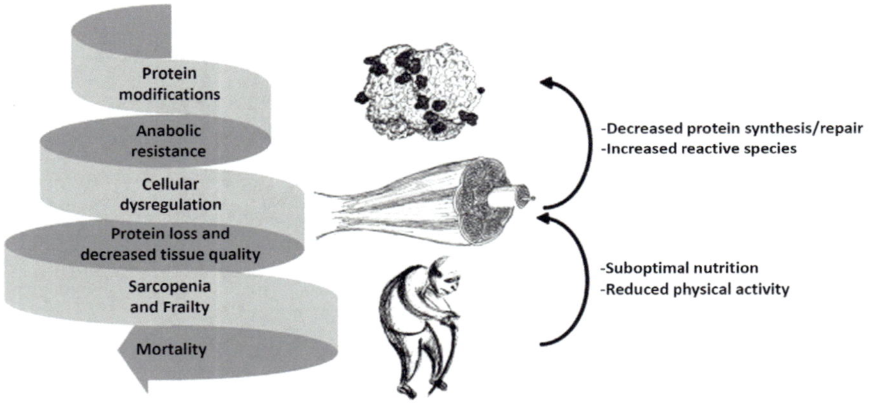

Figure 2.1. Protein metabolism in the elderly.

Source: https://ars.els-cdn.com/content/image/3-s2.0-B9780128021675000074-f07-03-9780128021675.jpg.

Definition of Protein Metabolism

Protein metabolism is a physiological process that entails the synthesis, breakdown, and utilization of proteins within the body. Essentially, protein metabolism incorporates two core pathways: anabolism and catabolism. Anabolism characterizes the biological synthesis of proteins from amino acids, the building blocks of protein that are crucial for cellular growth, maintenance, and repair. Catabolism, on the other hand, refers to the degradation of proteins into amino acids, which can either be used as energy sources or be converted into other biological compounds. This dynamic equilibrium between protein synthesis and degradation is particularly important in older individuals since aging alterations have the potential to interfere with the integrity of these metabolic processes, leading to alterations in body composition and heightened vulnerability to malnutrition and functional impairment. Establishing a clear understanding of protein metabolism is imperative when formulating nutritional strategies unique to the elderly population. The need for the inclusion of protein metabolism in geriatric nutrition arises due to the high prevalence of malnutrition among the elderly, particularly with acute medical illnesses such as hip fractures. Research shows that such patients tend to exhibit an impaired protein diet and, as a result, may not meet their dietary requirements, further deteriorating their general health (Malafarina et al., 2017). Malnutrition not only lowers protein turnover but also leads to adverse effects like prolonged recovery times and increased mortality. Because aging has been characterized by loss of muscle mass and strength over time, or sarcopenia, adequate protein-calorie intake becomes exponentially greater. Thoughts on the sources, how often they are taken, and the quality of protein in the diet become crucial to educating older adults with the necessary information to preserve their muscle function and health. Besides, the elderly gastrointestinal system presents particular challenges that significantly influence protein metabolism, forming an important interface between food digestion, absorption, and nutrient availability (Rémond et al., 2015). Changes in gastrointestinal function during aging can disrupt mechanical food breakdown, slow down gastric emptying, and undermine chemical digestion of proteins. These alterations render the efficiency with which older individuals are able to utilize protein from food unassailable, highlighting the importance of individualized nutrition treatments that account for such body changes. Metabolism of protein within a geriatric diet requires the building of specialized dietary guidelines that work in coordination with the altered digestive activity among the elderly. These suggestions must consider not only how much protein is ingested but also the density of the nutrients and general dietary pattern in an effort to most effectively sustain maximum health outcomes and recovery for this vulnerable population.

Significance of Protein to Geriatric Nutrition

The significance of protein to geriatric diets is emphasized by the growing incidence of malnutrition in older populations. Adequate protein intake is necessary throughout the aging process since it's necessary to maintain muscle mass, strength, and overall well-being. Aging is normally preceded by sarcopenia, a condition of decreased muscle mass and compromised physical function. Studies have demonstrated that low protein intake exacerbates this condition, leading to decreased mobility, fall risk, and quality of life. In particular, intervention from multidimensional assessment is able to customize nutrition intervention to address the unique needs of health issues in the older patient. According to a case report, nutrition management derived from Comprehensive Geriatric Assessment (CGA) is essential in the prevention and management of malnutrition and further validates the application of protein diets throughout the golden years of life to prevent adverse health consequences as well as promote longevity and functional autonomy (Park et al., 2025). Aside from defending muscle mass, protein also serves a vital function in the metabolic health of the elderly. Protein has been recognized to play an important part in the immune system, wound healing, and other metabolic processes. Since protein metabolism declines with age, elderly individuals become susceptible to a variety of complications. There were significant correlations between preoperative modified geriatric nutritional risk index (mGNRI) scores and survival outcomes in elderly surgical patients, showing the significance of measuring and optimizing nutritional intake, especially protein intake, before invasive interventions. This would mean that higher protein content can enhance recovery rates and overall health conditions among the elderly, thus validating the necessity for dietary adjustment unique to the special requirements of this population (Tsai et al., 2024). Furthermore, protein intake increase is essential in preventing refeeding syndrome, a life-threatening condition that may arise in individuals receiving nutritional rehabilitation. As the majority of the elderly have feeding issues due to dental issues, cognitive disturbances, or gastrointestinal upsets, tailored nutritional care with preferred protein consumption becomes of paramount significance. It is possible to reduce the risk of refeeding syndrome while keeping the elderly well-nourished without harming them by utilizing a slow process of protein and caloric intake. Coherent strategies, including education and well-structured guidance for carers, can improve nutrition status at discharge and lead to overall quality of life. Strategic re-prioritization of dietary needs to ensure sufficient protein improves recovery in hospitals but also allows older individuals to maintain their health and independence in life (Park et al., 2025) (Figure 2.2).

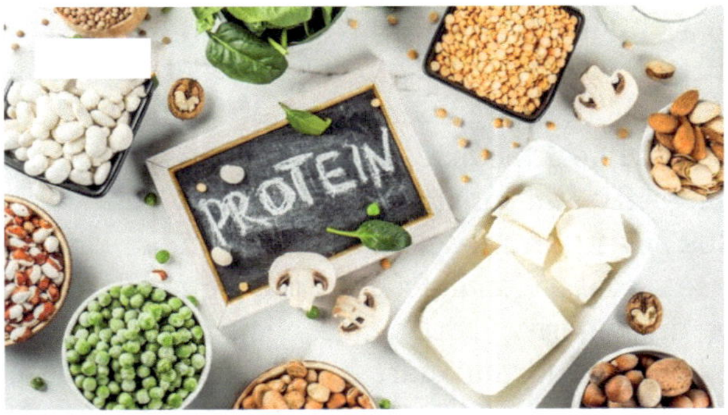

Figure 2.2. High protein foods for the elderly.

Source: https://blog.senocare.in/high-protein-foods-for-elderly-senocare-clg4t6gi6383421kowp8o6je44/.

2.1. The Role of Protein in the Body

The role of protein in the body is varied, including essential functions of great significance to general health, particularly in the elderly. Proteins are the building blocks of tissues in the body and are involved in the structure and function of muscles, bones, skin, and organs. They are responsible for the synthesis of enzymes and hormones, which regulate various physiological processes. In elderly patients, the necessity of adequate protein intake increases even more, as the alterations that take place with age can lead to loss of muscle mass (sarcopenia) and diminished strength. Adequate protein supply prevents not just physical strength, but also accelerates recovery from injury and surgery, such as hip fractures. Hence, it is crucial to provide optimal amounts of protein to geriatric patients for maintaining their functional independence as well as overall well-being. Protein metabolism knowledge is vital while determining the nutritional needs of the aged. Digestion is significantly influenced by aging and loses its effectiveness in absorbing and digesting nutrients, further complicating protein synthesis in the body. The older gastrointestinal tract may experience decreased motility and secretion of digestive enzymes, impairing effective hydrolysis of protein to functional amino acids. Thus, old people often exhibit an inadequate nutritional supply, which is linked to severe health outcomes, including malnutritional disorders with very high prevalence rates among geriatric patients. As reflected by emerging studies, malnourished patients who have developed disorders like hip fractures demonstrate lower recovery outcomes, which depicts the significance of learning about protein metabolism in this population (Malafarina et al., 2017). It can be enhanced to utilize proteins and overall health conditions by reversing these declines in old age through proper dietary interventions. More importantly, the consequences of malnutrition in the elderly are not just limited to muscle health; it has multisystem consequences to all organ systems, like nervous, musculoskeletal, cardiovascular, immune, and dermal systems. As older individuals find it hard to meet their protein needs, individualized dietary plans are required. These policies must consider alterations in the aged gastrointestinal tract and provide dietary advice focused on the bioavailability of nutrients. This emphasis on personalized nutritional approaches is highly critical in avoiding malnutrition complications, which have been shown to escalate mortality in elderly patients who are injured or undergo surgery (Rémond et al., 2015). By integrating nutritional education and practical dietary solutions, medical professionals are able to effectively address these problems and promote a healthier aging process among the aged population (Figure 2.3).

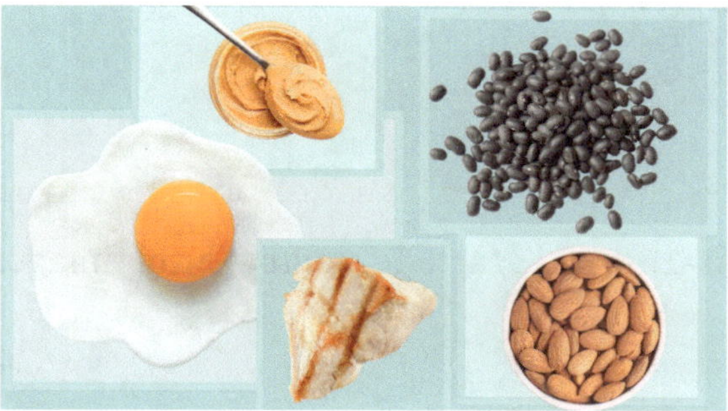

Figure 2.3. Role of protein in the body.

Source: https://images.everydayhealth.com/images/diet-nutrition/what-is-protein-guide-alt-1440x810.jpg?sfvrsn=5fac8ba1_5.

2.1.1. Functions of Proteins in Cellular Processes

Proteins play a crucial role in supporting cellular processes required to provide health and homeostasis. In gerontological nutrition, proteins' dual roles are more significant to study, particularly since the elderly population becomes highly susceptible to metabolic disorders and overall health diseases. Proteins not only constitute structural cell elements but also enzymes, which catalyze biochemical reactions to help in processes such as digestion and energy production. Signaling proteins are also crucial in cellular communication to cause cells to respond appropriately to internal as well as external stimuli. In aging, decreased protein synthesis can trigger a cascade of physiological impairments, thereby pointing to the importance of adequate protein intake in aging individuals to maintain muscle mass, satisfy metabolic demands, and avoid chronic diseases. During aging, the physiological changes in the body can have deleterious effects on protein metabolism, leading to significant health issues. Sarcopenia, which consists of muscle mass and strength reduction, is a prime example of protein insufficiency resulting in a condition among the elderly, with consequences of decreased mobility and increased frailty. The loss of muscle quality is known to alter the interaction between muscle and adipose tissue, causing a negative growth in fat mass that infuses fat into muscle fibers and thus compromises their contractility. This indicates the need for sufficient protein consumption to counteract age-associated muscle loss and augment physical function. In effect, proteins play a key role in combating the adverse consequences of aging, offering a method of preservation of lean body mass and general functional status in older individuals (Carter et al., 2019). Besides, aging influences not only protein metabolism but also the effectiveness of the gastrointestinal system, which may lead to malnutrition in the elderly. Because the aging process involves changes in digestive mechanics, nutrient uptake may be disrupted and compromise protein bioavailability. Impaired gastrointestinal effectiveness can further exacerbate malnutrition and engender a high risk for various health complications like cardiovascular disease and immune deficiency. Therefore, proper nutritional strategies specific to the special challenges of geriatrics are crucial in ensuring the best protein nutrition. Such guidelines need to emphasize the inclusion of nutrient-dense foods that ensure the highest protein availability while considering the special functional impairment of the aging gut. By attending to these nutritional requirements, healthcare professionals can make a significant difference to the nutritional needs of the elderly and limit the risks of malnutrition (Rémond et al., 2015) (Figure 2.4).

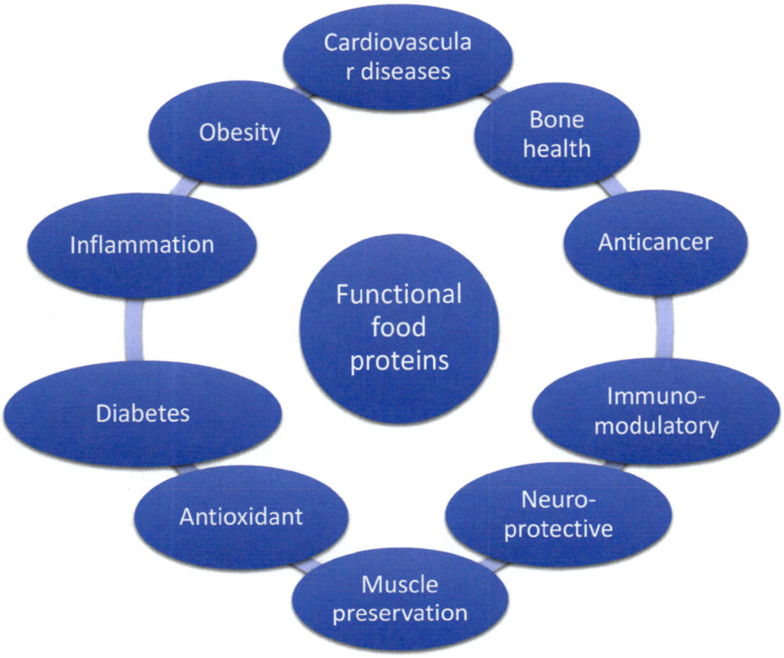

Figure 2.4. Functions of proteins in cellular processes.

Source: https://www.mdpi.com/nutrients/nutrients-16-02323/article_deploy/html/images/nutrients-16-02323-g001.png.

2.1.2. Importance of Proteins for Muscle Maintenance

The role of proteins in muscle maintenance cannot be exaggerated, particularly in the context of aging populations. As individuals age, skeletal muscle mass and strength tend to decline, a phenomenon known as sarcopenia. This degeneration is closely linked to inadequate protein intake and decreased muscle protein synthesis rates. Proteins are vital macromolecules composed of amino acids, which are the building blocks for muscle tissue. A high-quality protein-rich diet not only allows the preservation of lean body mass but also speeds up physical activity recovery. Further, sufficient protein intake may lead to improved muscle quality that promotes physical functioning in older adults, thereby less the chance of falls. It is therefore necessary to include sufficient protein in the older adults' diet for muscle health and well-being. In examining the special requirements of protein intake among the elderly, it is clear that the conventional nutritional guidelines may not be sufficient. It has been established from studies that older adults can gain some benefit from higher intakes of protein to properly stimulate muscle protein synthesis. The current recommendations are for the consumption of approximately 1.2–1.5 grams of protein per kilogram of body weight for this group in an effort to counteract the degenerative impact of aging on muscle tissue. Also, evenly distributing protein consumption throughout the day has the most anabolic effect because the body can use protein more efficiently when ingested in small doses in more frequent servings. Such a dietary strategy not only maintains muscle but also overall metabolic well-being, which is very important in aged populations. Thus, personalized protein advice plays an important role in ensuring proper nutritional status for the elderly. Protein metabolism underlying physiological processes also plays a pivotal role in muscle maintenance, particularly in geriatric care. With advancing age, the effectiveness of the anabolic signaling pathways that ensure muscle repair and growth diminishes, like the fibroblast growth factor signaling pathway, which is fundamental to muscle homeostasis. Dysregulation of these pathways could lead to decreased muscle resilience and susceptibility to injury and chronic disease. Therefore, protein consumption becomes paramount not only in maintaining muscle mass but also in adding to these essential physiological processes. Secondly, treatment such as the addition of exercise, resistance training in particular, combined with adequate protein intake, can significantly aid muscle preservation efforts. By adopting a holistic strategy that combines optimal nutrition and physical exercise, older individuals are better able to counteract loss of muscle mass with age, hence improving quality of life as well as functional independence (Ambrosetti et al., 2020; Xie et al., 2020).

2.1.3. Proteins as Enzymes and Hormones

The ubiquitous role of proteins as enzymes and hormones is significant in physiological homeostasis, particularly in the elderly. Enzymes, which are special proteins, catalyze the metabolic reactions that allow energy formation and nutrient breakdown to make it possible to utilize the food intake of elderly people in an efficient manner. With increasing age, loss of digestive efficiency is generally accompanied by malnutrition and a greater risk of chronic diseases. An aging gastrointestinal system contains reduced mechanical and chemical digestion mechanisms, which can compromise nutrient absorption. This condition emphasizes the necessity of diet recommendations that include protein-rich foods, which enhance not only the performance of enzymes but also the fight against the effect of aging on nutrient absorption (Rémond et al., 2015). Understanding the interaction of proteins and metabolic functions enables interventions to enhance the quality of nutritional consumption among older adults. Hormones, another of the vital functions of proteins, govern numerous body functions, including metabolism, immune response, and stress response. Hormonal balance is, therefore, important to be sustained during geriatric nutrition, all the more so in light of the altered hormonal responses that ensue as a result of aging. For instance, insulin, a hormone released from a protein, is involved centrally with the metabolism of glucose; insulin resistance in the elderly is widespread, and in most instances, it leads to complications such as diabetes and cardiovascular disease. Protein metabolism thus becomes fundamental to understanding, since proper intake can ensure hormone activity and production. Recent evidence emphasizes the importance of specialized nutritional diets to increase protein intake, which can potentially reverse hormonal dysregulation found in older people and maintain overall health (Pasini et al., 2015). Hence, diet modification based on protein can play a significant role in maintaining hormonal health in older patients. The process of aging normally leads to a weakening of enzymatic and hormonal function, which adds to the risk for malnutrition and secondary complications that follow. Given how complex these biological processes are, there is a need to integrate knowledge of protein metabolism and its requirements into geriatric nutrition. Proteins, in their dual functions of enzymes and hormones, are at the interface of metabolic well-being, determining everything from nutrient uptake to resistance to disease. By means of strategic nutritional interventions focusing on high-quality protein sources, healthcare workers can substantially lower the prevalence of malnutrition in older individuals. Such a strategy not only focuses on the optimal intake of proteins but also tries to maintain the functional capacity of enzymes and hormones, thereby facilitating healthier aging and reducing the burden of age-related diseases (Pasini et al., 2015; Rémond et al., 2015) (Figure 2.5).

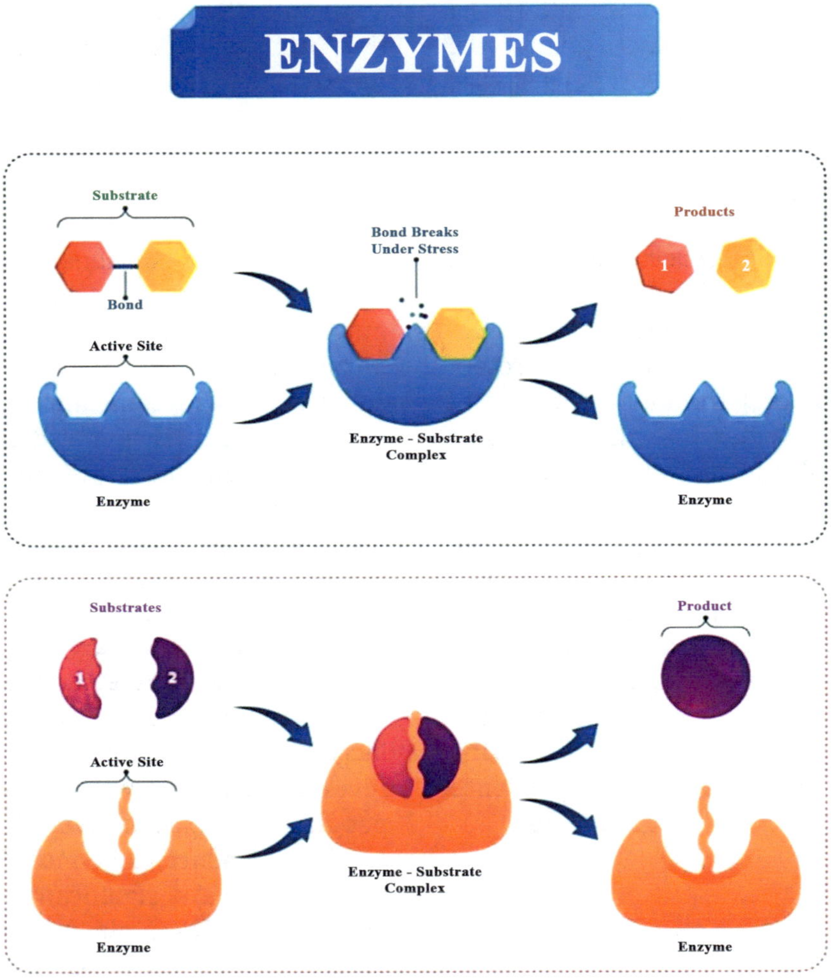

Figure 2.5. Proteins as enzymes and hormones.

Source: https://endoconsult.b-cdn.net/wp-content/uploads/enzymes-structure-and-mechanism.jpg.

2.2. Changes in Protein Metabolism with Age

With advancing age, profound alterations in protein metabolism occur that are highly relevant to understanding nutritional requirements in the geriatric phase. Almost a truism is the loss of body fat mass or sarcopenia which not only affects physical function but also metabolic processes overall. This loss of muscle is associated with a decrease in the ability of the body to synthesize new proteins, primarily due to decreased hormonal signaling and slower cellular processes. Therefore, older adults may require increased protein consumption to efficiently stimulate muscle protein synthesis, and therefore, caregivers and clinicians must provide adequate dietary protein to this age group. Studies indicate that the RDA for protein is too low for older people and suggest an individualized nutrition guideline considering such metabolic changes (Cryan et al., 2019).

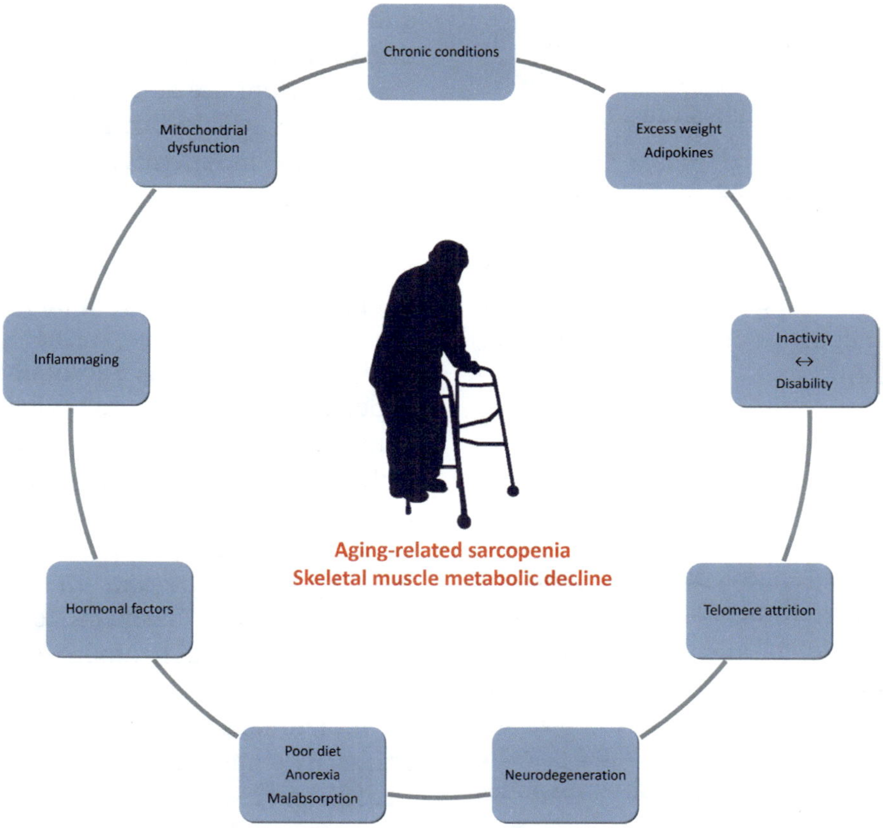

Figure 2.6. Inactivity and skeletal muscle metabolism.

Source: https://pub.mdpi-res.com/ijms/ijms-21-00592/article_deploy/html/images/ijms-21-00592-g001.png?1580925286.

The value of protein quality also grows as individuals move further along in life. Not all proteins make equal contributions to muscle maintenance and well-being; therefore, the source of dietary protein can play a significant role in health. Animal proteins, which contain the complete amino acid profile, are more likely to be effective in inducing muscle protein synthesis than most plant proteins that may lack one or more of the essential amino acids. But a balanced diet, including both, is well capable of satisfying certain nutritional needs, particularly in people who may have dietary limitations or preferences. The implementation of strategies involving high-quality protein sources is critical in the maintenance of muscle mass and healthy metabolism among older people, finally leading to improved quality of life (Rosa et al., 2017). The interplay between protein metabolism and gut microbiota also points out the complex physiological changes with aging. Studies have begun uncovering connections between protein digestion and health of the gut, which implicates microbiomes in nutrient metabolism and absorption. As gut microbiota diversity reduces with aging, it can compromise the metabolic pathways employed in protein fermentation and amino acid synthesis. This dysbiosis could lead to inflammation and other age-related diseases, complicating the nutritional situation in older individuals. Therefore, it is crucial to understand these intricate interactions in an attempt to develop integrated nutritional approaches not only for protein requirement fulfillment but also for gut health, thereby guaranteeing the overall well-being of the aging population (Cryan et al., 2019) (Figure 2.6).

2.2.1. Decreased Muscle Mass and Strength

Sarcopenia, this lost muscle strength and mass, is a critical issue in the geriatric patient population. It results from a multifactorial interaction of factors, including hormonal alterations with increasing age, physical inactivity, and inadequate dietary consumption. As age advances, the naturally occurring reduction in muscle protein synthesis is multiplied by a diminished response to protein intake from the diet, resulting in a lowering of the overall muscle mass. This, in turn, further deteriorates the ability for activities of daily living, contributing to the vicious cycle of physical decline. Treatment of sarcopenia with intensified nutritional therapy is critical in maintaining muscle preservation and overall well-being among the elderly, particularly in the area of protein metabolism and efficiency of diet treatment. The most significant aspect in the treatment of low muscle power and mass involves the observation and improvement of protein intake among the elderly. Research indicates that a majority of older people shortchange themselves on protein, which is essential for the repair and rebuilding process in muscle. The Recommended Dietary Allowance (RDA) for protein is too low for some older people who would be served better by consuming at higher levels, particularly in conjunction with co-existing illnesses or the recovery periods. Dietary interventions to increase protein intake, as well as distribution and timing throughout the day, can lead to dramatic improvements in muscle strength and mass. Appropriate dietary interventions not only inhibit sarcopenia but also play a key role in supporting independence and quality of life in the elderly, and therefore, including these dietary factors within the management of the aged is crucial. Furthermore, the consequences of muscle weakness and thinning extend beyond the physical to impact psychological and social components of aging. Sarcopenia patients will experience greater fall rates, fracture rates, and consequent hospitalization, which can lead to reduced mental well-being and loneliness. The intricate interconnection between malnutrition and muscle loss is presented as one explanation for why diagnostic and intervention methods must be refined early on to prevent further decline. The establishment of comprehensive nutritional assessments is vital for understanding an individual's dietary habits and nutritional status. By employing systematic risk screenings, health professionals are in a position to implement timely interventions, not only for muscle preservation but also for overall quality of life, a testament to the emphasis laid by the literature Reber et al. (2019) and Ambrosetti et al. (2020) on a multidisciplinary model for treating the multifaceted problems of geriatric nutrition.

2.2.2. Altered Protein Synthesis Rates

The aging process greatly affects protein metabolism, particularly through altered rates of protein synthesis. As age progresses, the efficiency of processes involved in muscle tissue construction and repair decreases due to various causes, including hormonal changes and reduced physical activity. Such changes may lead to a decrease in aggregate muscle protein synthesis, which is crucial in maintaining muscle function and mass. Interestingly, the digestive system also undergoes significant changes that promote such downward trends in levels of protein synthesis. Mechanical food breakdown, reduced gastrointestinal motility, and abnormal digestion limit the flow of nutrients, which can stretch malnutrition within the older population even longer, thus impairing their ability to synthesize proteins needed for body functions (Rémond et al., 2015). In addition, the clinical relevance of altered rates of protein synthesis in older diets is considerable given the occurrence of sarcopenia, the age-related loss of muscle mass and strength. Sarcopenia is a major disease that makes the elderly vulnerable to frailty, falls, and other comorbidities. According to scientific evidence, adequate protein consumption is reported to reverse most of the deleterious sequelae of aging and provide optimal health outcomes. For optimal maintenance of muscle function, the suggestions are 1.0–1.2 g protein per kilogram of body weight per day in healthy older individuals and higher in those at risk for malnutrition or with chronic disease (Deutz et al., 2014). By increasing protein intake, aging can intensify their rates of muscle protein synthesis and reverse the effects of sarcopenia and associated loss of physical functioning. The interrelationship between various rates of protein synthesis in altered conditions and physical functioning is a significant topic in geriatric nutrition. There are observations suggesting that the convergence of adequate protein intake with regular physical exercise can reliably contribute to muscle mass maintenance and physical functioning in the aged. Exercise, and more importantly, resistance exercise, stimulates protein synthesis through several biochemical routes that maximize the efficacy of ingested dietary protein. Therefore, health professionals need to encourage not only nutritional but also physical activity interventions tailored to the older adult. By taking notice of these parameters, the issues brought about by malnutrition and aging may be reversed, and it is possible to give older adults the chance to optimize their protein metabolism and overall health (Deutz et al., 2014) (Figure 2.7).

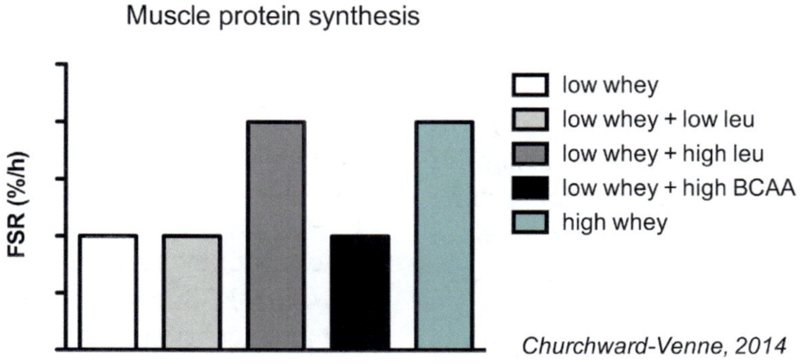

Figure 2.7. Protein synthesis rates.

Source: https://www.nutritiontactics.com/wp-content/uploads/2016/08/Churchward-Venne.jpg.

2.2.3. Impact of Chronic Diseases on Metabolism

Chronic diseases often interfere with the delicate balance of metabolic processes, significantly influencing nutritional requirements among the elderly. Diseases such as diabetes, cardiovascular disease, and chronic kidney disease not only alter macronutrient metabolism but also nutritional status in older adults. For instance, in diabetic individuals, insulin resistance can lead to compromised glucose metabolism, which requires some changes in carbohydrate and protein foods to maintain stable blood glucose levels. Consequently, the acknowledgment of such metabolic alterations is crucial for the development of dietary advice for the prevention of malnutrition and its related complications among the elderly, given that such individuals already have impaired nutrient absorption and utilization as a result of age-related changes in the stomach (Rémond et al., 2015). In addition to the direct influence on the metabolism of macronutrients, chronic illness also causes elevated nutritional needs and facilitates the loss of lean body mass. With advancing age, the majority of elderly individuals suffer from sarcopenia, which is a condition of loss of muscle mass and strength. Chronic disease exacerbates the condition by inducing systemic inflammation and metabolic stress, thus raising protein requirements indirectly. Thus, nutritional therapy to enhance protein intake is required to support the health of muscles and combat the adverse metabolic consequences of aging and chronic disease. Understanding these dynamics is key to promoting effective geriatric nutrition strategies for overall health and functional independence (Rémond et al., 2015). The interplay of chronic diseases with metabolism also becomes evident in the complex association with biomarkers of nutritional status. Lack of knowledge concerning these markers is a barrier to the development of effective dietary interventions among the elderly. Biomarkers can offer valuable information on nutrient bioavailability and the elderly's unique physiological requirements, showing how chronic conditions influence metabolic rates and nutrient use. Additionally, the identification and validation of these biomarkers can advance our understanding of malnutrition impact on disease and aging, ultimately informing healthcare practitioners in developing individualized nutrition recommendations to maximize geriatric health outcomes. Attainment of these needs will be a key determinant in improving the quality of life for elderly people with chronic illnesses and related metabolic complications.

2.3. Recommended Protein Intake for Older Adults

Recommended older adult protein intake has altered significantly in recent years, as it is increasingly recognized that ever before how protein affects health and function in this population. Aging is more often linked to the loss of muscle mass and strength that occurs naturally with aging, also known as sarcopenia, a condition that can increase greater risk of falls, fractures, and mobility issues. Studies show older adults require more protein than the standard recommended dietary allowance (RDA) of 0.8 grams per kilogram of body weight. The PROT-AGE study group recommends average daily intake at least in the range of 1.0 to 1.2 g protein per kilogram of body weight per day. Both endurance- and resistance-type exercises are recommended at individualized levels that are safe and tolerated, and higher protein intake (ie, ≥1.2 g/kg body weight/d) is advised for those who are exercising and otherwise active. Most older adults who have acute or chronic diseases need even more dietary protein (ie, 1.2–1.5 g/kg body weight/d). Older people with severe kidney disease (i.e., estimated GFR <30 mL/min/1.73m^2), but who are not on dialysis, are an exception to this rule; these individuals may need to limit protein intake. Older adults face unique challenges to protein digestion and absorption due to the aging GI tract, and individualized methods are thus crucial in ensuring proper intake of required nutrients. Alterations in gut motility, secretion of digestive enzymes, and intestinal wall function can hamper efficient protein assimilation. As such, knowledge of these alterations in physiology is vital to designing dietary guidelines that, in addition to suggesting increased protein consumption, provide for the intake of proteins of high biological value. Engaging older individuals in nutrition interventions that consider these factors can make a health improvement outcome easier by avoiding malnutrition, prevalent in this population. Finally, making sense of protein intake data and gastrointestinal health can actually make an impact on the nutritional status of older adults, allowing for quality-of-life improvement and survival (Rémond et al., 2015).

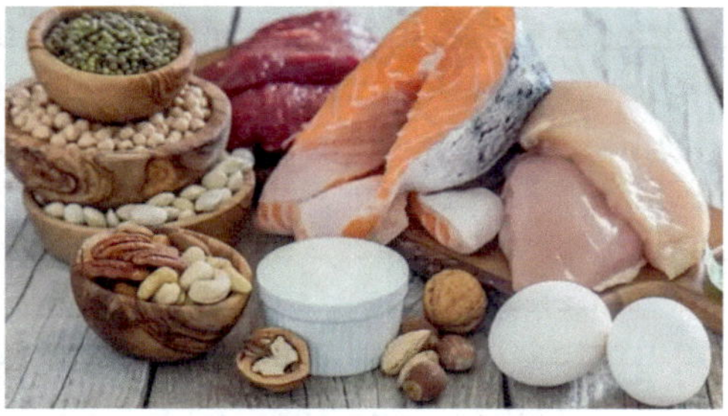

Figure 2.8. Protein intake for older adults.

Source: https://kajabi-storefronts-production.kajabi-cdn.com/kajabi-storefronts-production/file-uploads/blogs/13388/images/616041-d2b-7570-a654-3f0c623daed_57b8617-5152-beac-eeff-14e2f387b67_uTCWarfiRjeGBnSsKIVX_protein_meal_for_the_elderly_1_1_.webp.

The importance of adequate protein intake among elderly individuals is the prevalence of malnutrition among vulnerable groups, such as postoperative patients, like those undergoing operations for hip fractures. Older hip fracture patients, studies have shown, are likely to have compromised nutritional status that aggravates underlying deficits and heightens hospital complication rates and functional recovery following injury. For instance, malnutrition has a great impact on recovery results, and as is evident in research that revealed elderly patients have a very high prevalence of malnutrition at about 18.7% according to the Mini-Nutritional Assessment. The issue emphasizes the central role of global nutritional interventions supportive of protein priority intake, as reversal of nutritional status improves recovery and minimizes mortality among such patients (Malafarina et al., 2017). Meeting protein needs and creating focused nutritional interventions are critical aspects of geriatric care, which help ensure older individuals can stay independent and enjoy a good quality of life (Figure 2.8).

2.3.1. Daily Protein Requirements Based on Age and Health

The human requirement for protein differs significantly by age and health status, as they have to fulfill the changing metabolic requirements of the body throughout life. Generally speaking, healthy adults should consume approximately 0.8 grams of protein per kilogram of body weight. But it is normally greater in older individuals due to such reasons as muscle mass loss and changes in protein metabolism with age. Increased protein consumption with growing older, especially among the aged, is vital to prevent sarcopenia, a continuous reduction in skeletal muscle mass and strength. Research indicates that the older age group can benefit from additional protein consumption, with recommendations of 1.0 to 1.2 grams per kilogram of body weight for maintaining muscle mass and general well-being. This adjustment contributes to the success of better mobility, strength, and even recovery from illness, which are aspects of utmost importance in geriatric nutrition. Diseases also have a significant role in determining protein needs because patients with chronic diseases usually require a higher amount of protein than those with no diseases. For instance, conditions like diabetes, kidney disease, and metabolic disorders demand careful management of protein intake. In individuals with renal diseases, protein needs could be lower due to decreased renal ability to clear protein metabolism waste products. In contrast, patients recovering from trauma or surgery can be told to eat more protein considerably since protein is essential in the healing and repair of tissues. Additionally, the role of gut microbiota, which is influenced by dietary protein and health status, indicates that a focus on protein diversity and quality will be crucial in facilitating overall health outcomes, indicating that the digestibility and origin of protein can affect the absorption and utilization of essential amino acids (Ríos-Covián et al., 2016). Also, the overlap between protein intake and the gut microbiota points to the complex relationship between diet, health, and age. An unbalanced diet replete with high-grade sources of protein not only results in the preservation of muscle but also in promoting diversity and functionality of gut microbiota. The gut microbiota plays a central role in fermentation processes resulting in short-chain fatty acids (SCFAs), which are beneficial for colon health and potentially have a determining impact on nutrient uptake and metabolism (Cryan et al., 2019). In older adults, a balanced gut microbiota through proper intake of protein can regulate immune responses and metabolic processes, thus ensuring improved health outcomes. Awareness of these dynamics offers a complete understanding for personalizing dietary advice and intervention to optimize protein synthesis and general well-being as individuals grow older.

2.3.2. Differences in Protein Needs for Active vs. Sedentary Seniors

The difference in protein need between active and sedentary older adults is partly due to differences in muscle metabolism and overall energy expenditure. With age, muscle mass is lost, a condition known as sarcopenia, which both impairs physical function as well as quality of life. Active older adults, those who engage in regular exercise with resistance exercise and aerobic exercise, experience less blunted muscle mass loss, since these exercises activate muscle protein synthesis. On the other hand, their sedentary counterparts may have their muscle loss rate accelerated, hence an increased protein requirement to sustain muscle and strength. Moreover, protein consumption is critical in preventing sarcopenic obesity, where muscle breakdown follows with the development of fat, thereby necessitating energetic men and women to consume more proteins in an effort to nullify these effects while continuing to stay active, while subjecting inactive aging individuals to the destructive power of aging (Passaro et al., 2018). Activity level also affects the day's pattern and timing of protein intake, with active older adults usually having to plan more carefully. Research demonstrates that spreading protein intake across meals evenly can achieve maximum muscle protein synthesis, particularly in older adults who engage in frequent physical activity. Sedentary individuals, though, may not require as much planning because their total muscle growth and maintenance are less compromised by the rates of muscle protein breakdown. Active older adults, in contrast, are more likely to require consuming higher quantities of high-quality proteins such as lean meats, dairy, and vegetables because they engage in heavy exercise that would necessitate sufficient amino acid availability for recovery as well as muscle repair. Therefore, protein intake modulation aligns with energy demand as well as promoting long-term physical health and functional independence among aging populations (Frontera, 2019). Additionally, the implications for health due to insufficient protein intake among sedentary elderly can be particularly devastating. Insufficient protein has been associated with a range of conditions, including weakened immune response, impaired wound healing, and increased frailty, making this vulnerable population susceptible to adverse outcomes. On the other hand, active older adults who have adequate protein have a lower risk for such conditions since their diets are linked to better health. Therefore, attainment of protein needs through tailored nutrition intervention is imperative in the elderly, with emphasis on the distinction between requirements in active and sedentary older people. This focus on personalized nutrition can improve the quality of life of older adults and enhance the quality of life, as a result, highlighting the importance of these nutritional differences in recommendations (Passaro et al., 2018) (Figure 2.9).

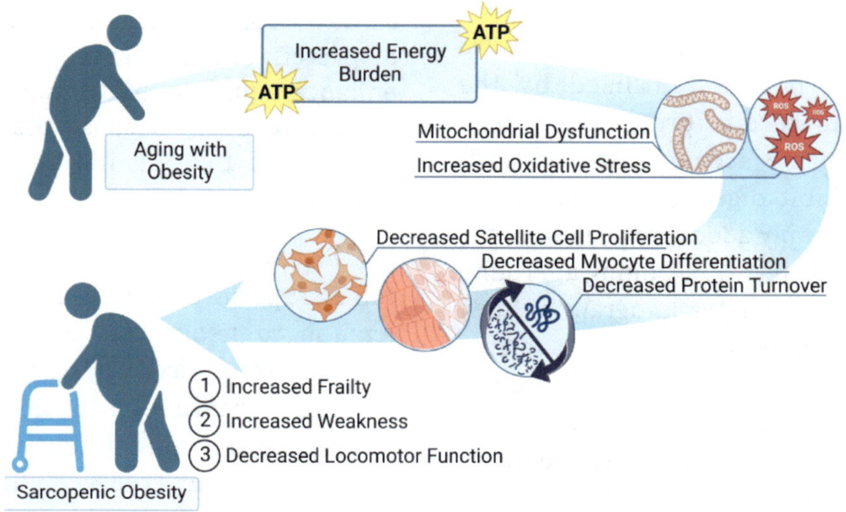

Figure 2.9. Sarcopenic obesity

Source: https://www.metabolismjournal.com/cms/10.1016/j.metabol.2023.155639/asset/721eedf7-13db-4c73-b753-4b62db816be9/main.assets/gr1_lrg.jpg.

2.3.3. Sources of High-Quality Protein

High-protein foods are extremely essential to provide the nutritional needs of the geriatric population, as these include essential amino acids to provide muscle mass and health. Animal-based protein foods, such as meat, fish, eggs, and milk, are generally considered superior because they contain entire amino acid profiles. These proteins have all nine amino acids that are essential and cannot be synthesized by the body, thus enabling important physiological processes, such as enzyme production and tissue repair. In older adults, the inclusion of sources such as lean meats and fatty fish not only aids muscle health but also brings other nutrients such as omega-3 fatty acids, which have been associated with decreased inflammation and increased cognitive function, making them vital for upholding quality of life in aging populations. Beyond animal sources, plant protein, while tending to be lower in certain essential amino acids, can be a significant contributor to the diet of elderly individuals when utilized effectively. Legumes, nuts, seeds, and whole grains can provide sufficient protein when utilized in mixed combinations, enhancing protein quality overall. Research has indicated that high-protein diets that incorporate plant and animal protein sources could be associated with better health in elderly people since they can assist in maintaining muscle and enhancing metabolic function. Incorporating legumes, for example, not only serves the protein requirement but also provides dietary fiber, which is significant in the functioning of the digestive system, something generally impaired in the elderly. Therefore, a balanced intake of proteins can be achieved by the integration of both quality animal and complementary plant proteins. In addition to the quantitative amino acid content, protein quality also involves considerations based on digestibility and bioavailability. Studies show that the digestibility of protein foods varies from animal sources to plant sources and affects their contribution to fulfilling protein needs among older adults.

For instance, proteins from animals are more easily absorbed and utilized by the body compared to certain proteins found in plants, which may be accompanied by anti-nutrients that inhibit digestion. In particular, it is important to supply adequate protein in the planning of geriatric nutrition, aiming at around 1.2–2.0 grams of protein per kilogram of body weight to reverse muscle wasting associated with aging. Hence, understanding the sources of good-quality protein and their respective contributions forms the core of the development of dietary guidelines that facilitate maximum health in the aged population and ensure they meet their personal nutritional requirements (Li & Wu, 2023; Jiang et al., 2024).

2.4. Consequences of Inadequate Protein Intake

Poor protein consumption among the geriatric population has serious effects on health, primarily due to its adverse effects on muscle function and muscle mass. With aging, muscle strength decreases naturally with age, a condition referred to as sarcopenia, further exacerbated by poor protein intake. Muscle loss will lead to loss of strength and mobility and increase the vulnerability to falls and fractures, which are serious conditions among the elderly. Moreover, muscle atrophy implications go beyond physiological boundaries; they will enable a cycle of dependence and reduced quality of life. If protein intake does not provide for the body's needs for repair and synthesis, particularly when in a state of illness or stress, risk for malnutrition increases, further compounding older adults' health profile (Rémond et al., 2015). In addition to physical effects, inadequate protein consumption can impact other organ systems, including the immune and cardiovascular systems. Malnutrition in the form of protein-energy wasting has been found to enhance vulnerability to infections and longer disease recovery because the immune system is impaired through the absence of essential nutrients.

Furthermore, disturbed protein metabolism can disrupt the balance of cardiovascular health, leading to heart failure and other chronic diseases. It requires a systemic comprehension of these interdependencies, as the older population is more likely to have multiple conditions concurrently. It is now apparent that protein nutrition is not merely an issue of dietary equilibration but also a mandatory criterion of care in geriatric medicine for promoting resistance to age-disease (Gama-Axelsson, 2014). The psychological effects of inadequate protein intake must also be valued because nutritional deficiencies can impair mood and cognitive function. The relationship between nutrition and mental state is well established, and protein plays a role in the production of neurotransmitters that regulate mood and cognition. Inadequate dietary status can exacerbate feelings of depression or anxiety and decrease overall well-being further in elderly groups. As the geriatric population is also found to be lonely and socially isolated, with an additional impact of inadequate diet intake, intervention becomes critical in managing not only protein requirement but also social support. Tailored dietary advice that considers the unique physiological changes that happen during aging can help improve nutritional status and general physical and mental well-being in older adults (Rémond et al., 2015) (Figure 2.10).

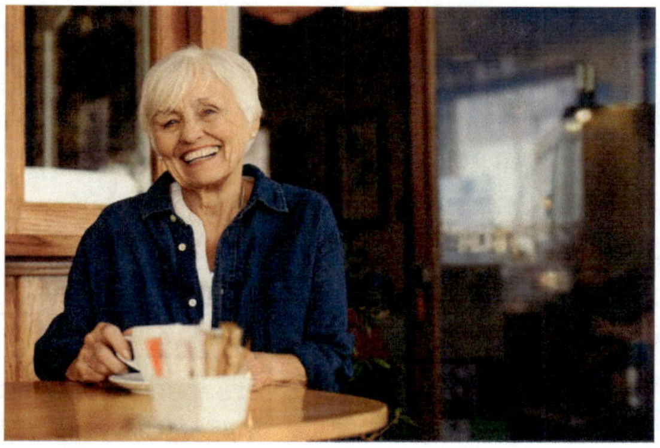

Figure 2.10. Protein intake for the elderly.

Source: https://geediting.com/wp-content/uploads/2025/05/independent-90s.png.

2.4.1. Risk of Sarcopenia and Frailty

Aging is not an easy thing when it involves a lot of sarcopenia and frailty, which are on the rise among older people. Sarcopenia, which entails the loss of muscle mass and strength, not only contributes to physical disability but also poses an increased risk of fractures, falls, and other adverse health effects. Conversely, frailty has been defined as a multifaceted syndrome that is linked with compromised physiological reserve and heightened vulnerability to stressors. The presence of these two conditions together tends aggravate the underlying medical conditions, leading to a synergistic effect on quality of life in older adults. Given that malnutrition is common among them, it is important to know how protein metabolism helps minimize such risks in the development of effective geriatric nutritional interventions.

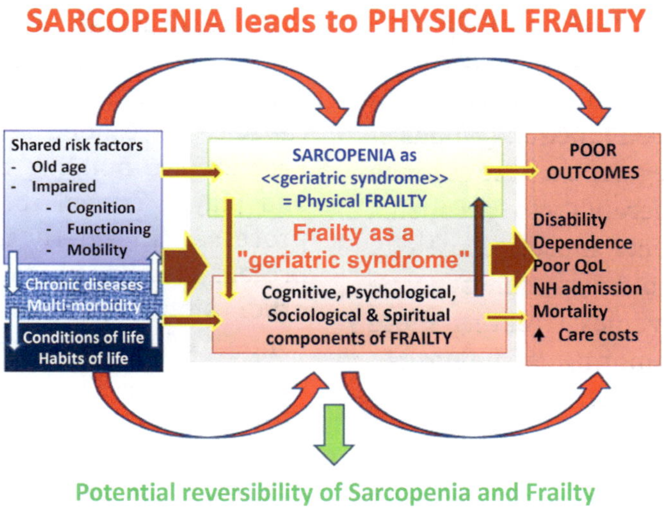

Figure 2.11. Sarcopenia: a useful paradigm for physical frailty.

Source: https://ars.els-cdn.com/content/image/1-s2.0-S1878764913000442-gr1.jpg.

Systematic interventions for both sarcopenia and frailty via personalized diets can improve the functional capacity and quality of life in older adults. Malnutrition is an important etiological factor for both sarcopenia and frailty, particularly in chronic diseases such as cirrhosis. The American Association for the Study of Liver Diseases emphasizes that inadequate nutrient consumption may initiate muscle wasting and frailty syndromes, thus creating a vicious cycle of deterioration (Lai et al., 2021). In elderly populations, inadequate protein consumption leads to considerable suppression of muscle protein synthesis, leading to compromised muscle quality and quantity. Moreover, other nutritional imbalances like vitamin and mineral deficiencies would further drive the onset of sarcopenia and frailty and therefore reinforce the overall health status of the aged. Nutritional evaluations and interventions directly targeted at the geriatric patient's specific requirements not only stand to rectify these conditions but also open doors for better recuperation and immunity to acute diseases. Furthermore, physical inactivity, compounded by age and chronic illness, is also central to frailty and sarcopenia development. Immobilized patients in situations like COVID-19 are most vulnerable; prolonged bed rest will result in rapid wastage of muscle tissue and impaired function (Woods et al., 2020). The lack of a regular exercise regimen also exacerbates the vulnerability to sarcopenia since it negatively affects muscle elasticity and strength, making older patients prone to falls and other syndromes. Treating these conditions calls for promoting an integrated approach combining nutritional intake and physical training. Engagement in exercise and resistance training, coupled with adequate protein, is able to effectively maximize muscle synthesis, counteract the effects of sarcopenia, and enhance well-being in geriatrics. It is thus vital to deal with the interlinked variables of diet and physical activity to lower the threats of sarcopenia and frailty within the geriatric population (Figure 2.11).

2.4.2. Impaired Immune Function

The interaction between geriatric nutrition and immune status is critical, especially among older individuals whose immune response is often decreased due to age. Impaired immune function can result from inadequate protein intake, which is required to develop antibodies and other immune molecules that protect against infection. With age, the effectiveness of the gastrointestinal tract (GIT) declines, impacting the intake, digestion, and absorption of basic nutrients, including proteins. Functional modifications in the elderly GIT and structural adjustments discourage the maximal bioavailability of nutrients, which in turn hastens malnutrition. Researchers note that malnutrition not only aids in the decline of immune function but also heightens the risk for pathologies of numerous organ systems, including even the immune system itself (Rémond et al., 2015). The circular dependency of this relationship underlines the requirement to address nutritional deficiencies to promote immune integrity and overall health in the geriatric population. Nutritional deficiencies, particularly in protein, can dramatically impair the immune system's capacity to respond adequately to pathogens. Proteins are building blocks of immune cells and play a crucial role in cellular signaling processes. In elderly individuals, inadequate protein metabolism can disrupt cytokine and other signaling molecule synthesis in the context of immune responses. Moreover, as aging progresses, comorbidities and chronic inflammation can further weaken immune effectiveness and thus become essential to put a strong focus on ideal protein food sources in this age group. The increment in the quantity of protein considered, along with the understanding of the altered function of GITs due to aging, can highly improve the uptake of nutrients and hence promote a stronger immune system in elders. Therefore, it is crucial to provide dietary recommendations considering such changes for malnutrition prevention and immune well-being improvement (Rémond et al., 2015). In addition, the significance of biomarkers in the assessment of nutritional status and immunity cannot be overlooked in geriatric care. Biomarkers can unveil functional changes associated with nutritional status and specify subjects at risk for malnutrition even prior to clinical onset. For instance, measurement of individual protein synthesis and immune biomarkers can guide individualized nutritional interventions. This cannot only help preserve immune competence but also enhance the quality of life in older age. The convergence of dietary intervention aimed at protein intake and biomarker profiling offers new opportunities for intervention. As the global aging population grows, it is more crucial to have comprehensive nutrition plans in a position that encompass and mitigate the risk of impaired immune function.

2.4.3. Effects on Recovery from Illness and Surgery

Illness and surgery recovery in aged patients are significantly influenced by protein metabolism and nutritional status. The older patients can experience compromised recovery due to physiological changes related to aging, such as sarcopenia, which refers to the continuing loss of muscle mass and strength (Larsson et al., 2018). Reduced muscle mass can inhibit recovery after surgery by leading to a longer hospital stay and a higher likelihood of developing complications such as infection or immobility. There should be proper intake of proteins for the retention and healing of muscle tissue; thus, achieving nutritional needs through adequate protein consumption is pivotal in geriatric medicine. It has been proven that higher dietary protein consumption can enhance muscle synthesis and alleviate the impact of sarcopenia, thereby enhancing recovery outcomes in surgical procedures. In addition, difficulty in swallowing or dysphagia also presents a major barrier to proper nutritional intake in older adults recovering from surgery (Baijens et al., 2016). The condition can potentially lead to severe complications such as malnutrition and dehydration, which are themselves well evidenced to further compromise recovery processes. The complex combination of factors related to age is generally seen to result in decreased oropharyngeal swallowing response, causing aspiration risk and resulting in respiratory infection. Given the fact that old patients will have multiple comorbidities, oropharyngeal dysphagia management is important in order to ensure adequate supplementation of nutrients during the course of recovery. Adequate diagnostic procedures and interventions, such as modified diets or swallowing treatment, can improve nutritional supply and overall outcomes in recovery, highlighting the essence of a multidisciplinary practice in geriatric medicine.

Finally, the impact of protein metabolism on recovery is not only in the synthesis of muscle alone but also has a vital role in the immune process and the healing of wounds. Older patients usually have a reduction in immune response, which can compromise their recovery from disease and surgery efficiently. Protein nutrition within safe limits increases the synthesis of immunoglobulins and other immune mediators, thus augmenting the body's defense function against infection and wound healing. The association between nutrition and immunocompetence establishes the imperative for a successful nutritional plan with special reference to protein requirements in geriatric nutrition. Here, personalized dietary interventions that consider personal likes and dislikes, swallow ability, and overall state of health are key to optimizing recovery and improving the quality of life for older adults in postoperative states (Figure 2.12).

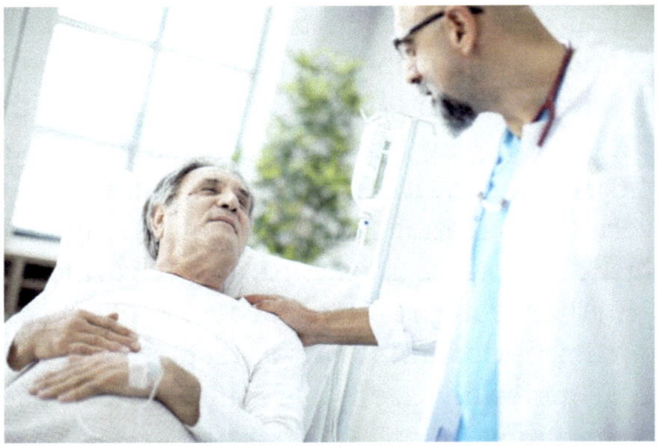

Figure 2.12. Effects on recovery from illness and surgery.

Source: https://radiusanesthesia.com/wp-content/uploads/2018/07/Smaller-elder-pic.jpg.

2.5. Protein Supplementation in Geriatric Nutrition

As a person gets older, maintaining muscle strength and mass becomes increasingly important to overall health and functional independence. Studies have established that sarcopenia, which is the gradual loss of skeletal muscle, typically begins at the advanced stage of middle age and accelerates in old age. The risk factor in Sarcopenia includes an increment in falls, disability, and mortality. In an effort to stop such adverse effects, protein supplementation became a prominent intervention in geriatric nutrition. Research indicates that older people might need greater protein consumption than younger individuals in order to adequately stimulate muscle protein synthesis. Through providing a sufficient amount of essential amino acids, protein supplements can help maintain muscle mass, increase functional ability, and enhance quality of life among this group, thus specifically dealing with the issues caused by aging and related illnesses. Moreover, beyond muscle preservation, the benefits of protein supplementation in older adults extend. Ideal protein intake is also associated with greater immune function, especially significant with the heightened susceptibility of the elderly to infection and chronic disease. The current evidence suggests that sarcopenia may exacerbate the immunocompromising of the body, and nutritional strategies are hence a pillar in the prevention of such risks. Additionally, conditions such as Alzheimer's and other forms of dementia, with which older adults may be suffering, have the potential to complicate matters of nutritional requirement and consumption. Treatment of such zones of health requires broad general knowledge of proteins' function in muscle support and immunology. Long-term nutrition innovations, like personalized protein supplementing regimens, can thus be critical to enhancing the health condition and well-being of older people in the wake of such varied challenges. The nutrition environment for older people has further deteriorated under the shadow of the COVID-19 pandemic, which has highlighted the group's vulnerabilities in stark relief. Their immobilization due to hospitalization, as well as the physical inactivity caused by quarantine practice, has threatened their general health, including aggravating conditions brought about by aging (Woods et al., 2020).

Taking such situations into consideration, an effective nutrition approach promoting protein supplementation may be a critical countermeasure. Factors such as loss of appetite, altered metabolism, and decreased protein digestion, typical among the aged, may necessitate the utilization of supplementary protein sources to avoid deficiency. Coupled with effective dietary education and counseling, protein supplementation can significantly contribute to the maintenance of muscle integrity, immune status, and overall well-being in age groups affected by the pandemic as well as in the future (Figure 2.13).

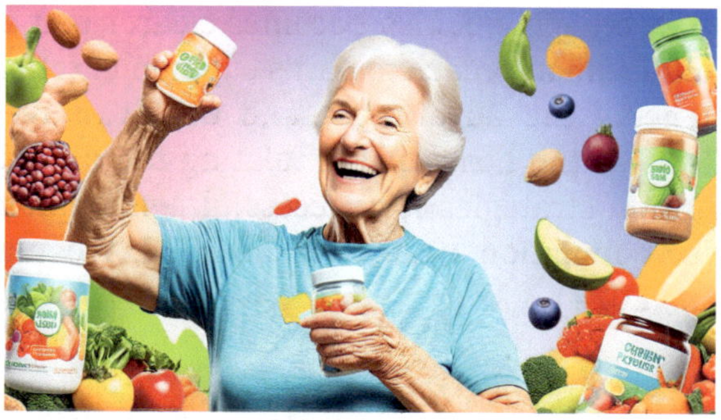

Figure 2.13. Protein supplementation in geriatric nutrition.

Source: https://greatsenioryears.com/wp-content/uploads/2024/02/senior-friendly-protein-drinks-image.jpg.

2.5.1. Types of Protein Supplements Available

Protein supplements are today very critical in addressing the nutritional requirements of older people, especially given the challenge they encounter in accessing their protein dietary requirements. Some of the accessible protein supplements are whey, casein, soy, and pea protein. Whey protein, a dairy-derived protein, is rich in essential amino acids and has high biological value, making it the preferred muscle synthesis option. Casein, a dairy-derived protein, offers slow digestion and time-release of amino acids, which may prove beneficial for overnight muscle recovery support. In elderly individuals, who are regularly beset by sarcopenia, it has been recommended that the intake of such quality protein supplements be increased to reverse muscle wasting and to aid overall health, thus alleviating malnutrition-related problems and their associated risks, particularly on gastrointestinal function in elderly individuals (Rémond et al., 2015). Another popular option is plant protein supplements such as soy and pea protein, ideal for individuals who just so happen to be lactose intolerant or following a vegetarian or vegan diet. Soy protein is also unique in that it contains a complete amino acid profile, thereby an excellent substitute for animal-based protein sources. On the other hand, pea protein is also gaining popularity due to its hypoallergenic property and digestibility, hence it is even more ideal for older people who may have sensitive stomachs. The substitutes not only guarantee the provision of macronutrients but also help with weight management, which is crucial in obesity-related disease prevention in older people. Utilization of plant-based protein supplements in the diet of older adults can hence be pivotal towards ensuring appropriate consumption of nutrients as well as addressing the diverse dietary requirements of the population (Volkert et al., 2019). Apart from these conventional substitutes, there are protein products specifically designed for incorporation into geriatric diets and often supplemented with vitamins and minerals to maximize their overall performance. They tend to supply more protein per serving to correspond with the higher needs of aging people. Others can have other added nutrients such as fiber, omega-3 fatty acids, or antioxidants as added support for the nutritional status of older individuals. Because older people lack appetite, such supplemented forms can be a useful aid in avoiding malnutrition as well as in maintaining sufficient muscle mass. Through the targeting of the specific needs of older populations, these individually tailored protein supplements offer a preventative approach to nutrition that can yield significantly improved quality of life and overall health outcomes (Rémond et al., 2015).

2.5.2. Benefits and Risks of Supplementation

The addition of nutritional supplements has become increasingly popular in the elderly, as a majority seek to boost their levels of protein in an effort to support the increased demands necessary for maintaining muscle and overall health. A big benefit of supplementation is the potential to assist in adding more protein consumption, essential for older adults who lose muscle strength and mass, a condition known as sarcopenia. Protein supplements can fill the gap for individuals who are unable to access their nutritional needs through food only. Furthermore, they can provide a convenient alternative for individuals with inadequate appetites or chewing and swallowing issues to make it easier to incorporate required nutrients into their diets. By addressing these issues head-on, supplementation may improve the nutritional status of the elderly, promote healthier aging and potentially better their quality of life. Despite the advantages of supplementation, some potential risks must be entertained, the most important of which is the potential for adverse side effects when used improperly. The elderly could also be at a greater risk of the negative effects of certain supplements, such as gastrointestinal distress or interactions with drugs. For example, too much dietary protein puts too much strain on kidney function, particularly in the presence of underlying kidney disease. Moreover, the lack of controls in the supplement industry has problems with the purity and effectiveness of products that have led to unsuspected health issues. Older adults and caregivers themselves should be informed that not all supplements are the same, and proper assessment of certain health conditions and nutritional needs must first be accomplished before any form of supplementation is introduced to their treatment program. Nutritional science's dynamic nature continues to unfold the nuances of benefits and risks of supplementation in the elderly. Recent research stresses the necessity of personalized nutrition intervention according to specific conditions like genetics, health status, and special dietary requirements. Personalized strategy may enhance the effectiveness of supplements while minimizing risks, particularly if interventions are guided by healthcare professionals. Additionally, the study of functional foods and their synergistic effect with conventional supplements further supports the potential for improved health outcomes in the geriatric population. As the scientific community keeps enhancing its understanding of protein metabolism and its impact on aging, it also becomes clearer that an equilibrium approach towards supplementation, balancing the advantages and disadvantages, will be at the heart of formulating the optimal nutrition strategies for successful aging among older populations (Karlic et al., 2022; Woźniak et al., 2024).

2.5.3. Guidelines for Incorporating Supplements into Diet

The manufacture of good guidelines to incorporate dietary supplements into the diet of the geriatric patient is of great importance, especially because the growing old population tends to experience protein metabolism disorders. Aging brings about changes in the physiological functions of elderly people, such that there is low protein synthesis capacity and impaired nutrient absorption, which can lead to deficiencies. Supplements, particularly those rich in essential amino acids, can be utilized strategically to supplement protein intake and preserve muscle and overall health. Evidence indicates that targeted supplementation not only rectifies such deficiencies but also diminishes the risk of malnutrition, a prevalent condition in the elderly with hip fractures (Malafarina et al., 2017). Thus, creating an extensive supplementation plan to meet individual needs is essential to maximize dietary interventions and ensure improved health outcomes for the elderly. In creating supplement guidelines for consumption, dietary restrictions and preferences need to be considered, as are typically found in the geriatric population. Older adults will have compromised swallowing capacity for pills or may have some dietary restrictions that will restrict them from using standard supplements. Offering protein supplements in liquid or powder formulas is an option that enables people to intake more protein without so much as altering their existing eating habits. Furthermore, the supplementation plan must aim at foods or commodities that improve nutrient bioavailability, considering the declining efficiency of the aging gastrointestinal tracts in nutrient absorption (Rémond et al., 2015). Therapy decisions must be framed based on dietary assessment and health status, such that healthcare providers are able to ensure that the chosen supplements are sufficient to fulfill nutritional needs. To maximize the utilization of dietary supplements in geriatric nutrition, ongoing monitoring and assessment of dietary intake and health status are necessary. Periodic checks can allow early detection of any changes in nutritional status and facilitate adjustment of the supplementation regimen as needed. It should include a multidisciplinary panel that consists of dietitians, pharmacists, and medical professionals to enhance the utility of such guidelines by considering everything that affects the health and lifestyle of the elderly. Further, education on proper supplement usage and an increased awareness of their interactions with prescribed medications are imperative. Through the establishment of robust guidelines that promote safe and effective use of supplements, health professionals can make a significant contribution towards the improved nutritional status and overall well-being of the elderly (Figure 2.14).

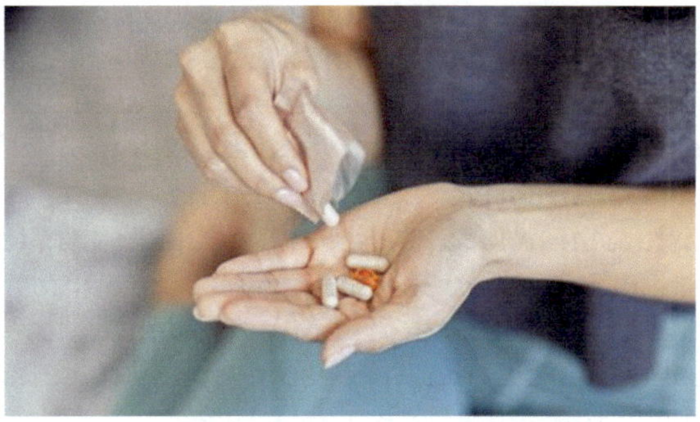

Figure 2.14. Incorporating supplements into the diet.

Source: https://external-content.duckduckgo.com/iu/?u= https%3A%2F%2Ftse2.mm.bing.net% 2Fth%3Fid%3DOIP.yAqfJwZplb THUJ QVyVjx1AHaE8%26r%3D0%26pid%3DApi &f=1&ipt= 313bcccd39c9ddb4913bf273fe1f f6e84e3f51a67fef00523d62f0c8f2bc8bc5.

2.6. Dietary Strategies to Enhance Protein Intake

The elderly face unique challenges with regard to protein intake, and this calls for adopting strategic dietary interventions. Older people are inclined to experience gastrointestinal tract changes that impair the absorption of nutrients, leading to an increased risk of malnutrition and its associated health complications. The aim of enhancing protein consumption means that dietary approaches must target the utilization of high-quality protein foods that are more absorbable and digestible. For instance, the combination of yogurt, eggs, fish, and legumes can provide the required amino acids and prevent gastrointestinal discomfort to a moderate degree. Such dietary sources not only facilitate protein consumption but also maximize nutrient bioavailability. By synchronizing nutritional strategies with the body's changes at old age within the gastrointestinal system, we can help minimize the dangers of protein deficiency among the elderly, ultimately resulting in better health, as well as enhanced quality of life, particularly as highlighted in the results of how the aging gastrointestinal systems affect nutritional statuses (Rémond et al., 2015). In addition to the selection of quality protein sources, frequency and portion size at meals are vital in maximizing overall protein intake in the elderly. It has been discovered that spreading protein intake over multiple meals throughout the day may optimize muscle protein synthesis, which is reduced during aging. Therefore, using interventions that allow more frequent, smaller portions might be particularly beneficial to the elderly who are unable to manage large portions. For example, adding a protein-containing snack like nuts, cheese, or protein bars between meals can effectively increase total daily protein intake. Furthermore, palatability and texture modification, by either cooking technique or added flavorings, can stimulate hunger, enabling older adults to more effectively meet protein needs. By promoting these eating habits, we are able to combat malnutrition and its consequent effects, like those seen in geriatric patients with hip fractures (Malafarina et al., 2017). Lastly, education and access are essential components of effective dietary planning for improving protein intake among elderly individuals. Many elderly individuals may be unaware of their personal nutritional needs and how they can be achieved through diet. Therefore, providing nutritional education can help them make appropriate choices about their food. Knowledge and motivation can be enhanced through community-based interventions, clinic visits, and measures like recipe books tailored to older adult nutritional requirements. Moreover, having access to inexpensive and easily available high-protein foods is very important, particularly in low-income neighborhoods where food security could be jeopardized. Collaborations with food banks or meal programs in the community can also provide access to healthy food options. By going beyond the single aspect of protein intake and addressing the interdependent factors of education and access, we can create a more supportive environment for older adults to develop optimal nutritional status throughout the life course (Rémond et al., 2015) (Figure 2.15).

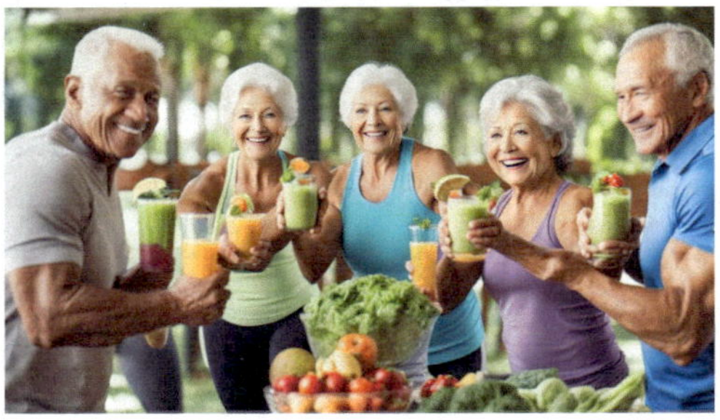

Figure 2.15. Protein shakes recommendations for the aging population.

Source: https://greatsenioryears.com/wp-content/uploads/2023/12/protein-shake-recommendations-for-aging-population-1024x585.jpg.

2.6.1. Meal Planning for Balanced Protein Distribution

Meal planning to achieve optimal protein distribution is increasingly being identified as a critical strategy in the field of geriatric nutrition, particularly when the elderly have peculiar metabolic needs. Protein maintains muscle mass, recovery, and maintenance of overall health in the elderly. With advancing age, the body's ability to synthesize proteins diminishes, leading to increased protein requirement through diet. Therefore, meal plans should not only address the total amount of protein consumed but also how it is spaced throughout the day. Distributing protein evenly over meals optimizes the anabolic response, and this goes further to improve muscle protein synthesis and physical function in the elderly, reversing sarcopenia or muscle waste that occurs with aging. Having several protein sources in well-planned meals can also help distribute proteins evenly. Animal proteins such as lean meat, fish, and dairy foods are complete proteins because they all contain all the essential amino acids. Plant foods such as legumes, nuts, and whole grains are incomplete proteins but can be combined to yield complementary protein profiles. Utilizing both sources in creating meal plans not only increases protein consumption but also diversity of nutrients, which is essential to malnutrition prevention, a condition prevalent among the elderly. Effective meal planning must also consider individual taste, individual health, and any dietary requirements that limit sources or kinds of protein, to promote customization to the fullest in order to ensure compliance and satisfaction with eating practices. In order to further enhance the efficiency of meal planning in the elderly, it is important to institute mechanisms to counter usual challenges towards meeting the prescribed protein intake. These may include difficulty in swallowing or chewing, decreased appetite, and lack of access to nutritious food. The incorporation of protein-dense, simple-to-process food and beverage products into meals and snacks, such as smoothies with added protein powder or yogurt, may assist in supplementing protein requirements without overburdening the patient. In addition, collaboration with health care professionals, including dietitians, may assist in individualized recommendations that are in accordance with evidence-based geriatric practice. For instance, routine malnutrition screening has been recommended to identify people at risk and appropriately target dietary interventions, which can ultimately address improved health outcomes in older individuals (Schindler et al., 2016; Volkert et al., 2019).

2.6.2. Importance of Protein-Rich Snacks

In the context of geriatric nutrition, protein-rich snack provision is paramount in averting the risk of age-related loss of muscle mass and overall health. With increasing age, human beings experience physiological alterations that can affect their ability to absorb and metabolize nutrients efficiently, particularly protein. Snack foods high in protein can offer a convenient means of augmenting daily consumption, compensating for the hardships resulting from decreased appetite and slowed gastrointestinal function, common among elderly people. By ensuring protein needs are met through snacks, older adults are better positioned to positively contribute to muscle anabolism and maintain functional independence, subsequently reducing the risk of falls and frailty associated with malnutrition, a concern brought into prominence by the escalating burden of age-related illnesses (Rémond et al., 2015). Protein snacks may also enhance food compliance in patients with particular dietary protocols. Geriatric patients are often faced with complex diet limitations due to underlying disease states, leading to frustration and a decrease in overall food intake. Protein-enriched snacks allow freedom and flexibility, enabling easier integration of needed nutrients with minimal disruption to their diet. More recent studies have suggested that higher protein intake in the form of readily available foods can lead to improved satiety and thus favorably influence overall caloric intake. Besides, studies show that snacks rich in protein and other macro- or micronutrients have the potential to enhance nutrient absorption, thus helping aging people who may have difficulty with bioavailability (Ostan et al., 2018). Furthermore, the social role in enjoying protein-rich snacks cannot be ruled out in relation to geriatric nutrition. Food is not only a physiological requirement but also a social occasion that provides the potential to reduce loneliness and enhance emotional health among older individuals. Shared eating times have the potential to create community ties and facilitate intergenerational interaction.

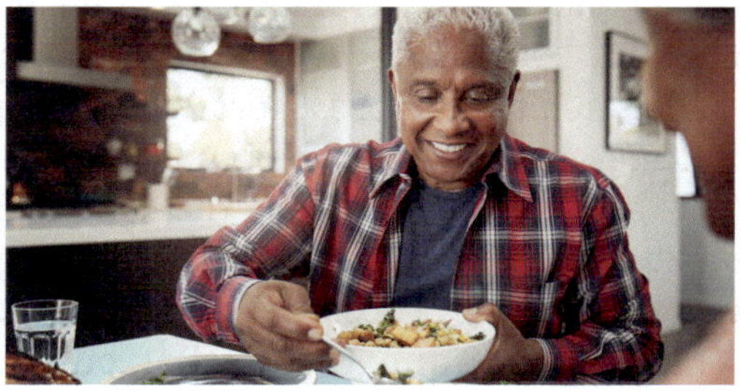

Figure 2.16. Protein rich foods for the elderly.

Source: https://www.onemedical.com/media/images/96.original.png.

The delivery of appealing protein snacks therefore, contributes to not only physical but also psychological health, lending support to an integrated model of aging. The inclusion of protein-rich snack foods in everyday lives can therefore be an effective intervention, addressing both nutritional deficiencies and enhancing the quality of life for older people. As the aging population continues to increase, effective and enjoyable nutritional options cannot be overstressed, calling for personalized dietary recommendations and interventions to achieve optimal healthy results (Rémond et al., 2015) (Figure 2.16).

2.6.3. Role of Hydration in Protein Metabolism

Hydration plays an important role in protein metabolism, particularly with regard to geriatric diets. The aging process tends to bring about extreme alterations in physiological conditions, both in the intake and in the absorption of nutrients, which are essential to maintain protein homeostasis. Adequate hydration is essential in older individuals in order to facilitate enzymic reactions during protein synthesis and degradation. Water is used as a substrate for substrates and enzymes to facilitate key biochemical reactions in organs and muscle tissues. When hydration is compromised, protein metabolizing function is compromised, hence potential for increased muscle loss and malnutrition. All this highlights the importance of understanding how hydration impacts nutritional status generally, especially in elderly people whose requirements may be fairly diverse from those of younger people. Maintenance of optimal hydration can help reduce the negative effects of aging on protein metabolism and result in greater health benefits for the elderly. Prevalence of dehydration among older adults is a major challenge to effective protein metabolism. In research, dehydration was found to exacerbate natural health problems in addition to reducing the quality of life among the elderly. Physical and mental deterioration associated with aging is likely to result in diminished perception of thirst as well as impair maintenance of adequate fluid intake. This deficiency in turn is likely to interfere with proper physiological processes for protein metabolism, i.e., utilization and utilization of amino acids. Further, evidence has been found to confirm that caregivers play a very crucial role in ensuring the hydration of elderly people, again highlighting the need for specific interventions within care settings. By promoting environments that facilitate hydration, healthcare providers can do a great deal to enhance the efficiency of diets, pushing protein metabolism and alleviating malnutrition danger prevalent in elderly populations. In light of what the data say regarding the aging gastrointestinal tract, special attention should be devoted to considering the effects of hydration on protein metabolism. Alterations in the mechanical and chemical digestion process in older age limit the efficiency of nutrient absorption, compounding their nutritional requirements (Rémond et al., 2015). Hydration levels influence these digestive processes and hence, monitoring and management must be performed cautiously. Efficient fluid intake not only aids in the absorption of nutrients but also aids in transporting amino acids to tissues where they can be used for repairing and constructing muscles. Also, optimal hydration can permit metabolic waste elimination, thereby providing an efficient metabolic environment. Adding consideration of hydration to dietary counseling recommendations for the elderly population can best meet the underlying challenges of protein metabolism in this group. This combined strategy is important in preventing malnutrition and promoting wellness with aging.

SUMMARY

Geriatric nutritional requirements and protein metabolism must be considered in an attempt to combat the widespread prevalence of malnutrition among the elderly. With increasing age, there are very significant alterations in the gut that interfere with effective absorption and utilization of the required nutrients, e.g., proteins. All such alterations result in reduced bioavailability of the nutrients, and this again increases the risk of malnutrition and consequent morbidity. It becomes essential to bridge the gap between aging-related gastrointestinal dysfunction and nutritional strategies, hence tailoring interventions to the elderly's specific requirements. Optimal nutritional counseling that takes into consideration the structural changes of the aging body plays a crucial role in enabling proper protein intake, ultimately contributing to improved health outcomes and overall quality of life in the elderly, as presented in the present literature (Rémond et al., 2015). In addition, it has been discovered that older age is associated with a decline in such markers of nutritional status, as expressed through the lower body weight, body mass index, and serum albumin of older patients. The relationship between nutritional deficiencies and old age serves to underscore the necessity of intensive assessment techniques that scrutinize not merely protein intake but the overall nutritional status of older patients. Through identifying the intricate interactions of age, chronic illness, and functional impairment on nutritional indicators, caregivers can construct nutritional intervention strategies that are capable of addressing these deficits more effectively. That malnutrition in older people is generally underdiagnosed is recognized, and thus there is a necessity for health professionals to incorporate frequent monitoring of nutritional status into geriatric care pathways (Forster & Gariballa, 2005). Lastly, protein metabolism and nutritional requirements in the elderly must be tackled on a multi-pronged level that combines nutrition interventions, regular assessments, and patient and caregiver education. To address the increasing aging population, healthcare systems must adapt more to meet the nutritional requirements of the elderly collectively. This would involve developing targeted dietetic products that respond to the physiological changes that accompany aging, thus enhancing the bioavailability of nutrients and considering factors such as the psychological, economic, and social determinants of food choice. Highlighting the interconnectedness between aging, nutrition, and health outcomes will enable us to devise effective measures to minimize the occurrence of malnutrition, ensuring better health throughout the later stages of life and enhancing overall quality of life among the geriatric population.

It is essential to comprehend the nuances of protein metabolism to provide the elderly with their nutritional requirements. With aging, alterations in the gastrointestinal tract significantly influence nutrient digestibility and absorption and hence leave them susceptible to malnutrition. The decline of mechanical and chemical processes in the elderly gastrointestinal tract diminishes the effectiveness with which the nutrients are absorbed and digested. This reduction in function is not just a biological issue; it is associated with other health conditions in various organ systems such as the nervous system, the musculoskeletal system, the cardiovascular system, the immune system, and the integumentary system. Hence, it becomes necessary to define the nutritional recommendations considering the gastrointestinal changes to avoid the commonality of malnutrition in older individuals and thus improve the quality of their life and overall health status (Rémond et al., 2015). In addition to ensuring adequate protein intake, sarcopenic obesity offers yet another challenge to geriatric nutrition. Sarcopenic obesity, the simultaneous occurrence of obesity and sarcopenia, complicates the implementation of the standard procedure for the body composition and functional strength of older persons. Evidence is in favor of the fact that not only lifestyle intervention, most notably a selective increase in the intake of protein, but also exercise therapy could serve synergistic roles against this disorder. While current evidence has shown limited reversibility of body fat percentages, improvements in muscle strength and physical function following adequate exercise regimes have been noted. Interventions combining nutritional strategies, including high protein consumption, with organized physical exercise are thus a possible avenue in the reversal of sarcopenic obesity in older adults (Theodorakopoulos et al., 2017). Lastly, effectively treating the elderly's protein metabolism and nutritional needs has to be accomplished by a process of dimensions. Establishing extensive mechanisms that not only entail augmenting dietary protein intake but also taking note of the physiological and pathological changes that occur due to age has to be accomplished. The identified nutrient intake and utilization knowledge gaps in the chapter demonstrate the necessity of performing additional research to establish successful dietary interventions. By advancing our understanding of the complexities of geriatric nutrition, healthcare workers can improve their ability to construct more efficient interventions that will increase the physical strength and well-being of elderly individuals. By implementing such measures, the incidence of malnutrition and related illnesses will be reduced in this at-risk population, ultimately preserving their autonomy and health (Rémond et al., 2015; Theodorakopoulos et al., 2017).

A CLOSER LOOK

FRAILTY AMPLIFIES THE EFFECTS OF AGING ON PROTEIN METABOLISM

Frailty amplifies aging's effect on protein metabolism, illustrating an important intersection of biological decline and nutrition risk. Frailty is a clinical syndrome of the older adult characterized by loss of strength, endurance, and physiological function that heightens susceptibility to illness, falls, and functional deterioration. Frailty can have one of its greatest impacts upon protein metabolism, which inherently declines with increasing age. As individuals grow older, their bodies become less efficient at synthesizing protein, leading to muscle wasting (sarcopenia) and reduced physical performance. When frailty is present, this inefficiency is further magnified (Figure 2.17).

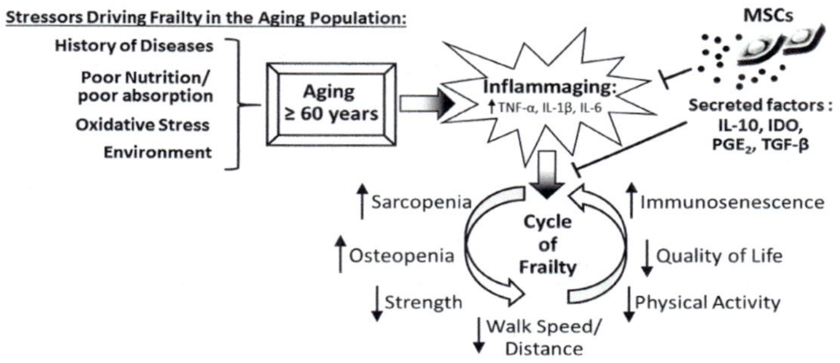

Figure 2.17. The role of stressors, aging, and inflammation in frailty and the effects of mesenchymal stem cells. As individuals grow older, several stressors (poor nutrition, diseases, oxidative stress, and environmental factors) increase the inflammaging process, leading to frailty.

Source: https://www.researchgate.net/publication/319400650/figure/fig1/AS:533568973094912@1504224164342/The-role-of-stressors-aging-and-inflammation-in-frailty-and-the-effects-of-mesenchymal.png.

Frailty enhances muscle protein degradation and decreases the efficiency of the body in using dietary protein, a process known as anabolic resistance. Therefore, even when older adults consume adequate protein, muscles will not respond by increasing or maintaining tissue. Inflammation, hormonal imbalance, and disorders that are usually associated with frailty make this dysregulation of protein metabolism even more adverse. The consequences are extensive: increased risk of falls, delayed recovery from illness or injury, decreased mobility, and elevated mortality.

In reversing these results, frail older individuals require higher-quality protein intake equally divided between meals and at times more than the normal recommended dietary allowance (RDA) for protein. Supplementing the diet with resistance or strength training will enhance protein utilization and facilitate muscle synthesis. Early nutritional management, medical evaluation, and lifestyle changes are critical to reversing the vicious cycle of frailty and protein inefficiency. It is knowledge of protein metabolism and its interaction with frailty that will assist in preserving independence and optimizing health span in the elderly.

REFERENCES

1. Alzheimer's Association. (2023). 2023 Alzheimer's disease facts and figures. *Alzheimer's & Dementia, 19*, 1598–1695. https://doi.org/10.1002/alz.13016 (accessed on 12th July 2025).
2. Ambrosetti, M., Abreu, A., Corrà, U., Davos, C. H., Hansen, D., Frederix, I., Iliou, M. C., et al. (2020). Secondary prevention through comprehensive cardiovascular rehabilitation: From knowledge to implementation. 2020 update. A position paper from the Secondary Prevention and Rehabilitation Section of the European Association of Preventive Cardiology. *European Journal of Preventive Cardiology, 28*, 460–495. https://doi.org/10.1177/2047487320913379 (accessed on 12th July 2025).
3. Szychowska, A., & Drygas, W. (2022). Physical activity as a determinant of successful aging: a narrative review article. *Aging clinical and experimental research, 34*(6), 1209–1214. https://doi.org/10.1007/s40520-021-02037-0(accessed on 12th July 2025).
4. Pasini, E., Aquilani, R., Corsetti, G., & Dioguardi, F. S. (2015). Malnutrition and Gut Flora Dysbiosis: Specific Therapies for Emerging Comorbidities in Heart Failure. *BioMed research international, 2015*, 382585. https://doi.org/10.1155/2015/382585(accessed on 12th July 2025).
5. Baijens, L. W. J., Clavé, P., Cras, P., Ekberg, O., Forster, A., Kolb, G., Leners, J. C., et al. (2016). European Society for Swallowing Disorders–European Union Geriatric Medicine Society white paper: Oropharyngeal dysphagia as a geriatric syndrome. *Clinical Interventions in Aging, 11*, 1403–1428. https://doi.org/10.2147/cia.s107750 (accessed on 12th July 2025).
6. Theodorakopoulos, C., Jones, J., Bannerman, E., & Greig, C. A. (2017). Effectiveness of nutritional and exercise interventions to improve body composition and muscle strength or function in sarcopenic obese older adults: A systematic review. *Nutrition research (New York, N.Y.), 43*, 3–15. https://doi.org/10.1016/j.nutres.2017.05.002(accessed on 12th July 2025).
7. Deutz, N. E., Bauer, J. M., Barazzoni, R., Biolo, G., Boirie, Y., Bosy-Westphal, A., Cederholm, T., Cruz-Jentoft, A., Krznariç, Z., Nair, K. S., Singer, P., Teta, D., Tipton, K., & Calder, P. C. (2014). Protein intake and exercise for optimal muscle function with aging: recommendations from the ESPEN Expert Group. *Clinical nutrition (Edinburgh, Scotland), 33*(6), 929–936. https://doi.org/10.1016/j.clnu.2014.04.007(accessed on 12th July 2025).
8. Schindler, K., Themessl-Huber, M., Hiesmayr, M., Kosak, S., Lainscak, M., Laviano, A., Ljungqvist, O., Mouhieddine, M., Schneider, S., de van der Schueren, M., Schütz, T., Schuh, C., Singer, P., Bauer, P., & Pichard, C. (2016). To eat or not to eat? Indicators for reduced food intake in 91,245 patients hospitalized on nutritionDays 2006-2014 in 56 countries worldwide: a descriptive analysis. *The American journal of clinical nutrition, 104*(5), 1393–1402. https://doi.org/10.3945/ajcn.116.137125(accessed on 12th July 2025).
9. Volkert, D., Beck, A. M., Cederholm, T., Cruz-Jentoft, A., Goisser, S., Hooper, L., Kiesswetter, E., Maggio, M., Raynaud-Simon, A., Sieber, C. C., Sobotka, L., van Asselt, D., Wirth, R., & Bischoff, S. C. (2019). ESPEN guideline on clinical nutrition and hydration in geriatrics. *Clinical nutrition (Edinburgh, Scotland), 38*(1), 10–47. https://doi.org/10.1016/j.clnu.2018.05.024(accessed on 12th July 2025).
10. Ostan, R., Guidarelli, G., Giampieri, E., Lanzarini, C., Berendsen, A. A. M., Januszko, O., Jennings, A., Lyon, N., Caumon, E., Gillings, R., Sicinska, E., Meunier, N., Feskens, E. J. M., Pietruszka, B., de Groot, L. C. P. G. M., Fairweather-Tait, S., Capri, M., Franceschi, C., & Santoro, A. (2018).

Cross-Sectional Analysis of the Correlation Between Daily Nutrient Intake Assessed by 7-Day Food Records and Biomarkers of Dietary Intake Among Participants of the NU-AGE Study. *Frontiers in physiology*, *9*, 1359. https://doi.org/10.3389/fphys.2018.01359(accessed on 12th July 2025).

11. Rémond, D., Shahar, D. R., Gille, D., Pinto, P., Kachal, J., Peyron, M. A., Dos Santos, C. N., Walther, B., Bordoni, A., Dupont, D., Tomás-Cobos, L., & Vergères, G. (2015). Understanding the gastrointestinal tract of the elderly to develop dietary solutions that prevent malnutrition. *Oncotarget*, *6*(16), 13858–13898. https://doi.org/10.18632/oncotarget.4030(accessed on 12th July 2025).
12. Carter, C. S., Justice, J. N., & Thompson, L. (2019). Lipotoxicity, aging, and muscle contractility: Does fiber type matter? *Boston University*. https://open.bu.edu/bitstream/2144/40625/7/carter_justice_thompson_Lipotoxicity_paper_04302019.pdf (accessed on 12th July 2025).
13. Cryan, J. F., O'Riordan, K. J., Cowan, C. S. M., Sandhu, K. V., Bastiaanssen, T. F. S., Boehme, M., Codagnone, M. G., et al. (2019). The microbiota-gut-brain axis. *Physiological Reviews*, *99*, 1877–2013. https://doi.org/10.1152/physrev.00018.2018 (accessed on 12th July 2025).
14. De Rosa, S., Samoni, S., Villa, G., & Ronco, C. (2017). Management of chronic kidney disease patients in the intensive care unit: Mixing acute and chronic illness. *Blood Purification*, *43*, 151–162. https://doi.org/10.1159/000452650 (accessed on 12th July 2025).
15. Forster, S., & Gariballa, S. (2005). Age as a determinant of nutritional status: a cross sectional study. *Nutrition journal*, *4*, 28. https://doi.org/10.1186/1475-2891-4-28(accessed on 12th July 2025).
16. Frontera, D. E. (2019). Age-related smell changes and their effects on the health status of older Americans. https://core.ac.uk/download/226778712.pdf (accessed on 12th July 2025).
17. Gama-Axelsson, T. (2014). Assessment and monitoring of nutritional status in chronic kidney disease patients. https://core.ac.uk/download/70341025.pdf (accessed on 12th July 2025).
18. Guseva, J., Vasiliev, A., Maksimov, N., & Bagdasarian, E. (2025). Balanced protein nutrition of fish is a key factor in high-quality fish products. *BIO Web of Conferences*. https://www.semanticscholar.org/paper/0333cd6d017eeded749f72a4a52949710de5ea3e (accessed on 12th July 2025).
19. Gutiérrez Rodríguez, A. (2019). Diagnosis of some diseases through biomarkers. https://core.ac.uk/download/288157992.pdf (accessed on 12th July 2025).
20. Jiang, X., Song, Z., Li, C., Hu, X., Ge, Y., Cheng, L., Shi, X., et al. (2024). Effects of dietary lipid levels on the growth, muscle fatty acid and amino acid composition, antioxidant capacity, and lipid deposition in mirror carp (*Cyprinus carpio*). *Animals: an Open Access Journal from MDPI*, *14*. https://www.semanticscholar.org/paper/aa8c6ccaa9199fd9a58a4e43611599e49a5863a5 (accessed on 12th July 2025).
21. Karlic, H., Krammer, U. D. B., & Haslberger, A. (2022). Nutritional supplements for athletes and personalization; a short review. *Functional Food Science*. https://www.semanticscholar.org/paper/63dd8090d861abe74d68f2ba9ed4d6dc68ba1165 (accessed on 12th July 2025).
22. Lai, J. C., Tandon, P., Bernal, W., Tapper, E. B., Ekong, U. D., Dasarathy, S., Carey, E. J., et al. (2021). Malnutrition, frailty, and sarcopenia in patients with cirrhosis: 2021 practice guidance by the American Association for the Study of Liver Diseases. *Hepatology*, *74*, 1611–1644. https://doi.org/10.1002/hep.32049 (accessed on 12th July 2025).

23. Larsson, L., Degens, H., Li, M., Salviati, L., Lee, Y. I., Thompson, W. J., Kirkland, J. L., et al. (2018). Sarcopenia: Aging-related loss of muscle mass and function. *Physiological Reviews, 99*, 427–511. https://doi.org/10.1152/physrev.00061.2017 (accessed on 12th July 2025).

24. Li, P., & Wu, G. (2023). Amino acid nutrition and metabolism in domestic cats and dogs. *Journal of Animal Science and Biotechnology, 14*. https://www.semanticscholar.org/paper/53aac7183f850c0d80df78e96fb50e1760d5a598 (accessed on 12th July 2025).

25. Malafarina, V., Reginster, J. Y., Cabrerizo, S., et al. (2017). Nutritional status and nutritional treatment are related to outcomes and mortality in older adults with hip fracture. https://core.ac.uk/download/pdf/212756692.pdf (accessed on 12th July 2025).

26. Miller, C. G. (2017). Dehydration in nursing home residents: A meta-analysis of causes of dehydration, implications, and those most at risk. https://core.ac.uk/download/84674618.pdf (accessed on 12th July 2025).

27. Novikova, V. P., Zavyalova, A. N., Yakovleva, M., Strukov, E. L., Kukes, I. V., & Lunegov, T. D. (2025). Assessment of mass spectrometric indicators of organic acids metabolism in children with sarcopenia on the background of protein-energy insufficiency. Pilot study. *Acta Biomedica Scientific*. https://www.semanticscholar.org/paper/540502030d421f8c66bfdfd87e25531fd9734904 (accessed on 12th July 2025).

28. Park, D., Shin, A., & Park, Y. (2025). Nutrition intervention for older patients based on comprehensive geriatric assessment: A case report. *Clinical Nutrition Research, 14*, 91–99. https://www.semanticscholar.org/paper/75815418aa0b497e93771369eaf805f333172235 (accessed on 12th July 2025).

29. Reber, E., Gomes, F., Vasiloglou, M. F., Schüetz, P., & Stanga, Z. (2019). Nutritional risk screening and assessment. *Journal of Clinical Medicine, 8*, 1065–1065. https://doi.org/10.3390/jcm8071065 (accessed on 12th July 2025).

30. Ríos-Covián, D., Ruas-Madiedo, P., Margollés, A., Gueimonde, M., Reyes-Gavilán, C. G. de los, & Salazar, N. (2016). Intestinal short chain fatty acids and their link with diet and human health. *Frontiers in Microbiology, 7*. https://doi.org/10.3389/fmicb.2016.00185 (accessed on 12th July 2025).

31. Tsai, Y., Tsai, M. H., Chang, G. H., Tsai, M., Huang, E. I., Lu, C. H., Hsu, C. M., et al. (2024). Prognostic importance of modified geriatric nutritional risk index in oral cavity squamous cell carcinoma. *Scientific Reports, 14*. https://www.semanticscholar.org/paper/d3b9b4aafc646a05cbe8e76013258bfce5c9dc74 (accessed on 12th July 2025).

32. Woods, J. A., Hutchinson, N. T., Powers, S. K., Roberts, W. O., Gómez-Cabrera, M. C., Radák, Z., Berkés, I., et al. (2020). The COVID-19 pandemic and physical activity. *Sports Medicine and Health Science, 2*, 55–64. https://doi.org/10.1016/j.smhs.2020.05.006 (accessed on 12th July 2025).

33. Woźniak, K., Hedesz, P., Żuk-Łapan, A., Jung, M., Gardian-Baj, M., Popczyńska, J., Doryń, A., et al. (2024). Nutrition strategies for optimizing performance and health in young athletes. *Journal of Education, Health and Sport*. https://www.semanticscholar.org/paper/96561ed643b196926d03734c5ac8dac12cb2f392 (accessed on 12th July 2025).

34. Xie, Y., Su, N., Yang, J., Tan, Q., Huang, S., Jin, M., Ni, Z., et al. (2020). FGF/FGFR signaling in health and disease. *Signal Transduction and Targeted Therapy, 5*. https://doi.org/10.1038/s41392-020-00222-7 (accessed on 12th July 2025).

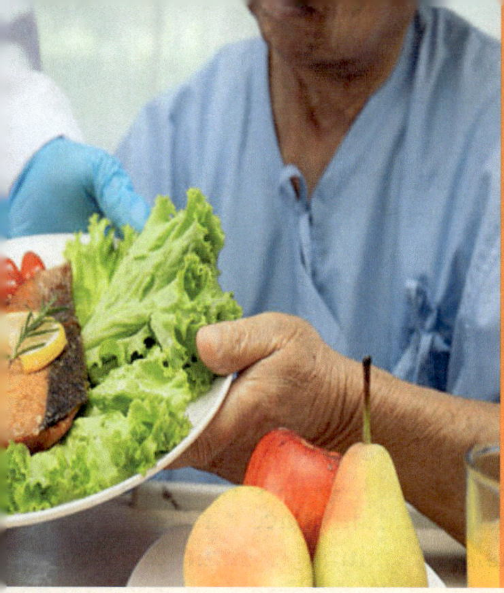

Chapter 3

CARBOHYDRATE, FAT, AND FLUID REQUIREMENTS IN OLDER ADULTS

Contents

Introduction

It is ever more critical to address the nutritional requirements of aging older adults as populations globally are aging. Aging introduces physiological changes necessitating the re-evaluation of dietary intake with a focus on carbohydrates, fats, and fluids. These macronutrients play a key role in promoting health, preventing chronic diseases, and overall well-being. Specific dietary guidelines to accommodate the specific needs of elderly people must not just emphasize adequate caloric value but also the appropriate quality and balance of macronutrients supplying energy, maintaining muscle, and maximizing intellectual functions. The challenge lies in creating guidelines that are at the same time practical and effective in addressing the complicated nutrition context of the older population and in requiring that the nutrition system has to be resilient and adaptive to individual health status and lifestyle. With respect to carbohydrate requirements, the digestibility and glycemic value of varying sources of carbohydrates have to be considered because older adults can react with their bodies in various ways to these foods. The intake of complex carbohydrates such as whole grains, vegetables, and fruits is particularly beneficial due to the excellent fiber content that promotes digestive function and has the potential to ensure a stable blood glucose. As Fusch et al. (2009) recommend, with increasing age, changes in metabolism could contribute to altering the fluid and nutrient needs in older adults; a fine balance of the kinds of carbohydrates is therefore an integral part of health in this group. Furthermore, increasing intakes of fiber also have a direct correlation with reduced risk of the formation of metabolic syndrome, particularly significant in the elderly who may have an increased risk due to decreased physical activity and aging. Of equal concern are the dietary fats, as fats also serve purposes other than providing energy; they serve significant roles in ensuring brain function and endocrine balance. Older adults should place emphasis on the intake of healthy fats, such as in avocados, nuts, and fatty fish and minimize saturated and trans fats that may cause cardiovascular diseases. Adequate hydration also becomes an essential factor in meal planning among the elderly because the sense of thirst diminishes with age. The recommendations of Carlson et al. (2007) fall within this need, where specific strategies for fluid consumption to counteract dehydration frequently require intentional actions. In conclusion, a general understanding of carbohydrates, fat, and fluid requirements is necessary to design optimal dietary interventions towards enhancing the quality of life in the elderly (Figure 3.1).

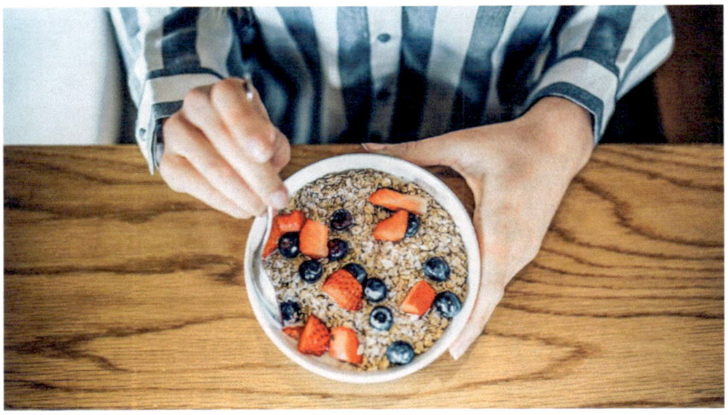

Figure 3.1. Carbohydrate, fat, and fluid requirements in older adults.

Source: https://i0.wp.com/images-prod.healthline.com/hlcmsresource/images/topic_centers/2020-6/oatmeal-berries-bowl-1296x728-header.jpg?w=1155&h=1528.

Importance of Nutrition in Older Adults

Nutrition is the essence of maintaining the health and well-being of elderly people, as the ageing process triggers various physiological changes to nutritional needs. With ageing, metabolic changes, digestion, and absorption efficiency lead to a rising vulnerability to malnutrition. Mechanical food breakdown and gastrointestinal (GIT) motor activity undergo catastrophic decline, impairing the body's ability to take in appropriate nutrients. These changes manifest in ineffective nutrient acquisition, which gives rise to a closer assessment of effective nutritional interventions considering the functionality of the aging GIT. Individualized nutritional advice taking a center stage role, healthcare professionals reduce the morbidity of malnutrition, thus optimizing older adults' quality of life. Thus, it becomes necessary to address these changes in nutrition in order to combat the health issues that are associated with insufficient nutrition among this vulnerable group (Rémond et al., 2015). Older adults require an equal intake of macronutrients—carbohydrates, fats, and protein—to support their overall health and functional ability. Carbohydrates are a source of energy, whereas fats are needed for the production of hormones and nutrient absorption. This group will often need higher-quality sources of these macronutrients to fight disease in aging and maintain body function. Nutritional strategies need to be concerned not just with quantity, but with quality as well, encouraging whole grains, healthy fats, fruits and vegetables with high nutrient content. Fluid intake should be considered as well, since elderly individuals are at greater risk for dehydration, which can exacerbate disease conditions such as cognitive impairment and cardiovascular disease. Awareness of the nutritional value of nutrient-dense foods alongside adequate fluid consumption is crucial to the promotion of vigor and longevity in older individuals (Hansen et al., 2023). Resolution of older people's nutritional needs effectively requires a multi-pronged approach involving dietary education, community, and individualized care planning. Engaging this group in a discussion of healthy eating behavior can promote the reinforcement of their awareness and compliance with nutritional strategies. Community initiatives that provide services, such as grocery store shopping assistance or meal preparation course instruction, help to empower older adults to make healthier food choices. Health workers should also encourage the use of nutritional supplements when necessary to supplement deficiencies in nutrition consumption, especially where food consumption can be hampered by causes like decreased appetite or difficulty with mastication. As the population continues to age progressively, it is crucial that their unique nutritional requirements are recognized and given priority. Through the implementation of these steps, we can enable healthier, more productive aging for older individuals, while preventing malnutrition and chronic disease (Rémond et al., 2015).

Overview of Macronutrients: Carbohydrates, Fats, and Fluids

Carbohydrates, fats, and fluids are all important macronutrients, each having its own unique functions in the nutritional needs of older people. Carbohydrates serve as the primary source of energy, particularly for cerebral functions and general physical activity. In this age group, it is crucial to highlight complex carbohydrates such as whole grains, fruits, and vegetables, which ensure sustained release of energy and dietary fiber required by the body. However, studies indicate that the majority of older people struggle with sustaining proper carbohydrate consumption, which can lead to lower energy levels and vulnerability to malnutrition (Fabiani et al., 2024). Additionally, it is important to note the role of carbohydrates in cognitive function since proper energy supply enhances processes vulnerable to aging. Fats are a macronutrient that is important in various body functions, like the absorption of fat-soluble vitamins (A, D, E, and K) and providing essential fatty acids. With the consideration of the fact that aging adults are susceptible to age-related changes in metabolism and body composition, the fats consumed should be of special concern regarding their quality and quantity. Healthier sources of fat, such as avocados, nuts, seeds, and olive oil, contribute to cardiovascular function and can decrease inflammation (Deane et al., 2017). Saturated consumption of fat in excess increases conditions, but the correct balance between omega-3 and omega-6 fatty acids can maintain muscle function and enhance overall health in aging groups. Incorporation of such sources of nutrition will have notable implications for health status and lifespan. Fluid intake is often overlooked, but it plays a key role in the overall health of elderly people. Hydration has a significant role in many physiological processes, including digestion, blood flow, and the regulation of body temperature. Particularly, elderly people can have trouble with mechanisms of thirst and kidney function, which are more susceptible to dehydration (Fabiani et al., 2024). As a result, it is important to promote frequent fluid intake throughout the day with a focus on water and fluids that are capable of restoring electrolytes. Inadequate fluid status may cause negative effects, such as impairment in cognitive function and kidney function, and for that reason, it is crucial to implement dietary habits that promote adequate fluid intake. Generally speaking, knowledge of the balance and interconnected nature of carbohydrates, fats, and fluids is important in maintaining optimal health among older individuals (Figure 3.2).

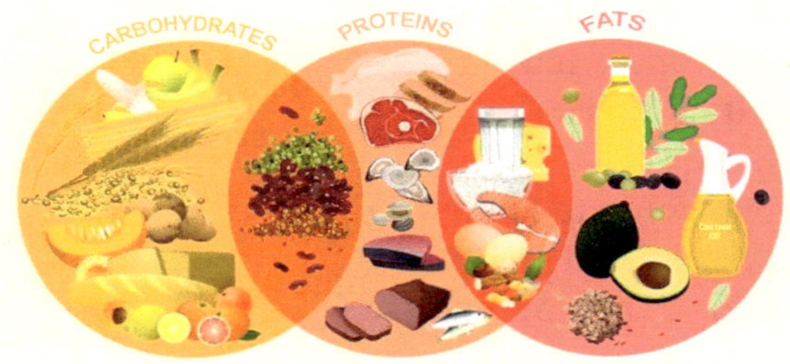

Figure 3.2. Macronutrients: Carbohydrates, fats, and fluids.

Source: https://avitahealth.org/wp-content/uploads/2022/03/macronutrients.jpg.

3.1. Understanding Carbohydrates

Understanding carbohydrates is required to be able to comprehend the nutritional needs of the elderly because these macronutrients are the source of energy for the body. The carbohydrates are either simple or complex, with simple carbohydrates composed of sugars, while complex carbohydrates are made up of starches and fibers. For the aged, the consumption of complex carbohydrates is particularly beneficial as they break down slowly and are low on the glycemic index, facilitating the maintenance of normal blood glucose levels. A diet of whole grains, fruits, and vegetables can prevent diseases that are common in this group, such as diabetes and heart disease. Therefore, a well-balanced understanding of the sources of carbohydrates and their respective benefits is necessary in the formulation of dietary recommendations promoting health and well-being among the elderly. Moreover, the quality of nutrition derived from the consumption of carbohydrates is critical in determining the health condition of the elderly. Consumption of refined carbohydrates and processed foods could have deleterious effects on the health of older individuals, such as obesity, insulin resistance, and inflammation. Conversely, intact forms of carbohydrates contain essential nutrients like vitamins, minerals, and dietary fiber, all of which offer positive gut health and metabolic activity. The fiber contained within intact foods helps the process of digestion and can reduce the occurrence of gastrointestinal diseases, which are common in geriatric patients.

In addition, a diet high in fiber carries the advantage of satiety, which helps maintain body weight in a more effective manner. As such, emphasized in diet intervention specific to the needs of aging groups are the consumption of good quality sources of carbohydrate. These relate directly to the health objectives of this population. The inclusion of carbohydrates in aging populations' diets is with optimal regard to both changing energy and carbohydrate needs. Care should be taken to balance carbohydrate intake with activity level, as older individuals decrease their activities and this may alter energy requirements. To optimize nutritional status, registered dietitian nutritionists (RDNs) need to assess individual eating behavior to ensure older individuals receive sufficient amounts of carbohydrates to facilitate daily activities while not ingesting excess calories. Carbohydrate education is important; learning to make healthy and unhealthy sources distinctions can assist in arming older adults to make successful food decisions. Ultimately, adopting an individualized approach of carbohydrate consumption—one that takes into consideration individual needs and health status—will prove key to the overall health and resilience of older adults in maintaining both physical and cognitive health during aging (Figure 3.3).

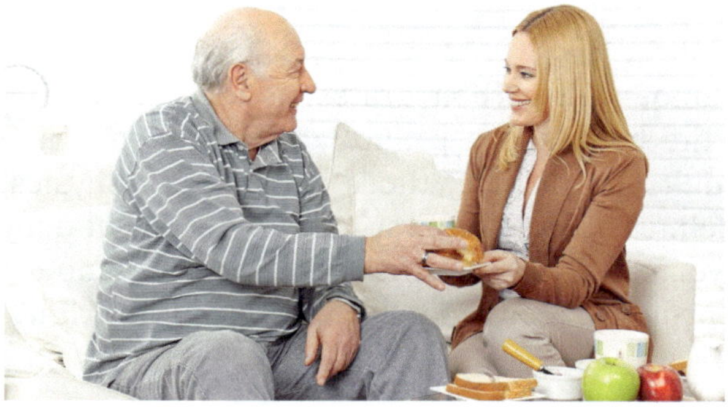

Figure 3.3. Older adults should know about eating bad carbs.

Source: https://integrishealth.org/-/media/blog/21-q4/oyh_bad-carbs.ashx?revision=d5abdb59-3fdd-4b23-8e02-57484fae5e24.

3.1.1. Role of Carbohydrates in Energy Production

Carbohydrates are a key player in energy production as the body's primary fuel, particularly under circumstances of intense exercise. For older adults, the role of carbohydrates increases with the changes associated with age and affecting energy metabolism. With muscle loss and decreased metabolic rates that accompany aging, proper consumption of carbohydrates is crucial to maintain energy needs. Carbohydrates are metabolized to glucose, which organs and muscles utilize for energy, maintaining levels of physical activity and overall well-being in the elderly population. Furthermore, a high-carbohydrate diet may act as a protective factor against muscle loss and aid in the management of prevalent illnesses among the elderly, with the encouragement of an active and independent life. As individuals mature in old age, physiological adjustments of carbohydrate utilization demand immense dietary care. Inadequate carbohydrate intake can be related to energy deficiencies, diminished activity in activities of daily living, and a higher risk of diseases such as frailty and obesity. In particular, optimal carbohydrate consumption among older adults typically ranges between 45% and 65% of total daily calories. This macronutrient is not only a ready source of energy but also plays a role in the regulation of protein and fat metabolism, emphasizing its integral role in the nutrition profile. Changing sources of carbohydrate toward whole grains, fruits, and vegetables enhances nutritional intake and provides dietary fiber, which plays a critical role in gut health, especially in the elderly who are prone to gastrointestinal motility disorders. Also, education regarding carbohydrate consumption is emphasized by various studies on knowledge gaps in nutrition awareness. Recent research illustrates how increasing nutrition awareness among various populations, including the elderly, is associated with optimal food decisions, which in turn contribute to better health outcomes. For instance, as established in Ekesa et al. (2017), education relating to food security and nutrition can empower one to make healthy decisions. Moreover, the effect of carbohydrate intake on sporting performance, as elaborated on in

Heikkilä (2020), suggests the significance of optimized nutrition for maintaining activity levels, central to older adult health and ageing. This data also highlights the necessity of targeted nutritional interventions aimed at carbohydrate needs in older adult populations to promote healthy ageing (Figure 3.4).

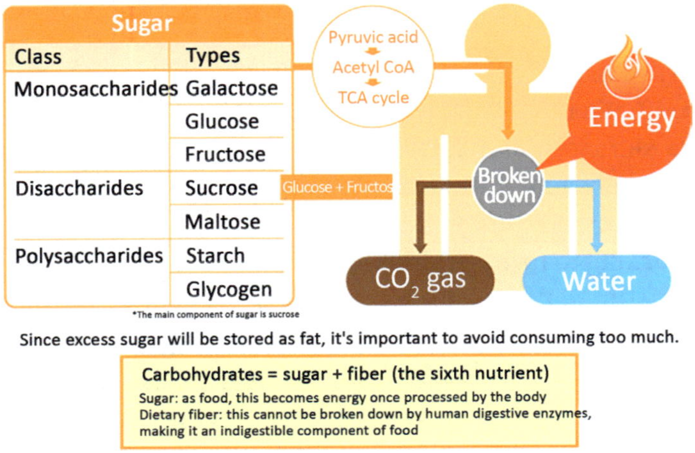

Figure 3.4. Carbohydrates: an efficient energy source.

Source: https://www.otsuka.co.jp/en/nutraceutical/about/nutrition/sports-nutrition/essential-nutrients/img/carbohydrates_im01.png.

3.1.2. Recommended Carbohydrate Intake for Older Adults

It is crucial that the older person has an adequate amount of carbohydrates, as they are one of the main sources of energy supporting function in the body and a prime factor in maintaining optimum health and function in old age. For older adults, particularly those with limited physical activity, a good balance is necessary. Nutritional guidelines usually suggest that 45%–65% of daily total caloric intake should be derived from carbohydrates. This is sufficient to provide enough energy but does not exclude a combination of nutrient-dense foods that are utilized to contribute to overall well-being.

Focus on the intake of complex carbohydrates such as whole grains, legumes, and vegetables, which are nutrient and fiber-rich, can enhance gastrointestinal health and reduce chronic disease risk common to this age, and even more in patients with impaired glucose tolerance, metabolic syndrome, or type 2 diabetes. Provided attention is given to the typical metabolic alterations seen with aging, carbohydrate recommendations then need to be tailored. Some older people will have decreased insulin sensitivity or alterations in glucose metabolism, which will complicate their carbohydrate requirements. Care must ensure food selection emphasizes low glycemic index carbohydrates that release more stable amounts of glucose and can treat diseases like diabetes. Moreover, the quality of the nutrients in carbohydrates cannot be left out; as research on the nutrient quality of bread and cereals has demonstrated, adhering to standards such as the ≤10:1 carbohydrate: fiber ratio can ensure enhanced overall health in older adults (Ghodsian & Madden, 2018). Moreover, the incorporation of dietary strategies with diverse sources of carbohydrates can be advantageous for appetite and energy. Older people can be supported through meal planning based on carbohydrate-fiber-rich foods, as this may lead to increased satiety and improved weight control. For instance, a study emphasizes the effectiveness of calorie-restricted diets compared to low-carbohydrate diets for long-term weight maintenance, suggesting that more efficient carbohydrate management might also provide healthy body weight among older adults (Brown, 2014). By placing high-quality sources of carbohydrates at the top and considering dietary requirements, older people can make the most out of their carbohydrate intake to improve their health and well-being.

3.1.3. Sources of Healthy Carbohydrates

Access to healthy carbohydrates is essential in ensuring that older individuals' dietary requirements are met as they struggle with the complexities of aging and associated health complications. Whole grains such as brown rice, quinoa, and whole wheat bread are rich in healthy carbohydrates and offer not only energy but also essential nutrients and dietary fiber.

The fiber obtained from these foods adds to the health of the individual's digestive system, which is typically compromised in the elderly due to physiological changes in the gastrointestinal system. Increased intake of fiber is also associated with a lower risk of constipation and other gastrointestinal diseases, prevalent among the elderly. Also, the intake of good carbohydrates will help to regulate weight and maintain a consistent energy level, hence supporting overall physical and mental well-being during the aging process. Vegetables and fruits are another essential source of good carbohydrates. These are abundant in functional vitamins, minerals, and antioxidants that are of prime significance in fighting oxidative stress and inflammation, which are elevated in the elderly. The variable texture and flavor of fresh fruits and vegetables may also enhance greater food intake, which is necessary due to the evidence of high rates of malnutrition among this group. Research indicates that well-balanced meals with fruit and vegetables of many different colors can lead to profound health advantages, like enhanced immune systems and enhanced brain function. Because older people may have decreased appetite and altered taste perception, creative food preparation highlighting the natural sweetness of fruits and the vibrant colors of vegetables can motivate them to participate in their own meal planning, thus resulting in appropriate caloric intake and nutrient acquisition. Legumes like beans, lentils, and chickpeas provide great amounts of good carbohydrates as well as protein and dietary fiber, thus being very beneficial to older individuals.

Apart from providing long-term energy, they are also beneficial in the preservation of muscles and body strength, which are both crucial in this age bracket. Moreover, the glycemic index of legumes is low, which promotes maintaining stable blood sugar levels, decreasing the occurrence of insulin resistance and type 2 diabetes, illnesses prevalent in the elderly. Incorporating legumes into a regular diet has been shown to improve cardiovascular health through cholesterol reduction in the blood and improved cardiovascular events. Because elderly people are coping with other nutritional deficiencies due to gastrointestinal tract changes and decreased nutrient absorption, legumes are an outstanding diet intervention that is perfectly adapted to their carbohydrate needs while overall nutritional status is enhanced, therefore fulfilling the risk factors associated with malnutrition and its health implications (Rémond et al., 2015; Malafarina et al., 2017) (Figure 3.5).

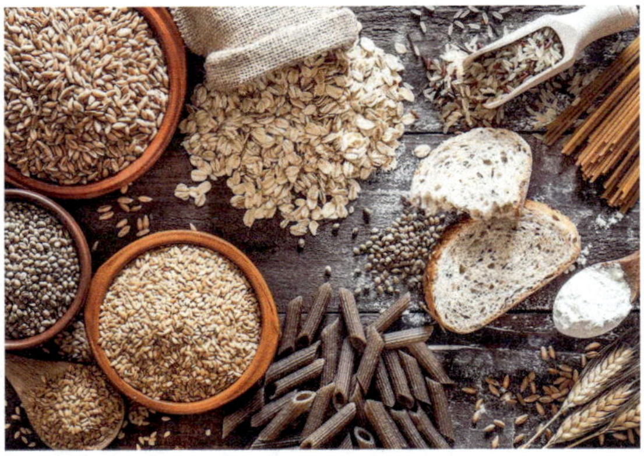

Figure 3.5. Healthy carbs.

Source: https://assets.clevelandclinic.org/transform/LargeFeatureImage/05385860-aa1c-4d70-96a4-c515cb380d15/various-whole-Grain-Carbs-835833518-770x533-1_jpg.

3.2. The Importance of Fats

Fats are an important part of meeting the nutritional needs of older individuals, necessitating a multifaceted appreciation of their importance. Fats are not only a dense source of energy, delivering approximately nine calories per gram, but they also facilitate the absorption of fat-soluble vitamins A, D, E, and K. Adequate levels of these vitamins in older individuals are necessary for immune system function, bone strength, and eyesight. Because metabolism declines with age, the incorporation of healthy fat from nuts, seeds, and fish can add to energy demand without adding to the excess calorie load associated with carbohydrates.

The composition of fat intake is also important; unsaturated fats, for instance, have been shown to increase lipid levels, hence decreasing cardiovascular risk, which is a common problem in older adults as they are at higher risk for heart disease. Another significant role of dietary fats is their role in brain health in elderly individuals. Scientific research indicates that certain fatty acids, including omega-3 fatty acids found in fish oil, have the ability to counteract the risk of reduced brain function and improve brain health overall.

These essential fats contribute to neuron function and synaptic plasticity, two elements involved with memory and cognitive function. As older adults may be at a greater risk of developing neurodegenerative illnesses like Alzheimer's, it is important to determine the function of adding omega-3 sources of food to their diets. However, it is also important that older adults balance how much fat they intake while considering the overall diet, since excessive intake of saturated fats has been linked to negative health impacts, such as elevated inflammation and higher chronic disease rates. In a discussion of the nutritional value of fats, it is important to touch on their impact on overall dietary patterns, especially when framed in the context of elderly health.

Diets high in healthy fats—such as those derived from the Mediterranean diet—have been found to be beneficial in lowering the risk of cardiovascular disease and increasing the overall longevity of an individual. This pattern is typically characterized by modest intake of fats, primarily from foods that provide beneficial fatty acids, such as olive oil, fatty fish, and avocados. Also, body synthesis of fat when in a caloric-restricted state further indicates the necessity to have a steady intake of fat in favor of preserving well-being. Hence, in older adults, fat should not only be considered as a food to be limited but as an essential component of a balanced diet that enhances health and well-being throughout aging, according to the latest nutritional research (Hester, 2017; Ghodsian & Madden, 2018) (Figure 3.6).

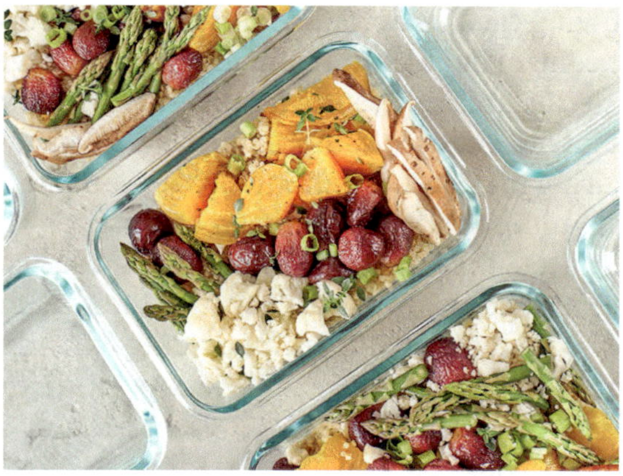

Figure 3.6. Healthy high carb foods.

Source: https://media.post.rvohealth.io/wp-content/uploads/sites/3/2022/07/high_carb_beet_quinoa_732x549_thumb.jpg.

3.2.1. Types of Fats and Their Functions in the Body

Understanding the types of fats and their function in the body is important for the supply of proper nutrition to aged people. The three primary types of fats are saturated, unsaturated, and trans fats. Saturated fats, which occur in animal foods and certain tropical oils like coconut oil, are associated with body functions through the provision of energy and allowing for the absorption of fat-soluble vitamins (A, D, E, K). Excess consumption of saturated fats has also been associated with cardiovascular disease, so balancing these fats in the diet is necessary. Unsaturated fats, found in vegetable oils, nuts, and fish, are essentially heart-healthy and have anti-inflammatory properties that can help reverse the aging risks. To understand how these fats function is to have a foundation for creating appropriate dietary advice for older individuals in an attempt to enhance their overall well-being. Fats not only supply energy; they play a critical role in maintaining the composition of cells and the production of hormones. Phospholipids, a category of fat, are significant as components of the cell membrane, keeping it fluid and intact, something also necessary as people grow older because the dynamics of the cell membrane can be compromised. Omega-3 and omega-6 fatty acids, in contrast, are precursors to messenger molecules utilized in inflammatory processes and thought. A diet high in unsaturated fats has been found to improve brain function, reduce the incidence of neurodegenerative diseases, and improve cognitive abilities among the elderly. In accordance with dietary guidelines, the emphasis on adding healthy fat to the diet of the elderly can have significant health benefits, pointing to its inclusion in the elderly's diet. Furthermore, consideration of fat consumption must address the possibility of an influence on common chronic conditions among elderly populations, such as obesity and diabetes. Knowledge of these associations enables clinicians to create dietary plans that will optimize positive health effects. For example, where the risk of overindulgence in saturated fats necessitates caution, a balanced perspective depicts the contextual benefit of adding moderate amounts of the same to a balanced diet. As indicated in research on eating habits, including a variety of fats in one's diet provides the necessary nutrients without subjecting one to the weight of chronic illnesses like cardiovascular issues if done in moderation. Hester (2017) and Tan et al. (2019) provide some insight into dietary frameworks that may help develop effective modules of nutrition relevant to these considerations for aged individuals, making fats a major consideration in individualized dietary measurements.

3.2.2. Recommended Fat Intake for Older Adults

In the case of using the recommended intake of fat among elderly individuals, it is notable to record the quiet role being played by fats in food in an individual's general well-being. Elderly individuals experience a change in metabolism and body composition and require an appropriately balanced diet that has the right amount of fat. Dietary guidelines generally propose that fats provide 20%–35% of total caloric intake to elderly individuals, with no more than 10% of total energy intake coming from saturated fatty acids and no more than 1% of total energy intake from *trans*-fatty acids from both industrially produced and ruminant animal sources. This suggestion stems from the observation that healthy fats, including those contained in avocados, nuts, and olive oil, are capable of improving heart health and brain function, both of which are important as one grows older. Furthermore, the knowledge of what kind of fat one is eating is significant since unsaturated fats are preferred to saturated and trans fats, the latter of which are associated with heightened cardiovascular disease and other medical issues. Additionally, increased fat intake may be necessary, taking into consideration the function of fat-soluble vitamins in older individuals. These include vitamins A, D, E, and K, and these rely on fat from the diet to be metabolizable by the body for well-being and health. Given that older individuals will often have malabsorption syndromes, fat intake may help avoid deficiency states from arising that might otherwise decrease well-being and health. Furthermore, quality rather than quantity in the proposed intake would be highlighted; incorporation of omega-3 fatty acid sources, which have both been proven to reduce inflammation and improve brain function, can be a significant factor in overall dietary adequacy. A better understanding of these factors directs healthcare clinicians and caregivers in developing nutrition plans specifically for this group. While the focus on fat intake is important, considerations must also be made in the overall scheme of macronutrient balance for the elderly diet. That includes the consumption of carbohydrates and protein, which gives synergistic action among these macronutrients to render healthy results. Older individuals typically require more protein to preserve muscle function and mass, thereby impacting the proportion of daily caloric intake from fat. Regular drinking of water is also essential, enabling better metabolic processes involving these macronutrients. Overall, proper diet control in older individuals should involve a precise balance between carbohydrates, proteins, and fats to set up a comprehensive approach to ensuring maximum health with age. Compliance with guidelines from nutrition researchers can guarantee that aging adults obtain adequate macronutrients, which will ensure their quality of life and lifespan, emphasizing the dual importance of quantity and quality in dietary fat intake (Carlson et al., 2007; Fusch et al., 2009) (Figure 3.7).

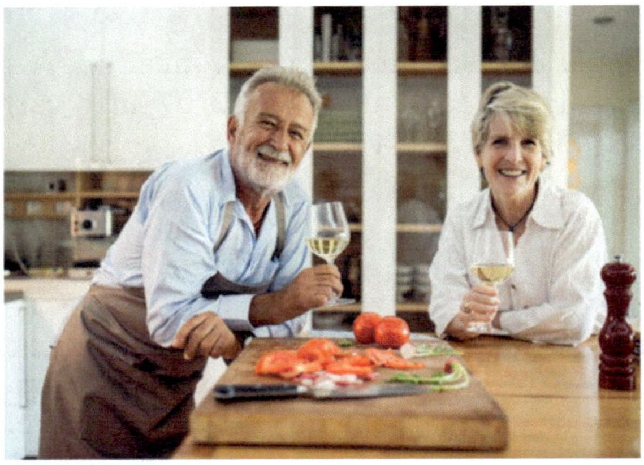

Figure 3.7. Healthy diet foods for older adults.

Source: https://www.gerdhelp.com/wp-content/uploads/2019/08/Senior-Nutrition-Guide.jpg.

3.2.3. Healthy Fat Sources and Their Benefits

The role of healthy fat intake in fulfilling the nutritional requirements of aged people cannot be overemphasized. Fats are important for several physiological processes such as production of hormones, nutrient absorption, and storage of energy. As age advances, the metabolism rate of the body decreases, and hence there is a need to have good fat sources such as avocados, nuts, seeds, and olive oil in the diet. These foods provide monounsaturated and polyunsaturated fats, which also happen to be good for heart health through the reduction of cholesterol levels and avoidance of cardiovascular illnesses.

Healthy fats can assist in fat-soluble vitamins (A, D, E, and K) absorption, which is required to maintain overall general well-being and health in aging individuals. Thus, including these sources in regular meals can have profound effects on nutritional response and aid in regulated aging processes. Furthermore, the health benefits of healthy fats are not limited to cardiovascular response to also encompass cognitive function and inflammatory control. Evidence suggests that omega-3 fatty acids, which are also found in high concentrations in fatty fish such as salmon and flaxseeds, may have a function in maintaining cognitive capabilities and alleviating the threat of neurodegenerative diseases common among elderly populations. Moreover, the anti-inflammatory effects of omega-3s can counteract the impacts of chronic inflammation that accompanies old age. On the other hand, despite coconut oil's frequent promotion as a healthy fat, the presence of saturated fatty acids in coconut oil raised issues about cardiovascular risk even in the context of an otherwise balanced diet that is plant-based. Thus, the understanding of the nuances of the different sources of fats allows older adults to make informed dietary choices that enhance long-term health and vitality (Hester, 2017). It also requires attention to calorie consumption, especially in older individuals who will have decreased appetite and changed metabolism. For this group, the energy density of healthy fat can be helpful in keeping them energized without food overload. Educational nutrition is essential, though, so that fats have a positive effect on general eating habits, especially when solving widespread deficiencies. Proper counseling can empower older individuals to achieve balance by complementing healthy fats with adequate amounts of carbohydrate and protein to meet their macro and micronutrient requirements. Establishing a multidimensional nutrition strategy is essential, focusing on how healthy eating can turn around the threats of aging as well as enhance the quality of life (Fusch et al., 2009).

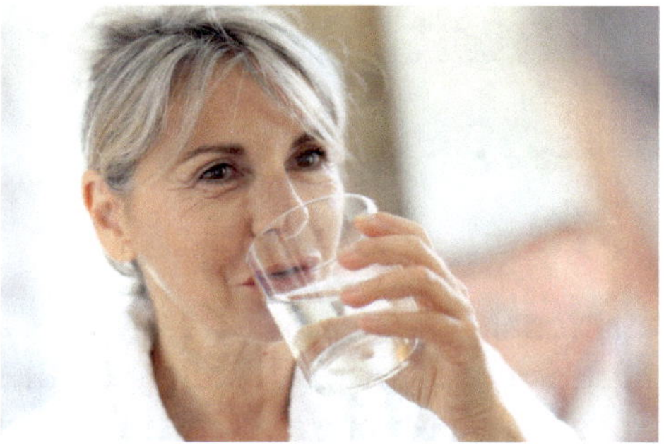

Figure 3.8. Healthy ways to increase your fluid intake.

Source: https://www.roswellpark.org/sites/default/files/styles/1600x800/public/cancer_fluid_intake.jpeg?itok=ENlpGBW2.

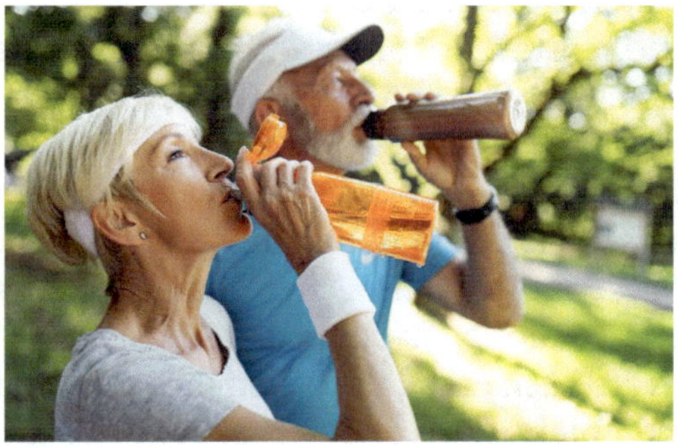

Figure 3.9. Importance of hydration for older adults.

Source: https://silverleafeldercare.com/wp-content/uploads/2022/10/senior-couple-drinking-water_1200x800.jpg.

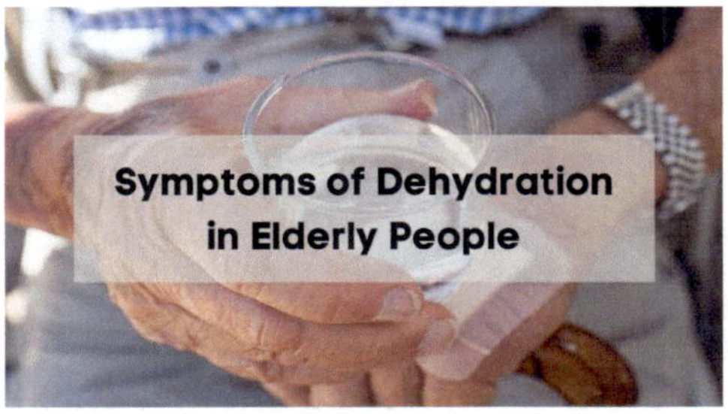

Figure 3.10. Symptoms of dehydration in elderly people.

Source: https://bermanlawyers.com/wp-content/uploads/2022/06/Symptoms-of-Dehydration-in-Elderly-People-1024x576.jpg.

3.4. Nutritional Challenges Faced by Older Adults

The nutritional profile varies greatly with aging, resulting in a plethora of challenges likely to impair overall well-being and health. Among the most significant sources of such challenges is the rise in physiological alterations accompanied by aging, such as decreased basal metabolic rate and altered digestive function. These changes can lead to reduced appetite and decreased subsequent food intake, with difficulty in meeting the required energy requirements and nutritional status of older adults. This deficiency is particularly of concern as older adults may be prone to maladies like sarcopenia, due to insufficient protein and caloric intake, leading to loss of muscle strength and function. In addition, the presence of socio-economic determinants, i.e., living alone or financial limitations, can aggravate such dietary deficiencies, thus making it a complex issue of inter-dependent factors requiring appropriate interventions (Nor et al., 2008). Another important characteristic of nutritional issues in the elderly is the need for macronutrients, i.e., carbohydrates and fats.

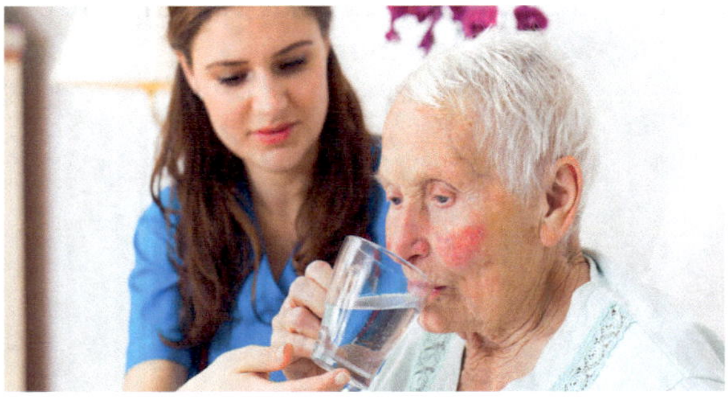

Figure 3.11. Common nutritional challenges within the older generation.

Source: https://www.clinicaleducation.org/wp-content/uploads/header-image-commonnutritionalchellenges-1024x512.jpg.

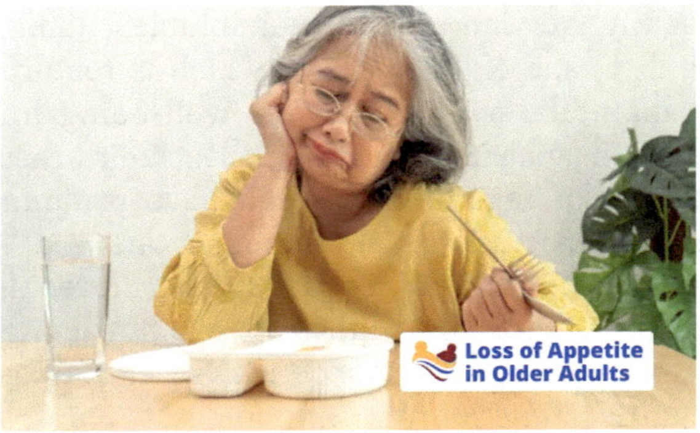

Figure 3.12. Loss of appetite in older adults.

Source: https://i0.wp.com/familycaregiversonline.net/wp-content/uploads/Loss-of-Appetite-in-Older-Adults_FISM.png?resize=645%2C400&ssl=1.

Although carbohydrates are a major source of energy, elderly individuals may have difficulty with the amount and quality of carbohydrate intake. Most of them prefer convenience foods that are easy to prepare and are made from refined carbohydrates, yet are low in nutrients and fiber. This transition causes elevated blood sugar levels and results in metabolic problems and further complicating their condition. The consumption of dietary fats is also a problem. Aging can necessitate changes in fat consumption due to cardiovascular health concerns, which can lead to baseless conclusions about eliminating all fats. Healthy fats, especially from the kind found in avocados and fatty fish, positively affect cognition as well as heart health and do not need to be eliminated completely from the diet of older populations (Heikkilä, 2020). Fluid intake is another critical but often overlooked problem in older individuals. Many individuals in this age group may not be able to feel their thirst properly, resulting in chronic dehydration, which puts them at risk for urinary tract infections, kidney stones, and other morbidities. Furthermore, dehydration can also play a profound role in cognition and aggravate the underlying diseases, such as heart disease and diabetes. It should be remembered that older people require adequate hydration to maintain their physiological functions, particularly because they can experience changes in renal function that affect fluid balance as well. Encouraging routine daily fluid consumption, both beverages and foods with water content, can prove to be a successful approach to this dilemma and the overall health state of community-dwelling elderly (Nor et al., 2008) (Figure 3.11).

3.4.1. Common Dietary Restrictions and Their Impact

Restrictions on the diet are placed regularly for various health reasons, especially among the older population who will probably have comorbid illnesses to be addressed accurately nutritionally. Low-sodium diets among hypertensives, low-sugar diets among diabetics, and gluten-free diets among those suffering from celiac disease are examples of typical restrictions. These dietary modifications can impose a significant effect on the overall carbohydrate, fat, and fluid requirements of these patients. For instance, elderly individuals following a low-sodium diet will need to seek alternative foods so that they acquire enough nutrients without risking their health. Furthermore, other dietary restrictions will demand the inclusion of high-fiber carbohydrates and healthy fats to maintain energy and metabolism, which is critical for this age group. Admitting the applicability of such dietary changes is essential to improve longevity and lower chronic disease risk in elderly people. Being vegan is another type of dietary restriction that is gaining popularity because of the health advantages it includes. Evidence confirms that a plant-based diet can lower obesity, heart disease, and type 2 diabetes risk, hence being a suitable choice for the elderly who need to improve their health conditions. However, individuals embracing a vegan way of life should exercise caution when it comes to specific nutrient deficiencies that may arise as a result of avoiding animal foods. For instance, the intake of key nutrients like calcium and protein is challenging unless one is well-instructed about their sources from plants. Despite such challenges, a well-formulated vegan diet can be nutritionally sufficient and capable of disease prevention and management for long-term diseases. Therefore, understanding food restrictions and their implications becomes vitally significant in guiding older adults to achieve and maintain appropriate nutrition without compromising their health objectives (Hester, 2017). Dietary management, particularly for heart health, requires well-thought-out interventions.

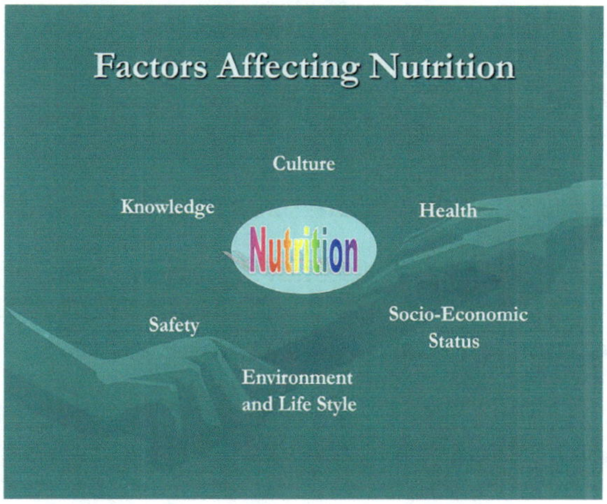

Figure 3.13. Factors affecting nutrition.

Source: https://image.slideserve.com/1296738/factors-affecting-nutrition-l.jpg.

Research suggests innovative diet manipulation beyond salt and fluid restriction to maximize cardiac performance in older patients with cardiovascular disease. Specifically, the addition of heart-healthy fats and an equilibrated amount of carbohydrate intake can positively influence fluid balance and cardiovascular function. Diets that are high in omega-3 fatty acids, for instance, have been found to be protective against cardiovascular diseases, while structured calorie intake is required in keeping with proper weight and overall health. Even liquid caloric consumption is accounted for to avoid dehydration, especially among older people. As food habits undergo change, the integration of such information into food guidelines can help to create sustainable, health-fostering food habits that suit the unique needs of an older age group (Butler, 2016).

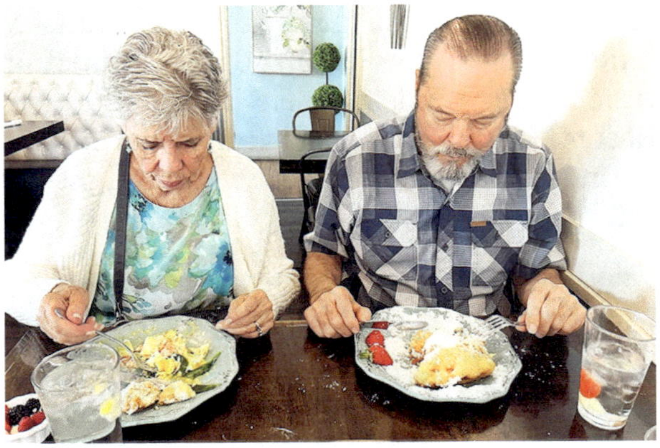

Figure 3.14. Nutritional needs in older adults.

Source: https://assistedlivingcarenm.com/wp-content/uploads/2022/05/NutritionNeeds_AssistedLivingCare_NM_TX_Blog.jpg.

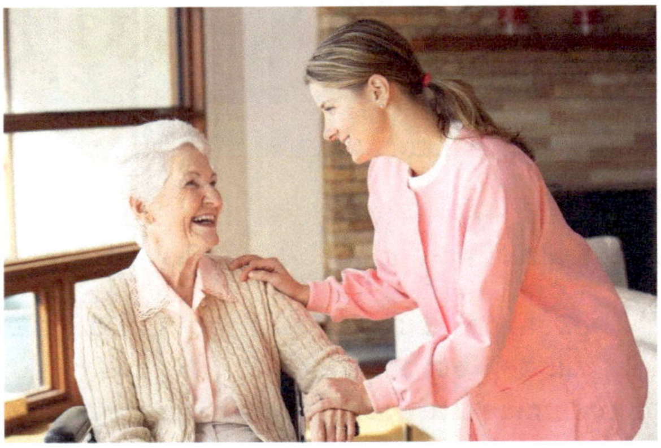

Figure 3.15. Mini nutritional assessment (MNA).

Source: https://www.mna-elderly.com/sites/default/files/styles/960px_width/public/2021-09/104-850x567.jpg?itok=DYS9TMjS.

3.4.2. Importance of Individualized Nutrition Plans

The importance of individualized nutrition plans for older adults cannot be overstated, given that individualized nutrition plans are specific to address the unique health and dietary needs of this group. Aging is typically associated with physiological changes that may have a significant effect on metabolism, digestion, and nutritional requirements. For instance, as one ages, the ability to metabolize and utilize nutrients can slow down, necessitating individualized dietetic interventions based on the patient's status, level of activity, and personal food habits. This personalized approach not only enhances dietary compliance but also the health and quality of life of elderly adults, thereby making the establishment of personalized nutrition plans imperative in addressing their requirements for carbohydrates, fats, and fluids in the context of the chapter Carbohydrate, Fat, and Fluid Requirements in Older Adults (Cioara et al., 2018). The incorporation of individual nutrition regimes is especially essential for the elderly who reside with long-term diseases such as diabetes or cardiovascular disease. The management of the former could require close attention to macronutrient intake, particularly carbohydrates and fats, in a bid to gain the optimum health outcome. Evidence indicates a wide gap in tailored nutritional interventions for older individuals with type 1 diabetes and suggests a higher degree of specificity in diet that acts on their unique position. With personalized nutrition recommendations, healthcare providers can better address the tailored nutritional needs for comorbidities while providing education in self-management strategies that empower older adults to be healthy (Sarteau et al., 2024). By recognizing the subtlety of the nutritional requirements of older adults, health care systems can enhance the quality of treatment available to this vulnerable population. Furthermore, the development of an expert system for nutrition care that is patient-centered can address limitations in existing dietary recommendations. The expert system can utilize the nutrition care process ontology, a simplified model to evaluate eating habits and identify signs of malnutrition among older patients. Utilizing technology to create tailored intervention plans with nutrition education, dietary prescription, and ordering of food based on particular diseases can improve compliance with dietary recommendations and prevent nutritional deficiencies. This method facilitates a more nuanced understanding of the dietary trends in older individuals, facilitating the implementation of effective nutritional interventions that promote better well-being and disease prevention (Anghel et al., 2018). Lastly, the emphasis on individualized nutrition plans is still key to promoting healthier aging trajectories among older adults, with their dietary needs taken care of with accuracy and empathy.

3.5. Strategies for Improving Nutrition

In addressing older individuals' nutritional needs, imposing certain interventions becomes a must for enhancing intake of carbohydrates, fats, and fluids. One of the most significant strategies includes designing and implementing comprehensive nutritional guidelines within RAC settings. These guidelines focus on routine screening and assessment of nutrition, thus enabling health care workers to identify individuals at risk of malnutrition. Early identification of such factors can lead to tailored nutritional interventions that not only address food preferences but also health conditions prevalent among the elderly. Multidisciplinary team involvement ensures that such interventions are holistic, combining dietary adjustments with educational components that promote healthy eating habits. This systematic approach can reduce the adverse impact of malnutrition on health and enhance the quality of life in this vulnerable group (Agarwal et al., 2016). Another key aspect of improvement in nutrition among the aging population is strengthening the consumption of nutrient-dense foods. Selecting foods with high levels of essential carbohydrates, healthy fats, and water is crucial. Breakfast cereals and breads, especially those that qualify for the ≤10:1 carbohydrate: fiber ratio, have been found to provide considerable nutritional benefit.

These foods tend to be lower in sugars and unhealthy fats, therefore contributing positively to a healthy diet while delivering the required energy and fiber (Ghodsian & Madden, 2018). Education on these foods for older adults should highlight their ease of access and preparation. Introduction of these foods into an individual's routine diet can assist in increasing dietary adherence and improving positive healthy outcomes overall, aiding a habit of good nutrition that can be maintained in the long term. Lastly, hydration is essential in preventing dehydration, a common problem for older adults, particularly those with compromised thirst perception or mobility impairment.

Interventions to improve hydration could include having water and other fluids made available and reminding patients to have fluids on a regular basis throughout the day. Another approach is to make fluids more appealing by flavoring them or providing several drink choices. Healthcare providers must also be trained to evaluate patients' hydration regularly, thereby allowing for early intervention. This multi-faceted approach not only addresses the imperative of adequate fluid intake but also promotes co-operation among caregivers and families to assist older adults in maintaining optimal hydration levels, which is positive for their welfare and health stability (Agarwal et al., 2016) (Figure 3.16).

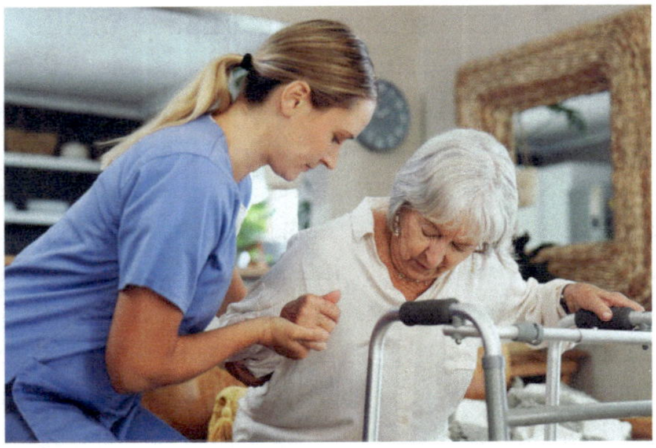

Figure 3.16. RNs face heightened pressure under new rules in aged care.

Source: https://assets.contenthub.wolterskluwer.com/api/public/content/2761282-nurse-with-elderly-patient-f84fe27a41?v=31dc37f5.

3.5.1. Meal Planning and Preparation Tips

Effective meal planning among older adults is crucial, particularly in their ability to get their carbohydrate, fat, and fluid needs. A comprehensive meal plan should first consider the individual's nutritional requirements and their dietary requirements. Introducing a variety of whole grains, fruits, and vegetables can help maximum carbohydrate intake while incorporating fundamental vitamins and minerals (Cioara et al., 2017). Additionally, the inclusion of healthy fats, such as those found in nuts, seeds, and oily fish, not only provides flavor but also provides nutrients that are integral to heart health, which is particularly important for the older age bracket. Caregivers and older individuals can effectively prevent the onset of malnutrition by taking time to make well-balanced meals, with all food choices contributing positively to health outcomes. Meal planning methods can also make cooking more efficient while encouraging nutritional adherence. A useful method is batch cooking, where larger quantities of healthy meals are prepared and stored in the refrigerator or freezer for future use. Not only is it time-efficient, but it also prevents sudden acts of unhealthy eating. Employing freezing as a preservation method retains the nutritional value of prepared meals, enabling older adults to have access to homemade meals even on days when cooking appears challenging. Moreover, using simple recipes that feature seasonal produce can encourage dietary variety while reducing the risk of monotony in daily meals. Strategically positioning the kitchen for easy access to commonly used ingredients can also make food preparation easier, allowing mealtime to be a source of pleasure rather than a chore. Finally, hydration cannot be omitted from meal planning for the elderly. Regular intake of fluids must be promoted since dehydration leads to severe health issues. Older people should try to incorporate high fluid content foods like soup and fruit into meals. Taking a bottle of water is an effective nudge to drink regularly during the day. Moreover, the addition of herbal tea or flavored water may enhance fluid intake without violating personal preference for taste (Cioara et al., 2017). Adding reminders or alarms is suggested to support habits of hydration. Collectively, these actions not only supplement the overall nutrient supply of carbohydrates, fats, and fluid intake but also improve the overall quality of lifestyle, allowing older people to remain independent and improve their health.

3.5.2. Importance of Community Resources and Support

Community resources and support are an essential contribution to the life of this group in the nutrition area, such that this group is able to meet their carbohydrate, fat, and fluid requirements effectively. Growing older tends to bring about physical, social, and economic challenges that can hinder access to required nutritional information and food sources. Community programs, including Meals on Wheels programs, senior centers, and nutrition classes, provide not just food but also knowledge on dietary guidelines geared towards the elderly. Such programs help to combat diseases such as obesity and malnutrition through promoting proper macronutrient intake and awareness, crucial in sustaining health and preventing chronic illnesses. Furthermore, such programs can effectively address the unique fluid needs of older adults whose physiological maturation may affect fluid balance and hydration levels, thus pointing to community support in optimizing nutrition across different environments (Pirotin et al., 2014). Interdisciplinary teamwork among healthcare providers, caregivers, and community agencies assists in ensuring the nutritional well-being of older adults. The interdisciplinary team ensures that patients receive personalized guidance based on their individual medical circumstances and life settings. Community health screenings and education can enable older people to take charge of making healthy food choices. For instance, elderly patients generally require modified carbohydrate and fat consumption to manage diabetes or cardiovascular illness. Not only is community integration helpful in supporting such patients in adapting to diet, but it also assists in bringing a feeling of belonging and attachment, important for psychological well-being. Such an environment encourages active participation of older adults in health care management and meal planning, reducing the complications of nutritional deficiency (Seleznev-Ivolga, 2024). Beyond the presence of food and nutrition education, an appreciation for community support involves building a global system aimed at sustaining older adults' social and nutritional requirements. Meeting with local farms, food banks, and nutrition professionals has the ability to yield sustainable measures to deal with food insecurity and poor diet intake. Nutrition advocacy and awareness campaigns also raise the degree of concern in the community about the dietary needs of the elderly. By adopting concerted efforts to enhance the nutritional landscape for the elderly, communities have the ability to raise overall health outcomes in addition to quality of life. Good support systems can absorb the adverse effects of stress and loneliness, ultimately fostering the importance of community resources in the task of meeting the nutritional needs of older individuals (Pirotin et al., 2014) (Figure 3.17).

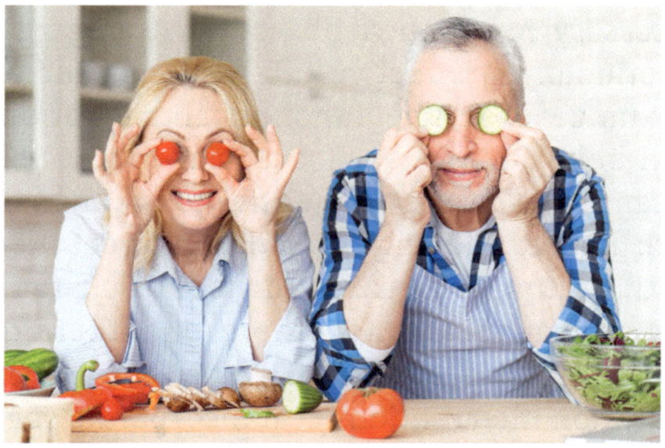

Figure 3.17. Enhance the nutritional well-being of older adults.

Source: https://genuineglobalcare.com/wp-content/uploads/2023/03/nutrition-guide-for-older-adults.jpg.

3.5.3. Encouraging Social Eating and Engagement

Encouraging social eating and involvement of older people is necessary to help them meet their carbohydrate, fat, and fluid requirements, but also to support a sense of community and well-being. Social eating situations, such as mealtimes and group meals, can have a significant role in enhancing the nutritional intake of older people. Sharing a meal can lead to increased consumption of food and increased diversity of diet, as individuals consume more when sitting together in a meal context. Social processes have been shown to influence the choice of food and preference, and thus, environments that facilitate interaction and warmth in the context of meals must be created. By promoting these social eating habits, health care workers may help combat nutritional disorders and overall pleasurable eating in the elderly, with dinner no longer being an occasion for mere sustenance but also an activity involving social integration and involvement. Social eating can also be employed as a treatment method in trying to combat the widespread complication of malnutrition in the elderly. When individuals dine together, not only will they be more likely to consume the necessary macronutrients, but also engage in emotionally productive interactions that can maximize cognitive function and emotional well-being. Being such a social component, it can be especially beneficial for individuals with limited mobility or those who eat alone because it gives a reason for food preparation and exchange among others and therefore boosts overall nutritional status. Nutrition education interventions that incorporate social dining experiences can further expand these advantages so that older people can learn healthier eating while enjoying the delight of eating as a socializing experience. Implementing particular programs that facilitate socialization and nutrition knowledge can create opportunities for creating healthier eating habits among this group. Also, do not forget the psychological aspect of social consumption because this is important in solving eating behavior among older people. Isolation and loneliness are typical situations that lead to incorrect nutrient intake, so it is necessary to engage this category of people socially. Studies have shown that when individuals feel like belonging to a group, their motivation to consume a proper diet rises significantly. By imagining mealtime as a social occasion, caregivers and healthcare workers can make older adults feel a sense of belonging and purpose. This is particularly crucial in interventions concerning carbohydrate, fat, and fluid consumption because social interactions can facilitate the learning of healthier habits and food selections. These initiatives are augmented by studies that have revealed social support structures significantly impact the adherence to dietary recommendations, and subsequently, overall health and quality of life among older adults (Baubérot et al., 2018; Heikkilä, 2020).

SUMMARY

In the investigation of carbohydrate, fat, and fluid requirements among older adults, it is critical to note the great role personalized nutrition plays in promoting health and longevity among older adults. As a person ages, physiological requirements alter, and food content needs to be adjusted to prevent complications that ensue with malnutrition and chronic disease. Evidence indicates that older individuals are at risk for nutritional deficiencies, and these deficiencies can lead to adverse effects such as unintentional weight loss and heightened risk of infection and hospitalization. Systematic nutrition strategy through frequent screenings and individualized meal planning can fix these problems and improve the health condition and well-being among the elderly significantly, highlighting the importance of frequent monitoring and intervention strategies (Agarwal et al., 2016). In addition, carbohydrates, fats, and fluids must not only be treated as macronutrients but as a part of a comprehensive nutritional plan aimed at keeping the nutritional status of the elderly optimum. Due to higher metabolism and appetite alterations with age, even this group of patients may find it difficult to meet their energy and nutrient needs from their normal diets. The use of food and nutrition plans based on individual energy needs and dietary practices of older adults can be helpful in promoting better health. Maintenance of appropriate fluid status is particularly critical, since dehydration is a significant risk for older adults, which in the majority of instances results in deteriorating cognitive function and increased hospitalization rates. Hence, balanced macronutrient consumption and fluid intake become essential in developing effective dietary advice for the elderly (Brown et al., 2014). Lastly, the consolidation of dietary requirements and interventions among the elderly underscores the importance of a multidisciplinary approach to the prevention of malnutrition and related health problems. Collaboration among health professionals, dietitians, and carers is necessary in creating seamless care plans that address the individualized needs of the elderly. Successful implementation of these plans relies on understanding the complexities surrounding food intake, mental processes during eating, and social processes involved with eating meals. Through supporting an environment that optimizes appropriate nutrition and hydration, stakeholders will be able to create an immense effect on health outcomes for older individuals, such that they not only live longer but also enjoy an enhanced quality of life. Hence, consistent research and advocacy of appropriate dietary practices is necessary in order to address the evolving nutritional needs of the elderly (Agarwal et al., 2016).

Knowledge about the exact nutritional needs of older people is an important key to enhancing health and avoiding chronic illness. As far as carbohydrate consumption is concerned, studies have found that well-balanced intake of complex carbohydrates in foods like whole grains, fruits, and vegetables is essential. These foods not only give the body the necessary nutrients but also help maintain the health of the digestive system, which can become a boon for elderly people with constipation and other digestive problems. Furthermore, the elderly are also susceptible to metabolic and energy requirement changes, for which their intake of carbohydrates has to be treated with some care. Emphasizing a combination of carbohydrate sources will keep the elderly from lacking in terms of energy requirements, but also equip them with the required vitamins and minerals to meet optimal levels of health. Fat intake also has a key function in the older population's nutritional needs, especially concerning brain activity and cardiovascular well-being. Research suggests that the intake of healthy fats, such as from avocados, nuts, and fish, can make a significant difference to overall health. They help with keeping inflammation levels in check and enhancing cognitive function, which are both vital elements in aging populations. Interestingly, higher awareness has been observed of the adverse effects of trans fats and certain saturated fats incorporated in processed foods. Consequently, dietary advice increasingly emphasizes the importance of the selection of unsaturated fats over saturated fats. The modification serves the purpose of considering certain specific nutrition advice, encouraging elderly individuals to give due importance to eating sources of desirable fats while limiting sources of unwanted fats in their diet. Hydration is another extremely significant factor influencing the well-being of older adults, as many have fluid consumption problems. Physiological changes with aging can influence the physiology of thirst, and hence, hydration could be poor. It is therefore necessary to promote fluid intake at regular intervals throughout the day, including water and other fluids like juice and milk, and moderation in caffeine and sweet drinks. Older adults are particularly vulnerable to dehydration, which can complicate underlying medical conditions, such as kidney function and cognition. In addition, proper levels of hydration intake can augment metabolic function and overall energy. With these points in consideration, healthcare providers are forced to heighten awareness about fluid requirements so that nutritional counseling is considered based on the individual's nutritional needs along with physiological aspects of aging regarding hydration status (Butler, 2016; Stephen et al., 2017).

A CLOSER LOOK

HYDRATION REQUIREMENTS FOR OLDER ADULTS

Hydration needs for older adults disclose that proper fluid balance becomes more and more important as age progresses, but harder to achieve. As one gets older, the sense of thirst decreases, so older adults might not feel thirsty even when they need fluids. At the same time, age-related alterations of reduced renal function, decreased total body water, and utilization of medications such as diuretics also may increase the risk for dehydration. Conditions such as diabetes or dementia can further obscure hydration status. Dehydration in older adults can lead to serious complications, including confusion, urinary tract infections, constipation, low blood pressure, and even falls (Figure 3.18).

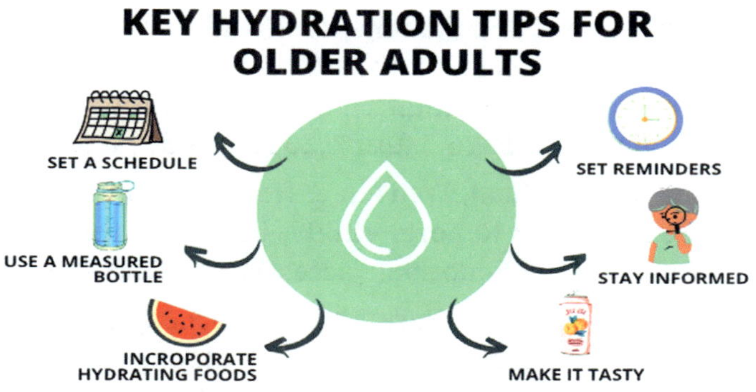

Figure 3.18. Hydration for older adults.

Source: https://secondwindmovement.com/wp-content/uploads/2023/12/hydration-tips.png.

Most older adults need 1.6–2 liters (6–8 cups) of fluid a day, but this can be influenced by health, activity, and season. The best fluid is water, but milk, soups, tea, fruit, and vegetables with high water content, such as watermelon, cucumbers, and oranges, also count towards fluid intake. Fluids need to be taken throughout the day, especially if mobility or cognition is impaired.

Hydration measures among older adults include the use of daily water-drinking reminders, offering preferred beverages, and assessing urine color as a rapid indicator (light yellow being optimal). In long-term care settings, caregivers play a key role in assisting with fluid access and looking for signs of dehydration. Proper hydration aids to aid digestion, heat control, joint lubrication, and brain function and is thus a key element of healthy aging.

REFERENCES

1. Mohammad Nor, Noor Safiza and Khor, Geok Lin and Shahar, Suzana and Kee, Chee Cheong and Haniff, Jamaiyah and Appannah, Geeta and Rasat, Rahmah and Wong, N. F. and Zainuddin, Ahmad Ali and Ab Rahman, Jamaluddin and Abd Talib, Ruzita and Yusoff, Ahmad Faudzi (2008) The Third National Health and Morbidity Survey (NHMS III) 2006: nutritional status of adults aged 18 years and above. Malaysian Journal of Nutrition, 14 (2). pp. 1-87. ISSN 1394-035X(accessed on 12th July 2025).
2. Agarwal, E., Isenring, E., Marshall, S., Miller, et al. (2016). Optimizing nutrition in residential aged care: A narrative review. https://core.ac.uk/download/196601588.pdf (accessed on 12th July 2025).
3. Alexy, A., Armstrong, A., Aufderheide, B., Badaloo, B., Bagnasco, et al. (2010). EFSA Panel on Dietetic Products, Nutrition, and Allergies (NDA); Scientific Opinion on Dietary reference values for water. https://core.ac.uk/download/13780775.pdf (accessed on 12th July 2025).
4. Cioara, Tudor and Anghel, Ionut and Salomie, Ioan and Barakat, Lina and Miles, Simon and Reidlinger, Dianne and Taweel, Adel and Dobre, Ciprian and Pop, Florin (2018) Expert System for Nutrition Care Process of Older Adults. Future Generation Computer Systems, 80. pp. 368-383. DOI https://doi.org/10.1016/j.future.2017.05.037(accessed on 12th July 2025).
5. Carlson, Andrea & Lino, Mark & Juan, WenYen & Hanson, Kenneth & Basiotis, P. Peter, 2007. "**Thrifty Food Plan, 2006**," CNPP Reports 42899, United States Department of Agriculture, Center for Nutrition Policy and Promotion. (accessed on 12th July 2025).
6. Baubérot, A., Drouard, A., Grisoni, A., Reckwitz, A., Rochedy, A., Stanziani, A., Warde, A., et al. (2018). Supplementing food for health: Practices amongst French adults aged 60 to 75 years. *Agritrop*. http://agritrop.cirad.fr/589499/1/LEPILLER-CAZES-VALETTE-Supplementing-Food-Post-Print-2018.pdf (accessed on 12th July 2025).
7. Fusch, C., Bauer, K., Böhles, H. J., Jochum, F., Koletzko, B., Krawinkel, M., Krohn, K., Mühlebach, S., & Working group for developing the guidelines for parenteral nutrition of The German Society for Nutritional Medicine (2009). Neonatology/Paediatrics - Guidelines on Parenteral Nutrition, Chapter 13. *German medical science : GMS e-journal*, *7*, Doc15. https://doi.org/10.3205/000074(accessed on 12th July 2025).
8. Shauna Pirotin, Christina Becker and Patricia B. Crawford (2014). Looking beyond the marketing claims of new beverages: Health risks of consuming sports drinks, energy drinks, fortified waters, and other flavored beverages. University of California at Berkeley, Atkins Center for Weight and Health . https://core.ac.uk/download/75778515.pdf (accessed on 12th July 2025).
9. Rémond, D., Shahar, D. R., Gille, D., Pinto, P., Kachal, J., Peyron, M. A., Dos Santos, C. N., Walther, B., Bordoni, A., Dupont, D., Tomás-Cobos, L., & Vergères, G. (2015). Understanding the gastrointestinal tract of the elderly to develop dietary solutions that prevent malnutrition. *Oncotarget*, *6*(16), 13858–13898. https://doi.org/10.18632/oncotarget.4030(accessed on 12th July 2025).
10. Brown, H. (2014). An analysis of the Weight Watchers and Atkins diets: The effects of calorie restriction and nutrition levels. https://core.ac.uk/download/129590383.pdf (accessed on 12th July 2025).

11. Stephen, A. M., Champ, M. M., Cloran, S. J., Fleith, M., van Lieshout, L., Mejborn, H., & Burley, V. J. (2017). Dietary fibre in Europe: current state of knowledge on definitions, sources, recommendations, intakes and relationships to health. *Nutrition research reviews*, *30*(2), 149–190. https://doi.org/10.1017/S095442241700004X(accessed on 12th July 2025).
12. McCoy, S. M., Campbell, K. L., Lassemillante, A. M., Wallen, M. P., Fawcett, J., Jarrett, M., Macdonald, G. A., & Hickman, I. J. (2017). Changes in dietary patterns and body composition within 12 months of liver transplantation. *Hepatobiliary surgery and nutrition*, *6*(5), 317–326. https://doi.org/10.21037/hbsn.2017.01.12(accessed on 12th July 2025).
13. Cash, Sean B. & Cortus, Brett & Goddard, Ellen W. & Han, Alice & Lerohl, Mel L. & Lomeli, Jose L., 2005. "**Integrating Food Policy with Growing Health and Wellness Concerns: An Analytical Literature Review of the Issues Affecting Government, Industry, and Civil Society**," Project Report Series 24056, University of Alberta, Department of Resource Economics and Environmental Sociology.(accessed on 12th July 2025).
14. Dodd, F., Haskell-Ramsay, C., Jackson, P., et al. (2020). Acute and chronic effects of multivitamin/mineral supplementation on objective and subjective energy measures. https://core.ac.uk/download/305121296.pdf (accessed on 12th July 2025).
15. Fabiani, H., Lestarina, L., Sutanto, L. B., et al. (2024). Overview of fluid and macronutrient intake, knowledge and attitudes, and eating behavior among private university medical students in Jakarta. https://core.ac.uk/download/617868276.pdf (accessed on 12th July 2025).
16. Hansen, E. (2023). Advertising sports nutrition practices to adolescent athletes: A poster series. https://core.ac.uk/download/573443301.pdf (accessed on 12th July 2025).
17. Heikkilä, M. (2020). Nutrition knowledge and skills among young endurance athletes. https://core.ac.uk/download/286389712.pdf (accessed on 12th July 2025).
18. Hester, E. R. (2017). The benefits and concerns of veganism in women's health. https://core.ac.uk/download/58824999.pdf (accessed on 12th July 2025).
19. Ghodsian, B., & Madden, A. M. (2018). Evaluating the ≤10:1 wholegrain criterion in identifying nutrient quality and health implications of UK breads and breakfast cereals. *Public health nutrition*, *21*(6), 1186–1193. https://doi.org/10.1017/S1368980017003718(accessed on 12th July 2025).
20. Malafarina, V., Reginster, J. Y., Cabrerizo, S., et al. (2017). Nutritional status and nutritional treatment are related to outcomes and mortality in older adults with hip fractures. https://core.ac.uk/download/pdf/212756692.pdf (accessed on 12th July 2025).
21. Butler T. (2016). Dietary management of heart failure: room for improvement?. *The British journal of nutrition*, *115*(7), 1202–1217. https://doi.org/10.1017/S000711451500553X(accessed on 12th July 2025).
22. Deane, C. S., Wilkinson, D. J., Phillips, B. E., Smith, K., Etheridge, T., & Atherton, P. J. (2017). "Nutraceuticals" in relation to human skeletal muscle and exercise. *American journal of physiology. Endocrinology and metabolism*, *312*(4), E282–E299. https://doi.org/10.1152/ajpendo.00230.2016(accessed on 12th July 2025).
23. Saravia, L., & Jenelle. (2025). Examining the influence of sports nutrition counseling on collegiate athletes. https://core.ac.uk/download/657353610.pdf (accessed on 12th July 2025).

24. Sarteau, C., Ercolino, G., Fruik, A., et al. (2024). Nutritional status, dietary intake, and nutrition-related interventions among older adults with type 1 diabetes: A systematic review and call for more evidence toward clinical guidelines. https://core.ac.uk/download/619687422.pdf (accessed on 12th July 2025).
25. Seleznev-Ivolga, E. (2024). Nutritional support and rehydration therapy for adult patients in need of palliative medical care. https://core.ac.uk/download/620847628.pdf (accessed on 12th July 2025).
26. Tan, G. S. (2019). Nutrition education modules for nurses. https://core.ac.uk/download/227994105.pdf (accessed on 12th July 2025).
27. Ekesa, B.; Johnson, V.; Kennedy, G.; Nabuuma, D.; Van den Bergh, I.; Ocimati, W. (2017) A community resource persons' training guide: improving food and nutrition security through banana-based farming systems and foods. Scripta Horticulturae 19, 74 p. ISBN: 978-94-6261-146-7(accessed on 12th July 2025)

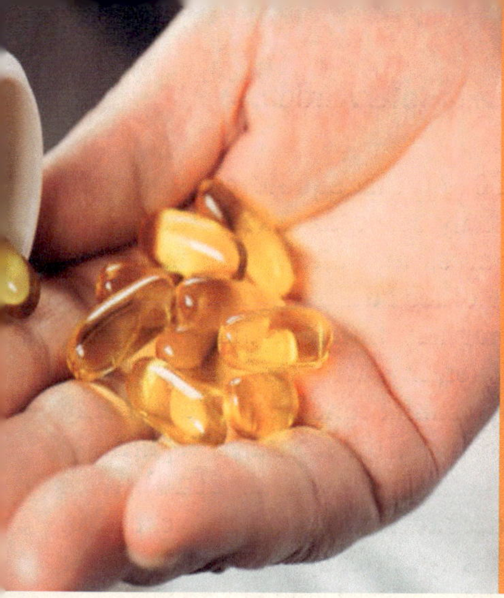

Chapter 4

VITAMIN NUTRITION IN OLDER ADULTS

Contents

Introduction

Due to the population aging process around the world, the nutrition of older adults has gained more attention, particularly regarding vitamins. These are critical vitamins, and they have a key role to play in sustaining health and preventing most of the age-related diseases. Among them are some, such as B12, folate, and vitamin D, which are required for sustaining maximal physiological functions, including mental status, immunity, and erythropoiesis. However, elderly individuals do face challenges that can negatively affect their vitamin status, including reduced diet intake, changed metabolism, and compromised nutrient absorption. Thus, consideration of the specific vitamin needs of this age group becomes critical to facilitating longevity and enhancing quality of life. Present research places significant emphasis on the need to assess dietary intakes and biomarkers to determine vitamin sufficiency among older adults. For instance, research indicates that iron, folate, and vitamin B12 deficiencies are highest in the elderly, typically due to inadequate food consumption as well as a host of physiological obstacles to nutrient consumption (Pillay, 2017). Inadequate consumption can lead to anemia and other related medical complications that only serve to exacerbate issues for older adults. Therefore, there is a need to identify dietary sources and alternative means of enhancing the bioavailability of such essential nutrients to provide older adults with the vitamins they need to maintain health and well-being. Vitamin D is another key nutrient that is usually deficient in this population and has been associated with several health outcomes, such as bone mineral content, muscle strength, and overall immune function. Professional consensus is that being adequately supplied with serum 25-hydroxyvitamin D levels is central to older adults, regardless of debate over the optimal amounts needed for optimum health (Lanham-New et al., 2010). With increasing occurrences of vitamin D deficiency and its associated conditions, such as rickets, in some regions, policymakers should develop universal dietary policies specifically tailored for older adults. Besides, promoting lifestyles and dietary interventions may take central stage to address the pervasive nutrient inadequacies, thus enhancing the health trajectory of the elderly (Figure 4.1).

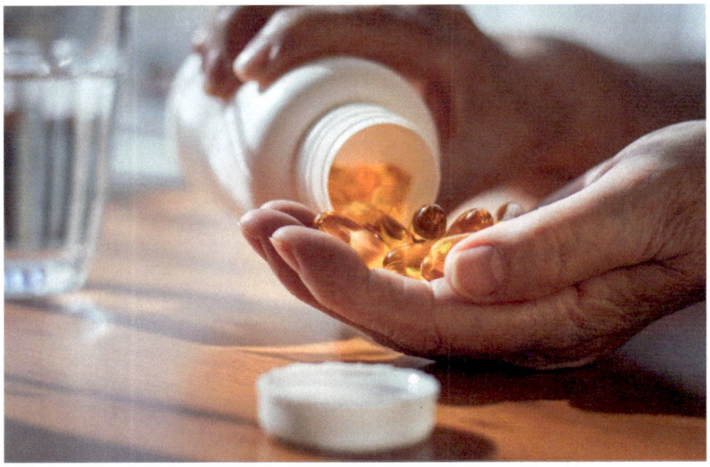

Figure 4.1. Vitamins for seniors to protect brain, eye, and bone health.

Source: https://images.squarespace-cdn.com/content/v1/5d9f65d12a10d4166969add0/1594846633344-S0BDB81JTOV0YW4MDBIK/best+vitamins+for+seniors+3.jpeg.

Definition of Vitamins and Their Importance

Vitamins refer to organic molecules required in normal physiological functions to carry out important roles in metabolism, immune function, and maintaining overall health in place. They are also classified into two categories: water-soluble and fat-soluble vitamins. Water-soluble vitamins like the B-complex and vitamin C are involved in energy metabolism and red blood cell synthesis, whereas fat-soluble vitamins A, D, E, and K are vital to well-being through their role in vision, bone maintenance, and antioxidant action. The importance of these micronutrients becomes particularly clear in the elderly, as the nutritional needs could change according to variations in dietary intake, absorption, and metabolism. The changing dynamics demand understanding of the precise functions of vitamins and their repercussions in age-related diseases, thereby underlining the critical need for proper vitamin intake among them. Research has illuminated the intricate relationship between vitamin status and mental function, particularly with B vitamins. Epidemiological data have demonstrated that levels of optimal B vitamins, such as folic acid (B9), pyridoxine (B6), and cobamides (B12), correlate with cognitive health in older individuals. Conversely, low levels of B vitamins have been linked with high levels of homocysteine, a marker of cognitive decline and neurodegenerative disease. Despite pervasive research, randomized control trials (RCTs) have provided mixed findings regarding the effect of B vitamin supplementation on behavior. However, a rise in B vitamins and a fall in homocysteine has been consistently observed, corroborating the hypothesis that, while a single supplement may not in fact induce apparent cognitive benefit, it does have significant impacts on biological indicators of impaired aging and cognition, and further research is needed (Reay et al., 2013).

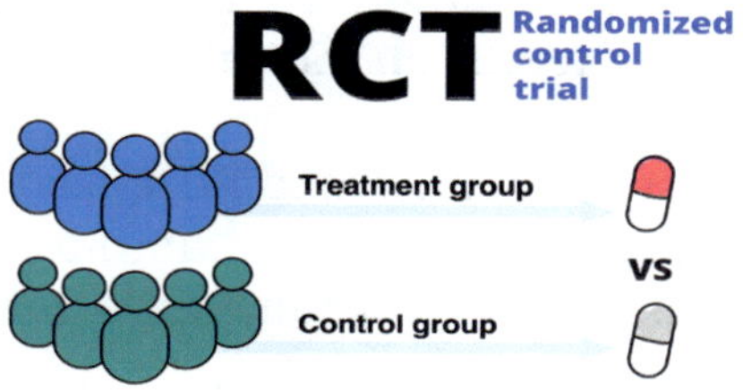

Figure 4.2. Randomized control trial (RCT).

Source: https://i.ytimg.com/vi/mWfjbmRZowM/maxresdefault.jpg.

As older individuals experience physiological changes, the aging gastrointestinal tract (GIT) negatively impacts nutrient absorption and bioavailability, with direct implications for vitamin status. Contributing factors for these shifts are decreased gastric acid secretion, alteration of motility, and reduced efficiency of intestinal nutrient absorption. Hence, elderly individuals are prone to exacerbated malnutrition, which can worsen the condition of various organ systems, including nervous, musculoskeletal, cardiovascular, immune, and integumentary systems (Rémond et al., 2015). This complex interaction of aging with the availability of nutrients calls for targeted dietary interventions to neutralize malnutrition and facilitate nutrient intake in the elderly. It is important to realize the functionality of the aging GIT and how this affects nutritional vitamin usage, emphasizing the necessity of complete dietary information, acknowledging these age-associated changes and improving general health and wellbeing in this susceptible population (Figure 4.2).

Overview of Nutritional Needs in Older Adults

As people age, their nutritional requirements significantly change due to the alterations in physiology, which are features of the aging process. One of the most significant aspects of the nutritional needs of older adults is the increased need for many nutrients, which are most important in maintaining health and preventing chronic disease. The older gastrointestinal system experiences morphologic and functional alterations that can compromise the capacity for digestion and absorption of nutrients, resulting in increased vulnerability to malnutrition. This is also worsened by physical changes like reduced appetite, compromised taste, and difficulty processing food, leading to inadequate intake of required nutrients. Therefore, there is a critical need for individually focused dietary interventions that consider such changes while promoting appropriate nutrition among elderly people, hence benefiting their longevity and well-being (Rémond et al., 2015). Vitamin B12 is particularly important in older people because the deficiencies can cause disabling neurological and cognitive dysfunction. Hormonal and physiological alterations that occur in the gastrointestinal tract during aging, including atrophic gastritis and decreased stomach acid secretion, often disrupt proper absorption of vitamin B12. To remedy this issue, new measures have been attempted, including the distribution of fortified foods via national programs to increase vitamin B12 intake in the elderly. One such measure is a study assessing the impact of a program implemented in Chile, which found supplementation with vitamin B12-fortified foods had results that were not conclusive for raising plasma B12 (Albala et al., 2013). This highlights the necessity of ongoing attention to adjusting dietary programs to be more effective in the specific needs of older individuals and to offer information to ensure sufficient vitamin status in later life. In addition, the overall nutrition setting for the elderly must encompass an assortment of micronutrients necessary for the maintenance of essential health. Nutritional guidelines suggest that older adults require higher intakes of vitamins D and K, and of micronutrients like calcium and magnesium, to support bone health and prevent osteoporosis. Adequate intake of protein is also necessary for the maintenance of muscle mass and strength, which slowly decline with age. These nutritional requirements are compounded further by risks of nutritional deficiency from chronic illness and drugs that can interfere with nutrient intake. Complete knowledge of the older individual's nutritional needs based on up-to-date research and evidence-based practice is still, therefore, important to ensure health and optimize quality of life as individuals age (Rémond et al., 2015).

4.1. The Role of Vitamins in Aging

With increased age, physiological changes in the gastrointestinal system have significant effects on the metabolism and absorption of vitamins. Aging is generally accompanied by a mechanical and functional decline in the efficacy of the gastrointestinal tract, which affects not only the process of food digestion but even the availability of nutrients per se. This decline can result in malnutrition, a prevalent condition among elderly individuals. Malnutrition increases vulnerability to other states of health, including those of the nervous, musculoskeletal, and cardiovascular systems. To respond to this, there is a need to create dietary guidelines considering the unique functional capacities of the aging gastrointestinal tract, so that the elderly are able to achieve optimal nutrient intake. Their inclusion in nutrition programs would be a major determinant of health and longevity among this population, emphasizing the urgency for tailored nutritional strategies to correct for the changes brought about by aging (Rémond et al., 2015). Vitamins also play a central role in cognitive function among the elderly, particularly B vitamins, which have been extensively studied for their therapeutic applications. Epidemiological evidence shows that maintaining adequate levels of the B vitamins is linked with cognitive status, and studies have demonstrated that elevated homocysteine levels, an indicator of disturbed one-carbon metabolism, are predictive of cognitive impairment. While RCTs have tested supplementation with B vitamins, results have commonly been inconclusive regarding behavioral improvement. Despite this, there is always resurfacing evidence that enhancing B vitamin status and reducing homocysteine will avert some of the risks associated with atypical aging. This indicates that while the direct benefits of supplementation are not observable in behavior, shared biochemical benefits warrant further investigation into personalized approaches and dosage peaks (Reay et al., 2013). Hence, the role of vitamins in aging is more than mere supplementation; it involves an understanding of the intricate relationship between need and intake in aged people. Current literature indicates the need for further research into the manner in which various vitamins operate in the context of aging tissue, and their impacts on metabolic pathways. As populations grow older, the impact of vitamin deficiency increases, highlighting the requirement for in-depth nutritional screening in clinical populations. In addition, improved education in food choice has the ability to allow older people to make well-informed decisions that optimize their health. With the advancements in the field, there is a necessity to give top priority to eliciting evidence-based recommendations based on the particular needs of the older population, leading to improved health outcomes and quality of life (Figure 4.3) (Rémond et al., 2015).

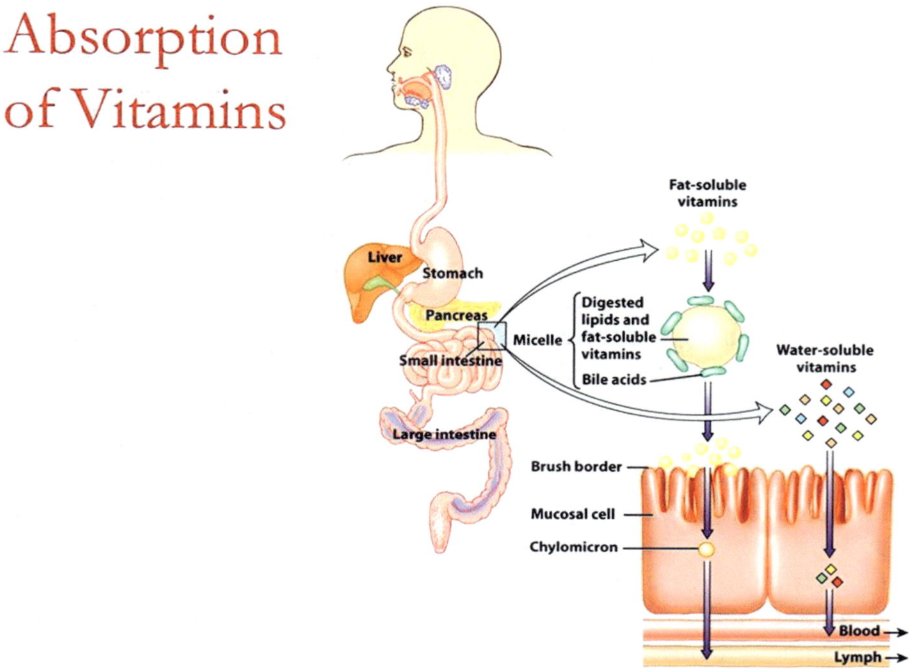

Figure 4.3. Absorption and metabolism of essential nutrients for aging.

Source: https://livhealthylife.com/wp-content/uploads/2018/10/AbsorptionofVitamins.jpg.

4.1.1. Impact of Vitamins on Immune Function

Age has a significant impact on immune response, predisposing to a state known as immunosenescence. This refers to the way in which immune response progressively diminishes over a period of time, making older individuals more vulnerable to chronic disease and infection (Rémond et al., 2015). Vitamins play a crucial role in immune function modulation, and certain vitamins, such as vitamins A, C, D, and E, are particularly vital in ensuring immune integrity. These vitamins are implicated in various biochemical reactions that enhance immune defense functions, including immune cell proliferation, antibody production, and cytokine secretion. Deprivation of one of the vitamins can lead to impaired immune capability, underlining the importance of adequate vitamin status in this age group. It is hence imperative to find out how to maintain vitamin nutrition in this group to improve their immune status, along with overall health. The relationship between food vitamin consumption and immune status is of particular relevance against the background of physiological changes associated with age. Aging alters the gastrointestinal tract, thus preventing nutrient uptake, which in turn can further exacerbate vital vitamin deficiency (Rémond et al., 2015). For instance, reduced gastric acid secretion and the altered gut microbiota composition can lead to influence vitamin B12 and other water-soluble vitamins' bioavailability. Moreover, since older people often have impairments such as loss of appetite or nutritional restrictions, proper eating behavior must be ensured. Dietary interventions for proper vitamin consumption can reverse the immunocompromised state with aging. Taking dietary advice suited to the needs of older adults is thus vital to enable them to achieve immune function safely. In addition to the immediate impacts of vitamins on the functioning of immune cells, there is also renewed recognition of how antioxidants protect against oxidative stress, as found in elderly populations. Vitamins C and E are both powerful antioxidants, with the ability to sweep up reactive oxygen species that have the potential to cause damage to cells and tissues, including those of the immune system (Maijó et al., 2013). Oxidative damage may be further accumulated to be responsible for the frailty and inflammation that occur frequently among elderly patients. Therefore, enhancing the intake of such vitamins through dietary or supplemental means has a twofold role: enhancing immune capacity while concurrently counteracting oxidative damage. Additional research is warranted to establish optimal dosages and sources of these nutrients and to create evidence-based interventions that improve vitamin nutrition and its resultant impact on immune function in older people.

4.1.2. Vitamins and Cognitive Health

The interaction of vitamin intake and cognitive performance in the elderly is a key area of investigation, reflective of the greater context of the impact of nutritional deficiencies on the elderly. In particular, certain vitamins such as B-complex vitamins are essential to maintain cognitive performance and overall brain well-being. A deficiency in vitamin B12, for instance, has been found to be related to cognitive impairment, including memory loss and increased vulnerability to dementia. This association is particularly relevant as older individuals have a high risk of acquiring a deficiency in vitamin B12 due to impaired absorption and dietary shortages. As malnutrition levels rise among older individuals, it is increasingly important to realize what role these vitamins play in avoiding cognitive impairment and achieving optimal brain function with age. Having an appropriate diet must take top priority to sustain mental vigor. Complicating matters further, the aging GIT poses special challenges to nutrient uptake. Changes in the GIT, including decreased motility and alterations in digestive processes, hinder the effectiveness of nutrient absorption. Since GIT is less efficient in breaking down and absorbing vitamins, the elderly are more prone to deficiencies, which can cause further cognitive decline and make them vulnerable to neurodegenerative disorders. It is significant to address the knowledge deficit regarding the nexus between GIT changes and nutritional absorption to enable effective dietary interventions tailored to this population. Overcoming these barriers will enable healthcare clinicians and caregivers to offer more effective dietary interventions that are proactive in mitigating the nutritional hazard of aging (Rémond et al., 2015). Moreover, attempts at fortifying food with essential vitamins such as vitamin B12 can go a long way in enhancing cognitive function among older people. Results of intervention, including the one conducted in Chile, have shown that while fortified food increases serum levels of vitamin B12, it may not necessarily ensure ideal nutritional status independently. This is a sign that while supplementation with fortified foods is a step in the right direction, there is a call for an improved method with consideration of guidelines on food and holistic nutrition programs (Albala et al., 2013). The methods should consider the multifaceted nature of malnutrition in the aged and look to offer nutrient-dense foods for diet which support cognitive functions and well-being. By aligning public health policy with access to nutrients, we can more effectively manage the cognitive health requirements of the elderly population (Figure 4.4).

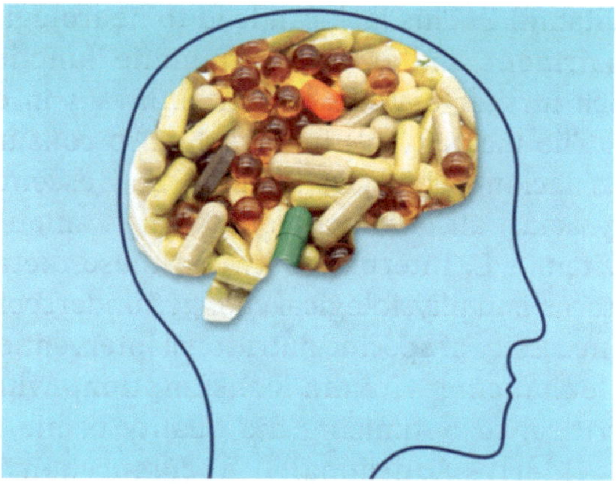

Figure 4.4. Cogitating cognitive health supplements.

Source: https://niemagazine.com/wp-content/uploads/2023/05/CognitiveHealth-940x400-1683826305.jpg.

4.1.3. Vitamins and Bone Density

The relationship between vitamins and bone density is of special interest for older adults, who are at a higher risk for osteoporosis and associated fractures. As aging continues, the ability of the body to absorb and utilize necessary nutrients diminishes, contributing to the risks of inadequate vitamin intake. Vitamins D and K have gained much attention due to their roles in calcium absorption and bone metabolism, respectively. Vitamin D facilitates intestinal calcium absorption, which is crucial in assisting to maintain bone density. Vitamin D deficiency can lead to mineralization impairment in bones and thereby increase fracture risk among the aging population. Moreover, an understanding of the mechanisms through which aging affects nutrient utilization can help in framing dietary recommendations for the older population. Malnutrition treatment via adequate vitamin intake is important for enhanced health benefits and preservation of skeletal health in older populations, as defined in current research on gastrointestinal aging that puts stress on issues of nutrient absorption (Rémond et al., 2015). Vitamin D is particularly important to the elderly since not only is it involved in the absorption of calcium, but it also appears to directly influence muscle strength and function. While many have associated higher levels of vitamin D with stronger bones, evidence regarding a direct effect on strength in muscles is less unified. Wright et al. (2018) find that increases in serum 25-hydroxyvitamin D are associated with increased muscle strength in some populations, though the results do not apply consistently across age.

As muscle strength is a key component in fall prevention and balance, the optimal status of vitamin D could play a two-fold role in muscle and bone health. Consequently, interventions on vitamin D supplementation could be a core component of health interventions for enhancing functional capacity as well as reducing the risk of falls among the elderly, ensuring skeletal as well as physical health. In addition to vitamins D and K, the impact of other vitamins on the bone cannot be overlooked. Vitamin C, whose role is implicated in collagen synthesis, has its function in the structural integrity of the bone tissue and can enhance bone density as it possesses antioxidant activity. Studies show that adequate intake of vitamin C is linked to greater bone density, especially in postmenopausal women, who experience dramatic hormonal changes affecting bone health. Vitamin B12 also has a significant function in DNA synthesis and metabolic processes, benefiting bone cell function. In older adults, B12 deficiency can lead to numerous health issues indirectly affecting bone status. Thus, a systems or overall approach to vitamin nutrition, e.g., one highlighting multiple vitamins—may offer synergistic enhancement of bone density, with the ultimate benefit of reducing the incidence of osteoporosis fractures in this population at risk (Figure 4.5).

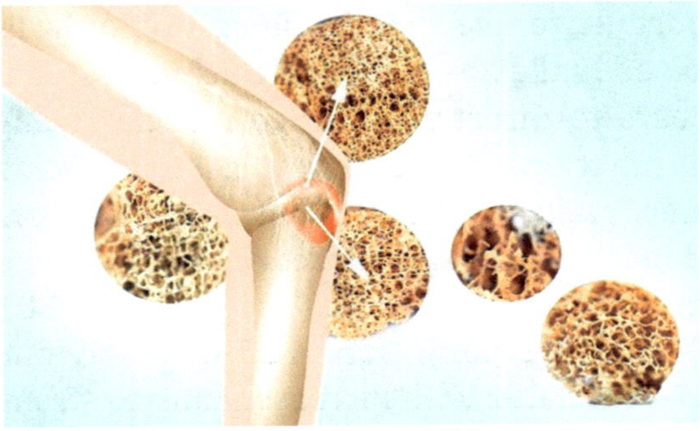

Figure 4.5. Bone density affects height.

Source: https://increaseheightblog.com/wp-content/uploads/2023/08/Bone-Density-Affect-Height-1.jpg.

4.2. Common Vitamin Deficiencies in Older Adults

With aging, physiological changes significantly affect the absorption and metabolism of essential vitamins, with a higher risk of deficiency. Common deficiencies among elderly people are vitamins B12, D, and E. Vitamin B12 is necessary for nerve function and DNA synthesis and red blood cell formation, but older people have decreased secretion of gastric acid that prevents the absorption of this vitamin from food sources. Vitamin D deficiency also accelerates age-related bone density losses, leading to increased risk of fractures and osteoporosis. This vitamin is produced most commonly by sunlight on the skin, which may be reduced in older adults by loss of mobility or increased time spent indoors. Thus, vitamin D deficiency can have severe health effects, and proper intake by this group is becoming more crucial. In addition to B12 and D, vitamin E deficiency is also of concern among the elderly because this antioxidant is important in protecting cells against oxidative stress. With advancing age, a decline in the body's ability to absorb fats occurs, and this interferes with the ability to absorb fat-soluble vitamins such as vitamin E. This lack can lead to neurological impairment and impaired immune function, which further distorts health pathways in old age. The majority of the elderly also consume diets lacking fruits, vegetables, and essential fatty acids, all of which contain high amounts of vitamin E. Interplay between these dietary patterns and physiological changes underscores the necessity of specific nutritional interventions for enhancing vitamin consumption, which is critical to optimizing the quality of life for the elderly. Additionally, a comprehensive understanding of the gastrointestinal tract of the aging population and its role in nutrient absorption is necessary to address the occurrence of vitamin deficiency. Aging leads to alterations in gastrointestinal motility, enzyme secretion, and intestinal mucosal integrity, all of which are characteristics that diminish the bioavailability of essential nutrients.

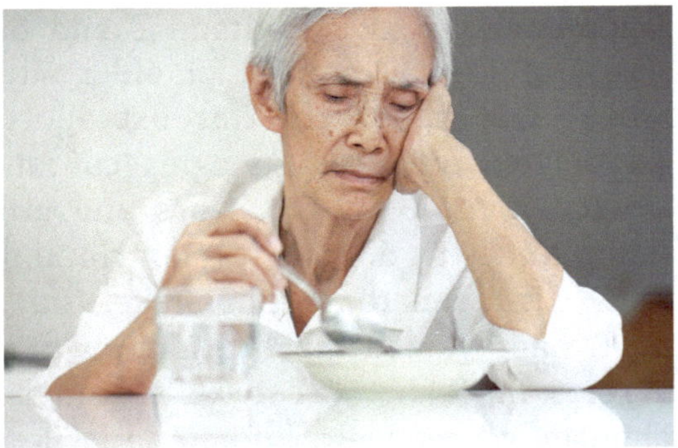

Figure 4.6. Signs of nutritional deficiency in elders.

Source: https://fromthehearthomecaresc.com/wp-content/uploads/2023/08/AdobeStock_565284537-min-scaled.jpeg.

This reduction may contribute to malnutrition and compound conditions like cognitive impairment as well as compromised immune function, as highlighted by recent studies. Therefore, successful nutritional recommendations and education interventions must be able to educate older adults about the necessary nutrients that they are probably lacking and recommend ways of optimizing their nutrient supply. Through coordination of these multi-dimensional strategies, the risk of vitamin deficiency can be reduced, ultimately leading to better health status in older adults (Rémond et al., 2015; Hester, 2017) (Figure 4.6).

4.2.1. Vitamin D Deficiency and Its Consequences

Vitamin D deficiency is a serious health issue among older adults, primarily due to the fact that it plays a vital role in maintaining bone density and preventing osteoporosis. Aging weakens the ability of skin to synthesize vitamin D from sunlight, along with other factors such as reduced mobility and food restriction. Thus, deficient vitamin D levels may result in a compromised skeletal system and heightened susceptibility to fractures and falls, which pose significant issues within elderly populations. In addition, the improper consumption of insufficient amounts of vitamin D is usually found with a lack of consuming proper nutritional sources, establishing an intersection of dietary deficiency and physiological loss that highlights the necessity for extensive dietary recommendations addressed specifically to the elderly. Filling such gaps in nutrition is imperative, since the implications of vitamin D deficiency go beyond skeletal well-being to the overall quality of life in older adults. In addition to its role in skeletal health, vitamin D has also been linked to a variety of systemic health outcomes of health concerning elderly individuals. The current evidence indicates that vitamin D deficiency may be linked to the risk of cardiovascular disease, cognitive dysfunction, and immune dysfunction. This broader spectrum of effects stems partly from vitamin D's role of control over inflammation and cellular function and suggests that maintaining optimal levels may serve to cushion against a spectrum of ill health associated with aging. The interconnectedness of these results underscores the importance of preventive nutrition strategies, particularly in an older group increasingly vulnerable to chronic diseases. Vitamin D status responded to fortification and diet could have significant long-term health impacts, suggesting dietary intervention is a central element in an overall healthcare strategy in older age, in encouraging healthier aging. As the population of older adults grows, so does the imperative to treat vitamin D deficiency.

Recent studies illustrate that malnutrition, i.e., both vitamin deficiencies, is surprisingly prevalent in older adults, often the result of decreased nutrient absorption and altered dietary habits. Because vitamin D deficiency may initiate a spectrum of disease, from musculoskeletal disease through enhanced infection susceptibility, special nutritional education and intervention programs must be at the top of the agenda for this group. Such successful strategies should include the promotion of foods and supplements fortified with vitamin D and programs within the community to increase safe sun exposure. By overlaying public health strategies against the specific nutritional needs of older adults, we are able to deliver improved health outcomes and create improved quality of life for this vulnerable segment of the population toward improved aging and longevity (Figure 4.7).

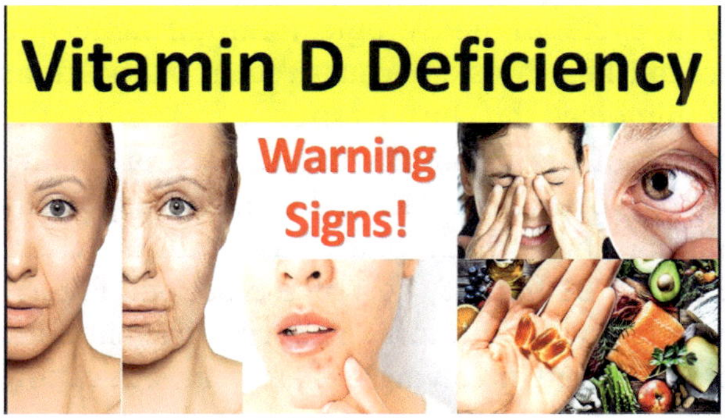

Figure 4.7. Signs and symptoms of vitamin D deficiency.

Source: https://i.ytimg.com/vi/0pr_lze0LhU/maxresdefault.jpg.

4.2.2. Vitamin B12 Deficiency and Neurological Effects

Vitamin B12 is an essential nutrient that plays a significant role in neurological functioning, particularly in the elderly, who are more likely to develop a deficiency through age-related physiological changes or nutritional deficiencies. With advancing age, vitamin B12 absorption becomes impaired due to reduced production of stomach acid and alteration in intestinal flora, resulting in decreased bioavailability of this very essential vitamin. This deficiency can manifest as a range of neurological symptoms, including cognitive impairment, mood disturbances, and peripheral neuropathy. Importantly, even mild deficiency in B12 has been found to predispose to neurodegenerative illness like Alzheimer's, again highlighting the importance of adequate vitamin B12 in maintaining cognitive function in aged individuals. In addition to its effect on cognitive ability, vitamin B12 deficiency can be a factor in severe neuropathological changes that have a detrimental effect on the quality of life of elderly individuals. The symptoms can include loss of memory, loss of balance, and coordination in locomotion, which can lead to falls and other issues. Furthermore, patients suffering from chronic diseases, including diabetes and gastrointestinal illnesses, may also be vulnerable to a vitamin B12 deficiency due to malabsorption or dietary restriction, leading to a cycle of neurological impairment and greater health risk. Because recent publications emphasize the importance of B12 in the health of the brain, the assessment of dietary sources of vitamin B12 in the elderly, especially among those with plant-based diets where B12 can be limited, becomes essential. Elderly deficiency in vitamin B12 requires holistic management involving assessment, education, and supplementation as indicated. There are also several fortified foods and supplements that provide bioavailable sources of B12, and these could become a key factor in the prevention of cognitive impairment and neurological health. Public health interventions to promote awareness of the significance of vitamin B12, with targeted efforts among high-risk groups, could also serve to improve general health status. With the complex interplay between nutrition and brain health, it is essential that healthcare professionals regularly check and monitor the vitamin B12 status of older adults to take effective interventions and maximize brain health across the life course (Pirotin et al., 2014; Hester, 2017) (Figure 4.8).

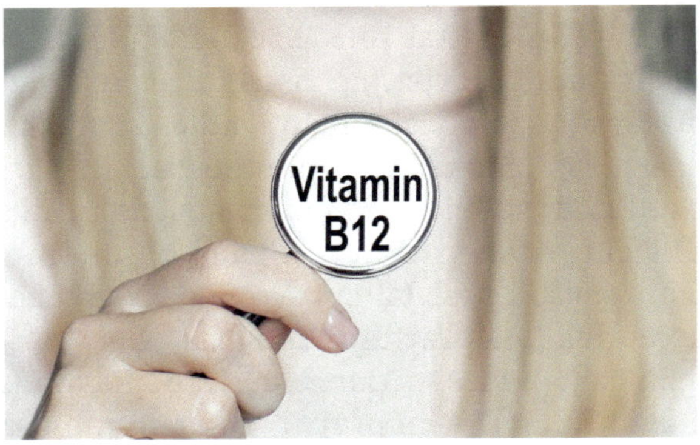

Figure 4.8. Vitamin B12 deficiency and neurological effects.

Source: https://cdn.healthyreads.com/wp-content/uploads/2023/06/Vitamin-B12-Deficiency-In-Older-Adults7.jpg.

4.2.3. Vitamin C Deficiency and Its Impact on Skin Health

The significant role that Vitamin C plays in the health of skin cannot be exaggerated, particularly for older individuals who may be exposed to increased vulnerability to deficiency. As a vital nutrient, Vitamin C has a very important function in collagen synthesis, a structural protein found within the dermal layer of the skin. Insufficiency of this vitamin results in diminished synthesis of collagen, which is linked with wrinkle development, sagging, and poor healing. This is particularly observed in the elderly because natural aging adds to an additional decline in skin elasticity and resilience. Lastly, Vitamin C deficiency can not only adversely affect physical integrity but also the functional integrity of the skin, emphasizing the importance of effective supplementation in the dietary intake of older subjects. Also, Vitamin C is a potent antioxidant with protective effects against environmental stress and oxidative damage. Older people are often exposed to such harmful factors throughout an entire lifetime of exposure to the sun and lifestyle problems, leading to greater susceptibility to skin damage, i.e., photoaging. Inadequate Vitamin C levels would enhance the susceptibility of the skin to such factors, and the result could be more instances of skin disorders, i.e., dryness, erythema, and even skin cancers.

Through preservation of the skin's barrier function and triggering repair mechanisms, optimal Vitamin C intake is central in preventing such adverse effects. Considering this reality, proper dietary Vitamin C intake in elderly individuals becomes a fundamental public health goal to optimize the overall skin health and general well-being. In addition, the broader implications of Vitamin C deficiency on the elderly adult's skin well-being, particularly psychosocial well-being, should be noted. Decline in skin integrity as a result of inadequate Vitamin C could lead to negative psychological impacts, including lower self-esteem and the development of depression. The visible signs of aging, in conjunction with dietary deficiency, can lead to an unfavorable body image, which affects social relationships and overall well-being. There is a pressing need for targeted public health campaigns highlighting the importance of Vitamin C and foods that contain it, particularly among older adults. Since health practitioners advocate for holistic approaches to nutrition, the addition of Vitamin C-containing foods and potential supplementation strategies must be emphasized in a bid to foster the physical and psychosocial aspects of skin health in older people.

4.3. Sources of Vitamins for Older Adults

As older adults become older, their nutritional needs vary significantly, and their sources of vitamins must undergo review. One of the major challenges is the decline in the functioning of the gastrointestinal tract (GIT) that could lower nutrient absorption, leading to potential deficiencies in essential vitamins. The decline can limit the mechanical breakdown of food, together with worsening gastrointestinal motor function and chemical digestion of nutrients. Therefore, older adults may struggle to obtain required levels of vitamins through diet only, which makes them susceptible to malnutrition, which is responsible for a number of health issues, including impaired cognitive function and weakened immunity. Therefore, the understanding of this relationship between aging and GIT function plays a crucial role in developing effective dietary advice for improving vitamin nutrition among the elderly (Rémond et al., 2015). In light of these limitations, there is a need to identify appropriate sources of vitamins in the elderly. Foods that are nutrient-rich, such as leafy greens, fruits, nuts, and whole cereals, should take precedence in their diets due to the richness of vitamins and minerals in these foods. Fortified foods and beverages can also play a significant role in complementing the elderly's vitamin consumption. These fortified foods, occasionally containing supplemented vitamins like D and B12, can help bridge the gap when nutritional intake from natural foods is insufficient. Furthermore, convenient-access alternatives in the form of fortified juices or milk alternatives can encourage healthier meals in older adults who may have decreased appetites or be incapable of preparing meals, ultimately reducing the prevalence of malnutrition among this group (Pirotin et al., 2014). The best intervention strategies to optimize the sources of vitamins in the elderly should be multi-pronged and include altering diets along with supplementation, wherever necessary. Health professionals must decide the individual's specific nutritional needs and provide tailored programs using whole foods along with supplements if necessary. Collaboration with dietitians can provide personalized meal plans that seek to improve the bioavailability of vitamins. In addition, public campaigns should promote education on the importance of having a balanced diet, highlighting the role of vitamins in maintaining health and promoting long life among the elderly. These strategies that are based on systems will not only enhance vitamin nutrition but also encourage the older adults to eat healthily and significantly enhance their overall health while reducing age-related disease due to nutritional disorders (Rémond et al., 2015) (Figure 4.9).

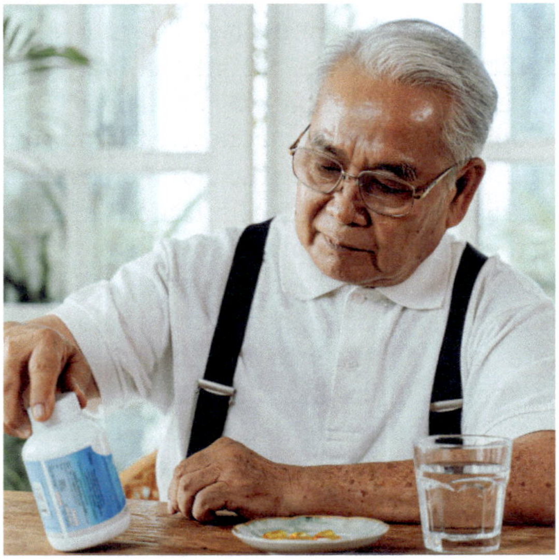

Figure 4.9. Vitamin C and older adults.

Source: https://easylivingfl.com/wp-content/uploads/Untitled-design-48.png.

4.3.1. Dietary Sources of Essential Vitamins

Food sources of vital vitamins are crucial for the well-being and life quality of the elderly. Vitamins are needed as a person grows older because their nutritional requirements shift with age, and their diet needs to be rich in varied vitamins to combat the appearance of aging. Vital vitamins such as A, C, D, E, and K are predominantly found in fruits, vegetables, whole grains, and lean protein. For instance, green vegetables like spinach contain a lot of vitamins A and K, whereas citrus fruits are full of vitamin C. Fatty fish, fortified milk items, and eggs also provide critical vitamin D and B vitamins. The complex interplay of the various vitamins is accountable for numerous physiological events, including immune function, bone health, and mental function. Offering a diverse intake of these sources of vitamins could then be prioritized in preventing the frequent occurrence of deficiencies among the elderly. Elderly people can experience some conditions that inhibit their ability to consume the correct vitamins, particularly for their nutrition. Reduced appetite, impaired taste perception, and gastrointestinal changes often hamper the intake of needed nutrients. The older gastrointestinal system, consistent with Rémond et al. (2015), experiences a decrease in the effectiveness of mechanical and chemical digestion, which may result in malnutrition. Older individuals can thus be supported by intervention on nutrient-dense foods. Also, fortified foods and supplements alleviate deficiencies, particularly vitamins B12 and D, which play key roles in sustaining neurological and skeletal health. A tailored eating plan, with the addition of these fortified foods, can counteract nutrition deficiencies caused by metabolic and digestive changes that come with age. Taking fortified foods has also emerged as a major role in supplying older individuals with nutritional needs, one of a broader pattern in food sources. Fruit juices and plant milks are fortified with vitamins, making as easy supplements to enhance vitamin intake. These fortified beverages typically contain added nutrients like vitamins A, D, and B12, thereby providing an easy means of achieving dietary requirements. However, elderly people and caregivers must also critically review the nutritional content and potential sugar levels in these foods to ascertain that they are enhancing rather than compromising overall well-being. Educational programs can be beneficial in making individuals aware of natural as well as supplemented vitamin sources, emphasizing the importance of having a combination of sources included in daily diets. Judicious selection of food can be useful in optimizing vitamin nutrition, thereby leading to enhanced health in elderly populations.

4.3.2. Role of Supplements in Vitamin Intake

The increased prevalence of malnutrition in the elderly underscores the importance of efficient methods of encouraging uptake of vitamins, particularly with the use of food supplements. Aging can have a negative impact on the gastrointestinal tract, which has a secondary impact on nutrient digestion and absorption. For instance, the mechanical and chemical breakdown of food is reduced, leading to inadequate acquisition of nutrients. As suggested in the literature, there is still an enormous gap in understanding how these changes are associated with nutritional deficiencies and their overall effect on health status, as well as the development of related pathologies on organ systems like cardiovascular and musculoskeletal health (Rémond et al., 2015). Consequently, the addition of vitamins as supplements to the diet of older adults can be an effective intervention that reverses the risks from such alterations in nutrient metabolism that occur in aging. Supplementation with vitamins has emerged as an important aspect of managing the health of older individuals, especially considering their special nutritional needs. A majority of elderly people have a hard time getting sufficient recommended dietary allowances (RDAs) from diet alone, either due to dietary restrictions or loss of appetite. Supplements play an important role in creating this nutritional gap, particularly by providing key vitamins that would otherwise be missing in their diet. For instance, vitamin D and calcium supplementation play an important role in ensuring strong bones and preventing the onset of osteoporosis, a condition prevalent among the elderly. Also, because of the growing consumption of fortified beverages, one needs to critically analyze their place vis-à-vis traditional supplements. Even though such drinks may contain some vitamins, their overall health impact, particularly regarding added sugar and calories, needs to be addressed with caution to ensure that they assist positively as part of the food package in the diets of older people (Pirotin et al., 2014).

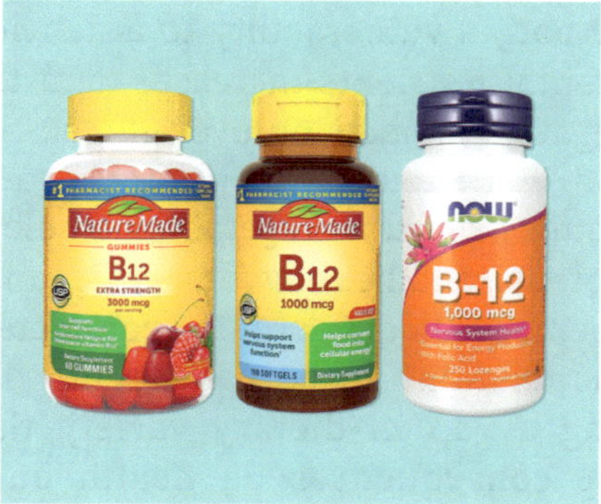

Figure 4.10. Vitamins supplements.

Source: https://hips.hearstapps.com/hmg-prod/images/gh-b12-supplements-64ecb5b714be4.png.

Lastly, the strategic application of vitamin supplements must be tailored to individual needs, considering the specific deficiencies and medical conditions of the elderly. Medical providers must conduct in-depth assessments to ascertain which vitamins are best suited based on one's own diet and lifestyle. Adequate education on the correct supplementation is crucial in order not to over-count on supplements, which can generate unwanted side effects or create nutrient imbalances. Moreover, ongoing research is required to identify biomarkers for the evaluation of nutrient bioavailability and overall risk for malnutrition among this population. With the development of guided dietary interventions, including supplements, in combination with physician appointments, older adults can maximize their vitamin intake and enhance their quality of life while navigating life's difficulties in old age (Rémond et al., 2015) (Figure 4.10).

4.3.3. Importance of a Balanced Diet

A balanced diet is required to promote optimum health, particularly in older individuals who might have specific nutritional requirements. As body metabolism decreases with increasing age, the body's vulnerability to a deficiency of fundamental nutrients increases, and this can have negative impacts on overall well-being. A balanced diet should incorporate a variety of food groups like fruits, vegetables, whole grains, lean proteins, and healthy fats. Fruits and dairy have been revealed in studies conducted with older populations to be consistently lacking, revealing a gap in dietary variety that has negative consequences on health outcomes (Schmir, 2018). Not only is a balanced diet necessary for general physical health, but also for enhancing cognitive function and reducing the risk of chronic disease, placing it at the top of the agenda of nutritional care for older populations. An adequate diet has a significant impact on preventing malnutrition, a common state among older people, caused by physiological changes related to aging. The gut, as it ages, undergoes various changes affecting nutrient intake, digestion, and absorption. These physiological changes can weaken the body's ability to uptake necessary nutrients, thus raising the stakes for malnutrition and its resulting health issues, including impaired immune system function and muscle loss (Rémond et al., 2015). Malnutrition impacts extend beyond the individual's health and can influence quality of life by increasing disease vulnerability and physical disability. Accordingly, a balanced diet addressing these factors should be given top priority in nutritional interventions for older people to effectively combat such risks. Additionally, the encouragement of a balanced diet is not merely a matter of food choices; it also entails recognizing the nutritional needs that are unique to older adults. With age, people may lose appetite or experience altered taste perception and so might fail to ingest adequate nutrients on a daily basis. Nutritional standards should thus consider the individual needs of this group in order to develop appropriate food plans and food products that can supplement their health to the desired level, considering the functionality of the gastrointestinal system of the elderly (Rémond et al., 2015). Elderly individuals are typically also facing psychological and social challenges, which can impact their diet. Through the encouragement of a culture that not only provides nutritional education but also facilitates social eating, caregivers and health workers can enhance adherence to healthy eating, ultimately improving overall health in older adults.

4.4. Challenges in Vitamin Absorption

The intricate process of vitamin absorption becomes increasingly problematic for elders due to physiological changes associated with aging. As the age of the gastrointestinal tract advances, its efficiency in nutrient uptake decreases, leading to complications that significantly affect vitamin bioavailability. For instance, alterations in gastric acidity, decreased intestinal motility, and a gradual decrease in mucosal surface area are all factors that add up to dysfunctions of nutrient uptake. In fact, vitamin B12 absorption, which is greatly dependent on intrinsic factor secretion by the gastric mucosa, can be reduced, adding to the risk of deficiency among elderly people. Thus, an understanding of these physiological alterations is necessary in order to meet nutritional needs and utilize effective diets that maximize vitamin uptake among elderly individuals. In addition, malabsorption syndromes make the nutritional picture of elderly individuals more complex, exacerbating underlying deficiencies. Recently stressed, mechanical and chemical digestion of food, intestinal wall function, declines with age and may lead to failure of effective intake with augmented risks for malnutrition. All these changes are part of a vicious cycle in which impaired nutrient absorption enhances disease progression, potentially involving multiple organ systems, i.e., cardiovascular and immune systems.

Thus, their resolution is critical to developing dietary guidelines and interventions specifically designed to address the unique needs of older adults, ensuring adequate vitamin intake and general well-being. Socioeconomic determinants and eating habits typical among many older people also blur the picture of vitamin intake. For many among them, financial constraint prevents access to quality food high in essential vitamins, such as vitamin B12. Secondly, cognitive impairment or physical disability is likely to impede proper meal planning and preparation, leading to less than adequate dietary choices. For instance, the shortcomings of food fortification programs must be evaluated, and results revealing that even well-designed intervention may not sufficiently improve vitamin B12 status in elderly people, as depicted under Chile's national program (Albala et al., 2013). Thus, an integrated strategy that connects knowledge of physiological, psychological, and socio-economic determinants is most important in countering the problem of vitamin absorption and eventually improving better health outcomes for the elderly (Rémond et al., 2015) (Figure 4.11).

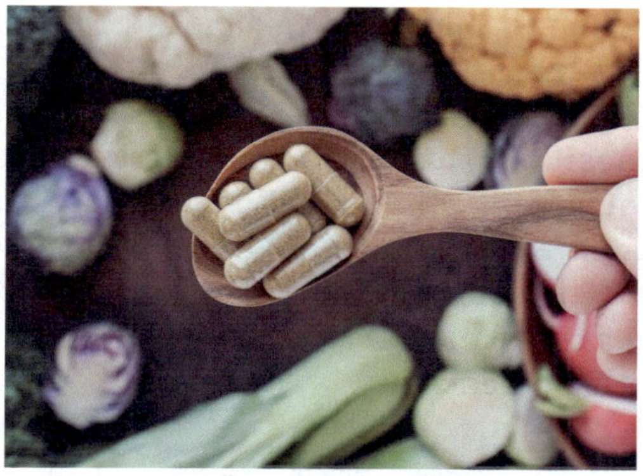

Figure 4.11. Increase vitamin absorption.

Source: https://www.besthealthmag.ca/wp-content/uploads/2019/11/how-to-increase-vitamin-absorption.jpg.

4.4.1. Age-Related Changes in Digestion

With ageing, the functioning of the gastrointestinal tract (GIT) is subject to several functional deteriorations that significantly impact nutrient digestion and absorption. The breakdown of food mechanically lowers in efficiency, as well as alterations in gastrointestinal motility, leading to quicker transit times within the gastrointestinal tract. Such a reduction could hinder the ability of the body to digest and utilize essential nutrients, which leads to an insufficient level of essential vitamins and minerals that are imperative for the promotion of health among older adults. The implications are profound because the reduced functionality of the older GIT to deliver sufficient nutrients could exacerbate the risk of malnutrition, increasingly regarded as a silent epidemic of older adults. Such alterations become significant in recognizing the need for certain dietary management based on the specific physiological requirements of the group (Rémond et al., 2015). Aging is further complicated by the loss of numerous digestive juices, like stomach acid and digestive enzymes. Not only do these structural changes become inefficient in food breakdown, but they also diminish nutrient availability, particularly for the absorption of critical vitamins like B12, folate, and minerals like calcium and magnesium. Research demonstrates that individuals over the age of 75 have significantly lower levels of important nutritional markers than their younger counterparts, and there is a clear correlation between advancing age and nutritional deficiency.

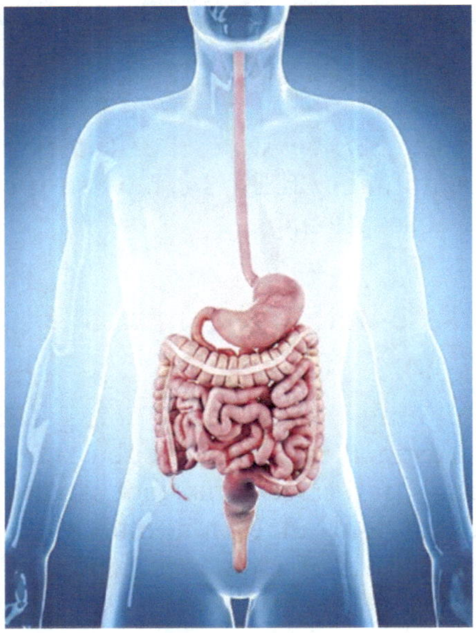

Figure 4.12. Digestive changes with aging.

Source: https://i2.wp.com/hospitalnews.com/wp-content/uploads/2018/09/iStock-490480750.jpg?fit=360%2C480&ssl=1.

This decrease in biochemical indicators of nutritional status is of particular interest within the aging context, where adequate consumption of vitamins is of highest significance to maintain health overall and decrease the risk associated with age-related pathology. Along with these physiological changes happening, they underscore the necessity for specific nutritional strategies (Forster & Gariballa, 2005). In addition, the social and psychological complications of aging are also likely to make the nutritional process in the elderly more complex. For the most part, individuals are able to develop weaker appetites or simply not perform normal meal preparation for a range of cognitive or physical impairments. This can lead to consuming inadequate diets that further contribute to the risk of malnutrition. With the knowledge of the interplay between aging, digestion, and nutrition, it becomes essential to maintain health and functional autonomy among the aged. As far as addressing these challenges is concerned, dietary intervention must address not only the functional impairment of the GIT but also the general socio-economic determinants of older individuals. Implementing evidence-based dietary recommendations and interventions tailored to the elderly's unique needs can enhance their nutrient intake and quality of life substantially (Rémond et al., 2015) (Figure 4.12).

4.4.2. Medications That Affect Vitamin Absorption

The intricate relationship between medications and vitamin absorption is one that is increasingly in the spotlight, particularly for older adults who frequently have several chronic conditions. Certain medications have a significant interference effect on the absorption of basic vitamins, leading to deficiencies that aggravate geriatric diseases. Proton pump inhibitors (PPIs), which are commonly prescribed for acid reflux disease, can lead to interference in the absorption of vitamin B12 and magnesium, essential for neurological and muscular functions. Antibiotics can also disturb gut flora, interfering with the absorption of fat-soluble vitamins like A, D, E, and K. As elderly patients are more reliant on a multiplicity of drugs, awareness of what happens when these interact with each other is critical in elderly nutrition therapy and health care. Alongside this, natural aging progressively impairs gastrointestinal function, which makes it more difficult to properly absorb nutrients. The chemical transformation in the aging gastrointestinal tract and mechanical transformation decrease its efficiency in nutrient absorption, and this latter necessitates the need to address proper drug handling in aged persons (Rémond et al., 2015). To the degree that antacids and other medications that change gastric pH impact the solubility of vitamins, particularly those employing an acidic pH medium to achieve the best absorption, there is a considerable impact. Thus, healthcare providers ought not only to monitor the use and demand for such drugs but also to consider dietary changes or supplementation to prevent potential deficiencies that can occur due to their use. The interaction between drug and nutrient consumption necessitates a holistic approach to ensure proper vitamin nutrition. Lastly, vitamin absorption requires an ongoing conversation among caregivers, patients, and medical providers to maintain nutrition as a key component of healthy living. Teaching practices must be implemented to inform older adults about how their medications influence nutritional intake and encourage an open-minded approach to meal preparation. For example, patients taking long-term drugs that will impede the absorption of vitamins can be assisted with customized diets or vitamin supplementation such that the nutritional needs of patients are met without exacerbating the underlying medical illnesses. With the implementation of the knowledge of aging gastrointestinal tracts' mechanisms and dietary interventions alongside drug therapy, a holistic approach can be provided, ultimately resulting in enhanced quality of life as well as health outcomes in older adults (Hester, 2017).

4.5. Recommendations for Vitamin Intake

Emphasis on personalized vitamin consumption recommendations among older adults cannot be overemphasized, given the unique physiological changes that accompany aging. As one ages, the ability of the body to metabolize and absorb essential vitamins diminishes, which frequently leads to deficiencies. Older individuals, particularly, are faced with various nutritional requirements for vitamins based on elements such as decreased dietary intake, altered gastrointestinal tract function, and specific diseases. The guidelines need to stress essential vitamins like D, B12, and folate, essential for bone health, mental function, and overall energy levels. It is important to involve health professionals to revise and standardize these guidelines so that elderly individuals can receive proper nutrition to maintain their well-being, and such efforts could help counter the quickly increasing number of seniors suffering from malnutrition. Also, there needs to be more awareness of the role of vitamin D, particularly in skeletal health and immunity, among elderly people. The Rank Forum on Vitamin D indicates that serum 25-hydroxyvitamin D (25(OH)D) levels over 25 nmol/l are what is advised on the matter of public health. Nevertheless, the majority of older people lack such levels due to having access to too little sunlight and diet. Rethinking dietary reference values, as per the forum, is important, and a policy of sufficient vitamin D intake over the lifespan should exist in regions where sunlight is poor. With evidence having established the adverse effect of poor intake of vitamin D on bone health and susceptibility to chronic illnesses, certain supplementation regimens may function as effective interventions in sustaining the well-being of the elderly, such that their vitamin D status is consistent with existing guidelines (Lanham-New et al., 2010). It is also important to consider not only physical but also psychological health outcomes associated with the intake of vitamins. Research has established that inadequate fruit and vegetable consumption, a critical source of vitamins, can be linked with increased rates of depression and anxiety among aging adults. For example, research indicates that high intakes of fruits and vegetables will have beneficial effects on mental health and self-worth, highlighting the multi-faceted benefits of adequate vitamin consumption. Hence, whereas fruit and vegetable portions are needed to fulfill vitamin A and C requirements, they can also contribute to mental health, which is equally crucial to quality of life in elderly populations. Through the promotion of comprehensive nutritional education and enhanced access to nutrient-rich foods, a unified approach can be created to target both physical health and mental health in older generations (Figure 4.13) (Miller et al., 2019).

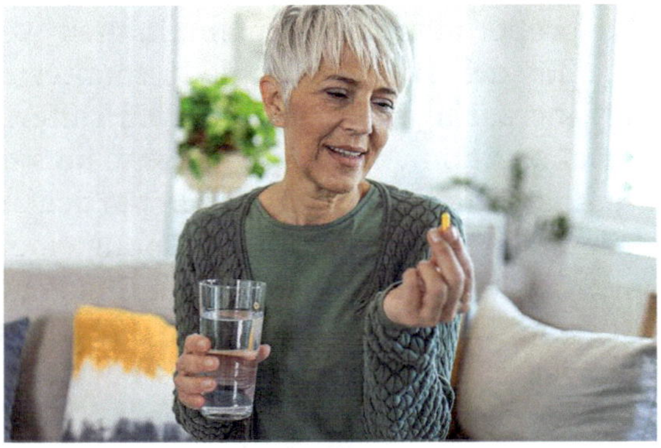

Figure 4.13. Recommendations on vitamins for older adults.

Source: https://www.harmonyhomehealth.com/wp-content/uploads/2024/02/woman-taking-medication.jpg.

4.5.1. Daily Vitamin Requirements for Older Adults

With increasing age, daily vitamin requirements of people alter significantly because of some alterations in the physiological and metabolic functions with time. Specifically, elderly individuals are known to exhibit decreased efficiency in nutrient absorption, which can be caused by gastrointestinal function changes. These modifications, such as reduced gastric acidity and reduced intestinal motility, disrupt the process of digestion and absorption of vital vitamins and minerals, ultimately culminating in deficiencies. As an illustration, vitamins B12, D, and folate play crucial roles in maintaining mental function and cardiovascular performance, and their adequate consumption is thus vital to the elderly. Without conscious effort to meet these nutritional needs, older adults will be increasingly vulnerable to malnutrition-related disorders such as cognitive impairment and impaired immunity, hence the significance of adherence to individualized dietary advice specifically tailored for this demographic category, as shown by research (Rémond et al., 2015). The establishment of customary vitamin requirements for the elderly is also made more complex by the action of chronic disease and drugs that most elderly individuals have in their bodies on a regular basis. Conditions such as diabetes, hypertension, and osteoporosis necessitate dietary adjustments that may decrease the absorption or utilization of specific vitamins. For example, individuals on certain diuretics may require additional potassium and magnesium to make up for loss of electrolytes. Besides, the vulnerability to polypharmacy in older adults increases vulnerability to nutrient-drug interaction, a condition that necessitates careful attention to diet. Nutritional education for older adults should encourage awareness of how such conditions and their treatment influence vitamin needs, eventually informing sound dietary choices. Equivalently, these specialty requirements can strongly counteract risks of age-related illness that are prevalent and contribute to overall quality of life in older adults, as described in many studies on nutrient intake for this demographic (Rémond et al., 2015). In addition to the physiological and health determinants of vitamin intake, the psychological and social determinants must also be considered. Older people typically have mobility limitations, financial constraints, and social isolation, all of which undermine access to healthy diets. Poorer mental health, with higher rates of depression and anxiety in older persons, can also complicate diet adherence and appetite for health food. Research has indicated that diet quality, especially fruit and vegetable consumption, is correlated with mental health in adults across all age ranges, unveiling an important connection that can influence the dietary habits of older adults as well. Improving means to enhance social interaction around food, such as community meal programs and workshops, can enable older adults to place a higher priority on their vitamin consumption while, at the same time, improving their mental health. Therefore, addressing both nutritional material needs and psychosocial barriers they face is essential in supporting the general well-being of the elderly.

4.5.2. Importance of Regular Health Check-Ups

Routine health check-ups are important for maintaining overall well-being, particularly in the elderly who may face age-related sickness issues. These regular check-ups not only aid in finding potential health issues prior to them becoming serious but also allow for health-care providers to provide opportunities for patient education in the form of lifestyle modification, e.g., diet. Since older patients often experience changes in metabolism and nutritional needs, regular checks allow their health-care providers to recommend appropriate diet modifications, e.g., supplementation of vitamin D or replacement of deficiencies that are prevalent among this group. Early detection of diseases such as diabetes or hypertension can lead to treatment that significantly improves quality of life, highlighting the central role that health check-ups play in preventive health care. Additionally, the advantage of health check-ups is not merely for instant health assessment, but it also builds a solid patient-physician relationship based on trust and communication. This report can get older adults to come forward and discuss some of the health problems that they might otherwise forget or downplay. For example, discussions on vitamins and mineral supplements can lead to tailored nutritional strategies towards improved health results. Evidence demonstrates that regularly visited patients in checks are more likely to be able to adhere to diet recommendations and nutritional guidance prescribed for them. By integrating health checks with dietetics advice, older adults can make informed decisions that are supportive of longevity and vitality, underlining the complementarity of health check-ups and dietary health. Finally, the psychological benefit of frequent health checks should not be overlooked, especially in relation to aging. Regular consultations make older adults feel more responsible for their health status and can contribute to reducing anxiety caused by potential health issues. Furthermore, such engagement also tends to result in beneficial support groups. Healthcare professionals can refer patients to community resources, nutritional services, and well-being workshops that enhance their healthy lifestyles. In particular, elderly individuals can gain benefits from initiatives focused on vitamin nutrition, which will lead to healthier profiles and reduce age-related risks. Thus, regular health check-ups are a significant aspect not just in the treatment and diagnosis of health problems but also in the ability of older individuals to lead healthier lives (Figure 4.14).

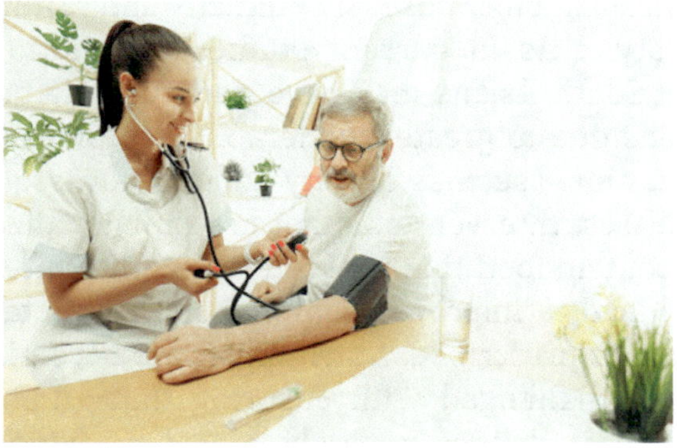

Figure 4.14. Importance of full body check-ups for senior citizens.

Source: https://lotusdiagnostic.com/wp-content/uploads/2023/03/Full-Body-Checkup.png.

4.5.3. Tailoring Vitamin Intake to Individual Health Conditions

The nutritional needs of older people are not generic; rather, they need an individualized approach considering particular health conditions. As age progresses, metabolic processes change, affecting the absorption and utilization of vitamins and nutrients in the body. This calls for a customized assessment of vitamin intake relative to prevalent diseases such as diabetes, osteoporosis, and cardiovascular diseases. For instance, elderly patients with type 2 diabetes may require adjustments in the number of vitamins for glucose metabolism and optimal energy levels. Vitamin supplementation specific to these unique health conditions not only manages symptoms but also enhances overall well-being and quality of life. Therefore, a comprehensive nutrition plan considering individual health profiles is critical to the promotion of enhanced health in older adults. Moreover, cultural background plays a role in food preference and food consumption behavior, which emphasizes the critical need to integrate cultural competence into nutritional intervention. Older adults with varying backgrounds are likely to have varying nutritional needs and food availability based on ethnicity and cultural lifestyle. As in current studies, populations like South Asians may have particular dietary needs due to greater vulnerability to pressure conditions, such as obesity and cardiovascular diseases. Interventions that are individualized to contain food that is of interest to the culture can lead to improved compliance with dietary changes prescribed. Nutritionists are becoming more challenged with ensuring that vitamin intake guidelines not only consider scientific findings but also resonate with the cultures of the patients they care for. This approach yields a more effective and compassionate pathway toward optimizing health in older adults. Finally, the relationship between proper vitamin intake and longer life is extremely significant in geriatric populations. Research into whole food diet plans illustrates that the correct proportion of vitamins will avoid age-related conditions of ill health. For elderly people, there may be tailored vitamin intake in the form of higher doses of specific vitamins like vitamin D and calcium to combat osteoporosis and improve bone strength. Also, adequate vitamin B12 intake is crucial to prevent cognitive function reductions and preserve neurological activity, perhaps preventing dementia. Since the number of elderly people is growing, healthcare providers must give top priority to management strategies that are responsive to physiological as well as lifestyle change so that vitamin nutrition is not only supportive of individual illness or disease states but also of enhanced quality of life. With thorough scrutiny and appropriate cultural intervention, the potential for health gain is significantly enhanced.

4.6. The Role of Healthcare Providers

Healthcare providers play a critical role in ensuring vitamin nutrition among older adults, addressing a group that often suffers from particular nutritional concerns. As physiological changes that accompany aging can affect the absorption and metabolism of nutrients, healthcare providers must conduct thorough assessments in order to be able to identify possible inadequacies in vitamins and minerals. Effective interventions are dependent on understanding the individual requirements of the age group, particularly in the context of dominant conditions such as osteoporosis and cardiovascular diseases. Providers need to be aware that there are certain ethnic groups with variations in nutritional requirements, therefore necessitating the tailoring of dietary information to suit the cultural backgrounds of patients under treatment. By patient-centered practice, the providers can become better at improving vitamin intake among the elderly, thereby resulting in healthier outcomes and a better quality of life. Furthermore, constant education and communication between healthcare workers and older adults is required in order to encourage adherence to recommended food intake habits. Healthcare workers not only have to instruct on the importance of vitamins but also give their patients valuable methods of how to incorporate these nutrients into their diet. This could include giving them easily accessible vitamin sources in the form of fruits, vegetables, and fortified foods or recommending the use of supplements if necessary. Moreover, they must provide resources for promoting self-management to support older adults in charge of their nutritional health. In vulnerable groups, like minority populations, culturally relevant education is even more critical. By using diet recommendations that consider patients' cultural food preferences and eating patterns, practitioners have the ability to produce a more collaborative partnership, improving compliance and subsequently overall health outcomes in older adults (Szczepura et al., 2011). Last, the strategic interaction of health systems and policies is essential in ensuring healthcare providers' work in optimizing vitamin nutrition in older people. Preventive and care-coordination-oriented evidence-based policies create an environment for solving the intricate problems of vitamin deficiency in this age group. Examples include ongoing screening programs against nutritional deficiency, which can enable early detection of the high-risk group and allow timely intervention. Besides, educational programs to increase the knowledge of healthcare professionals in terms of geriatric nutrition can further enhance their capacity to deliver effective nutrition counseling. As healthcare moves ahead, support for family caregivers also becomes imperative, as they may be involved with the eating habits of older individuals. Thus, an education-based approach, along with policy intervention and caregiver influence, can make a big difference in promoting the nutritional health of the aging population, such that they receive adequate vitamin nutrition in their later years (The Stern Center for Evidence-Based Policy, 2015) (Figure 4.15).

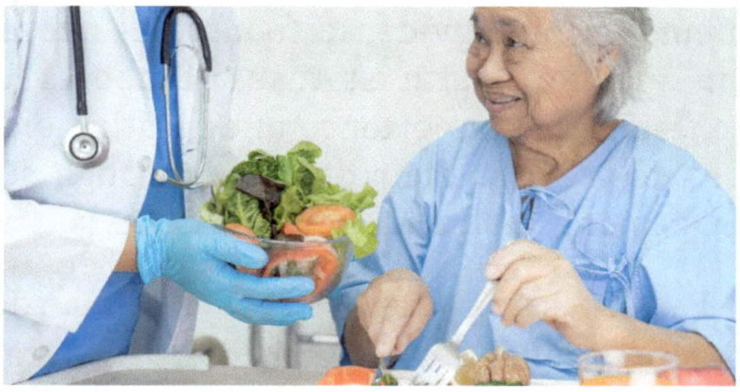

Figure 4.15. Benefits of an elderly nutrition program.

Source: https://cdn.growtha.dev/66503d1e5b67d304ddf7b32a/66543d6d3d498a2491a60fcc_660af9eeea363b47ad399c4b_Dessert%2520Spring25%2520(45).webp.

4.6.1. Educating Older Adults About Nutrition

The need to educate older people on nutrition is due to the special dietary needs and health issues they encounter with age. As one ages, one's body experiences physiological changes that affect nutrient uptake and nutritional needs in general. For example, older people tend to lose appetite or have difficulties accessing food, which contributes to poor nutrition. Food insecurity is prevalent among elderly populations in the United States, as they lack regular access to sufficient food required to maintain an active and healthy lifestyle. Food insecurity is associated with a variety of adverse health outcomes, including diabetes, depression, and cardiovascular disease, and thus deserves targeted nutritional education that can mitigate risks (Ziliak & Gunderson, 2014). By presenting nutritional education as part of the overall health care services for the elderly, professionals can help improve dietary intake and overall health in this high-risk group. Nutrition education is particularly crucial for elderly individuals who have chronic conditions such as diabetes, which necessitates an individualized approach to diet and food choice. Educational interventions have to equip these individuals to manage their conditions effectively through diet, high-protein, and energy-dense foods that address their specific health statuses. Diabetes UK emphasizes the importance of educating older adults to manage their diabetes through self-management, diet, and dietetic advice.

By assessing the risk of malnutrition and professional advice from health workers, dietetic interventions may be implemented to satisfy nutritional needs adequately (McClinchy, 2018). In this regard, facilitation education that integrates both nutritional knowledge and cooking skills may lead to improved health outcomes, together with enhancing the quality of life of many older individuals residing at home or care home settings. Along with direct educational interventions, older adults' nutritional literacy also depends on community involvement. Healthcare professionals, community groups, and families can implement interventions that create a setting of support for older adults to thrive. Nutrition education classes, cooking competency training, and social eating programs can strive to increase participation and enhance food security among older adults. Furthermore, by the use of local resources and partnerships, such programs have the potential to break down food access barriers, offering older adults not only information but also resources to make informed nutrition-related choices. These partnerships can then help break down negative effects of food insecurity and malnutrition for this population (Ziliak & Gunderson, 2014). As nutritional education rises to its rightful status as a high priority with communities, it will be the key to the health and wellness of older adults, enhancing overall wellness in the later stages of life.

4.6.2. Monitoring Vitamin Levels in Patients

Patient vitamin monitoring, particularly for older adults, is essential in avoiding malnutrition and addressing many of the health concerns that accompany advancing age. Aging affects the body's ability to absorb nutrients directly, which in turn may lead to deficiencies, particularly in vitamins like B12, D, and folate. When the GIT starts showing changes in its functioning, the mechanical and chemical digestion of food becomes slower, and one has to exert more effort to have an adequate amount of nutrients in the body. This inability to properly digest and absorb essential vitamins can induce or exacerbate chronic health conditions that are common among elderly populations, including cardiovascular disease and mental impairment. Regular monitoring of vitamin status not only serves to identify deficiencies but also helps tailor dietary interventions capable of reversing the health benefits of aging and optimizing health benefits in this vulnerable population (Rémond et al., 2015). Regular tracking of vitamin levels may inform the nutrition care routines used by practitioners to address malnutrition in the elderly population. Tracking may be done by various approaches, including blood work and dietary assessment, to estimate the patient's intake and physiological response to nutrient intake. Establishing an overall image of nutritional status in elderly patients allows the practice of evidence-based interventions to address specific deficiencies. One example of effective intervention is dietary modification, such as an increase in the consumption of fortified foods or supplements that provide necessary vitamins like B12 and D. Likewise, these assessments can identify the impact of non-medication interventions, such as structured exercise and diet counseling, on reducing the hazards of falls and fractures (Wilson et al., 2020). Personalized nutritional care, then, based on systematic monitoring, can enhance the health of older patients. Furthermore, the application of multidisciplinary teams in the treatment of vitamin deficiency plays a key role in ensuring holistic care for older adults. With the collaboration of dietitians, geriatricians, and other health workers, medical professionals can create holistic care plans that encompass not only nutritional needs but preventive interventions against common age-related diseases as well. The incorporation of educational methods also allows patients to make intelligent food decisions and have an active role in the maintenance of their health. This collaborative model not only enhances compliance with diet recommendations but can even significantly reduce the risk of complications arising due to nutrient deficiencies. Given the challenges posed by the aging GIT and the resulting threats of malnourishment, continuous monitoring and multidisciplinary interventions are essential in favor of optimal health for older individuals (Rémond et al., 2015; Wilson et al., 2020).

4.6.3. Collaborating with Dietitians for Personalized Plans

Collaboration between health care providers and dietitians is important in the development of personal nutrition plans for older adults, particularly in vitamin nutrition. Older adults tend to have special dietary issues due to changes in physiology, chronic diseases, and variations in activity. These issues need an integrated approach that meets not just individual nutritional needs but also includes modifications beneficial to their lifestyle. Through the incorporation of dietitians, medical doctors can make nutrition interventions evidence-based and targeted to the specific nutrient deficiency or excesses, which in this age group are typically prevalent. Thus, the incorporation of nutrition professionals considerably enhances the effectiveness of nutritional counseling, resulting in better health for the elderly through ensuring that their vitamin requirements are properly addressed in an age-specific manner. The role of a personalized nutrition strategy cannot be overestimated, particularly with reference to vitamin supplementation. Older people's diets tend to lead to deficiencies in vital micronutrients, making specific supplementation under medical guidance imperative. As borne out by current evidence, individuals with restrictive diets such as vegan or vegetarian can prove most vulnerable to shortages of nutrients. This renders it essential that dietitians conduct rigorous evaluations of older adults' diets and their corresponding state of health. Subsequently, dietitians can adjust dietary routine and recommend appropriate supplementation so as to minimize the risk of potential ill health effects due to low concentration of vitamins. Repeated communication among older adults and their dietitians can facilitate frequent monitoring that considers evolving health needs as they progress with age and therefore guarantee continued wellness. Furthermore, educational programs led by dietitians are crucial in enabling older individuals with the requisite knowledge to make informed food decisions. Culinary nutrition education programs can enhance eating behaviors among various groups, such as older individuals. With more direct involvement and education by additional registered dietitians, the probability of enhanced compliance with individualized nutrition protocols is also heightened. It is especially important in those groups where access to dietary advice may be limited. Merging culinary education with conventional nutrition instruction allows older people to be able to select healthier foods, thus reversing prevalent issues like inadequate micronutrient consumption. Therefore, coordination between healthcare practitioners and dietitians not only makes it possible to develop customized nutrition regimens but also promotes educational outreach critical to the improvement of the overall nutritional status among elderly populations (Figure 4.16).

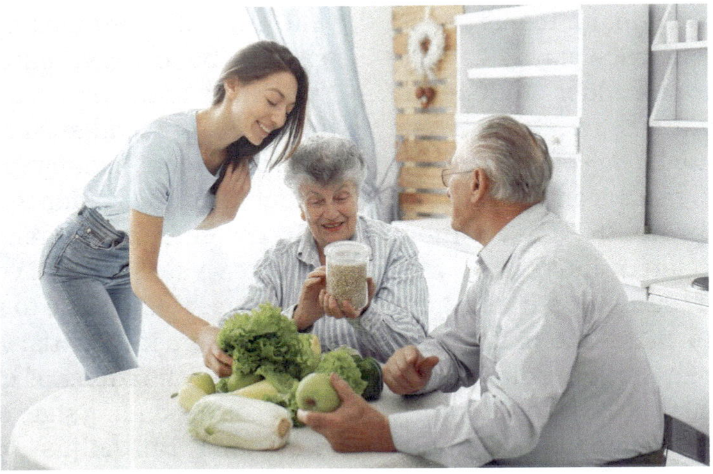

Figure 4.16. Role of dietitians in assisted living.

Source: https://cdn.prod.website-files.com/6674accd613ea976deacd057/66a09ec5d76c278c8e6b32c5_aaaaaaaa.jpg.

SUMMARY

The exploring of vitamin nutrition among elderly populations, it is important to identify the complex interaction between food consumption, micronutrient status, and resultant health outcomes in this vulnerable population. Because older adults undergo unique physiological alterations that can impair nutrient use and metabolism, their individual nutrient requirements are critical to providing optimal health. The identified deficiencies of vitamin D and zinc among older adults are a strong argument for the introduction of specific nutritional guidelines. These deficiencies can manifest into a range of various health disorders, underscoring the importance of treating them with dietary modification and potentially supplementation regimes. Furthermore, research suggests that a significant proportion of older subjects possess subnormal amounts of key nutrients, including zinc and vitamin D. For instance, data collected among older patients indicated that around 67% of them had plasma zinc in the deficient zone, highlighting an overriding focus on increased awareness of micronutrient intake during this phase of life. Studies also depict the impact of good eating habits, as shown by research indicating that good eating habits with proper nutrition augmented by vitamins and minerals enhance health significantly. Therefore, healthcare professionals and caregivers must attach great importance to nutritional assessment to allow shortcomings to be detected, thus enabling appropriate interventions to be taken that can reverse the effects of deteriorating health in correlation with increasing age, as confirmed by evidence in this field of study (Paterson, 1982). Finally, the implications of vitamin nutrition extend far beyond mere dietetic counseling; they encompass broader public health issues. The potential effects of nutrient deficiencies among the elderly reveal the importance of setting in motion comprehensive approaches and policies that ensure maximum nutrition for the elderly. An interdisciplinary partnership among healthcare professionals, policymakers, and communities is the key to ensuring access to foods with nutrients and proper diet education. As noted in analyses of zinc consumption and its physiological importance, synchronizing nutritional recommendations could be the most effective way to resolve the inconsistency of nutrient status in elderly people (Moran et al., 2012). Ultimately, vitamin nutrition optimization is an elementary measure to encourage longevity as well as quality-of-life improvement among the aged.

A comprehensive review of vitamin nutrition among the aged offers valuable information regarding the interaction between aging and nutritional needs. Aging has a profound impact on the gastrointestinal tract (GIT), which, in turn, impacts nutrient intake, digestion, and absorption. Structural and functional changes of the GIT can impair its efficiency, leading to a diminishment of the body's ability to provide adequate nutrition. This decrease is strongly related to an increased risk of malnutrition that can exacerbate health status in different organ systems, including the nervous, musculoskeletal, cardiovascular, immune, and cutaneous systems. All of these relationships need to be understood to overcome malnutrition and maintain overall well-being in the elderly, suggesting the necessity for personal dietary guidelines corresponding to this age group's specific physiological needs (Rémond et al., 2015). Besides, the prevalence of diabetes in the elderly demands focused efforts on nutritional care strategies. As diabetes becomes more prevalent among the elderly, its confluence with malnutrition is a problem that has become increasingly evident. The elderly, particularly the frail elderly, have a higher risk of adverse outcomes because of poor nutritional status stemming from various physiological and environmental factors. The revised nutrition standards published by Diabetes UK emphasize the importance of eating and education on self-management among older adults with diabetes. The guidelines recommend nutritional screening for the risk of malnutrition and also refer to the argument that dietitians must include high-energy and high-protein foods in the development of care plans (McClinchy, 2018). Through management of both diabetes and malnutrition, clinicians are able to improve health outcomes and quality of life in the elderly. Finally, managing vitamin nutrition in the elderly requires a multi-pronged approach with regard to the declining functionality of the aging GITs as well as the growing prevalence of diseases such as diabetes. The interaction between nutrient absorption and GIT integrity is the cornerstone of the need for differentiated dietary recommendations that are appropriate for the ageing population. In addition, there is a need to introduce certain interventions, particularly for the vulnerable groups of the population, to mitigate the dangers of malnutrition and the associated health issues. Such an integrative strategy, blending knowledge of the physical stresses of aging and the specific chronic illnesses, forms a foundation for developing effective nutrition intervention that promotes health and well-being in older adults (Rémond et al., 2015; McClinchy, 2018).

A CLOSER LOOK

VITAMIN D'S ROLE IN GUT HEALTH

Vitamin D's role in gut health is a growing area of research that highlights its relevance outside of bone metabolism. Traditionally known to be responsible for bone density in terms of calcium and phosphorus balance, vitamin D also has a significant immune modulation and barrier function in the gut. In the gastrointestinal tract, vitamin D modulates the immune function of the gut-associated lymphoid tissue (GALT), or protects against pathogens and is in harmony with healthy microbiota. It enhances the generation of antimicrobial peptides such as cathelicidin, which defend the gut lining against harmful microbes and keep the microbial community healthy (Figure 4.17).

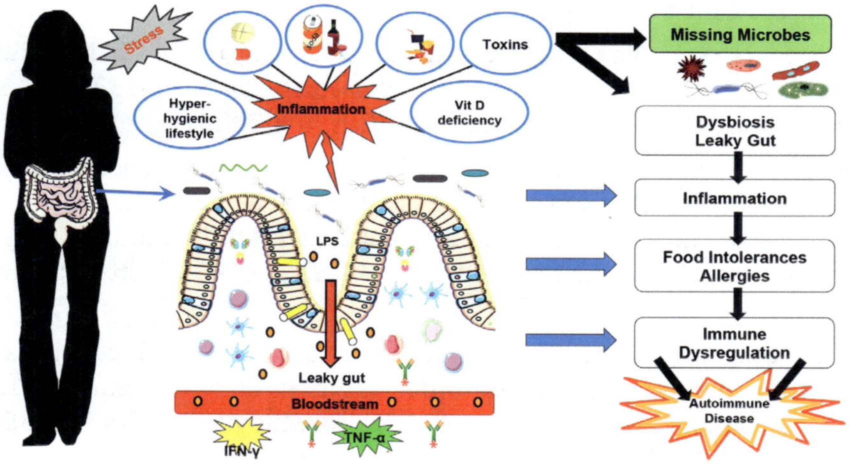

Figure 4.17. Vitamin D's role in gut health.

Source: https://www.frontiersin.org/files/Articles/215942/fimmu-07-00627-HTML/image_m/fimmu-07-00627-g001.jpg.

Vitamin D also contributes to the maintenance of the integrity of the intestinal epithelial barrier, the thin layer of cells covering the gut lumen and dividing it from the bloodstream. A strong barrier keeps "leaky gut" in check, where toxins and bacteria cannot penetrate into the bloodstream and threaten the onset of inflammation and chronic disease. Vitamin D deficiency has been correlated with disease conditions like inflammatory bowel disease (IBD), irritable bowel syndrome (IBS), and even metabolic diseases like obesity and type 2 diabetes—all with a gut health factor.

Moreover, vitamin D receptors (VDRs), expressed along the entire gastrointestinal tract, are involved in regulating the expression of genes that regulate inflammation, cell growth, and microbial composition. A good balance of gut microbiota for digestion, immune defense, and even mood regulation through the gut-brain axis is ensured by adequate vitamin D levels. Since it affects us so generally, getting sufficient vitamin D—be it through diet, sunlight, or supplements—is a fundamental place to start to improve gut health and overall wellness.

REFERENCES

1. Wilson, N., Hurkmans, E., Adams, J., Bakkers, M., Balážová, P., Baxter, M., Blavnsfeldt, A. B., Briot, K., Chiari, C., Cooper, C., Dragoi, R., Gäbler, G., Lems, W., Mosor, E., Pais, S., Simon, C., Studenic, P., Tilley, S., de la Torre, J., & Stamm, T. A. (2020). Prevention and management of osteoporotic fractures by non-physician health professionals: a systematic literature review to inform EULAR points to consider. *RMD open*, *6*(1), e001143. https://doi.org/10.1136/rmdopen-2019-001143 (accessed on 12th July 2025).
2. Wright, C. S., Laing, E. M., Pollock, N. K., Hausman, D. B., Weaver, C. M., Martin, B. R., McCabe, G. P., Peacock, M., Warden, S. J., Hill Gallant, K. M., & Lewis, R. D. (2018). Serum 25-Hydroxyvitamin D and Intact Parathyroid Hormone Influence Muscle Outcomes in Children and Adolescents. *Journal of bone and mineral research : the official journal of the American Society for Bone and Mineral Research*, *33*(11), 1940–1947. https://doi.org/10.1002/jbmr.3550(accessed on 12th July 2025).
3. Maijó, M., Clements, S. J., Ivory, K., Nicoletti, C., & Carding, S. R. (2014). Nutrition, diet and immunosenescence. *Mechanisms of ageing and development*, *136-137*, 116–128. https://doi.org/10.1016/j.mad.2013.12.003(accessed on 12th July 2025).
4. Moran, V. H., Stammers, A. L., Medina, M. W., Patel, S., Dykes, F., Souverein, O. W., Dullemeijer, C., Pérez-Rodrigo, C., Serra-Majem, L., Nissensohn, M., & Lowe, N. M. (2012). The relationship between zinc intake and serum/plasma zinc concentration in children: a systematic review and dose-response meta-analysis. *Nutrients*, *4*(8), 841–858. https://doi.org/10.3390/nu4080841(accessed on 12th July 2025).
5. Albala, C., Dangour, A. D., Lera, L., Sanchez, M., et al. (2013). Effectiveness of the National Program of Complementary Feeding for older adults in Chile on vitamin B12 status in older adults: Secondary outcome analysis from the CENEX Study (ISRCTN48153354). https://core.ac.uk/download/13115389.pdf (accessed on 12th July 2025).
6. Shauna Pirotin, Christina Becker and Patricia B. Crawford (2014). Looking beyond the marketing claims of new beverages: Health risks of consuming sports drinks, energy drinks, fortified waters, and other flavored beverages. University of California at Berkeley, Atkins Center for Weight and Health . https://core.ac.uk/download/75778515.pdf (accessed on 12th July 2025).
7. Boldt, P. (2019). Quality of life and health status of female and male vegetarian, vegan, and omnivorous endurance runners. https://core.ac.uk/download/237193446.pdf (accessed on 12th July 2025).
8. Rémond, D., Shahar, D. R., Gille, D., Pinto, P., Kachal, J., Peyron, M. A., Dos Santos, C. N., Walther, B., Bordoni, A., Dupont, D., Tomás-Cobos, L., & Vergères, G. (2015). Understanding the gastrointestinal tract of the elderly to develop dietary solutions that prevent malnutrition. *Oncotarget*, *6*(16), 13858–13898. https://doi.org/10.18632/oncotarget.4030(accessed on 12th July 2025).
9. Lanham-New, S. A., Buttriss, J. L., Miles, L. M., Ashwell, M., Berry, J. L., Boucher, B. J., Cashman, K. D., Cooper, C., Darling, A. L., Francis, R. M., Fraser, W. D., de Groot, C. P., Hyppönen, E., Kiely, M., Lamberg-Allardt, C., Macdonald, H. M., Martineau, A. R., Masud, T., Mavroeidi, A., Nowson, C., ... Williams, C. M. (2011). Proceedings of the Rank Forum on Vitamin D. *The British journal of nutrition*, *105*(1), 144–156. https://doi.org/10.1017/S0007114510002576(accessed on 12th July 2025).

10. Famakin, O., Gadhvi, D., Griffiths, C., Hull, S., et al. (2015). "Test me and treat me" – Attitudes to vitamin D deficiency and supplementation: A qualitative study. https://core.ac.uk/download/30698108.pdf (accessed on 12th July 2025).

11. Forster, S., & Gariballa, S. (2005). Age as a determinant of nutritional status: a cross sectional study. *Nutrition journal*, *4*, 28. https://doi.org/10.1186/1475-2891-4-28(accessed on 12th July 2025).

12. Galiani, Sebastian (2009) : Reducing Poverty in Latin America and the Caribbean, Documento de Trabajo, No. 88, Universidad Nacional de La Plata, Centro de Estudios Distributivos, Laborales y Sociales (CEDLAS), La Plata (accessed on 12th July 2025).

13. Marini, Alessandra and Gragnolati, Michele, Malnutrition and Poverty in Guatemala (January 2003). Available at SSRN: https://ssrn.com/abstract=636329Dr. James P. Ziliak University of Kentucky Dr. Craig Gundersen Baylor University (2021). The health consequences of senior hunger in the United States: Evidence from the 1999–2010 NHANES. Prepared for Feeding America. https://core.ac.uk/download/71365139.pdf (accessed on 12th July 2025).

14. Hester, E. R. (2017). The benefits and concerns of veganism in women's health. https://core.ac.uk/download/58824999.pdf (accessed on 12th July 2025).

15. Jasiuk, I., Kister, K., Krukar, K., et al. (2024). The importance of supplementation in vegan and vegetarian diets for adults. https://core.ac.uk/download/620863932.pdf (accessed on 12th July 2025).

16. McClinchy, J. (2018). Dietary management of older people with diabetes. https://core.ac.uk/download/287581385.pdf (accessed on 12th July 2025).

17. Miller, N. (2019). The association between fruit and vegetable consumption and mental health among young adults. https://core.ac.uk/download/215464247.pdf (accessed on 12th July 2025).

18. The Stern Center for Evidence-Based Policy (2015). The Stern Center for Evidence-Based Policy, 2015. The Stern Center for Evidence-Based Policy ("Stern Center"), University of Pittsburgh's Health Policy Institute. The Stern Center for Evidence-Based Policy, 2015(accessed on 12th July 2025).

19. Paterson, P. (1982). Zinc levels of hospitalized elderly. https://core.ac.uk/download/590879860.pdf (accessed on 12th July 2025).

20. Pillay, D. (2017). Intakes, adequacy, food sources, and biomarker status of iron, folate, and vitamin B_{12} in Māori and non-Māori octogenarians: Life and living in advanced age: A cohort study in New Zealand (LiLACS NZ): A thesis presented in partial fulfilment of the requirements for the degree of Master of Science in Nutrition and Dietetics, Massey University, Albany, New Zealand. https://core.ac.uk/download/158297897.pdf (accessed on 12th July 2025).

21. Reay, J., Riby, L., & Smith, M. (2013). B vitamins and cognitive performance in older adults: Review. https://core.ac.uk/download/9991207.pdf (accessed on 12th July 2025).

22. Schmir, C. R. (2018). A nutritional analysis of food menus offered at local older adult assisted living facilities. https://core.ac.uk/download/215520909.pdf (accessed on 12th July 2025).

23. Szczepura, A., Bhopal, R., Cappuccio, F., Connor, H., Duke, W., Foster, G., et al. (2011). Nutrition in an ethnically diverse society: What are some of the key challenges? https://core.ac.uk/download/44180.pdf (accessed on 12th July 2025).

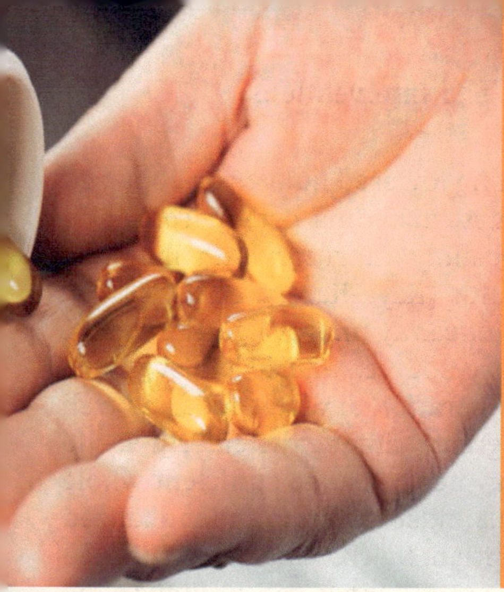

Chapter 5

MINERAL REQUIREMENTS FOR GERIATRIC NUTRITION

Contents

Introduction

The aging of the geriatric population carries with it unique nutritional needs, particularly with regard to mineral requirements. Physiological changes that occur with aging influence the nutritional needs of the elderly, and it is thus essential that the nutritional needs change accordingly. Calcium, magnesium, and potassium are essential minerals that play critical roles in bone health, regulation of blood pressure, and preservation of muscle function in the elderly. Further, the existence of age-related chronic illnesses typically necessitates a re-evaluation of eating patterns to ensure that the elderly adult is well fed. Research indicates that adequate consumption of minerals can enhance the overall quality of life among the elderly and hence justify the importance of tailored nutritional interventions within geriatric care (Lumbis, 2018). Recognition of the role of minerals in geriatric nutrition warrants an investigation into the special requirements of aging bodies. As metabolism decreases and the efficiency of nutrient absorption declines, deficiency risk increases. The essential minerals are not properly ingested due to numerous factors, including lowered hunger or impaired sense of taste. These deficiencies lead to a myriad of health issues, including osteoporosis and cardiovascular disease, that are prevalent among the elderly. Secondly, nutrition with minerals as part of a balanced diet is important in increasing overall health (Kaya-Karasu et al., 2018). Nutritional interventions that identify such changing needs will significantly improve geriatric care. To satisfy these mineral requirements adequately, adequate dietary sources and levels of intake recommendations require thorough knowledge. This requires consideration of whole foods as well as potential supplementation, given that eating practices will vary greatly among the elderly. While some older individuals may do well with fortified foods, others may not consume sufficient whole grains, fruits, or vegetables with significant minerals. Professionals must facilitate individualized nutrition screenings to identify nutritional gaps in mineral consumption. By creating individualized meal plans that include a variety of sources of crucial minerals, practitioners can minimize the health hazards associated with aging and promote maximum well-being and function in older adults throughout their later years (Lumbis, 2018).

Importance of Minerals in the Diet

The importance of minerals in the diet cannot be overstated, particularly if the nutritional needs of the elderly are considered. Minerals play many functions in the body, including supporting bone strength, smooth muscle function, and fluid balance. Proper intake of minerals by older individuals, who are prone to degenerative changes related to aging, will do much to prevent complications of osteoporosis and sarcopenia. Lack of important minerals like calcium and magnesium may lead to increased bone fragility, a higher risk of fractures, and complications. Thus, providing sufficient amounts of essential minerals to the elderly is an important aspect of nutrition planning that determines better indices of health and quality of life. Furthermore, the aging process naturally alters the efficiency of nutrient uptake in the gastrointestinal system. As described in recent literature, alterations in the structure and function of the aging gastrointestinal system can hinder the absorption of necessary nutrients, including minerals, raising the prevalence of malnutrition among the elderly (Rémond et al., 2015). Malnutrition, in turn, will exacerbate whatever medical conditions the patient has, leading to a cycle that is contrary to optimal health. For example, a deficiency of iron may lead to anemia, which has a severe effect on energy levels as well as mental abilities. Promoting mineral-rich foods appropriate to the altered digestive capacity in aging is very important in order to maintain health in geriatrics. Thus, rectification of mineral uptake and effectiveness of adoption of dietary regimens aimed at enhancing mineral bioavailability becomes exigent in geriatric nutritionetics. Also needed is knowledge of how minerals become incorporated into old people's diets, as their synergistic interactions with other nutrients need to be fully understood. Minerals do not function in isolation; rather, their uptake and metabolic action can be radically influenced by the presence of vitamins and other dietary components. For instance, calcium bioavailability may be enhanced by the presence of vitamin D, while excessive amounts of some minerals may inhibit the absorption of others. This renders the balancing of meal planning so critical in maintaining a diversity of food sources rich in beneficial minerals. With ample evidence demonstrating that malnutrition is correlated with adverse health outcomes, like higher post-fracture mortality, the incorporation of certain mineral considerations into nutritional therapy could have a significant overall effect in favor of elderly individuals (Malafarina et al., 2017). Ultimately, an integrated philosophy of geriatric nutrition with an emphasis on minerals as being one important aspect can lead to enhanced strength, recovery, and function in this high-risk population (Figure 5.1).

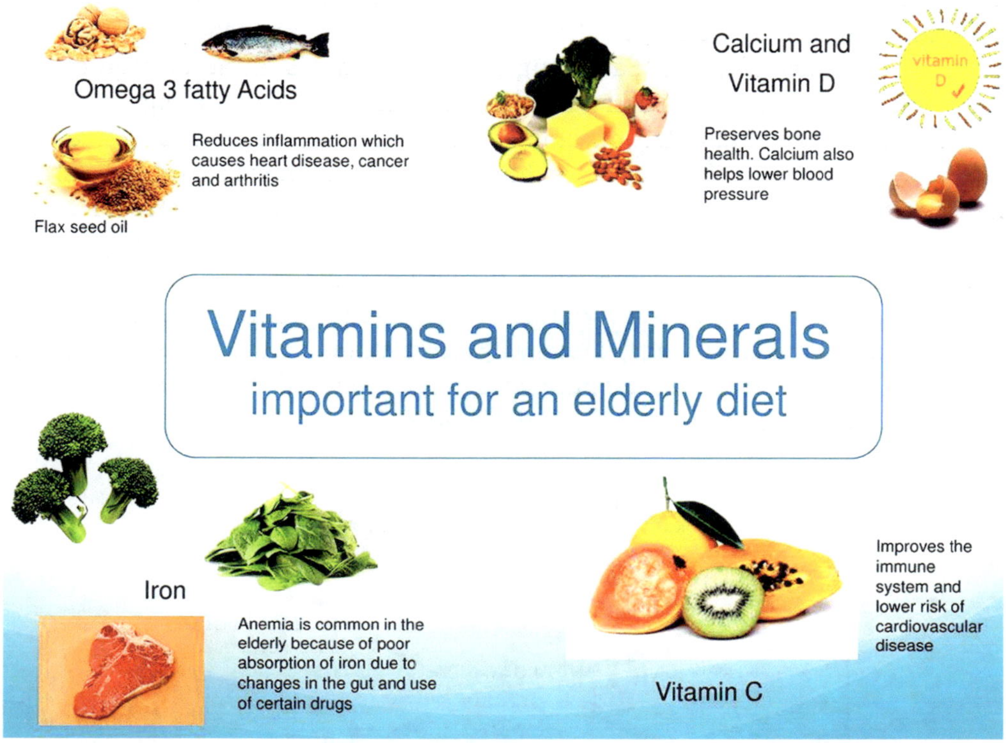

Figure 5.1. Vitamins and minerals are important for an elderly diet.

Source: https://slideplayer.com/slide/13059798/79/images/2/Vitamins+and+Minerals+importan t+for+an+elderly+diet.jpg.

5.1. The Role of Minerals in the Body

Minerals play a crucial role in fulfilling several physiological functions in the human body, particularly in the case of the elderly, who face a few challenges regarding the intake and absorption of minerals. Essential minerals such as calcium, magnesium, potassium, and iron are necessary not only for bone integrity but also for optimum functioning of the cardiovascular and nervous systems. The mineral absorption capacity of the gastrointestinal tract decreases with increasing age for a wide range of reasons, including decreased acid secretion in the stomach and alterations in gut motility. Such a decline can trigger the risk of mineral deficiency of minerals, thereby causing health complications in the form of osteoporosis, high blood pressure, and mental decline. Therefore, there is a need to understand how mineral metabolism is affected by aging so that targeted dietary interventions are designed to supply adequate levels of minerals in the aging population. Mineral deficiency effects go beyond physical health alone but include cognitive function and well-being as well. Evidence shows a striking correlation between anemia, commonly due to iron deficiency, and decline in cognitive function among the elderly. For instance, it was found in research among elderly Chinese that low hemoglobin levels had a significant correlation with poor cognitive function, illustrating the critical role played by iron and essential minerals in ensuring neurological health. Subclinical folate and vitamin B12 deficiencies further fuel the risks, as evidenced by research showing nearly 35% of the subjects studied were so deficient, which was associated with cognitive dysfunction. Thus, in maintaining cognitive status as well as quality of life, it is important that geriatric nutrition cover both macro and micronutrient needs. Satisfying older individuals' mineral requirements in their diets should thus involve complete dietary alterations unique to overcoming the obstacles of the elderly gastrointestinal tract. Malnutrition among older adults, as evidenced in recent literature, was prevalent and often the product of a combination of physiological and psychological issues, including the impaired capacity of the gastrointestinal system to adequately receive nutrients. The identification and incorporation of food sources rich in essential minerals, along with care for the digestive mechanisms of the elderly, can reverse the risk of malnutrition. New methods that focus on optimizing the bioavailability of such minerals are essential. Through enabling an awareness of such dynamics, nutritionists can craft dietary advice attuned to the needs of older individuals, ultimately resulting in improved health outcomes and improved resilience against age-related diseases (Alim et al., 2005; Rémond et al., 2015) (Figure 5.2).

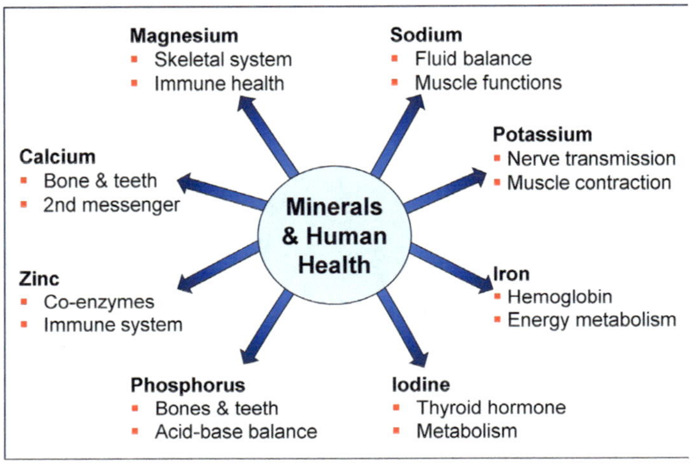

Figure 5.2. Minerals and human health.

Source: https://www.mdpi.com/nutrients/nutrients-17-00454/article_deploy/html/images/nutrients-17-00454-g001-550.jpg.

5.1.1. Essential Functions of Minerals

The roles of minerals in human nutrition extend past the basic dietary requirements; they are essential in maintaining various physiological functions, especially among the aged. Simple minerals such as calcium, magnesium, and potassium play significant roles in bone structure, cardiovascular functions, and neuromuscular processes. With age, the body experiences a decrease in mineral absorption and metabolism, leading to an increased risk of conditions like osteoporosis and hypertension.

This is compounded by the aging gastrointestinal tract that experiences mechanical and functional decline, inhibiting nutrient intake and absorption, leading to malnutrition among the elderly. Therefore, understanding the important functions of minerals is essential to developing dietary recommendations and interventions that take into consideration the unique nutritional needs of older adults, especially in order to support them in remaining at their best health and functional independence (Rémond et al., 2015). Zinc is an especially important mineral for cognitive function among older adults, a population of individuals who often experience declining cognitive capacity. Research has indicated that there are sufficient levels of zinc that will enhance cognitive function, with a more pronounced effect on memory and attention. A randomized controlled trial indicated that zinc supplements were useful for certain cognitive functions in older individuals, indicating a potential role in the preservation of cognition during aging. With the commonality of zinc deficiency in the aging population, this is both an issue and a challenge and opportunity for nutrition intervention. Secondly, the complexity of aging and nutritional well-being underscores the need for certain strategies in mineral supplementation, particularly zinc, for improved geriatric outcomes (Maylor et al., 2006). The prioritization of minerals like zinc can thus significantly impact the cognitive well-being of the elderly. Apart from cognitive as well as physical well-being, the implications of mineral ingestion go as far as influencing immune function and overall disease resistance. Such minerals as selenium, iron, and copper not only sustain enzymatic functions but also enhance the immune system, critical in older populations who typically show impaired immunity. Old individuals tend to show increased susceptibility to infection and inflammatory alterations and hence require adequate mineral consumption. The interaction of nutrition status and minerals with the aging immune system highlights the potential use of dietary interventions to avert health complications. Introducing holistic dietary regimens with adequate consumption of minerals can enhance health stability among the elderly, ultimately leading to the prevention of age-related illnesses and longevity. Therefore, constant research and validation of dietetic standards is essential in narrowing mineral requirements particularly for geriatric nutrition (Rémond et al., 2015) (Figure 5.3).

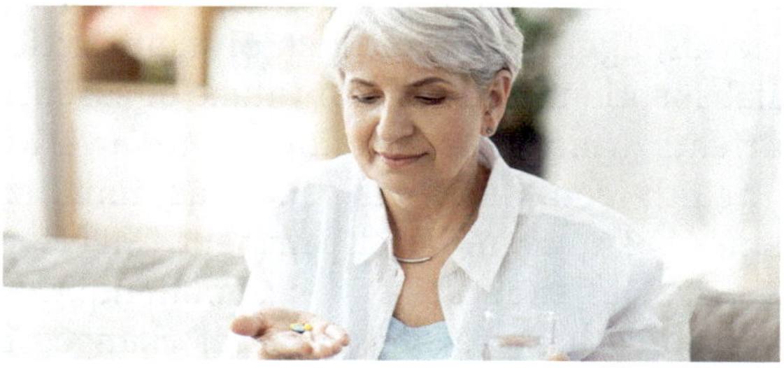

Figure 5.3. Importance of vitamins and minerals in seniors.

Source: https://cdn.megawecare.com/Featured- Images/vRrsaREXzhj 7uy4mNSOru BvI7eV7Q3HhzeRs1sCu.webp.

5.1.2. Impact of Minerals on Overall Health

The role of minerals in the general health of the elderly cannot be taken lightly, as they have a direct influence on various physiological functions. Such necessary minerals are calcium, magnesium, potassium, and zinc, which are engaged in important processes concerning bones, cardiovascular function, and immune protection. In geriatric medicine, an adequate supply of calcium is necessary to prevent osteoporosis, a condition that significantly enhances the risk of fractures. Additionally, magnesium is important for the functioning of muscles and energy metabolism, both of which are necessary for maintaining the mobility and independence of the elderly. Deficiency in these minerals can lead to a decline in health status, eventually impacting not just the physical functions but also the mental states of the elderly. Thus, an integrated approach to mineral needs must be followed to prevent age-related decline in health (Rémond et al., 2015). Moreover, the aging gastrointestinal tract is afflicted with numerous alterations that affect the use and absorption of these nutrients. Since elderly individuals are affected by mechanical as well as functional alterations in the gastrointestinal tract, the ability to assimilate minerals decreases. For instance, reduced gastric acid secretion can hinder the absorption of essential vitamins and minerals, aggravating the risk of malnutrition. Malabsorption leads to poor intake of essential nutrients, which in turn is linked with a variety of health complications, such as impaired immunity and cognitive impairment. Therefore, it is crucial that dietary recommendations accommodate these physiological changes by recommending mineral-based food sources to ensure maximum nutrient delivery and absorption among older adults. Improvement in knowledge of these factors will ensure enhancement in the nutritional status and health of elderly populations (Rémond et al., 2015). Geriatric malnutrition tends to present through a number of different indicators, most commonly the incidence of insufficient mineral consumption, which can significantly impact health outcomes. Evidence suggests that elderly people commonly experience nutritional deficiencies, especially in minerals, which could be related to increased mortality and worse recovery following illness or injury. For instance, a study on elderly hip fracture patients revealed that malnutrition has a strong negative impact on functional outcome, and the most crucial determinant is poor mineral intake. These findings indicate the urgent need for effective nutritional intervention strategies that aim at the inclusion of essential minerals in the diet of the elderly. By treating the consequences of mineral deficiencies and promoting general dietary changes, health care professionals can enhance outcomes for health and reduce the threats associated with malnutrition among older people.

5.1.3. Differences in Mineral Needs Across the Lifespan

During the human life span, mineral needs vary considerably, as is fitting with the changing physiological needs at different stages of life. During infancy and childhood, minerals such as calcium and phosphorus are required for the growth and development of the skeleton. Pregnant and lactating women also need greater mineral intakes, particularly for iron and calcium, to support fetal development and lactation. Conversely, with the onset of adolescence, the demand for minerals continues to increase due to more intense growth and hormonal activity. Notably, the demand for iron arises during menstruation in view of the gender-specific differences in the demands for minerals. These differences show that healthy intake of required minerals is the foundation of health and development at every age of life, providing a basis for nutritional treatments capable of addressing these unique needs effectively. As individuals age further, their mineral needs alter once more, primarily due to physiological factors affecting nutrient absorption and utilization. In the elderly, declining function of the gut microbiome can retard the effectiveness of mineral absorption, making them more susceptible to deficiencies. Iron, calcium, and magnesium are particularly relevant at this age as they play pivotal roles in maintaining healthy bones, functional muscles, and overall metabolic health. In addition, the greater burden of chronic diseases among the elderly population further increases the pace of mineral deficiency occurrence, making the geriatric population in dire need of an in-depth examination of their nutritional requirements. The call for targeted nutritional interventions becomes paramount, making it easier for caregivers and healthcare providers to enhance proper mineral intake to enhance overall quality of life among the geriatric population and thereby meet the specific needs of the group (Rémond et al., 2015). Finally, progress in learning about the needs of minerals in older people emphasizes the importance of specially formulated dietary advice that considers both physical and physiological changes. For example, the greater osteoporosis risk in postmenopausal women at a later age emphasizes the need for greater calcium and vitamin D consumption, which is crucial for bone strength. Similarly, nutrient availability may be undermined by aging, and dietary interventions need to be utilized in order to supply adequate intake levels through well-formulated nutrition. More practical interventions, such as fortified food and supplements tailored particularly for elderly people, can turn around the risk of mineral deficiency and malnutrition. It is a health requirement and a social issue that needs to be addressed since the aging population continues to grow. Hence, geriatric nutrition and policies based on research should take these differences in mineral needs throughout life into account in order to achieve the best possible health in older adults (Lumbis, 2018) (Figure 5.4).

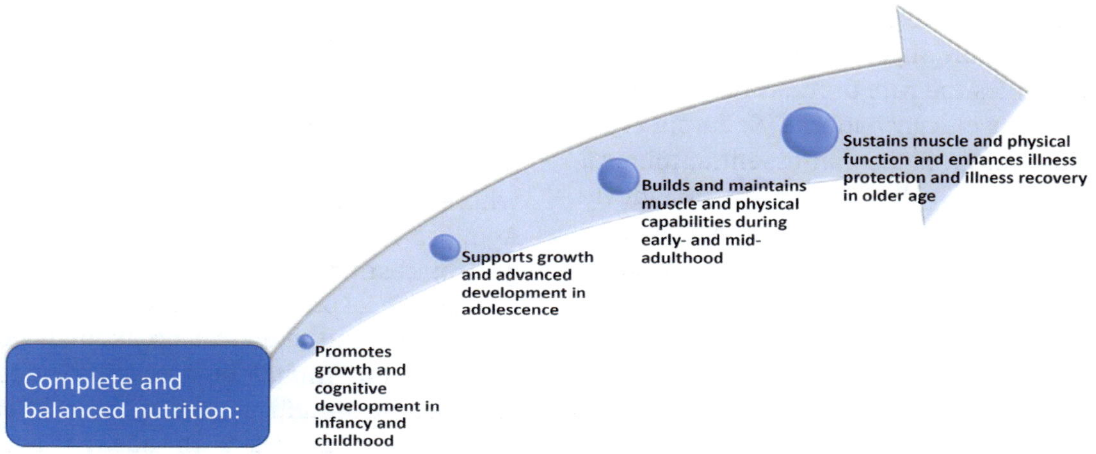

Figure 5.4. Good nutrition across the lifespan foundational for healthy aging.

Source: https://www.frontiersin.org/files/myhome%20article%20library/1113060/1113060_Thumb_400.jpg.

5.2. Common Mineral Deficiencies in the Elderly

Mineral deficiencies among the elderly pose a significant challenge to optimizing overall health and functionality. With age, there are physiological alterations that could impair the ingestion, digestion, and absorption of required nutrients. Precisely, the aging GIT is affected by mechanical and chemical changes that could have a strong impact on nutrient bioavailability. For instance, impaired GIT motility could reduce transit of food, whereas a compromised gastric acid secretory response can impair the digestion of minerals such as calcium and magnesium. This decrease in nutrient absorption can also be responsible for the increasing prevalence of malnutrition among the elderly, which is a risk factor for the onset of a range of chronic diseases in various organ systems (Rémond et al., 2015). As such, detection and correction of such deficiencies become a top priority in the design of effective dietary programs that can improve the nutritional well-being of the elderly. Calcium deficiency is one of the most common mineral deficiencies among older people, and it has intimate associations with osteoporosis and increased fracture risk in elderly people. Adequate calcium intake is not only essential for maintaining bone function but also for proper cardiovascular functioning and muscle contraction. Unfortunately, a majority of elderly individuals fail to achieve the optimal daily intake of calcium, perhaps even more due to dietary restriction or decreased consumption of dairy products and milk. The interaction of such effects as decreased appetite, gum disease issues, and certain medications may worsen this condition and consequently result in decreased levels of calcium. Furthermore, vitamin D deficiency, which plays a significant role in the absorption of calcium, typically aggravates the condition. The decreased ability of old skin to synthesize vitamin D from sun exposure also leads to this condition, creating a double-edged sword that hikes the rate of fractures and other illnesses among elderly patients (Setiarsih et al., 2016). Magnesium is also an essential mineral whose deficit is widely observed in elderly individuals. This mineral is an essential element of numerous biochemical processes, including protein synthesis, muscle and nerve function, and blood glucose maintenance.

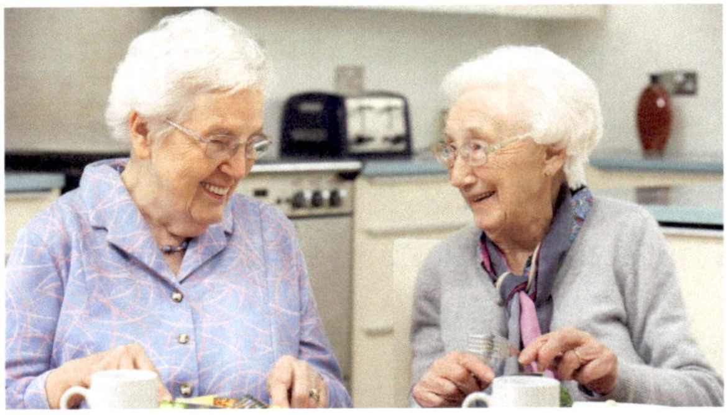

Figure 5.5. Common nutrient deficiencies in the elderly.

Source: https://www.topnoshmeals.com.au/wp-content/uploads/2023/05/image3-edited.jpg.

Deficiency can be due to a shortage of dietary intake or due to the aftereffect of common medications that block magnesium absorption. Symptoms of magnesium deficiency can be quite initially but lead to more forceful consequences such as muscle cramps, mental disease, and cardiovascular disease. Furthermore, interactions between magnesium and other nutrients of significance create a complex interconnection of deficiencies leading to synergistic health hazards. An integrated approach to geriatric nutrition should, therefore, address the importance of adequate intake of magnesium with other nutrients of utmost significance, resulting in better health outcomes for the aged (Rémond et al., 2015; Setiarsih et al., 2016) (Figure 5.5).

5.2.1. Calcium Deficiency and Its Consequences

Calcium has a core role to play in sustaining a large number of physiological processes, particularly in the geriatric population, where the risk of deficiency is heightened. Aging is inherently linked with alterations in gastrointestinal function that adversely affect calcium absorption. With the reduction in gut mechanical and chemical breakdown potential for food, nutritional bioavailability decreases and has profound implications for calcium intake. This decrease in absorption, along with potential dietary deficiencies, increases susceptibility to calcium deficiency in older adults. As such, suboptimal levels of calcium can initiate a number of health complications, from osteoporosis and fractures to further enhancing the quality of life as well as healthcare burdens overall. Therefore, it is necessary to understand the complex association of aging, mineral absorption, and nutritional requirements to meet the unique mineral requirements of aged individuals (Rémond et al., 2015). Also, the manifestations of calcium deficiency are not confined to skeletal health but influence other organ systems as well as overall health. Calcium deficiency may disrupt the parathyroid hormone (PTH) equilibrium, which is responsible for bone remodeling and maintenance. Low calcium levels result in increased secretion of PTH, attempting to maintain serum calcium at homeostasis. This process, however, can result in increased bone turnover, which is detrimental in older adults. There is some evidence that elevated levels of 1,25-dihydroxyvitamin D

(1,25(OH)2D), along with decreased levels of 25-hydroxyvitamin D (25(OH)D), also play a role in poorer bone density and increased fracture risk, as seen in studies among middle-aged and older adults (Akhter et al., 2013). Consequently, calcium deficiency pathophysiology becomes entwined with the dynamics of vitamin D metabolism, indicating the necessity to address the nutritional requirements of the elderly as a whole. Considering these features, addressing the calcium deficiency in the elderly should involve a multidimensional solution that includes food modifications and potential supplementation. Nutritional counseling should aim at calcium-rich foods of high digestibility, in line with functional changes of the aging gastrointestinal tract. In this manner, the intake of nutrients is optimized and malnutrition risk is minimized. Also, healthcare professionals must pay attention to the unique calcium requirements of the elderly; therefore individualized nutritional counseling should consider special needs and comorbidities. Regular monitoring of calcium and vitamin D levels can proactively manage deficiencies, thereby strengthening the bones and nutritional health of the aged (Rémond et al., 2015). Comprehensive interventions through education, nutritional care, and medical management can effectively go a long way in avoiding the dangers caused by the deficiency of calcium among the aging population (Figure 5.6).

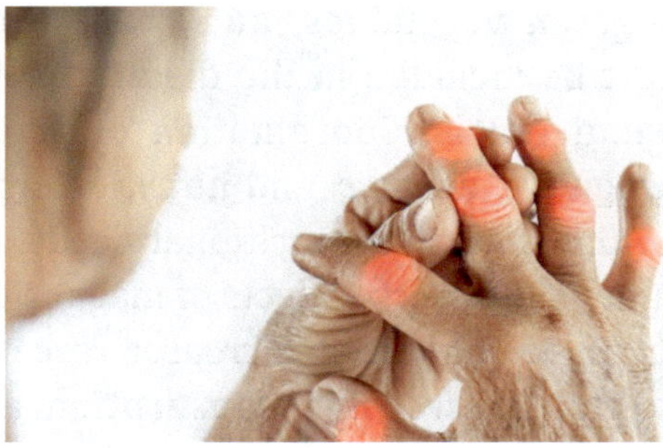

Figure 5.6. Calcium deficiency.

Source: https://ceylontoday.lk/wp-content/uploads/2025/05/2-detail-main-Calcium-Deficiency-1.jpeg.

5.2.2. Iron Deficiency and Anemia in Older Adults

Iron deficiency and anemia are severe nutritional problems in elderly populations, compromising their overall health and quality of life. With aging, the physiological changes in the gastrointestinal tract can compromise the absorption of nutrients, including iron. With declining gastrointestinal function, food mechanical and biochemical digestion becomes less effective, leading to inadequate nutrient intake and increased risk of malnutrition. Older people are most likely to develop iron deficiency against this backdrop, coupled with lifestyle factors such as dietary restriction, chronic illness, and polypharmacy that compromise their nutritional profile.

Addressing these challenges calls for comprehensive dietary interventions that consider the uniqueness of aging and loss of gastrointestinal function (Rémond et al., 2015). Anemia prevalence among the elderly is a significant concern, especially with loss of cognitive ability and life quality. Research has shown that the vast majority of the elderly population suffers from both iron deficiency anemia and vitamin deficiencies, such as folate and vitamin B12. A discussion of the correlation between anemia and intellectual functioning among elderly people showed that low hemoglobin in this age group was often accompanied by impaired cognitive functioning.

In the study under discussion, 22.9% of the population exhibited anemia, 5.7% being found to have iron deficiency anemia (Alim et al., 2005). The findings highlight the critical role played by iron levels in maintaining cognitive health, informing the need for targeted nutritional interventions to reverse the threats posed by anemia and promote mental vitality in older individuals. Remedial measures to improve iron levels and reverse anemia must be multi-disciplinary, including dietary recommendations alongside educational initiatives for older citizens. Encouragement of consumption of iron-containing foods such as lean meat, beans, lentils, and fortified cereals is essential in order to enhance iron intake. Furthermore, the inclusion of foods rich in vitamin C will significantly enhance iron absorption, providing a twin approach in the fight against deficiency. Given the major contribution of malnutrition towards changing the health of older adults, it is essential that they have biomarkers that can effectively assess dietary intake and nutrient status. Such interventions will not only give better health results but also help formulate individualized nutrition advice that may counter the functional impairments associated with aging (Rémond et al., 2015). Preemptive intervention for iron deficiency and anemia can make the geriatric population experience better health and quality of life.

5.2.3. Magnesium Deficiency and Health Implications

The clinical consequence of magnesium deficiency in the elderly is profound, with major effects on numerous physiological systems. Magnesium plays a critical role in numerous biochemical processes, including energy metabolism, protein synthesis, and muscle function, so adequacy is crucial to health in older adults. Because aging often is associated with changes in diet and nutrient utilization, individuals may be particularly vulnerable to deficiency. This insufficiency can lead to a chain reaction of health disorders, such as cardiovascular disease, osteoporosis, and neuromuscular diseases. Magnesium insufficiency's occurrence is even more deserving of attention because elderly individuals also often have multiple comorbid conditions that increase the risk of malnutrition, in accordance with findings showing that geriatric malnutrition is much more common than was previously thought and may add to increased health care costs as well as decreased quality of life (Agarwal et al., 2016). Moreover, the old gastrointestinal system could be another piece of the puzzle for difficulty in absorbing magnesium. Anatomical and functional decline within the digestive apparatus can slow nutrient absorption, including magnesium, leading to deficiency when dietary levels are insufficient. These changes of the gastrointestinal tract encompass decreased motility, altered secretion of digestive enzymes, and disturbed transport of nutrients through intestinal walls, all of which are of concern for nutrient bioavailability (Rémond et al., 2015). For such reasons, its detection and treatment are significant in geriatric nutrition because deficiency of this mineral can enhance other health problems that come with aging, including immune dysregulation and increased susceptibility to chronic diseases.

The management of targeted dietary regimens and nutritional screening has the ability to identify high-risk patients and direct appropriate magnesium intake. Overall, the management of magnesium deficiency as it exists within the context of geriatric nutrition is not only a possible means of improved individual health outcome but also a window to improve overall quality of life in the elderly population. Specific nutrient guidelines, for example, food sources of magnesium like leafy green vegetables, nuts, and whole grains, must be included in the dietary advice for aged individuals. Coordination of action among caregivers, doctors, and nutritionists is necessary to ensure that nutritional needs are met, and thus, the adverse effects of magnesium deficiency can be minimized. Increased research regarding biomarkers of malabsorption and undernutrition is also essential to institute effective interventions. By focusing on magnesium's role in the health of aging, we can facilitate a healthier aged population (Agarwal et al., 2016; Rémond et al., 2015) (Figure 5.7).

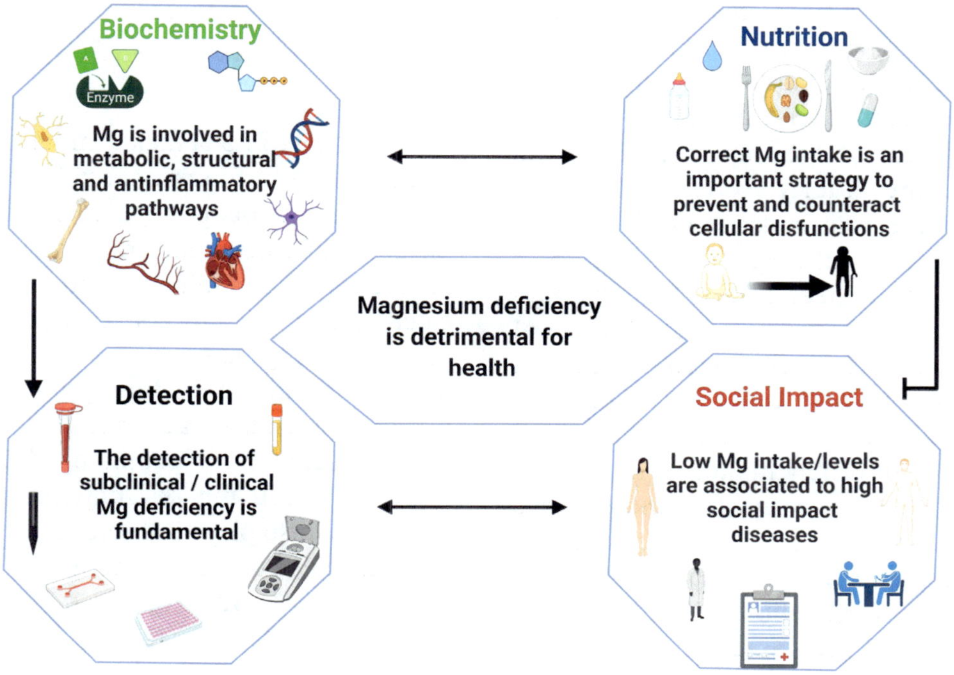

Figure 5.7. Magnesium: Biochemistry, nutrition, detection, and social impact of diseases linked to its deficiency.

Source: https://www.mdpi.com/2072-6643/13/4/1136#.

5.3. Recommended Daily Allowances (RDAs) for Geriatric Minerals

RDAs of minerals in older adults are important in maintaining overall health and minimizing widespread deficiencies associated with aging. With increasing age, alterations in physiology and nutrition can profoundly influence mineral intake and absorption. For instance, calcium and vitamin D are important in maintaining bone strength in the elderly, as impaired bone density leads to a higher frequency of fractures and osteoporosis. The RDAs suggest that older adults aim to consume approximately 1,200 mg of calcium and 800–1,000 IU of vitamin D daily to support bone strength. Other minerals such as magnesium, potassium, and zinc are also important for many bodily functions, such as muscle function, blood pressure regulation, and immune status. Proper levels of these minerals can play a large role in influencing outcomes and quality of life in this group. Iron and B vitamins are also significant in geriatric nutrition, particularly for energy level and cognitive status. Iron deficiency anemia is prevalent among the elderly, and it may compromise cognitive function and general well-being. The RDAs recommend a daily intake of at least 8 mg for men and 18 mg for women, reflecting varying needs on the basis of sex and physiologic factors. At the same time, micronutrients such as folate and vitamin B12 are significant as deficiency due to malabsorption could impair cognitive health. In one study determining cognitive impairment among elderly individuals, nearly 34.3% presented subclinical deficiency in folate, while several had vitamin B12 deficiency at a low level, predisposing them to cognitive impairment (Alim et al.,

2005). Keeping these problems in view, active nutritional assessment and interventions are essential to meet the unique mineral needs of the elderly population with maximum support for their physical as well as mental health. Agencies like the Elderly Nutrition Program (ENP) play a vital role in assisting in meeting such mineral needs through the provision of healthy meals that meet RDAs. The program effectively increases participants' intake of necessary nutrients, with improved overall dietary quality among the aged. Research indicates that participants in nutrition meal programs have noticeably higher mean intakes of all crucial minerals, except for zinc, on days when they are involved in such programs (Lin et al., 1999). While the nutritional gains are significant, the majority of participants' intakes remain below the recommended intake for minerals like vitamin D, calcium, and zinc. This illustrates the requirement for coupled nutrition education and encouragement of older adults towards the choice of mineral-rich foods beyond their meal program. Strategies improving awareness and facilitation of nutrient-dense foods in the household can further enhance the efficacy of planned programs, ultimately improving geriatric health outcomes (Figure 5.8).

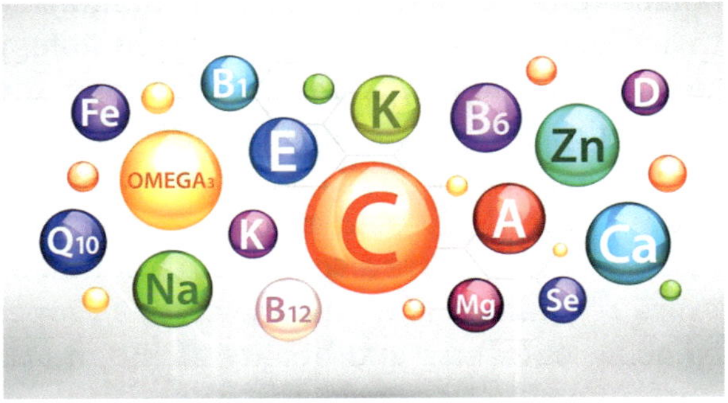

Figure 5.8. Recommended dietary allowances.

Source: https://cdn.shopify.com/s/files/1/0245/0722/0064/files/RDA_large.jpeg?v=1582174832.

5.3.1. Overview of Recommended Dietary Allowances (RDAs) for Key Minerals

Knowing the RDAs of major minerals is essential in fulfilling the nutritional needs of the aging population. As people age, there is a change in physiological need, and the body's capacity to absorb and utilize minerals reduces. Specifically, calcium and vitamin D are of pivotal concern in maintaining bone health, and RDAs suggest higher intake for aging persons to avoid osteoporosis and fractures. For instance, the RDA for calcium for people aged 51 years and above is 1,200 mg per day. Magnesium and potassium also play vital roles in cardiovascular and musculoskeletal health, so their RDAs are equally vital at 320 mg and 4,700 mg per day, respectively. It is essential that the elderly achieve these standards to prevent disease and maintain overall health. Iron is another critical mineral whose RDA has to be addressed with serious consideration in the older adult. Impaired absorption of iron and potential dietary inadequacy can lead to anemia in the elderly, exacerbate cognitive impairment, and affect quality of life. The RDA for iron in adult men is 8 mg, while women require 18 mg until menopause, after which their requirement goes down to 8 mg per day. The relationship between mental alertness and iron levels has been documented, with studies indicating that subclinical deficiency impacts mental alertness (Alim et al., 2005). Iron's function goes beyond simple hematological markers, bridging food intake to overall cognitive status. As such, it is critical to monitor and correct iron intake in this age group for the optimization of health outcomes and protection of cognitive status in geriatric populations. Zinc, an element that is crucial for many biochemical mechanisms, has gained attention within the realm of geriatric nutrition as a result of its bearing on cognitive status. Research has indicated that adequate zinc intake can be linked to improved memory and attention skills (Maylor et al., 2006). The

RDA for older adults for zinc is 11 mg for males and 8 mg for females, but there are numerous individuals who are not achieving these levels. Zinc deficiencies have been found to inhibit immune function as well as cognitive processes, and therefore, dietary change or supplementation is necessary in some people. The implications of zinc status on the health of older people need to be explored further, particularly for those with suboptimal mineral intake or underlying medical conditions that exacerbate deficiencies. Attainment of these mineral RDAs from an integrated perspective can help health workers better support the nutritional needs and well-being of the aging population.

5.3.2. Variations in Mineral Needs Based on Gender and Age

The age- and gender-related differences in mineral needs are part of the contributory factors in the determination of nutritional requirements in the elderly. With advancing age, physiological and metabolic functions of the body alter, and in the process, it also alters its mineral use and absorption efficiency. For example, the older population needs more diets of minerals such as calcium and magnesium for maintaining bones. Gender is also of primary significance, since postmenopausal women are more susceptible to osteoporosis due to decreased estrogen production, which in turn raises their need for calcium. Hence, identification of the individual mineral requirements of various genders is an important component in creating dietary guidelines for the geriatric population so that both men and women receive adequate nutrients to combat threats of age-related disorders. The efficiency of mineral absorption is also compromised by the alterations in the gastrointestinal system caused by aging, and these alterations also introduce additional barriers to providing nutrients. As highlighted in current studies, the aged gastrointestinal system exhibits decreased motility and alterations in digestive enzymes, resulting in impairment in the ability of the older population to absorb necessary minerals. This decrease in absorptive capability may then lead to the development of malnutrition, particularly in combination with poor dietary intake. Particularly, minerals like iron and zinc, which are necessary for immune functioning and overall health, can become sub optimally absorbed. Regulation of these variations in mineral need requires not only information regarding individual nutritional status but also techniques considering the age-related changes in gastrointestinal functionality (Rémond et al., 2015). Besides, the potential risk of sarcopenia in older individuals renders minerals important in maintaining muscle function and preventing functional loss. Sarcopenia is defined as muscle loss and weakening, which could compromise the capacity to carry out everyday activities. Research indicates that adequate consumption of minerals, including essential nutrients such as calcium and vitamin D, is essential for muscle function and maintenance of muscle mass (Burton & Sumukadas, 2010).

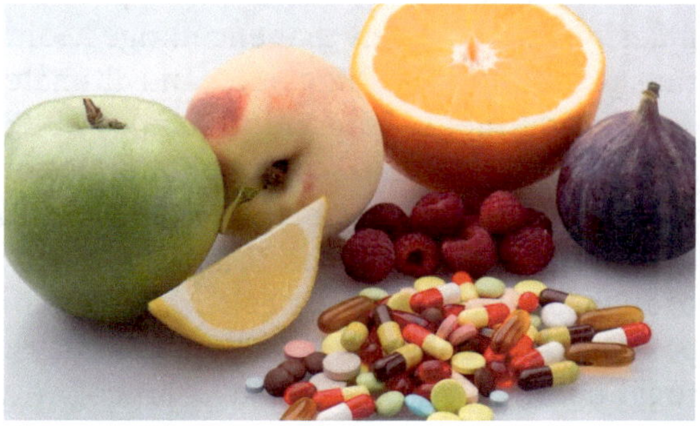

Figure 5.9. Does age or gender affect vitamin and mineral requirements.

Source: https://www.fitpaa.com/wp-content/uploads/2023/10/Untitled-design-2023-10-09T171648.109-jpg.webp.

Thus, not only are geriatric patients in need of changes in mineral intake based on age and gender, but nutritional interventions must also take these into account in order to help maintain overall muscular health. Not only does this help correct for mineral insufficiency, but enhances physical functioning in geriatric patients who are coping with the challenges of aging (Figure 5.9).

5.3.3. Importance of Consulting Healthcare Providers for Personalized Recommendations

Consultation with healthcare providers for personalized dietary advice plays a crucial role, particularly for elderly people who have unique nutritional problems. As a person grows older, their physiology changes in many different ways, affecting nutrient absorption and metabolism, particularly minerals. Healthcare providers can offer personalized advice based on these changes and assist geriatric patients in receiving their specific mineral requirements. An individualized approach is also supported by the realization that diet barriers among older adults may significantly differ depending on sociocultural, financial, and health factors. With a clear identification of such barriers, providers can design interventions that encourage healthy eating, prevent dietary difficulties, and ultimately enhance wellness (Bigando et al., 2023). Additionally, personalized recommendations from healthcare professionals extend beyond mere dietary suggestions, encompassing a thorough analysis of the health condition of a person. Different elderly individuals may be struggling with chronic disease or cognitive impairments, factors that make their nutritional requirements more challenging to meet. Interventions for frailty under combined care systems point out how powerful evaluation must take into consideration physical as well as psychological factors affecting nutrition. By using personalized dietary modifications based on medical evaluations, health care providers can ensure that their recommendations are in tune with the unique needs of each geriatric patient. Not only does this improve mineral intake, but it also results in better health outcomes and improved quality of life among the elderly (Uchmanowicz et al., 2025). Besides that, the role of a healthcare provider is not limited to first visits; ongoing consultation is an integral part of the adaptive needs of older patients. Nutrition is not static and varies with time due to numerous factors like changes in physical condition, drug-induced side effects, and personal preferences. Regular follow-ups with health practitioners allow for alterations in nutritional counsel, forming a dynamic and effective nutrition program. This proactive approach is critical in the prevention of deficiency and addressing future health complications as they arise. By establishing a patient-provider partnership relationship, an all-encompassing framework can be created that promotes maximum mineral intake and overall nutritional health in the geriatric population (Bigando et al., 2023; Uchmanowicz et al., 2025).

5.4. Sources of Essential Minerals

In geriatric nutrition, knowledge of sources of essential minerals is significant to ensure proper health among the elderly. These minerals, like calcium, magnesium, and potassium, play crucial roles in various physiological functions, including bone health, muscle contraction, and fluid balance. All these essential minerals occur abundantly in foods such as dairy, leafy green vegetables, nuts, and whole grains. For instance, milk is a dense source of calcium that is important for bone strength and the avoidance of osteoporosis, which is common among the elderly. By emphasizing such nutrient-dense foods, caregivers and nutritionists can also minimize the chances of deficiencies that are likely to arise from inadequate dietary intake, thus promoting healthier aging among the elderly. Therefore, a well-balanced diet that includes a diversity of mineral-fortified foods is a core component of geriatric nutrition plans. Throughout the process of aging, physiological changes may influence mineral digestion and metabolism, and thus, the nutritional status in the elderly becomes more intricate. Gastrointestinal alterations such as reduced gastric acid secretion and diminished enzymatic activity affect the body's digestion capacity and ability to absorb nutrients, exacerbating the risk of malnutrition among the elderly (Rémond et al., 2015). The alterations necessitate re-evaluation of dietary guidelines to address the unique requirements of this group. It is crucial that medical professionals provide dietary recommendations individualized to deliver sufficient quantities of minerals in the elderly through dietary sources and supplementary methods where required. It is also crucial in the development of effective dietary regimens to promote improved mineral absorption, therefore improving geriatric health and quality of life to offset the functional decline of the aging gastrointestinal system. The overlap of information regarding food sources of trace minerals and physiological alterations at advanced ages can result in comprehensive approaches in geriatric nutrition. Additionally, minerals like selenium and zinc responsible for immune function and wound healing, are commonly overlooked in older diets. Seashore food, pulses, and seeds are good sources of these trace minerals and need to be incorporated into the diet regularly. Educating older people and their caregivers about the nature and value of these food sources can empower them to make effective food choices. Additionally, since malnutrition is increasingly gaining recognition as a leading geriatric care issue (Lumbis, 2018), highlighting the intake of primary minerals through nutritious and flavorful foods can go a long way in mitigating risks of nutrient inadequacy/. With strategic planning for diet, practitioners can ensure that older people can achieve a balanced diet to enhance their health and life expectancy.

5.4.1. Dietary Sources of Calcium

Calcium is an important mineral that is vital for the maintenance of bone health, particularly in the elderly age group, who are at risk of osteoporosis and other bone disorders. Sources of calcium in foods are milk, leafy green vegetables, fish with bones, and fortified foods. Dairy foods such as milk, yogurt, and cheese are also among the most concentrated sources since they are extremely bioavailable in calcium. Leafy green vegetables such as kale and collard greens also provide calcium to the diet, although their concomitant oxalates will block absorption. Certain fish, such as sardines and salmon, also offer calcium together with healthy omega-3 fatty acids. Fortified foods, including some of these orange juice and cereals, are excellent alternatives for people who are lactose intolerant or have vegetarian diets. Ensuring adequate intake of these foods from the varied sources is crucial to ensuring bone health in older individuals. With age, nutrient absorption capacity, including calcium, can be compromised due to changes in the physiology of the gastrointestinal tract. Aging changes in digestion result in older people potentially failing to meet their requirements for calcium via dietary means alone, which increases the risk of deficiency. With an aging gastrointestinal system, there is decreased efficiency in the metabolic breakdown and absorption of key nutrients, which could increase the significance of intake of foods containing calcium. Research has indicated that a hyper-phosphorus diet combined with a low calcium-to-phosphorus ratio has a tendency to worsen the bone condition in the elderly. The situation, therefore, necessitates adequate planning of diets from the interactions of minerals. It is therefore essential to encourage older adults to prioritize calcium foods while regulating their total phosphorus intake. Attention to these food relationships is imperative for reducing osteoporosis risk and promoting overall health in older adults (Summers et al., 2020). In addition, access to calcium foods can be hindered by economic and social factors, which impact the nutritional status of the older adult. Malnutrition among this population is not only determined by body needs, i.e., the inability to chew or swallow, but also by mental impairment that will affect food preparation and food selection. Supplying older adults with information and access to choose and utilize sources of calcium from food becomes paramount in addressing these issues. Strategies such as educating people on the cooking preparation of leafy green vegetables, selecting fortified foods, and encouraging the consumption of dairy will enhance the consumption of calcium. Developing community efforts supportive of grocery shopping access or meal delivery can be an important intervention in mitigating these barriers. Balanced dietary suggestions that consider the specific needs of older people can contribute significantly to better well-being and prevention of malnutrition caused by insufficient consumption of calcium (Rémond et al., 2015).

5.4.2. Iron-Rich Foods Suitable for Older Adults

The nutritional needs of older people demand careful prioritization of iron-rich foods, which are essential to maintain well-being and prevent malnutrition. With increasing age, the capacity for nutrient absorption declines due to various physiological changes in the digestive system, decreasing iron bioavailability. The loss increases the likelihood of iron deficiency anemia and requires the diet to include good sources of iron. Lean red meat, poultry, and fish provide heme iron, which is better absorbed than non-heme iron found in vegetables. It, therefore, follows that an effective approach targeting animal and plant sources of iron can counter the nutritional needs of the elderly population towards improved health status and reduction of malnutrition vulnerability as stipulated in the research findings of Rémond et al. (2015). Other than animal iron, some legumes and leafy greens play an important role in the boost in the elderly's intake of iron too. For example, lentils, chickpeas, and spinach are not only rich in iron but also in fiber, as well as other nutrients crucial to good digestive health. With the addition of foods containing much vitamin C, such as citrus fruits or bell peppers, along with such plant sources, the utilization of non-heme iron is encouraged, which can rectify any such lack in the diet. By this synergistic action, the required amounts of iron are maintained in elderly individuals while they benefit otherwise by a diversified diet for nutritional health. The need for nutritional therapy aimed at preventing malnutrition underscores the importance of considering not only the quality of nutrients and the functionality of the food consumed by older people, in harmony with the results presented in Rémond et al. (2015), but also its role as a provider of iron, which cannot be overlooked in the field of geriatric nutrition. Poultry flesh is particularly helpful since it not only provides quality protein but also contains essential B vitamins as well as minerals, including iron, zinc, and copper. Poultry is more easily digested and contains less collagen than red meat, so it could be easier for older adults who have dental or gastrointestinal issues. Epidemiological studies indicate that the consumption of poultry in a nutritious diet is connected with different health benefits, including reduced obesity and chronic disease risk, prevalent among older adults. As highlighted in the literature, food containing iron like poultry, in a sufficient diet, increases the nutritional status of older people and improves the health condition of the elderly, as established in.

5.4.3. Foods High in Magnesium and Their Benefits

In the context of the elderly's nutrition, it is essential that one is aware of foods high in magnesium and their associated advantages to enhance the quality and well-being of the elderly. Leafy green vegetables, legumes, nuts, seeds, and whole grains are rich in magnesium. These foods, while being high in magnesium, a vital part of many physiological processes, also provide significant nutrients that have the capability to reverse the diminished physiological function typically experienced in aging. As the failing gastrointestinal tract in older people may be faced with decreased efficiency in nutrient absorption, the addition of foods high in magnesium can help reduce the risk of malnutrition and promote better general well-being in older generations. Meeting these dietary needs becomes especially important, as magnesium deficiency has been linked to adverse health effects, including osteoporosis and cardiovascular disease, which are prevalent in elderly people (Rémond et al., 2015). Magnesium is important for bone density and health, particularly for elderly individuals who are at higher risk for developing osteoporosis. Aging adults often suffer from a natural loss of bone mineral density that puts them at risk for fractures and other musculoskeletal issues. Incorporating magnesium-enriched foods such as almonds, spinach, and black beans into their diets not only provides their bodies with the mineral required for the maintenance of bones but also helps their bodies to absorb calcium, a key mineral for bone maintenance. Apart from this, the role of magnesium in protein synthesis and the regulation of muscle function is instrumental in ensuring the maintenance of mobility and physical functioning in older individuals. By default, promotion of the consumption of foods that are high in magnesium can go a long way in assisting in the preservation of functional capacity and overall quality of life in older individuals (Feskens et al., 2022). Additionally, the neuroprotective effects of magnesium must be addressed when planning a geriatric diet. It has been discovered through studies that adequate magnesium consumption can be beneficial in mitigating cognitive impairment typically found among older people and may decrease the risk for neurodegenerative diseases such as Alzheimer's. Avocados, dark chocolate, and whole grains can be employed to enhance magnesium content, and they can correct mood equilibrium and cognitive function. Moreover, magnesium has a calming effect on the nervous system that alleviates symptoms of depression and anxiety, diseases that tend to be common among the elderly. With the aging population and being exposed to intricate health complications, proper supplementation with magnesium through diet becomes an essential measure in guaranteeing mental well-being and cognitive resilience, thereby translating to healthier aging (Feskens et al., 2022).

5.5. The Impact of Medications on Mineral Absorption

The relationship between medications and mineral absorption is particularly critical in geriatric nutrition, as older adults frequently manage chronic conditions that necessitate the use of pharmacological interventions. Many commonly prescribed medications can interfere with the gastrointestinal (GI) tract's ability to absorb essential minerals, resulting in nutritional deficiencies that can exacerbate existing health issues. For instance, certain antacids that contain aluminum or magnesium may bind to dietary minerals such as calcium, iron, and phosphorus, ultimately impairing their bioavailability. Additionally, medications such as proton pump inhibitors (PPIs) and H2 receptor antagonists, which are used to treat acid-related disorders, have been shown to alter gastric acidity, thereby impacting the solubility and absorption of minerals like magnesium and zinc. As malnutrition poses significant risks to the elderly population, understanding these interactions is essential for developing effective dietary strategies that mitigate the impact of medications on mineral absorption (Rémond et al., 2015). Further complicating the relationship between medication use and mineral absorption is the growing body of evidence that highlights the age-related decline in gastrointestinal function. The aging GI tract naturally undergoes various changes that affect digestive processes, including decreased motility and altered enzyme secretion, which can diminish nutrient absorption capacity. Therefore, when combined with the effects of certain medications, these age-related changes can significantly increase the risk of micronutrient deficiencies in older adults. For instance, malabsorption of essential minerals can arise not only from direct drug-nutrient interactions or altered gastric pH levels but also from other aging-related dysfunctions. Moreover, a decline in the overall health status of older adults often leads to decreased dietary intake, further exacerbating deficiencies that can stem from both medications and the aging process itself (Maylor et al., 2006).

Furthermore, specific cases highlight the importance of monitoring mineral status in elderly patients undergoing pharmacological treatment. Research demonstrates that zinc supplementation, for example, may play a role in enhancing cognitive functions in older adults, yet its efficacy can be influenced by concurrent medication use, which could either enhance or antagonize its absorption. In a double-blind study focused on cognitive function in older adults, zinc showed positive effects on working memory and attention; however, these benefits were also accompanied by undesired interactions with certain dosages of the supplement. Implications for clinical practice underscore the necessity of scrutinizing medication regimens in geriatric patients to identify potential interactions that could adversely impact mineral status. Ultimately, more comprehensive approaches that integrate dietary assessments and medication management can optimize mineral absorption and support overall nutritional health in the elderly (Rémond et al., 2015).

5.5.1. Common Medications Affecting Mineral Absorption

The interaction between medications and the absorption of essential minerals is a critical area of concern in geriatric nutrition. Many elderly individuals are prescribed medications for chronic conditions such as hypertension, diabetes, and arthritis, which can inadvertently affect mineral absorption in the gastrointestinal tract. For instance, proton pump inhibitors (PPIs), commonly used to manage acid reflux and gastritis, can significantly reduce the absorption of important minerals like calcium and magnesium. This reduction is largely due to the decreased stomach acidity, which is necessary for optimal absorption of these minerals. As aging individuals often face altered gastrointestinal functionality, the interaction between medications and nutrient absorption becomes a vital consideration in their dietary management and overall health. Another common category of medications impacting mineral absorption comprises diuretics, frequently prescribed for heart failure and hypertension. While diuretics are effective in managing fluid retention, they can also lead to increased urinary excretion of vital minerals, particularly potassium and magnesium. The depletion of these minerals can have serious consequences, including muscle weakness, arrhythmias, and overall decline in health status, especially among older adults who may already be at a high risk for mineral deficiencies. With the elderly population facing both the challenges of aging and medication side effects, understanding the ramifications of these interactions is essential. Adequate medical oversight is thus imperative to balance the therapeutic benefits of these medications with their potential nutritional downsides. In light of these interactions, it is crucial for healthcare professionals to develop a comprehensive approach to the dietary and nutritional needs of older adults. Tailored dietary guidelines should map out the impact of common medications on mineral absorption, striving to mitigate malnutrition risks linked to both pharmacological treatments and physiological changes. Interventions might include targeted mineral supplementation or modifications in diet to enhance the bioavailability of key nutrients. Moreover, continuous monitoring and adjustment of medication regimens may be necessary to prevent nutrient depletion, ultimately leading to better health outcomes for the geriatric population. Given the increasing prevalence of malnutrition in this age group, it is vital to integrate nutrition management within the larger framework of geriatric care to ensure optimal health and quality of life for elderly patients (Cheung et al., 2013; Rémond et al., 2015).

5.5.2. Strategies to Mitigate Absorption Issues

Addressing the nutritional needs of the geriatric population necessitates a comprehensive understanding of strategies aimed at mitigating absorption issues. One significant approach involves tailored dietary modifications that account for the inherent physiological changes in the aging gastrointestinal tract, which include reduced motility and altered digestion. Consequently, the incorporation of easily digestible foods, such as those high in soluble fiber and low in fat, can facilitate smoother digestion and absorption of essential nutrients. Furthermore, small, frequent meals can be beneficial, as they lessen the burden on an aging digestive system and enhance nutrient bioavailability. This notion is particularly crucial, as effective absorption directly influences the overall health status of elderly individuals, potentially reducing the risk of malnutrition, which is increasingly prevalent in this demographic (Rémond et al., 2015). In conjunction with dietary strategies, the utilization of nutritional supplementation can play a pivotal role in compensating for the declining absorption capacity observed in geriatric populations. Specific attention should be directed towards micronutrient and macronutrient supplementation tailored to individual needs. For instance, supplements containing vital minerals such as calcium, magnesium, and vitamin D could be essential for addressing deficiencies that commonly arise in older adults. Additionally, the timing of supplementation can enhance its effectiveness; administering certain nutrients alongside meals may promote better absorption compared to isolated intake. Healthcare providers should conduct regular assessments to identify at-risk individuals and develop personalized supplementation plans, ultimately fortifying their nutritional status and reducing the incidence of associated health complications (Agarwal et al., 2016). Moreover, fostering a supportive environment that emphasizes both psychological and social factors can significantly enhance nutrient absorption in older adults. Engaging elderly individuals in social dining experiences can stimulate appetite and improve food intake, mitigating malnutrition risks. Furthermore, employing multidisciplinary teams to regularly monitor nutritional status and implementing educational programs on healthy eating practices can empower the elderly to make informed dietary choices. Such initiatives should also aim to educate caregivers about the unique nutritional requirements of older individuals and the importance of consistent nutrition screening. By creating a holistic support system encompassing proper dietary planning, monitoring, and social reinforcement, the likelihood of absorption issues can be significantly reduced, thereby enhancing the overall well-being of the aging population (Rémond et al., 2015).

5.5.3. Importance of Discussing Medications with Healthcare Professionals

The discussion of medications with healthcare professionals is a critical aspect of geriatric nutrition, particularly concerning the mineral requirements of older adults. As age-related physiological changes can significantly impact nutrient absorption and metabolism, healthcare professionals need to evaluate how various medications might interact with dietary minerals. Certain medications, for instance, can hinder the absorption of essential minerals such as calcium and magnesium, which are crucial for bone health and neuromuscular function. Understanding these interactions helps healthcare providers tailor nutritional advice and recommend dietary adjustments that mitigate potential deficiencies. Furthermore, by engaging in conversations about prescribed medications, older adults can voice their concerns and preferences, enabling a more personalized approach to their nutritional care. Additionally, discussing medications allows healthcare professionals to address polypharmacy, a common concern among the elderly. With many older adults taking multiple medications to manage various chronic conditions, there is a heightened risk for adverse drug interactions that may influence mineral status. For example, diuretics are often used to manage hypertension, but they can lead to increased excretion of potassium and magnesium, resulting in imbalances that adversely affect overall health. By advocating for open communication regarding medication regimens, healthcare providers can help ensure that patients receive appropriate guidance on managing their mineral intake. This collaborative approach not only mitigates risks associated with polypharmacy but also supports the broader aim of improving nutritional status in older populations, aligning with the recommendations for optimizing geriatric nutrition outlined in recent clinical guidelines (Volkert et al., 2019). Incorporating discussions about medications into routine healthcare practices fosters a more comprehensive approach to geriatric nutrition. Engaging older adults in conversations about their medications can reveal specific barriers to adequate mineral intake, such as side effects that deter proper nutrition. Furthermore, such discussions can enhance medication adherence by reinforcing the importance of nutrition in achieving health outcomes. Healthcare professionals, therefore, play a vital role in educating older patients about the implications of their medications on nutritional needs. As evidenced by guidelines emphasizing the necessity of individualized care (Volkert et al., 2019), these conversations become instrumental in tailoring nutritional interventions aimed at enhancing the well-being of older adults. By prioritizing these discussions, healthcare providers can implement effective strategies that address the unique nutritional needs of their patients, ultimately leading to improved health outcomes in the geriatric population.

5.6. Nutritional Strategies for Meeting Mineral Needs

Effective nutritional strategies for meeting mineral needs in geriatric populations must account for the unique physiological changes that occur with aging. As individuals age, their ability to absorb minerals can diminish due to altered gastrointestinal function and changes in metabolism. This necessitates careful planning of dietary intake to ensure adequate levels of essential minerals such as calcium, magnesium, and potassium. Incorporating a variety of nutrient-dense foods, including leafy greens, nuts, seeds, and dairy products, can help to meet these mineral requirements. Furthermore, fortifying foods with necessary minerals or utilizing supplements may also play a crucial role, particularly when dietary intake alone cannot meet the recommended daily allowances. By tailoring nutritional strategies to enhance mineral bioavailability, health professionals can help mitigate deficiencies that may detrimentally affect the quality of life in older adults. In combating malnutrition, particularly protein-energy malnutrition, it is vital to implement comprehensive approaches within community and residential aged care settings. Many elderly individuals face multi-morbidity challenges that complicate their nutritional status, leading to increased susceptibility to mineral deficiencies (Agarwal et al., 2016). Therefore, establishing routine nutrition screening and assessments in these environments is essential to identify at-risk individuals. Once malnutrition is detected, appropriate interventions can be deployed, such as introducing enriched foods and enhancing meal appeal through culinary modifications. This involves collaboration among caregivers, dietitians, and healthcare providers to ensure that elderly individuals receive balanced meals that meet their mineral and overall nutritional needs. By prioritizing these coordinated efforts, facilities can substantially improve the health outcomes of their residents and promote better dietary habits that support longevity. Finally, educational initiatives for both caregivers and the elderly are critical in understanding the importance of minerals in maintaining functional status and overall well-being. Care providers should receive training on the nutritional needs of the geriatric population, emphasizing the impact of mineral intake on common age-related health issues, such as bone density and cardiovascular health. Additionally, engaging elderly individuals in discussions around their food preferences and nutritional needs can lead to improved dietary compliance and satisfaction. Tools such as meal planning guides and interactive workshops can empower older adults to make informed food choices that align with their mineral requirements. By fostering an environment of awareness and support, communities can bridge the gap between nutritional knowledge and actual dietary practices, thereby addressing the mineral needs of geriatric individuals effectively (Lumbis, 2018).

5.6.1. Meal Planning for Balanced Mineral Intake

The best meal planning can ensure balanced mineral intake in elderly people, whose nutritional requirements are generally different than those of other age groups. As age advances, dietary needs undergo a shift that necessitates increased focus on specific minerals such as calcium, magnesium, and potassium. Calcium intake becomes significant in the aged, particularly, as it is involved with maintaining bone health in the geriatric group, where osteoporosis is prevalent. A well-planned meal plan might include a variety of dairy foods, greens, and fortified foods that are able to sustain the optimal mineral status. Moreover, consuming whole grains, nuts, and legumes could enhance the availability of magnesium and fruits and vegetables could deliver the potassium needed. By placing these factors at the top priority, meal planning not only corrects the nutritional deficiencies but also malnutrition, which is a significant problem in long-term care facilities (Volkert et al., 2019). The procedure of meal planning must also involve a combination of food sources so that a wide variety of minerals is present in the diet of older adults. For instance, the combination of red meat, chicken, and fish can provide valuable heme iron and vegetable foods provide non-heme iron. In elderly individuals who may find protein foods difficult or have limited food intake, meal planning according to these requirements becomes crucial. Caregivers and dietitians may appreciate a person-oriented approach, possibly involving the utilization of nutritional supplements where necessary, in further maximizing mineral intake. Food texture and flavor control may also enter the scene, since most elderly people have an impaired appetite or altered sense of taste and are less likely to consume nutrient-dense food. Although not solely focusing on each mineral separately, a holistic approach in terms of eating behaviour is deserved for meal planning. This involves not only giving sufficient intake of essential minerals but also respecting the interplay among various nutrients and their combined influence on health. As an example, the role of vitamin D in calcium absorption is particularly germane for older adults, who may have restricted exposure to sunlight. An eating plan rich in fruits, vegetables, whole grains, and lean protein promotes a synergistic interaction among minerals and other nutrients to ultimately result in better health outcomes. With the use of holistic meal planning strategies based on these principles, caregivers are able to allow older adults to achieve functional capacity, augment quality of life, and minimize the occurrence of nutrition-related complications (Volkert et al., 2019).

5.6.2. Importance of Hydration in Mineral Absorption

Hydration plays an important role in the absorption of required minerals, particularly in the elderly. As age progresses, physiological changes in the gastrointestinal system inescapably affect the way in which nutrients, including minerals, are absorbed. Adequate hydration permits normal functioning of the gastrointestinal tract by facilitating the mechanical disintegration of food and chemical digestion by way of effective enzymatic action. Hydration deficiencies have been said to lead to compromised digestive processes, which in turn compromise the absorption of vital minerals such as calcium, magnesium, and phosphorus, which are central to bone strength as well as general physiological homeostasis. This puts heavy emphasis on the role of hydration not only as a method of quenching thirst but as a fundamental component of nutritional planning among older adults that is designed to maximize mineral availability, which is essential for their health and well-being. Moreover, aging can result in decreased perception of thirst and altered kidney function, which makes appropriate fluid intake even more crucial among the elderly. With lower capability for hydration, the risk of malnutrition rises, as elderly people may not consume sufficient amounts of fluids to support mineral absorption effectively. Low levels of fluid intake can impair such minerals from dissolving properly inside the gut, thus leading to low bioavailability. Research has established that hydration not only influences food digestion but also nutritional status among the elderly, making it directly related to their quality of life. Therefore, hydration care becomes an essential part of dietary guidance that seeks to minimize deficiency and malnutrition risks in geriatric patients, standing firmly on their nutritional needs. Furthermore, certain minerals interact synergistically with hydration to enhance metabolic processes essential for the elderly. For instance, maximum absorption of calcium and phosphorus, which are essential for bone integrity, relies on proper hydration to maintain an ideal internal environment for nutrient utilization and absorption. Malnutrition, which remains a priority condition based on recent research, is exacerbated by deficiencies related to hydration, leading to increased susceptibility to a myriad of health problems, including impaired immune function and weakened muscular performance. Increased understanding of the mechanism through which hydration impinges on mineral absorption can guide age-specific diet planning. Meeting both hydration and nutrition requirements is paramount for preventing adverse health outcomes among the elderly, making it imperative that caregivers and clinicians pay more attention to the demand for fluid consumption alongside mineral-based diets among the elderly.

5.6.3. Role of Supplements in Geriatric Nutrition

The role of dietary supplements in geriatric nutrition is becoming regarded more and more as a valuable step towards addressing nutrient deficiencies that become prevalent with advancing age. The elderly will experience changes in the body, such as decreased absorption efficiency and altered metabolism, which will disrupt nutritional well-being. The group is likely to be pushed to receive RDAs from food and rely on supplements to provide needed vitamins and minerals. Not surprisingly, micronutrient supplementation will enhance therapeutic response, particularly with the management of chronic disease and increased overall health. Thus, healthcare professionals are encouraged to assess elderly patients' dietary habits on a regular basis and advise the inclusion of nutraceuticals in their diet as a way of maximizing beneficial effects and minimizing risk of deficiency, with complications or compromised quality of life arising therefrom. The specific mineral requirements of the elderly can be highly variable; thus, careful choice of supplements is crucial. For instance, calcium and vitamin D are relevant to bone health, particularly significant in elderly individuals who are at risk of osteoporosis. Additionally, magnesium contributes to cardiovascular disorder control, a common problem with aging. Current evidence indicates that the majority of older adults do not consume sufficient levels of these minerals, consequently suffering from various health issues. Supplements can compensate in these domains, giving elderly individuals the intake they require for healthy maintenance and function. Accordingly, demystification of these mineral requirements and promotion of appropriate supplementation can be crucial in enhancing geriatric nutrition practices and health among the elderly. Beyond the necessary vitamins and minerals, other nutrients such as omega-3 fatty acids have been the subjects of interest in geriatric nutrition. Aging has often been associated with increased inflammation and vulnerability to cognitive decline, for which omega-3 fatty acids can be beneficial. The evidence indicates the benefits of including these essential fats in the diet to support cardiac and brain function. Moreover, as highlighted in studies on animal populations, like aged dogs and cats, appropriate nutrition according to their specific requirements can greatly improve their quality of life and lifespan. It is the same in geriatric nutrition, where particular supplementation not only meets dietary requirements but also sustains maximum body function. It thus becomes a necessity to advocate for customized nutritional plans consisting of required supplements to promote geriatric health and improve the quality of life in aging.

SUMMARY

It is a complex problem to meet the mineral requirements in geriatric nutrition, which necessitates a holistic perspective of the different factors affecting nutrient intake and absorption among the aging. As individuals age, physiological changes such as shifts in gastrointestinal function and loss of appetite significantly impact their nutritional status. Physiological changes are the cause of higher prevalence of malnutrition, which, as seen in relevant literature, increases risk to health and decreases quality of life. Management of these conditions necessitates an intervention strategy that integrates dietary measures with an understanding of individual needs of old adults, ultimately aiming at optimizing their overall well-being and quality of life (Rémond et al., 2015). In addition, the integration of targeted nutritional therapy within care environments is important to avoid the consequences of malnutrition in older people. As highlighted in the study, the rate of protein-energy malnutrition is shocking among elderly care homes, where half of the residents can experience malnutrition. Malnutrition is more than an eating issue; it is associated with negative clinical outcomes, such as higher infection and hospitalization rates (Agarwal et al., 2016). Adding a robust nutritional regimen that entails consistent screening and evaluation can assist in early identification of susceptible individuals and direct particular interventions to satisfy nutritional needs as well as physiological barriers. Finally, a multidisciplinary approach is central in promoting effective nutritional care among geriatric populations. Inviting participation from healthcare professionals, dietitians, and caregivers in planning and executing holistic nutritional strategies not only improves individual health conditions but also promotes wellness culture among care environments. Prioritizing mineral requirements and demystifying causes of malnutrition enables stakeholders to manage the increasing number of the elderly more effectively. Consequently, the success of these initiatives will not only enhance the quality of life but also ensure a sustainable healthcare system that properly addresses the holistic needs of the elderly in different settings (Rémond et al., 2015; Agarwal et al., 2016).

When addressing the mineral requirements of the elderly, a basic understanding of the particular physiological alterations that take place in aged individuals is essential. With increasing age, alterations in gastrointestinal (GI) function, such as compromised efficiency of nutrient absorption and modification of intestinal motility, have a significant impact on mineral bioavailability. This diminishment in GI function will lead to malnutrition, which is responsible for many health issues prevalent among the elderly, including decreased immune response and vulnerability to chronic illnesses. It is thus crucial to come up with targeted dietary strategies that will take into consideration these changes to promote mineral nutrition among the elderly with a perspective to improve longevity and living standards. In total, an understanding of these physiological alterations is needed to direct the formulation of effective nutritional guidelines for the elderly. Aside from this, geriatric nutrition should also be concerned about the adequacy of particular minerals that contribute to health maintenance. These essential minerals, such as calcium, magnesium, and potassium, are particularly important because they are responsible for bone strength, cardiovascular function, and muscle upkeep. For instance, calcium supplementation is integral in reducing the risk of osteoporosis, whereas magnesium plays a critical role in neuromuscular conduction and cardiovascular health. Additionally, potassium assists in regulating blood pressure, which is important in preventing cardiovascular diseases prevalent among the elderly. Thus, being careful to see that geriatric diets are rich in such minerals, and others that promote overall health, is a significant topic under the nutritional management of the elderly. This will counterbalance aging-related illnesses and ensure functional independence in later life processes. Besides, to overcome malnutrition, it is imperative to balance a range of factors that impact dietary lifestyle among the elderly. Psychological impairments, budget constraints, and social problems may impair old age nutritional intake due to worsening the issue caused by inadequate mineral levels. Studies have shown that delaying excessive numbers of elderly people from food due to inferior food intake caused by these various factors. Therefore, complete dietary plans need to incorporate solutions considering not only the physiological aspects of old age but also the multifaceted challenges confronting older people in nutrient consumption. Interventions via dieting have to aim at enhancing mineral intake via fortified foods, supplementation, and nutrition education for optimal food selection. Essentially, there has to be an overall approach to meet the needs of minerals required in geriatric nutrition and contribute towards improved health outcomes among this population (Rémond et al., 2015; Lumbis, 2018).

A CLOSER LOOK

IRON NEEDS AND ANEMIA RISK IN THE ELDERLY

Iron is an essential mineral required for the production of hemoglobin, which carries oxygen in the blood, and for overall cellular function. In older adults, maintaining adequate iron levels is crucial, as both deficiency and excess can have significant health implications. Aging often brings changes in dietary intake, gastrointestinal absorption, and chronic medical conditions that can affect iron status. Reduced appetite, difficulties in chewing or swallowing, and diets low in iron-rich foods may contribute to inadequate intake. Additionally, chronic inflammation or conditions such as gastrointestinal bleeding can further compromise iron levels. Anemia, characterized by a reduced number of red blood cells or low hemoglobin, is common among the elderly and can lead to fatigue, weakness, impaired cognitive function, and decreased physical performance, significantly affecting quality of life.

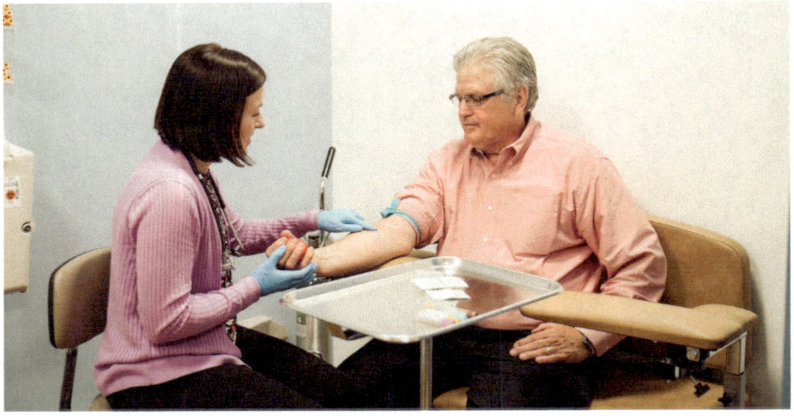

Source: https://www.onemedical.com/media/images/94.original.png

Detecting iron deficiency anemia early is important, as it is often reversible with dietary adjustments or supplementation under medical supervision. Sources of dietary iron include lean meats, poultry, fish, legumes, and fortified cereals. Pairing plant-based iron sources with vitamin C-rich foods can enhance absorption, while excessive intake of tea, coffee, or certain medications may inhibit it. Health professionals emphasize regular monitoring of hemoglobin and ferritin levels in older adults, especially those with chronic illnesses or on medications affecting iron metabolism. By ensuring adequate iron intake through a balanced diet and addressing underlying health conditions, the risk of anemia can be minimized, supporting optimal energy levels, immune function, and overall well-being in the elderly population.

REFERENCES

1. Setiarsih D, Wirjatmadi B, Adriani M. Bone Density Status and Vitamin D and Calcium Concentrations in Pregnant and Non-Pregnant Women. Makara J Health Res. 2016;20. (accessed on 12th July 2025).
2. Agarwal, E., Isenring, E., Marshall, S., et al. (2016). Optimizing nutrition in residential aged care: A narrative review. https://core.ac.uk/download/196601588.pdf (accessed on 12th July 2025).
3. Akhter, A., Giwercman, A., Annesley, A., Araujo, B., Bates, B., Bischoff-Ferrari, H., Boonen, S., et al. (2013). Active vitamin D (1,25-dihydroxyvitamin D) and bone health in middle-aged and elderly men: The European male aging study (EMAS). https://core.ac.uk/download/16458345.pdf (accessed on 12th July 2025).
4. Maylor, E. A., Simpson, E. E., Secker, D. L., Meunier, N., Andriollo-Sanchez, M., Polito, A., Stewart-Knox, B., McConville, C., O'Connor, J. M., & Coudray, C. (2006). Effects of zinc supplementation on cognitive function in healthy middle-aged and older adults: the ZENITH study. *The British journal of nutrition*, *96*(4), 752–760.(accessed on 12th July 2025).
5. Feskens, E. J. M., Bailey, R., Bhutta, Z., Biesalski, H. K., Eicher-Miller, H., Krämer, K., Pan, W. H., & Griffiths, J. C. (2022). Women's health: optimal nutrition throughout the lifecycle. *European journal of nutrition*, *61*(Suppl 1), 1–23. https://doi.org/10.1007/s00394-022-02915-x(accessed on 12th July 2025).
6. Volkert, D., Beck, A. M., Cederholm, T., Cruz-Jentoft, A., Goisser, S., Hooper, L., Kiesswetter, E., Maggio, M., Raynaud-Simon, A., Sieber, C. C., Sobotka, L., van Asselt, D., Wirth, R., & Bischoff, S. C. (2019). ESPEN guideline on clinical nutrition and hydration in geriatrics. *Clinical nutrition (Edinburgh, Scotland)*, *38*(1), 10–47. https://doi.org/10.1016/j.clnu.2018.05.024(accessed on 12th July 2025).
7. Bigando, A. (2023). The impact of personal barriers to incorporating the American Heart Association diet. https://core.ac.uk/download/588599824.pdf (accessed on 12th July 2025).
8. Rémond, D., Shahar, D. R., Gille, D., Pinto, P., Kachal, J., Peyron, M. A., Dos Santos, C. N., Walther, B., Bordoni, A., Dupont, D., Tomás-Cobos, L., & Vergères, G. (2015). Understanding the gastrointestinal tract of the elderly to develop dietary solutions that prevent malnutrition. *Oncotarget*, *6*(16), 13858–13898. https://doi.org/10.18632/oncotarget.4030(accessed on 12th July 2025).
9. Burton, L. A., & Sumukadas, D. (2010). Optimal management of sarcopenia. https://core.ac.uk/download/20453974.pdf (accessed on 12th July 2025).
10. Cheung, S. K. W., Cheung, T. C., Choi, P. T. F., et al. (2013). The Osteoporosis Society of Hong Kong (OSHK): 2013 OSHK guideline for clinical management of postmenopausal osteoporosis in Hong Kong. https://core.ac.uk/download/38026126.pdf (accessed on 12th July 2025).
11. Corsello, G., Cricelli, C., Ferrara, N., Ghiselli, M., et al. (2015). Role of poultry meat in a balanced diet aimed at maintaining health and wellbeing: An Italian consensus document. https://core.ac.uk/download/53302710.pdf (accessed on 12th July 2025).
12. Uchmanowicz, I., Faulkner, K. M., Iovino, P., Kwaśny, A., Surma, S., Magi, C. E., Jakubiak, G. K., Longobucco, Y., Janczak, D., Rak-Pasikowska, A., Czapla, M., & Uchmanowicz, B. (2025). Integrating frailty interventions into existing care models: a comprehensive approach to

enhancing patient outcomes in chronic disease management. *Frontiers in public health, 12,* 1518774. https://doi.org/10.3389/fpubh.2024.1518774(accessed on 12th July 2025).

13. El-Amin, A. (2023). Engaging the aging process: Unlock the fountain of youth. https://core.ac.uk/download/552889276.pdf (accessed on 12th July 2025).
14. Gulsah Kaya-Karasu, Peter Huntington, Christine Iben, Jo-Anne Murray (2018). Feeding and management practices for racehorses in Turkey. https://core.ac.uk/download/82893738.pdf (accessed on 12th July 2025).
15. Summers, S. C., Stockman, J., Larsen, J. A., Zhang, L., & Rodriguez, A. S. (2020). Evaluation of phosphorus, calcium, and magnesium content in commercially available foods formulated for healthy cats. *Journal of veterinary internal medicine, 34*(1), 266–273. https://doi.org/10.1111/jvim.15689(accessed on 12th July 2025).
16. Lin, J. C. (1999). The nutritional effects of the Elderly Nutrition Program: Title III-C for the Menomonie congregate-site meal program participants. https://core.ac.uk/download/5067537.pdf (accessed on 12th July 2025).
17. Lumbis, R. H. (2018). Nourishing dogs and cats through their twilight years. https://core.ac.uk/download/154422917.pdf (accessed on 12th July 2025).
18. Malafarina, V., Reginster, J. Y., Cabrerizo, S., et al. (2017). Nutritional status and nutritional treatment are related to outcomes and mortality in older adults with hip fracture. https://core.ac.uk/download/pdf/212756692.pdf (accessed on 12th July 2025).
19. Mohd Alim, J., Lee, X. K., Mokhtar Abu Bakar, N. A., et al. (2005). Anemia and cognitive function among Chinese elderly in old folks' homes. https://core.ac.uk/download/11490096.pdf (accessed on 12th July 2025).

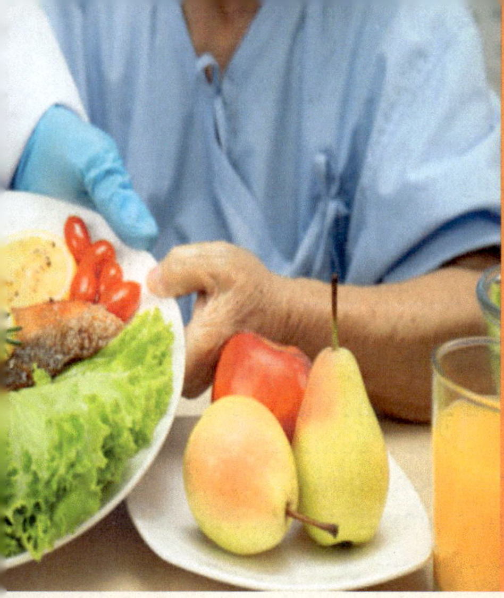

Chapter 6

TRACE METAL REQUIREMENTS FOR GERIATRIC NUTRITION

Contents

Introduction

The health and quality of life of elderly individuals are increasingly dependent on nutrition, with particular emphasis on trace metal requirements. With increasing age, physiological changes can regulate the ability of the body to absorb and utilize major micronutrients like trace metals, zinc, copper, and selenium. Notably, zinc is involved in a host of metabolic processes, immune function, and repair of cells; however, studies have indicated that the majority of older individuals can be lacking in this important micronutrient. Research has shown that even though plasma zinc levels reflect adequate intake at one point in time, older adults are challenged to maintain adequate levels, thus rendering trace metal needs in gerontology an area deserving of particular research (Paterson, 1982). This realization forces health care professionals to place great importance on dietary assessment and intervention so that the elderly are well cared for in their nutritional requirements. Trace metal involvement in the overall health of the elderly is more than just fundamental nutrient needs, as it involves intricate interactions with chronic diseases prevalent among this age group. For example, trace metal deficiencies would have an impact on magnifying the course of age-related illnesses, affecting outcomes that are associated with oxidative stress and inflammation. It is evident through research that sufficient trace element intake is not only beneficial but rather imperative in maintaining cognitive ability, immune status, and metabolic effectiveness in aging populations (Maitra et al., 2024). This aspect of nutrition is particularly essential in geriatric patient care, in which individuals may have several disease states simultaneously, and thus, the incorporation of the full scope of trace metal requirements must be considered in nutritional recommendations. Thus, determining the role of trace elements in the diet is paramount to the promotion of geriatric health and in solidifying the state of knowledge regarding nutrition in aging. Importantly, understanding the specific trace metal requirements in geriatric nutrition entails consideration of many factors, including geography, health status, and overall dietary patterns. Since evidence indicates the heterogeneity of trace metal requirements, it is clear that one-size-fits-all is inadequate (Maitra et al., 2024). For example, dietary intake fluctuates greatly based on local production, cultural beliefs, and individuals' individual health requirements. Therefore, identification of trace metal status through clinical measures, coupled with dietary questionnaires, is of utmost importance in individualized nutritional therapy to cater to the specific needs of the elderly. A well-designed program with food sources and bioavailability of such nutrients can significantly improve the nutritional condition in the elderly, eventually leading to improved health status and quality of life in the elderly (Figure 6.1).

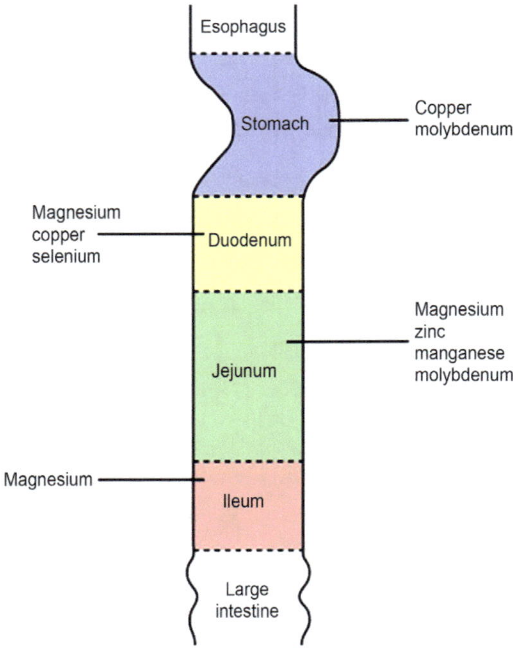

Figure 6.1. Trace metal requirements for geriatric nutrition.

Source: https://ars.els-cdn.com/content/image/3-s2.0-B9780128028964000158-f17-01-9780128028964.jpg.

Definition of Trace Metals

Trace metals, also referred to as trace elements, are vital micronutrients that are required in minute quantities, typically measured in micrograms, but also play vital roles in a variety of biochemical reactions at all phases of life. Though they are required in minute quantities, their impact on metabolism and health is great. Trace metals such as zinc, selenium, iron, and copper are of particular importance in geriatric nutrition due to their involvement in enzymatic reactions, immune response, and the function of the brain. Deficiency or excess of these trace metals will lead to pathologic effects, which highlight the significance of balanced dietary intake. The exact nutritional requirements of trace metals in the elderly to a large extent rely on particular medical states, dietary patterns, and ecological conditions, and thus, it is essential to promote awareness of their intrinsic roles in preserving health. Trace metals' definition transcends nutritional substance; it encompasses their biochemical roles in the human body. Trace metals are enzyme cofactors that facilitate the reactions central to protein synthesis, respiration, and DNA repair mechanisms. Zinc, for instance, supports immune function and has been associated with cognitive performance in some cases, while copper participates in energy metabolism and iron metabolism. Furthermore, selenium has been highlighted in recent studies as one possible protective factor against depressive disorders, particularly in certain populations (Sajjadi et al., 2022). This helps to emphasize the point that trace metals must not be thought about in isolation but rather in terms of contributions in complex nutritional regimens that enhance the well-being and health of elderly people. Diet-wise, trace metals can come from a variety of foods and emphasizing the importance of diet diversity for elderly people's nutrition. These trace minerals are abundant in nuts, seeds, whole grains, fish, and green vegetables, and thus, their maximum intake is made easy. Elderly individuals are prone to deficiencies as they have altered the rate of absorption and dietary patterns, and thus determining the very need for trace metals becomes important. Such deficits can be overcome with nutritional remedies or supplementation and would significantly improve health status, particularly in the control of chronic ailments and enhancement of cognitive function. Trace metal and general health interactions are a paradigm for the requirement of a holistic strategy to nutrition in geriatric care centers, such that elderly populations are adequately offered semi-structured instruction in the maintenance of trace metal homeostasis (Betz et al., 2023).

Importance of Nutrition in Geriatric Health

Dieting is a key part of maintaining health and well-being in the elderly because with age comes a series of physiological changes that influence dietary requirements. The GIT loses its function with increasing age, leading to altered digestion and nutrient uptake. The alterations influence the body's ability to absorb vital nutrients, eventually leading to malnutrition, which is alarmingly prevalent in the elderly. Malnutrition is more than suboptimal caloric absorption; it has the capability to predispose elderly individuals to a variety of health problems, such as cardiovascular, musculoskeletal, immune, and neurological. Knowledge of the interrelationship between aging GIT function and nutritional needs is, therefore, critical for formulating effective dietary advice for the prevention of malnutrition and for the promotion of health in elderly individuals (Rémond et al., 2015). The importance of trace metals such as zinc and copper in the nutrition of the elderly cannot be overstressed. The latest studies emphasize that wide proportions of the elderly suffer from suboptimal zinc status, which can affect immune function, cognitive function, and the healing of wounds adversely. In a trial assessing zinc nutriture in elderly subjects, 67% of the patients were found to have deficient plasma zinc levels, although a high rate claimed adequate dietary supply. These findings emphasize the complexity of trace metal metabolism and uptake among the elderly, which requires deliberate nutritional interventions that will enhance trace metal intake based on their specific physiological requirements (Paterson, 1982). Therefore, not only must dietary assessments be modified to address these precise trace metal requirements among elderly individuals, but so too must evidence-based guidelines. Furthermore, the interplay between nutrition and overall geriatric health is also connected to the overall effects of dieting on the quality of life. Enhanced dietary balance in regard to required nutrients, including trace metals, has been found to improve outcomes in regard to mobility, cognitive function, and longevity. In older people, nutrition not only sustains physical health but also psychological and social health—a crucial element that often takes a back seat in geriatric management. The well-designed nutritional interventions that enhance the intake of beneficial trace elements can lead to a significant reduction in the incidence of illness and hospitalization due to complications of malnutrition. This holistic approach is critical to ensuring that older adults not just live, but thrive in their golden years, enhancing overall quality of life and autonomy in self-maintenance (Rémond et al., 2015).

Overview of Trace Metal Roles in the Body

Trace metals play significant roles in numerous biochemical processes in the human body, facilitating critical body functions that are particularly crucial with increasing age. These substances, such as zinc, copper, iron, and selenium, are not only trace elements; they are constituents of the numerous enzymes and proteins essential to metabolic processes. Zinc, for instance, is a critical constituent of immune function, acting as a cofactor for over 300 enzymatic reactions. Trace metal deficiency, such as zinc, in aging populations can lead to compromised immune function, increased infection susceptibility, and wound healing impairment. Similarly, copper is required for the production of hemoglobin and collagen, both essential for maintaining healthy vascular function and tissue integrity. Loss of absorption and increasing nutritional requirements for these metals with advancing age further highlight the need for those specific nutritional strategies that are sensitive to these aging alterations. Iron, another obligatory trace metal, is utilized primarily for oxygen delivery as part of hemoglobin and myoglobin. With aging, the risk of developing iron deficiency anemia mounts due to declining dietary intake, drug-drug interactions, and changed intestinal absorption. Iron deficiency anemia can lead to fatigue, compromised cognitive function, and decreased physical ability, which are frequently ascribed to physiological processes of aging. Ensuring adequate iron status by diet or supplements becomes essential in older individuals. However, iron supplementation must be in moderation since excessive amounts are injurious and can cause oxidative stress and lead to chronic diseases of aging. Addition of iron-rich foods or iron-fortified foodstuffs to the diet of the elderly is thus a necessity towards optimal health and functional status. The role of selenium as a trace element in gerontological nutrition cannot be ignored because of its potent antioxidant action. Selenium is essential for the function of certain enzymes that protect cells from oxidative stress and inflammation and contribute to general health and disease prevention among older adults. Selenium deficiency has been linked to many diseases, including memory loss and susceptibility to infections. Moreover, studies have shown that selenium status may influence the development of certain chronic diseases and therefore, be a decisive factor to be considered under nutritional intervention. Therefore, health practitioners should promote diets rich in selenium-containing foods such as nuts, fish, and whole grains. With the growing geriatric population, it is increasingly important to comprehend these trace metal functions in the human body to achieve the optimum health benefits and enhance the quality of life in older individuals (Figure 6.2).

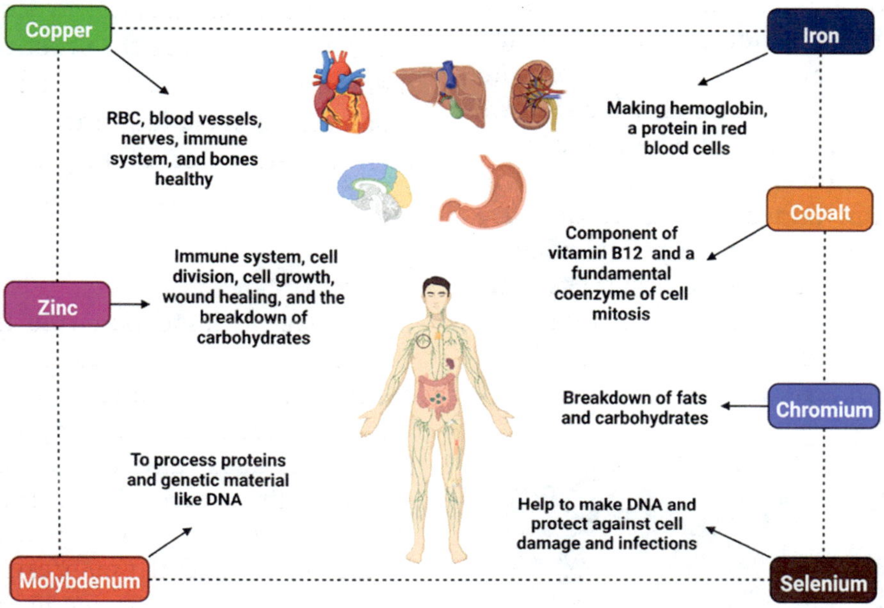

Figure 6.2. Role of trace elements in human health.

Source: https://www.researchgate.net/publication/366120563/figure/fig1/AS:11431281192027515@1695694633616/Role-of-trace-elements-in-human-health-Numerous-traceelements-are-necessary-for-the-body.png.

6.1. Common Trace Metals in Nutrition

The role of trace metals in nutrition is particularly targeted in geriatric age groups, where changes in physiology have tremendous potential to affect nutritional requirements. Important trace metals like zinc, copper, iron, and selenium play various roles in biological processes that are crucial in elderly subjects. Zinc, for instance, is critical to immune function, wound healing, and maintenance of skin integrity, something particularly vital in older patients whose bodies can be in compromised health (Paterson, 1982). Copper, in turn, facilitates iron metabolism and maintenance of connective tissues and neurological function. Trace element deficiencies will lead to exacerbation of currently existing issues, including increased susceptibility to illness and slower recovery from illness. Hence, knowledge and availability of adequate intake of these trace essential metals become utmost in improving health outcomes among the elderly population. Zinc, being one of the foremost trace elements, has plenty of significance in geriatrics, owing to its prevalence with respect to elderly nutrition. Through research on elderly populations, a surprising trend comes into view whereby most individuals exhibit poor dietary intake of zinc-containing foods, considering their apparent plasma sufficiency in zinc (Paterson, 1982). This disproportion indicates a potential gap between physiological needs and dietary habits, potentially leading to reduced well-being. Notably, zinc status influences the immune system and cellular repair processes, requiring regular evaluation and nutritional adjustment in geriatric patients. In addition, zinc bioavailability differs depending on food composition and interaction with other nutrients, which shows the complexity of providing effective zinc levels in geriatric nutrition. Interventions aimed at dietary education and supplementation are therefore needed to ensure optimal zinc in this population. Copper is yet another essential trace metal that has functions in numerous physiological processes, including antioxidant defense and mobilization of iron.

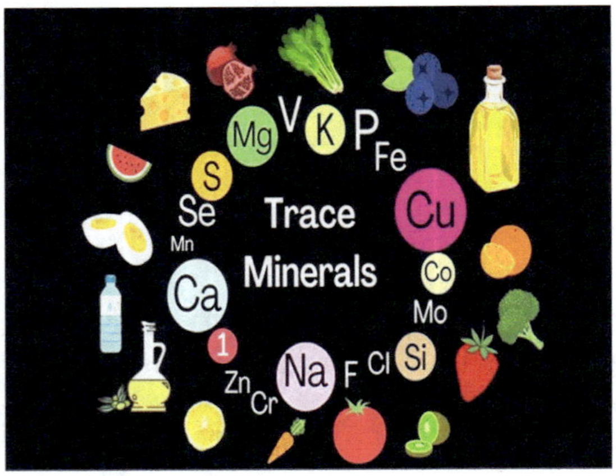

Figure 6.3. Trace minerals.

Source: https://www.water-for-health.co.uk/cdn/shop/articles/img-1697543824613_3adb1ae0-997b-437c-829a-e0b76854d049.jpg?v=1743503517&width=1024.

The daily recommended allowance for copper is low, but deficiencies are important in the elderly and most notably on cardiovascular function and cognitive processes. Moreover, the copper-zinc balance should be taken care of, as the surplus of one might lead to the deficiency of the other, hence complicating the nutrition scenario for the elderly. Notably, such interactions have to be considered in relation to overall dietary habits and overall well-being among the elderly. As demonstrated by increasing evidence for micronutrient interactions, an integrative approach to managing trace metal requirements is essential to aid longevity and healthy aging. Health practitioners should therefore provide high priority to nutritional assessments, including trace metal statuses, to offer well-targeted dietary recommendations for elderly individuals (Figure 6.3).

6.1.1. Iron

Iron plays an important role in the elderly's nutritional needs, making a substantial contribution to wellness and overall health. The iron needs of the body can vary as the individual ages, and it is essential to have foods modified accordingly. Iron is involved in synthesizing hemoglobin to transport oxygen in the blood, and if not present, it may lead to anemia. Older adult anemia can exacerbate various health conditions, like heart disease and can further cause mental impairment. As elderly people are prone to compromised iron absorption from changes in gastrointestinal function or consumption of certain medications, awareness of iron-rich foods like meat, legumes, and fortified cereals becomes necessary to effectively meet their nutritional requirements. In the consideration of iron's bioavailability in elderly individuals, consideration should be given to food sources of iron. Two forms of iron exist: heme and non-heme. Heme iron, as found in foods of animal origin, is absorbed more compared to non-heme iron, which is present in foods of plant origin. This is particularly observed in older individuals who are on restricted diets. Some dietary factors can also influence the absorption of iron. For instance, vitamin C-rich foods enhance the body's absorption of non-heme iron, whereas tannins present in tea and coffee hinder it. The optimal optimization of iron absorption among the elderly must not only consider iron levels in foods but also the impact of food habits and interactions on the absorption. This is a multifaceted approach that can reduce the risk of iron deficiency and associated diseases among elderly people. Secondly, iron supplementation of older adults' diets must be done with caution. While iron supplementation is beneficial for those with iron deficiency anemia, too much intake of iron can be detrimental, causing oxidative stress, as well as gastrointestinal disturbances. Older adults suffer more from susceptibility to side effects of supplements due to polypharmacy and varied physiological responses. Clinical assessment of individual iron status should be done by clinicians through the use of blood tests before recommending supplementation. Of particular note, research showed that a fish supplement of high-mineral content, such as carp, would not only enhance iron intake but also nutritional status in general to elderly populations (Kaliniak-Dziura et al., 2024). A well-balanced nutrition regimen considering both dietary consumption and potential supplementation is thus called for to maximize geriatric well-being in an era beset by increased susceptibility to nutritional deficiency (Figure 6.4).

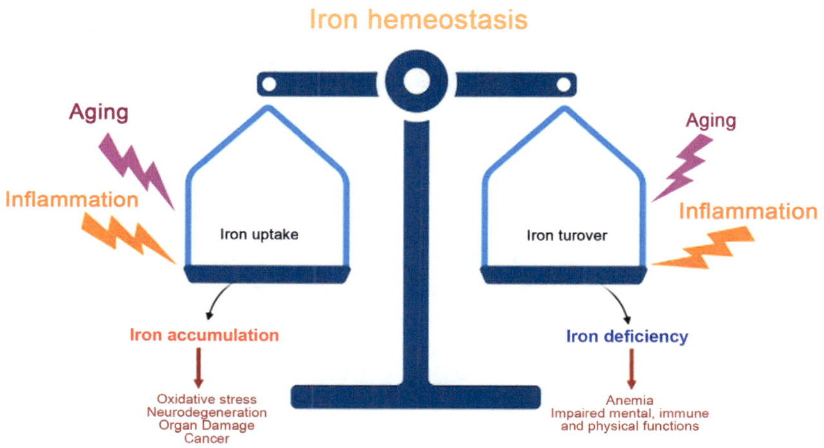

Figure 6.4. Iron homeostasis and organismal aging.

Source: https://ars.els-cdn.com/content/image/1-s2.0-S1568163721002579-gr1.jpg.

6.1.2. Zinc

The trace element zinc plays a crucial role in the geriatric nutrition regimen. In older individuals, the physiological deterioration of aging can greatly impair zinc uptake and metabolism. The gastrointestinal tract also undergoes some significant alterations, including reduced mechanical and chemical breakdown of food, which can affect the bioavailability of zinc and other nutrients. Since the aging body cannot break down and absorb essential minerals, the risk of zinc deficiency occurs. This shortage could exacerbate health status with age, like impaired immune function and impaired wound healing. Hence, understanding the specific needs of zinc among the elderly and how its consumption can be maximized is now crucial in preventing malnutrition and its resulting adverse effects, which range from chronic diseases to increased mortality (Rémond et al., 2015). Zinc also has many hormonal mechanisms that are needed to age successfully. It influences the synthesis and functioning of hormones that play a role in maintaining muscle mass and metabolic function. For instance, optimal zinc levels have been linked to improved insulin sensitivity and control of insulin-like growth factor-1 (IGF-1), both of which are extremely crucial for metabolic and muscle functions (Maggio et al., 2014). Consequently, sufficient dietary zinc supplementation is not only important for the prevention of deficiency-related disease but also for inducing an anabolic state conducive to muscle preservation and global physical function in older individuals. Such an association further underscores the importance of beneficial dietary interventions to increase zinc consumption in older individuals in order to optimize their overall nutritional status more effectively. The role of zinc in older adult nutrition extends beyond its link to chronic disease prevention. Low zinc status has been associated with several age-related diseases, including cognitive impairment, cardiovascular diseases, and susceptibility to infections. With sufficient zinc status, older adults can potentially reduce the severity and frequency of such diseases, translating to a better quality of life. Furthermore, food-based interventions involving zinc supplementation are able to tackle other nutrition deficiencies simultaneously as well, particularly among groups vulnerable to malnutrition. As with each study, increasingly convinced that trace metal status and health outcomes are closely linked, pressure to develop nutrition advice endorsing zinc supplementation or fortification as a pillar of geriatric dietary planning is ever more necessary (Rémond et al., 2015). By these avenues, health professionals can enhance the nutritional well-being of older adults and decrease the risks of zinc deficiency, thus fostering healthier aging (Figure 6.5).

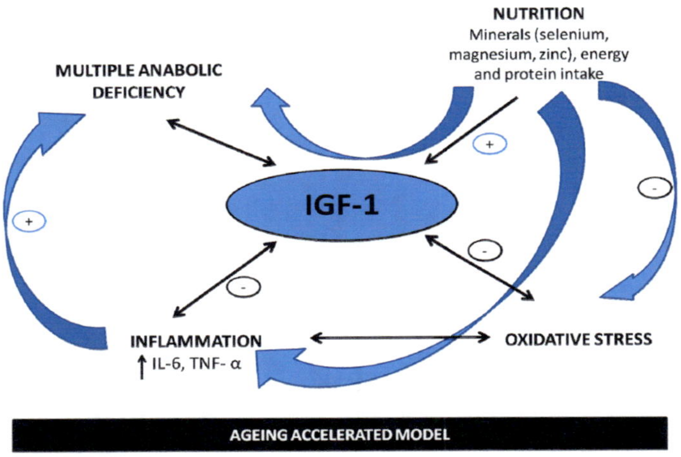

Figure 6.5. Insulin-like growth factor-1 (IGF-1), The crossroad of nutritional.

Source: https://pub.mdpi-res.com/nutrients/nutrients-05-04184/article_deploy/html/images/nutrients-05-04184-g001.png?1390370736.

6.1.3. Selenium

Selenium is a crucial trace metal with a significant role in many physiological processes, notably as an antioxidant to neutralize oxidative stress in the human body. Increased oxidative stress is observed among elderly populations, which may lead to chronic diseases such as cardiovascular disease and hypertension. Since older people are prone to changed metabolism and reduced efficiency in nutrient absorption, providing adequate selenium levels becomes a priority. It has been suggested that selenium supplementation will enhance immune function and may slow the incidence of a range of degenerative disorders with which aging is so commonly associated. With progressive nutrition planning for geriatric populations, inclusion of selenium in diets is necessary to attain optimal benefits and ensure longevity, as evidence by trace metals profound significance in the enrichment of geriatric diets. Selenium's bioavailability also rests on the sources of it in foods, which are primarily selenium-rich foods such as nuts, seafoods, and certain grains. The unequal selenium content of the soil in various regions of the world also contributes to the challenge of acquiring sufficient selenium from natural foods. In elderly people, who may be suffering from dietary restrictions or may have eating habits that limit the intake of foods containing selenium, supplementation is a viable solution.

Nutritional debates now focus on the need for personalized dietary recommendations for individual selenium requirements in light of age, health status, and lifestyle (Sgarbieri et al., 2017). Physicians are thus encouraged to assess selenium status as part of trace metal nutrients overall and promote an integrated therapeutic approach to elderly nutrition. In addition to the role of maintaining antioxidant defense mechanisms, selenium has been found to be involved in anti-inflammatory actions and its potential protective actions against specific cancers. Research points out how selenium can influence cancer pathway gene expression and its involvement in selenoprotein synthesis, which is crucial in cell repair functions. The elderly patient, already predisposed to cancer due to the loss of immunity with advancing age, can benefit immensely from adequate selenium intake as part of an overall dietary strategy for cancer risk reduction. Furthermore, as decreasing budgets and rising healthcare costs create a tight pinch on nutritional adequacy, selenium and other trace elements must have high priority in the diet management of the elderly patient to enhance quality of life. Supplying the aging population with adequate selenium, along with other nutrients, can maintain healthier aging and longer longevity (Niego et al., 2021).

6.2. Physiological Functions of Trace Metals

Trace metal and physiological functions interaction is quite significant in geriatric nutrition because aging adults will undergo alterations in nutrient absorption and metabolism. As the gastrointestinal tract (GIT) weakens, its ability to effectively digest and absorb essential trace metals like zinc, selenium, and iron decreases. Gastrointestinal motility and wall function changes hinder food digestion, ultimately reducing nutrient bioavailability. The decrease can lead to a deficiency that negatively impacts a myriad of body systems, from the immune, muscular, to cardiovascular health. Correction of these deficiencies through individually tailored dietary recommendations that take into consideration the unique functional decline in the aged GIT is central to health promotion and prevention of malnutrition in the elderly. There is a need for diet interventions to address foods that are rich in trace metals and consider the complex physiological principles that affect nutrient intake and absorption in the aged (Rémond et al., 2015). Trace metals have physiological functions that transcend minimal nutritional roles; they are components of numerous enzymic reactions and antioxidant protection systems against oxidative stress. Selenium, for instance, is an integral component of glutathione peroxidase, an enzyme that features prominently in cellular protective systems. Research has determined that selenium intake is not only critical to maintaining plasma levels but that plasma levels can be utilized as biomarkers for selenium status in older age groups. Interestingly, studies have shown that institutionalized elderly women have plasma selenium levels lower than those of their younger counterparts, which means that lifestyle considerations will be a more significant determining factor for trace metal reserves than age itself. Sufficient selenium intake can thus reverse the risk of oxidative damage and consequent chronic illnesses in elderly people (Ducros et al., 1997). The strong interdependence of trace metals and gerontological well-being calls for a profound understanding of their requirements. Because diet deficiencies can lead to morbidity and vulnerability to a myriad of diseases, geriatric nutrition needs to be addressed from an integrative approach by medical practitioners. This would entail not only the ingestion of trace metals but also consideration of lifestyle determinants that would affect their absorption and utilization. Interventions toward the resolution of such issues may include the ingestion of fortified food items or supplements suitable for the elderly. By integrating data on the physiological roles of trace metals with a profound knowledge of the nutritional needs of the elderly, medical practitioners are able to enhance the welfare of elderly individuals and reduce the incidence of age-related diseases efficiently (Rémond et al., 2015) (Figure 6.6).

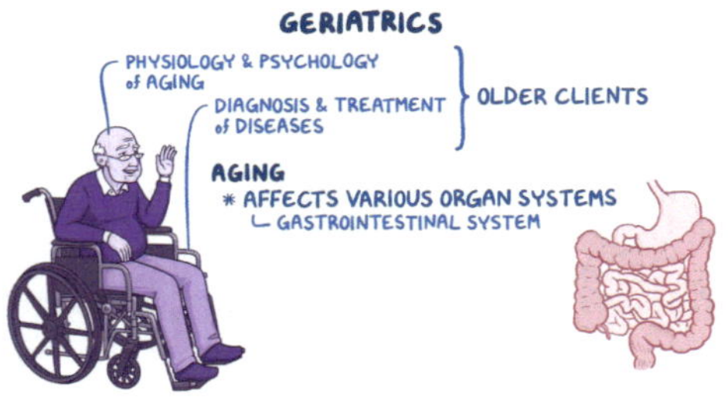

Figure 6.6. The gastrointestinal tract (GIT) deterioration of the geriatric population.

Source: https://www.osmosis.org/_next/image?url=https%3A%2F%2Fd16qt3wv6xm098.cloudfront.net%2FS3ZSCtjKRSWKOSSV5W20e_JVRFusUeUU%2F_.jpg&w=3840&q=75.

6.2.1. Role in Enzyme Function

Enzymes, like biocatalysts, play a significant role in the catalysis of metabolic processes that are critical to the preservation of health, particularly in the elderly. Trace metals such as zinc and copper play significant roles in influencing enzyme function as they are essential cofactors. Zinc, for example, is a component of the metalloenzyme structural complex, which are enzymes that rely on metal ions for their function. These metalloenzymes regulate a variety of metabolic activities, including DNA synthesis and protein metabolism, both of which are vital for aging individuals who experience physiological changes that can influence nutrient consumption and utilization. Earlier research has highlighted the significance of the interaction between zinc deficiency and compromised enzyme function, demonstrating a direct correlation between trace metal status and enzymatic activity, which assumes significance to avoid the risk of malnutrition among the elderly (Rémond et al., 2015). The aging gastrointestinal system undergoes many structural and functional changes that are likely to have an effect on nutrient absorption, including trace metals. With increasing age, the function of trace metal-dependent enzyme systems may decline, aggravating nutritional deficiencies. Studies have shown that individuals in advanced age groups are usually discovered to have suboptimal levels of trace metals such as zinc, which reflect the dysfunction of enzymes. This dysfunction of enzymic activity also restricts metabolic processes required for the maintenance of health and leads to an increased prevalence of malnutrition in older people. Specifically, the age-related changes in the gastrointestinal tract could hinder trace metal absorption, thus perpetuating a vicious cycle of suboptimal nutrient intake and compromised enzyme function (Paterson, 1982). In addition, measuring trace metal status is an important indicator of nutritional status in the elderly. The interaction of trace metals with enzymatic activity points to an important target for nutritional intervention. Through the adequacy of trace metals such as zinc and copper consumption, it is possible to enhance enzyme function and thus maximize overall metabolic efficiency and reduce malnutrition risk. Providing treatment for the nutritional requirements of the aged in order to meet their trace metal needs can stimulate enzyme activity and consequently, help contribute to basic health outcomes. Guidelines of strategic nutritional consumption targeting metal-consuming foods must be established to enhance the enzymatic deficiencies inherent in aging and support geriatric well-being (Rémond et al., 2015).

6.2.2. Contribution to Immune System Health

The immune function is highly interconnected with nutritional consumption, particularly trace metals that are essential for optimal immune status among the elderly. With increasing age, several physiological changes occur, which lead to altered nutrient intake and vulnerability to malnutrition. These changes are maximal in the gastrointestinal system, where mechanical and chemical food breakdown is compromised. Reduced nutrient availability can impair immune function, rendering an individual more prone to infection and disease. Coping with these nutritional deficiencies via dietary adjustments that consider the particular trace metal needs of the aging population can deflect some consequences of aging and maximize immune robustness and, ultimately, health outcomes.

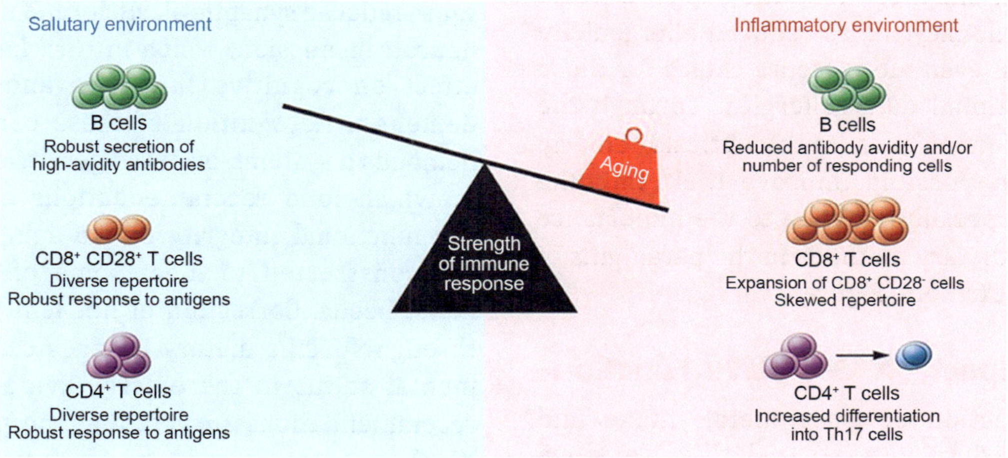

Figure 6.7. Contribution to immune system health.

Source: https://www.frontiersin.org/files/Articles/735151/fpubh-09-735151-HTML-r1/image_m/fpubh-09-735151-g001.jpg.

As a result of the increased susceptibility of the elderly, there is a need to come up with overarching diet standards that integrate determinants of nutrient uptake and overall health in this group (Rémond et al., 2015). Moreover, some trace metals, such as selenium and zinc, are crucial for the maintenance of immune system function. Zinc is involved in the growth and activation of immune cells, such as T lymphocytes and macrophages, that are necessary in the immune defense mechanism of the human body. Zinc deficiency can lead to weak immune functions and facilitate infections and autoimmune diseases in older individuals. Similarly, selenium exerts antioxidant effects that combat oxidative stress, which can compromise immune function in the long run. Studies show that proper selenium supplementation is linked with reduced morbidity and mortality in elderly individuals, which hints at its implication in the diet for elderly individuals. Upkeep of sufficient levels of these trace metals in the form of balanced diets or supplements needed can enhance immune function and limit the risk of age-related disease (Rémond et al., 2015). In addition to traditional sources of nutrition, novel dietary sources such as donkey milk provide viable alternatives for the augmentation of immune function in the elderly. Rich in bioactive molecules like lactoferrin, which regulates iron homeostasis and exhibits antimicrobial activity, donkey milk has a unique nutritional composition that would be extremely beneficial to the elderly.

The presence of critical proteins that facilitate immune functions suggests that the addition of this beverage to the diet of older adults may enhance their nutrient status, thereby assisting in enhanced immune support. Apart from this, donkey milk's reduced allergenicity makes it an even more secure choice for those with traditional dairy allergies. Through the consumption of such nutraceuticals, elderly people can possibly improve their immune potency, especially pointing to the importance of diverse dietary methods in the paradigms of geriatric nutrition (Figure 6.7).

6.2.3. Impact on Cognitive Function

The interaction of trace metal intake and cognitive performance in the elderly is of extreme importance since increasingly large numbers of elderly populations are experiencing cognitive decline. Trace metals such as zinc, copper, and selenium are all essential to neurological health and may be significantly influential on cognitive function. Zinc, for instance, is essential for synaptic processes and neurotransmitter release; deficiencies have been correlated with impaired learning and memory. Secondly, copper is involved in brain development and myelination; its deficiency might lead to neurodegeneration, which exacerbates age-related cognitive impairment. By supplementing geriatric patients with adequate amounts of these trace metals, healthcare providers might avert or slow cognitive impairment and enhance quality of life in older adults, facilitating enhanced mental health as well as functional capacity. The aging gastrointestinal tract (GIT) plays a major role in adsorbing trace metals, and its dysfunction has adverse effects on the cognitive function of elderly patients. With increasing age, changes in the GIT, such as reduced motility and changes in the intestinal microbiota, interfere with the maximum absorption of nutrients and cause malnutrition, primarily in the major trace elements (Rémond et al., 2015). Such malnutrition not only impacts physical health but also plays a vital part in the deterioration of cognitive functions.

For instance, trace metal deficiency can cause reduced synaptic plasticity and unbalanced neurotransmission, which in turn has a direct effect on cognitive functions and leads to dementia. Recognition of these complexities demands a systems-oriented geriatric nutrition in which food recommendations are set by the functional integrity of the aging GIT and are constructed to meet some of the trace metal needs. Correction of nutrient deficiency through specific dietary changes can enhance mental status in the elderly. Evidence-based recommendations suggest that the population of the elderly needs to be screened for malnutrition as a regular procedure so that early intervention may be assured (Volkert et al., 2019). Oral nutritional supplements coupled with food management and general nutritional advice may be used to improve the intake of trace metals in the aged population. Additionally, involving physical activity will also improve cognitive function through enhanced nutrient uptake and overall health. Together, promoting an environment where trace metal intake is optimized improves not only malnutrition prevention but also cognitive vitality support, thus ensuring the optimization of the health profile and quality of life in elderly populations.

6.3. Recommended Dietary Allowances (RDAs)

RDAs are a reference for levels of nutrient intake recommended to support the nutritional requirements of almost all healthy members of certain demographic groups. To older people, to whom there are special nutritional requirements due to the physiological alterations and enhanced incidence of chronic illnesses, such allowances are particularly significant. RDAs of trace metals such as zinc and selenium have been adjusted to take into consideration reduced absorption and altered metabolism frequently encountered among aged individuals. As illustrated by recent studies, ensuring that elderly individuals receive adequate quantities of their RDAs of these trace metals can fortify their immune system and overall well-being, considerations of relevance in the fight against the harmful effects of chronic disease endemic within this demographic. Zinc stands apart from the trace metals in the sense that it is involved in intricate functions in human physiology, particularly within elderly groups. It is required for many physiological processes, including regulation of the immune system, and is associated with increased risk of infection and impaired recovery from illness when the body lacks it. Recent research emphasizes that a deficiency in zinc can have a critical effect on health and thus meeting the RDA for this mineral matters in older individuals. Given that approximately one-third of the global population is estimated to be deficient in zinc, dietary sources cannot be overstressed. Also, choosing zinc supplementation is appropriate, since some organic forms of zinc have better absorption, increasing their efficacy in aiding the immune system in combating the rising health challenges of the elderly, particularly in light of global health emergencies established in recent studies (Majeed et al., 2021). Other than zinc, the contribution of trace metal interaction with cardiovascular health cannot be overlooked, particularly as cardiovascular disease ranks among the leading causes of mortality worldwide. Dietary habits play a critical role in controlling atherosclerosis and other cardiovascular diseases. Emphasis on vegetable diets with the addition of adequate trace metal intake can be a significant contributor to promoting geriatric nutrition by maintaining cardiovascular health and total vitality. Adjusting RDAs for trace metals according to the balance of macro- and micronutrients becomes imperative in the treatment of the elderly to ensure complete dietary interventions. Through intervening into the individual health needs of elderly people with individual RDAs, healthcare providers can better help this population use nutrition as a means to improve their health outcomes (Hever & Cronise, 2017) (Figure 6.8).

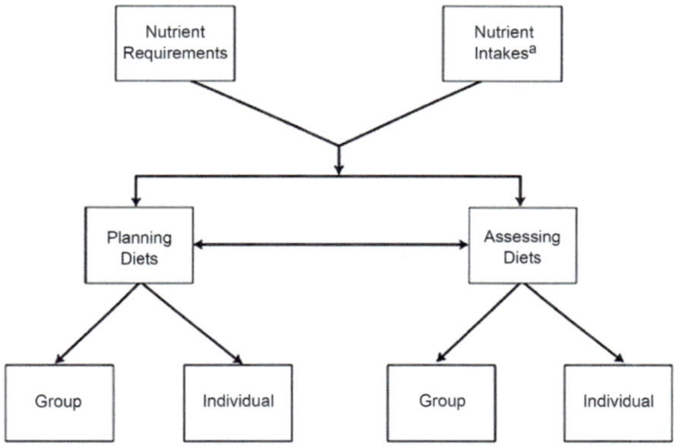

Figure 6.8. Uses of dietary reference intakes.

Source: https://nap.nationalacademies.org/openbook/0309069351/xhtml/images/p20003381g384001.jpg.

6.3.1. Age-Specific Requirements

The aging process calls for many physiological changes that significantly affect nutritional needs, particularly with trace metals such as zinc and copper. The gastrointestinal tract suffers a decline in function with age, which has an adverse effect on intake, digestion, and absorption of the required nutrients. The mechanical food breakdown is less effective, while the gastrointestinal motility changes may result in delayed transit times, thus compromising nutrient absorption efficiency. Such changes can lead to a compromised capacity of the older people to take up adequate amounts of trace metals necessary for the maintenance of general health.

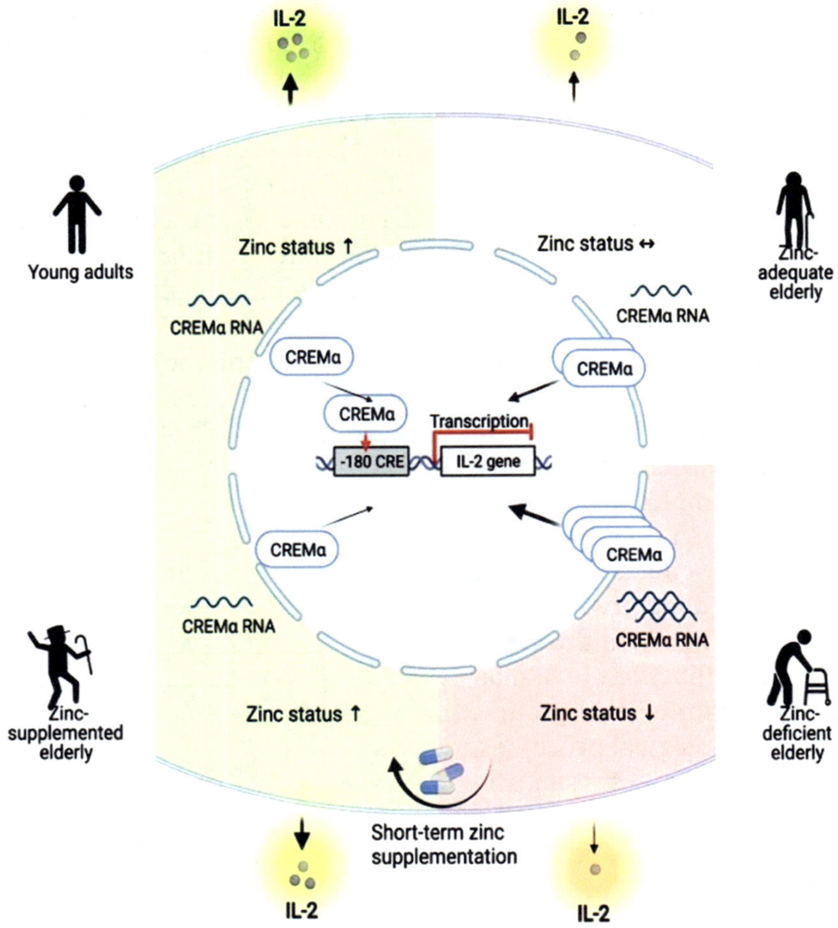

Figure 6.9. Zinc nutriture of the geriatric population.

Source: https://media.springernature.com/lw685/springer-static/image/art%3A10.1186%2Fs12979-022-00295-8/MediaObjects/12979_2022_295_Figa_HTML.png.

The impending risk of malnutrition thus becomes increasingly pertinent, as it has the potential to foretell the onset of pathologies involving various organ systems. Therefore, it is of extreme significance that these age-specific requirements are fulfilled with augmented dietary advice and nutritional interventions so as to prevent the threats of derangement in gastrointestinal function and resulting malnutrition (Rémond et al., 2015). Trace metals play a role in an array of biochemical processes and also help with immunity, bone strength, and mental processes. Zinc, for instance, plays a crucial role in immune system function and dermal health, while copper preserves iron metabolism and nervous system function. In a study of zinc nutriture in elderly patients, 67% were found to have plasma zinc values within the range for deficiency, even though most claimed to have adequate zinc-containing foods. Ironically, this situation is indicative of the possible difference between dietary consumption and biological availability secondary to changes in absorption potential in the elderly (Paterson, 1982). Simultaneously, the fluctuating copper: zinc ratios among these demographics need to be further researched, as they could point to subsisting diseases that are often found in the geriatric patient. In understanding these dynamics, it is clear that specialized dietary solutions reflecting the singular nutritional nuances of the elderly need to be implemented for the generation of enhanced health dynamics. To effectively address age-related requirements for trace metals, a coordinated strategy that combines both dietary and possibly supplementary methods is essential. Older people have reduced appetite, increased medication use, and chronic diseases, all of which contribute to suboptimal nutrient intake. Consequently, nutritional remedies will have to incorporate not just trace metal food sources with easily absorbed forms but also provide for the intake of food that is in conformity with the physiological and cultural tastes of the elderly. The evidence suggests that adding to the diet bioavailable sources of zinc and copper and measures designed to maximize gastrointestinal function can minimize the prevalence of malnutrition and its disorders. Development of practical nutritional recommendations from understanding the elderly gastrointestinal tract can thus be a basis for meeting geriatric nutritional needs, eventually improving overall health and quality of life of the group (Rémond et al., 2015) (Figure 6.9).

6.3.2. Gender Differences in Trace Metal Needs

Understanding the gender differences in trace metal needs is significant in the resolution of geriatric nutritional requirements. As per the studies, men and women were discovered to have unique body composition and hormone-dependent physiological requirements for trace metals such as iron, zinc, and copper. For instance, males will have more muscle tissue than females, and this can impact trace element distribution and need within the body. Women, particularly postmenopausal women, also experience extreme hormonal fluctuations, which can impact iron metabolism and zinc absorption, necessitating certain dietary adjustments. These gender-specific demands underscore the need for dietary assessments that are sensitive to these differences, and through this, potentially enhance health outcomes in older adults. In addition, gender-specific metabolic processes involved in trace metal utilization translate into different recommendations for diet. Women are especially vulnerable to iron deficiency, notably during periods of elevated physiological demands such as pregnancy and lactation, but also exposed to potential overexposure to zinc through supplementation. Zinc is required for wound healing and immune function, significant in the elderly; however, excess zinc may interfere with copper absorption, making trace metal balance challenging. In contrast, men might require more of certain trace metals due to their higher muscle mass and metabolic rates. This difference necessitates individualized nutrition regimens that consider such variations to optimize health and minimize risks of deficiency among the aged, as establishing equilibrated trace metal intake could make an enormous difference in overall well-being. Finally, the implications of such gender contrasts extend beyond clinical care to broader public health programs for geriatric nutrition. As trace metal deficiencies may exacerbate the prevalence of chronic ailments such as cognitive impairment and osteoporosis, understanding gender-specific needs for these minerals becomes essential in setting effective intervention strategies. Elderly-directed education should, thus, include understanding the varied needs and possible food sources of principal trace metals. Nutrition policy for the elderly should further incorporate the gender-sensitive framework to successfully enhance health outcomes. The health professionals can make their contribution towards sustaining and enhancing the quality of life of older persons by adopting gender-specific nutritional guidelines, so that nutrition interventions are kept in tune with the specific needs of women and men in their advanced age.

6.3.3. Variability Based on Health Status

In gerontological nutrition, the interface between trace metal needs and health status comes to the forefront as a matter of prime concern. Nutritional needs are vastly different among the elderly due to diverse health complications, impacting the absorption and metabolism of trace metals such as zinc, copper, and selenium. For instance, chronic diseases like cardiovascular diseases and diabetes can interfere with metabolic processes and necessitate corresponding changes in diet to realize optimal health outcomes. In addition, elderly people can also have differences in gut microbiota composition, which is vital for nutrient absorption and may also make trace metal bioavailability more complicated. Clinicians are therefore required to evaluate individual health conditions comprehensively to provide individualized nutritional interventions not only to meet baseline metabolic needs but also to meet the respective physiological needs of each elder. Furthermore, the role of trace metals in promoting immune function is even more notable because elderly people are more likely to get exposed to infections and chronic illnesses. Health status within the elderly population has the potential to affect the dosage and preparation of trace metals necessary to provide optimal immune function. For instance, zinc and selenium deficiency have been linked to impaired immune function, such that they become more vulnerable to illness. More importantly, some elderly people may have diseases affecting their dietary preferences or dietary intake for certain foods.

These further limit the intake of these trace metals, hence further deficiencies in these trace metals. With an excellent health report, personalized nutritional approaches facilitate the determination of deficits and supplementation wherever possible. This comprehensive approach not only enhances nutrient status but also increases the health resilience of older adults to disease, as the clinical significance of individual profiles of health is understood. Lastly, the interaction between trace metals and health conditions is also complicated by environmental variables and lifestyle. Socioeconomic differences play a critical role in affecting nutrient-dense foods, thereby compounding differences in trace metal status in older adults. Certain populations may lack sufficient access to quality foods rich in essential trace metals due to economic or geographic barriers, which can negatively impact their health outcomes. Moreover, environmental changes may further influence dietary patterns and nutrient composition, underscoring the need for a multi-faceted approach to geriatric nutrition. Successful interventions should not only consider the personal health status of older adults but also respond to societal determinants that influence nutritional access and equity. By combining information from both individual measurements and community health data, health professionals are able to promote dietary approaches that maximize trace metal intake in terms of the individual health situations of elderly patients, leading to enhanced health and quality of life for this high-risk population (Figure 6.10).

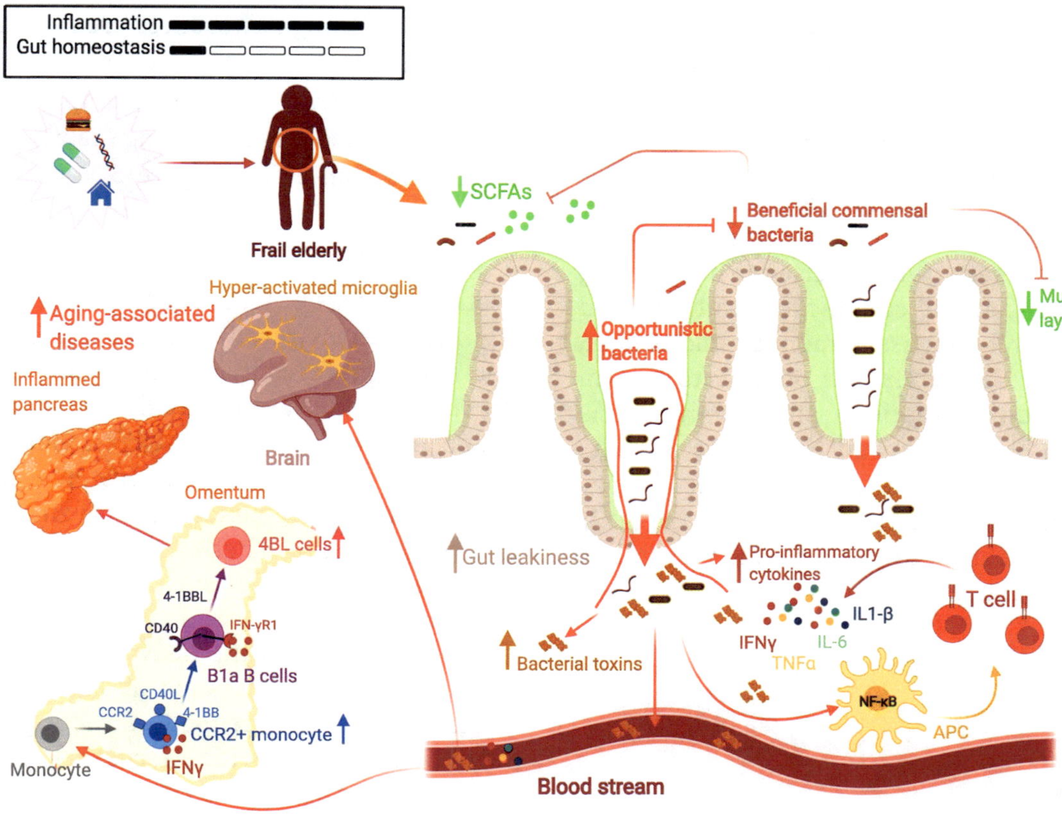

Figure 6.10. Gut microbiota as the key controllers of "healthy" aging of elderly people.

Source: https://media.springernature.com/lw685/springer-static/image/art%3A10.1186%2Fs12979-020-00213-w/MediaObjects/12979_2020_213_Fig3_HTML.png.

6.4. Sources of Trace Metals

The role of trace metals in the diet of the elderly cannot be overemphasized since they have several physiological functions. Food sources of trace metals such as zinc, copper, iron, and selenium are vital in ensuring the health of geriatric patients. Animal foods like meat, seafood, and dairy products are rich in trace metals and are likely to provide enhanced bioavailability relative to plant foods. Yet, eating habits among the elderly tend to change for reasons including loss of taste, dental disease, or financial factors, which might restrict their consumption of these essential nutrients. Therefore, the demand for dietary changes to consider the diminished capacity of aging gastrointestinal tracts to absorb these trace metals efficiently, as identified in literature on the subject of malnutrition among the elderly (Rémond et al., 2015), should be acknowledged. Apart from animal food sources, a range of foods of plant origin can meet the trace metal needs of the elderly when part of an adequate diet. Whole grains, legumes, seeds, and nuts provide essential minerals, but some of the plant sources do contain phytates that may inhibit absorption. For example, while crops like lentils and beans are rich in zinc and iron, availability may be hampered by phytates. To improve mineral absorption, it is recommended that such foods be accompanied by sources of vitamin C or by employing preparation techniques that lower phytate content, like soaking or fermenting. These efforts can counteract the ill effects of phytates, thereby enhancing dietary intake of trace metals important for geriatric well-being (Paterson, 1982). Trace metal status monitoring among the elderly will be critical in avoiding deficiencies that will complicate health-related conditions. Frequent assessment of zinc, copper, and other trace metals will be able to inform dietary recommendations and interventions based on a person's needs. Numerous patients under geriatric care could have poor dietary intake combined with alterations in their metabolism that modify their ability to utilize these basic nutrients.

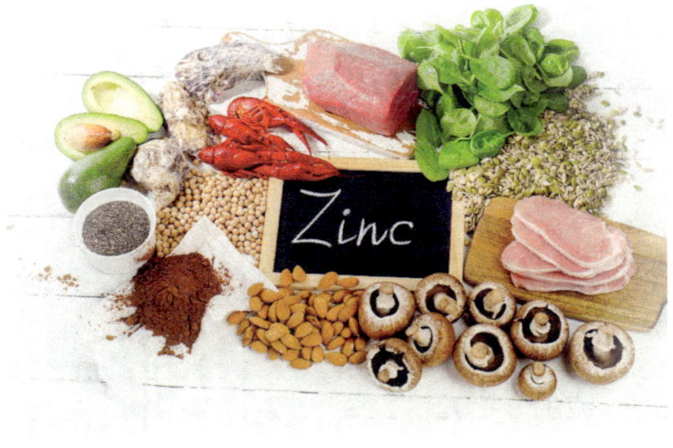

Figure 6.11. Significance of trace metals in the diet of the elderly.

Source: https://external-content.duckduckgo.com/iu/?u=https%3A%2F%2Fblog.ultimatelifespan.com%2Fwp-content%2Fuploads%2F2020%2F04%2FDepositphotos_140333796_original-scaled.jpg&f=1&nofb=1&ipt=b55f79ce0a5a5c16ab7c966805970d6e59f65bac40268482c2e24822f0f0b526.

As has been observed in one study, although most older adults had proper diets when it comes to zinc, there still was a significant proportion with insufficient plasma levels, which might be related to overall health deteriorations and malnutrition (Paterson, 1982). Bridging these gaps through awareness creation and the distribution of fortified food products can assist in enhancing trace metal consumption among older adults, thereby enhancing their nutritional status and well-being (Figure 6.11).

6.4.1. Dietary Sources.

Dietary sources of trace metals are of greatest significance in gerontic nutrition since the micronutrients are vital for numerous functions crucial in maintaining health in older age. Older individuals have lower appetites and nutritional diversity, so they are most likely to lack essential trace metals such as zinc, copper, and magnesium. These trace minerals are abundantly present in such foods as legumes, whole grains, seeds, and nuts. For instance, studies centered on the heavy mineral load of root and tuber crops such as cassava, sweet potato, and taro. These foods, besides providing carbohydrates, provide necessary minerals like zinc and manganese, meaning that the addition of such foods can help enhance the nutritional value of meals for the elderly, in turn addressing potential inadequacies of trace metals necessary for their health (Millena et al., 2024). The nutritional importance of bioavailable trace metals is underscored by the findings that certain foods have the potential to significantly increase mineral intakes among older individuals. Root and tuber crops contain high concentrations of minerals that have a significant degree of bioavailability, in which these nutrients can be successfully utilized and absorbed by the body. For instance, giant swamp taro intake has been linked to supporting zinc and manganese requirements, which are both critical to immune function and bone health. Additionally, nutritional compositions of these crops reveal that they carry impressive amounts of dietary fiber, which can support digestive health, another prime consideration in geriatric nutrition. Therefore, promotion of consumption of these mineral-rich crops can lead to increased dietary diversity and address the nutritional gaps prevalent among geriatric populations (Millena et al., 2024). Moreover, exploration of the contribution of dietary supplements, such as boron, emphasizes the incorporation of trace metal bioavailability and total health benefits among older age groups.

Current research has indicated that boron supplementation positively impacts mineral balance, through increased calcium and phosphorus content, crucial to bone density maintenance. By borrowing from avian nutritional research, the inclusion of boron in diets provided increased eggshell weight, thereby pointing towards the mineral's role in biological function and health. This information prompts additional studies on how similar methods can be applied to human nutrition, particularly in older people, to achieve maximum intake of major trace metals and promote overall health. Since older individuals may require mineral supplements as a complement to their trace metal needs, the incorporation of good dietary sources in their food plans is critical for enhancing their quality of life (Figure 6.12).

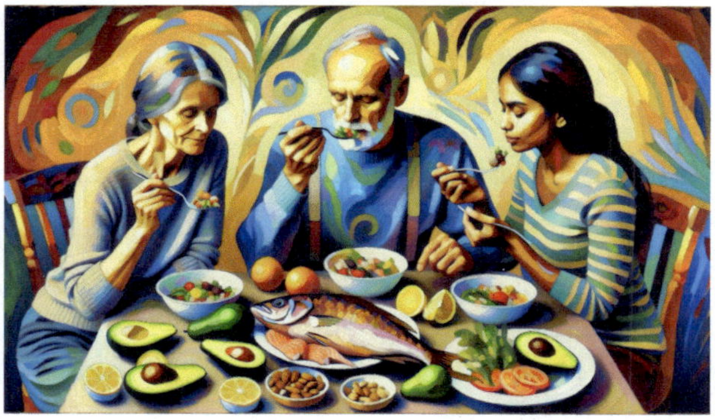

Figure 6.12. Nutrition for elderly.

Source: https://external-content.duckduckgo.com/iu/?u=https%3A%2F%2Fi.pinimg.com%2Foriginals%2Ffe%2Fc0%2F37%2Ffec037972b533907852f62055a067d1f.jpg&f=1&nofb=1&ipt=5093084a055017138ea1214fc4581f46c535821a5b738fa2d839be5c6f5e08fa.

6.4.2. Supplementation Options

The importance of supplementation alternatives to the achievement of trace metal requirements for a geriatric diet cannot be overstated. As one ages, the efficiency of the body in absorbing vital nutrients, including trace metals such as zinc, selenium, and copper, decreases. They play a critical role in various physiological functions like immune response, antioxidant protection, and enzyme activities. Supplements specifically designed for older adults are able to bridge the gaps offered by dietary lack, presenting adequate amounts of these necessary nutrients. Further, multi-nutrient supplements specifically designed for older adults often include trace metals with the ability to neutralize common age-related diseases, presenting a better nutritional balance. This does not merely inhibit deficiency but also enhances the overall health, presenting a more balanced health status within the geriatric population. The employment of natural substances, such as royal jelly, has been considered a reasonable option for supplementing geriatric nutrition. Royal jelly has been characterized by high protein, vitamins, lipids, and trace minerals content, which emphasizes its therapeutic potential. Its bioactive molecules, like 10-hydroxy-2-decenoic acid and other peptides, have demonstrated diverse health advantages. These functions range from immunomodulatory activity to neuroprotection, which could be particularly useful for elderly patients with age-related illnesses. Moreover, the capacity of royal jelly to enhance energy and function on a metabolic level guarantees that it can prove to be an effective supplement for geriatric subjects to guarantee nutritional adequacy as well as quality of life. Hence, integrating such new paradigms of supplementation would be a long way towards redressing the unique nutritional needs of senile populations. New technologies in wearable technology and telehealth promise to extend further how supplements are administered and monitored for geriatric nutrition. The integration of optical sensor systems is opening up new possibilities for personalized care, where there is real-time monitoring of nutrients and metabolic function.

This technology is in line with the increasing demand for individualized health interventions in aging since it allows clinicians to dynamically modulate supplementation strategy based on individual requirements. Through the use of data-driven information, elderly professionals can optimize trace metal supplementation in the elderly to give them precisely the nutrients necessary to manage their health effectively. Consequently, not only does this approach enhance adherence to supplementation regimes, but it also promotes an active style of geriatric care, confirming the central position of good nutrition in elderly groups (Junior et al., 2024; Oršolić & Jembrek, 2024).

6.4.3. Bioavailability of Trace Metals in Food

Trace metal food bioavailability is a major determinant of their nutritional status, particularly in geriatric groups. As age advances, there are gross changes in the gastrointestinal system which influence the uptake of nutrients, such as trace essential metals, such as zinc and copper. Aging leads to impaired functioning of the gastrointestinal tract with reduced mechanical breakdown, motility, and chemical digestion of food. Thus, such physiological changes can significantly reduce the efficiency with which trace metals are absorbed, increasing the risk of deficiency further, which can adversely affect health. Understanding these dynamics is critical in the development of dietary guidelines that will maximize trace metal consumption among older individuals, considering adequacy in nutrient bioavailability as a requisite to provide overall health as well as the prevention of malnutrition (Rémond et al., 2015). The interaction between food sources and the bioavailability of trace metals further complicates nutritional planning in the elderly. Certain foods enhance or inhibit the absorption of trace metals and thus food combinations need to be considered during meal planning. For instance, vitamin C enhances the absorption of non-heme iron, while phytates present in whole grains and legumes inhibit the bioavailability of zinc. The significance of such interactions becomes relevant in the case of geriatric nutrition, where food choice and limitation can limit the ingestion of significant metal sources. As research has shown, a proper diet that is rich in different food groups can counterbalance absorption limitations and allow for the attainment of requisite levels of trace metals and thus support the complex health needs of the elderly (Paterson, 1982).

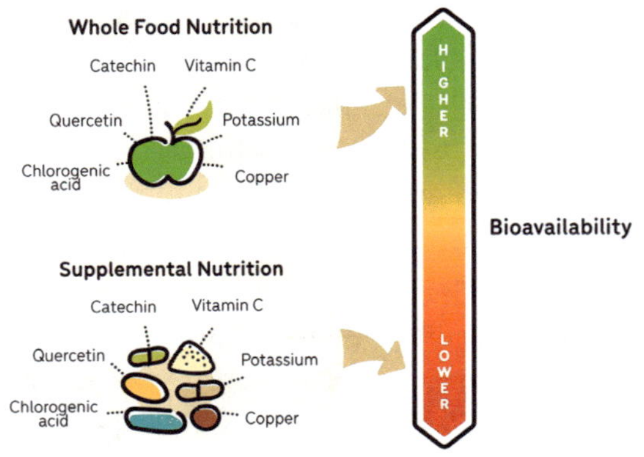

Figure 6.13. Bioavailability of trace metals in food.

Source: https://assets-global.website-files.com/5d6322f018659f07ac06321a/611dc250914adfde2b5e297b_Bioavailability-natural-vs-synthetic.jpg.

In assessing trace metal status in the elderly, a knowledge of both dietary intake and bioavailability is essential. It has been found that older subjects are frequently below recommended dietary allowances for trace metals such as zinc, an element crucial to immune function, and copper, an element crucial to cardiovascular health. Several factors, including the altered dietary habits and the greater prevalence of chronic diseases, can impact such metals' bioavailability among this population. For instance, a study identified that there was a high rate of older subjects with inadequate dietary intakes of zinc-rich foods, although some of them maintained normal plasma levels of zinc. Supplying elderly adults with the right, bioavailable forms of trace metals is essential for the sustenance of their nutritional needs and prevention of associated complications due to malnourishment (Paterson, 1982; Rémond et al., 2015) (Figure 6.13).

6.5. Deficiency and Excess of Trace Metals

The balance of trace metals is significant in ensuring optimal health, especially in the elderly who may suffer from some dietary restraints and physiological changes. A deficiency in trace metals such as zinc, selenium, and copper may influence overall health significantly. Trace metals play diverse critical functions in biochemistry, including immune function, antioxidant defense, and neurocognitive health. Lacking sufficient intake, elderly individuals will be exposed to suboptimal immune function, increased risk of infection, and impaired cognitive status, which may all have a significant bearing on their quality of life. Geriatric nutrition requirements also often must be modified due to variations in absorption and alterations in metabolism, which reflects the importance of maintaining specialized dietary guidance that can correct for these shortages while promoting well-being and longevity.

On the other hand, excessive use of trace metals can even lead to such health risks for elderly individuals. The population is particularly susceptible to heavy metals like lead, mercury, and cadmium, which could lead to long-term accumulation in the body and a negative impact on vital systems. For example, an overload of zinc causes dysfunction in the immune system and gastrointestinal difficulties, whereas excessive levels of selenium could result in selenosis with symptoms such as gastrointestinal disturbances, hair loss, and neuropathy. In addition, elderly individuals might suffer from impaired renal function, further impairing the body's ability to excrete excess metal, thereby raising the risk of toxicity. Therefore, an understanding of trace metal deficiency and excess is crucial in formulating dietary recommendations with a preference for healthy aging and the avoidance of subsequent diseases and disorders typical in old age.

Evidence indicates that certain biological markers, like DNA damage due to trace metal exposure, could better explain the connection between trace metals and cognitive state. The comet assays, which challenge DNA integrity, suggest that high levels of DNA damage have a significant association with cognitive impairment caused by both aging and environmental effects on trace metals. The same is particularly relevant to older adults, who can be demonstrated to have increased susceptibility to oxidative stress and cumulative biological damage, with resultant effects on cognitive functions relevant to daily performance and occupational functioning. The implications of these findings highlight the importance of bioactive nutrients in the diet that will offset oxidative stress and enhance cellular health, thereby enhancing the overall nutrition regimen for the elderly (López et al., 2022; Abreu et al., 2023). Precise understanding of trace metal requirements tailored to the unique needs of the elderly will ultimately enable caregivers and health professionals to be able to better serve older individuals in maintaining their well-being and mental coherence (Figure 6.14).

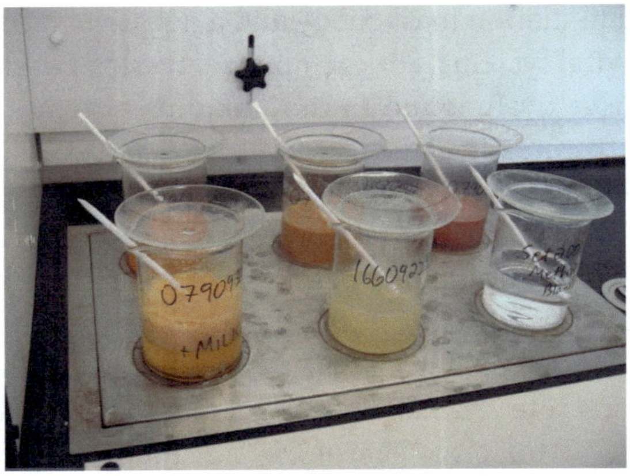

Figure 6.14. Deficiency and excess of trace metals.

Source: https://lab-training.com/wp-content/uploads/2015/07/IMG_0945-1024x768.jpg.

6.5.1. Symptoms of Deficiency

Older people's trace metal deficiency may have several symptoms, which create an immense burden on general health and well-being. The physiological changes within the gastrointestinal tract with advancing age interfere with nutrient uptake. Such alterations, such as reduced motility and efficacy in nutrient breakdown, add an immense risk of malnutrition with several deficiency symptoms. For example, zinc deficiency may result in compromised immune function, making one more susceptible to infections and impaired wound healing. Iron deficiency may cause anemia, as evidenced by fatigue and impaired mental function. Awareness of these symptoms is key to fulfilling the special nutritional requirements of aging and implementing dietetic interventions to mitigate deficiency and malnutrition risk in such a high-risk population (Rémond et al., 2015). Furthermore, trace metal deficiency is also considered to be involved in severe neurodegenerative diseases that are responsible for a considerable influence on cognitive performance in older individuals. Alzheimer's disease (AD) is one such disease that highlights the significance of micronutrients in protecting neural tissue from degeneration. Low consumption of trace essential metals such as selenium and magnesium has been associated with increased oxidative stress and inflammation in the brain. This is a worrisome discovery since deficiencies are likely to promote the state of cognitive decline among elderly people. Furthermore, low trace metal levels could cause disturbances in calcium homeostasis and energy metabolism, states that could trigger or exacerbate neurodegenerative disease (Staehelin, 2017).

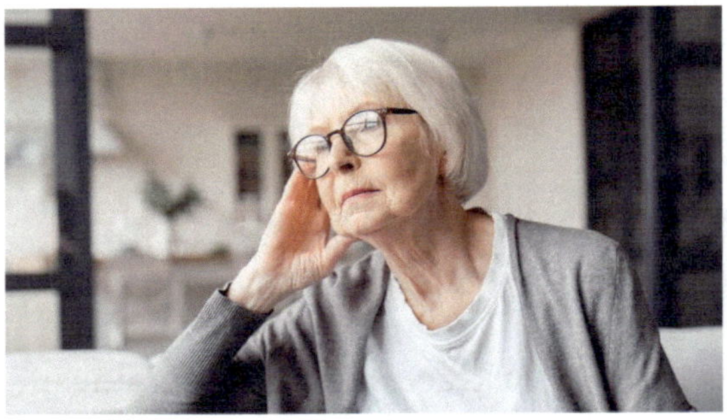

Figure 6.15. Common nutrient deficiencies in the elderly.

Source: https://www.topnoshmeals.com.au/wp-content/uploads/2023/05/image1-edited.jpg.

Therefore, the treatment strategy for geriatric nutrition needs to be oriented towards optimum trace metal intake in order to prevent these adverse symptoms. The impact of trace metal deficiency extends beyond individual wellness and into social behavior and healthcare policy. With the increasing prevalence of malnutrition among elderly populations, expressions of deficiency—deterioration of the immune system to dementia—can lead to mounting caregiver stress and healthcare costs. For instance, elderly people with deficiencies can be hospital readmitted continuously due to their compromised health. Correction of these deficiencies through targeted nutrition interventions is essential not only for improving individual health outcomes but also for reducing the economic load on healthcare systems. By maintaining that the elderly are given a balanced diet with all the required trace metals, healthcare practitioners can improve the quality of life for older individuals and encourage healthier aging, thus lowering the broader social impacts of malnutrition and its signs (Rémond et al., 2015) (Figure 6.15).

6.5.2. Health Risks Associated with Excess Intake

The absorption of trace metals, although essential in minimal quantities for the sustenance of health, leads to acute risks when consumption levels surpass tolerance levels. Trace metal consumption equilibrium in the elderly is crucial as the elderly have their metabolism altered and nutritional needs diverse. For instance, excessive consumption of metals such as cobalt, which is required in traces for normal physiological functioning, is harmful to health. It is evidence that trace metal-deficient regions must be supplemented in animal feed, but over-supplementation would be the reason for toxicity, with concerns for cobalt accumulation within the body. It becomes necessary to be aware of the thin boundary between taking sufficient and taking excessive trace metals, especially among the elderly, when trace metal consumption enters the toxic ranges even when consuming only dietary amounts (Khan et al., 2023). The fame of heavy metal deposition in marine food organisms highlights the inherent risk involved in trace metal consumption. For example, fish such as Catla catla, which are otherwise a healthy protein, can have lethal levels of metals such as lead, mercury, and arsenic due to environmental pollution. The health risks that come from exposure to such metals are of the greatest risk to elderly individuals, who may have impaired kidney functions or heightened vulnerabilities to neurological damage. With increasing intake of seafood, the chances for toxic accumulation within the system rise, particularly if the metals cross international safety levels. Consequently, consumption of fish from contaminated sources may lead to significant long-term non-carcinogenic and carcinogenic health risks, emphasizing the necessity for cautious dietary recommendations for the aged (Saleem et al., 2022). Moreover, the overall health impacts of trace metal excess consumption require a comprehensive risk assessment suitable for the elderly age group. Geriatric nutrition is not only about adequate consumption but also about avoiding trace metal toxicity. The nuances of certain medical conditions also complicate this scenario, as conditions like current medical conditions or other medications consumed concurrently can synergistically raise risk from overconsumption. By assessing both approximated weekly consumption and potential hazard quotients, medical professionals can create diet strategies that avoid overconsumption of metals. Implementing routine diet evaluation and establishing awareness regarding credible sources of safe food is of greatest significance in order to safeguard older people from the hazards of trace metal intoxication (Saleem et al., 2022; Khan et al., 2023).

6.5.3. Strategies for Maintaining Balance

Maintaining nutritional balance in geriatrics requires a multifaceted approach in consideration of the characteristic physiological alterations that accompany advancing age. With the gastrointestinal system undergoing ongoing functional impairment, it becomes increasingly challenging to attain adequate nutrient uptake. This is further aggravated by the risk of malnutrition that impacts various organ systems, like the musculoskeletal and nervous systems. It is thus essential to know how aging impacts trace metal ingestion and absorption. Successful interventions must involve formulating specialized dietary recommendations that take into consideration modification of digestion and nutrient bioavailability. Implementing these suggestions would not only help correct trace metal deficiencies but also reverse the general impact of malnutrition, thereby improving the health condition of the elderly population as a whole (Rémond et al., 2015). In addition to devising appropriate nutritional recommendations, the use of systematic malnutrition screening is critical for maintaining balance in the nutrition of the elderly. Regular testing can help identify those at risk, allowing early intervention with a diet modified accordingly. Evidence shows that mouth nutritional support, complemented with education programs, can further promote nutrient intake among the elderly. For instance, tailoring nutritional advice to suit people's tastes and lifestyles can significantly enhance adherence to eating patterns as advised. Also, this integrated approach confirms that nutrition prevention from malnutrition is not only based on dietary intervention but must also consider the social and psychological determinants of food intake. This multi-pronged strategy is also in line with the urgency of personalized nutrition interventions to counteract aging-related threats (Volkert et al., 2019). Lastly, the promotion of hydration in addition to proper nutrition is necessary for optimal health among older adults. Dehydration is a widespread concern among older adults that is often neglected amidst dietary concerns. Encouragement of adequate fluid consumption should be included as part of routine monitoring to support overall dietary guidance to meet both nutrition and fluid needs. Interventions like adjustment of food texture or intake of nutrient-filled fluids can encourage greater fluid consumption, particularly in the case of swallowing disorders. Moreover, one must recognize that, while weight management may be beneficial for some older individuals, specific assessments must direct any dietary restriction. Thus, an overall approach to dietary management, such as hydration, weight, and trace metal intake, is still key to maintaining nutritional balance in the elderly population (Volkert et al., 2019) (Figure 6.16).

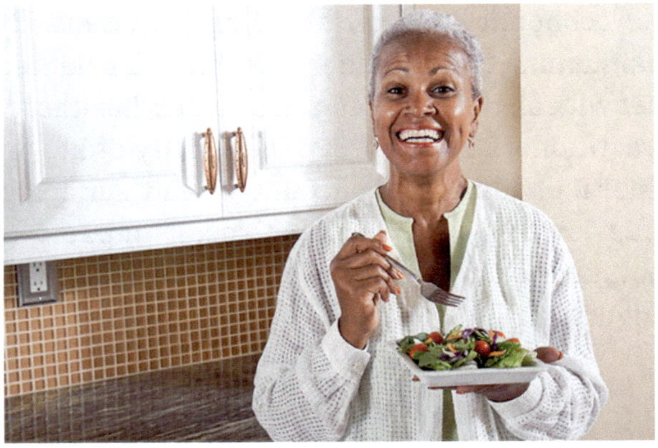

Figure 6.16. Importance of a balanced diet for the elderly.

Source: https://abbyseniorcare.com/wp-content/uploads/2021/06/senior-woman-eating-salad_800px.jpg.

6.6. Special Considerations for Geriatric Population

The elderly population presents special challenges that demand special considerations regarding nutrition, particularly trace metals. Physiological changes, such as diminished absorption and altered metabolism with age, can significantly affect their nutritional needs as individuals age. Furthermore, older adults typically have several comorbid diseases, which make food intake complex and necessitate individualized nutritional intervention. Trace metal deficiencies such as zinc and selenium have also been implicated in compromised immunity, heightened morbidity and mortality due to chronic diseases, and impaired cognitive function in this population. Hence, there is a need for healthcare professionals and nutritionists to adopt an integrative approach based on both lifestyle and biological determinants affecting older adults so that their trace metal requirements are met to yield optimal health benefits in various arenas of aging. Besides biological alterations, social and behavioral determinants also play an irreplaceable role in determining the dietary pattern of the elderly. For instance, decreased mobility and social isolation can restrict accessibility to sources of wholesome food, leading to poor intake of required trace metals. Family members and caregivers also come into the forefront, as they are capable of playing a significant role in the dietary intake of older adults. Education and enabling resources for older adults and their caregivers need to be leveraged to reclaim these social determinants of health. Coordination of support programs at the community level and personalized nutrition guidelines can promote better dietary habits that can reduce the likelihood of deficiency disorders in geriatrics. Nutrition consciousness strategies, particularly about trace metals, must be culturally acceptable and relevant to the heterogeneous populations in this group. Moreover, the encouragement of multi-domain interventions involving nutrition, physical activity, and education for health has been found useful in enhancing the quality of life among the elderly. Focused interventions have even been recently found to encourage successful counteraction of mild cognitive impairment (MCI) among the aging population, which is a key problem of geriatric health. The integration of holistic approaches encompassing not only nutritional needs but also lifestyle factors is critical for improving outcomes in health. It provides an opportunity for healthcare professionals to promote holistic geriatric nutrition delivery, emphasizing maintaining cognitive function as much as physical well-being. As emphasized in recent studies, the development of such multidomain interventions is not only beneficial but also inevitable, as they align with the multifactorial progression of health worsening in elderly individuals, representing in a way an active approach to caring for the elderly (Betz et al., 2023; Wu et al., 2023).

6.6.1. Changes in Metabolism with Age

During aging, very significant changes are seen in their metabolic processes, influencing both energy expenditure and nutritional requirements. Basal metabolic rate, which is normally the energy required for important physiological functions, gradually declines with increasing age. The decline results from a combination of factors like loss of lean muscle mass and endocrine regulation alterations. As such, elderly individuals will have lower caloric demand, which, when not well controlled, will result in weight loss and malnutrition. Apart from that, when metabolism declines, the efficiency of nutrient uptake and utilization also declines, particularly for trace metals critical to health. This necessitates a better understanding of the specific nutritional requirements of the elderly population in order to ensure they are supplied with essential micronutrients that promote optimal health and well-being, particularly against the backdrop of the increased vulnerability to chronic illnesses within this group (Cristina et al., 2021). Also, aging affects gastrointestinal function significantly, and this has a significant impact on nutrient absorption. The elderly gut is marked by reduced mechanical breakdown of food, reduced gastrointestinal motility, and compromised intestinal wall function, all leading to ineffective delivery of nutrients. These changes in physiology might lead to decreased trace metal absorption necessary for various enzymatic processes and overall well-being, such as zinc and magnesium. The metabolic slowdown with aging affecting gut health necessitates a geriatric nutrition plan that is strategic in its focus on the intake of nutrient-rich foods. A mechanistic strategy employing assessment and intervention methods with the aim of optimizing nutrient bioavailability can take center stage in turning around the adverse effects of metabolic slowing and dysgut function in the elderly (Cristina et al., 2021). Therefore, achieving nutritional needs becomes essential for reversing the threat of malnutrition evoked by such changes in metabolism. In addition, the psychological dimensions of aging also have the ability to multiply metabolic health and nutritional needs. Social isolation, financial troubles, and the psychological stress of chronic diseases all have the potential to suppress appetite and nutrient needs, exacerbating underlying metabolic disorders. As a result, older adults are burdened with a double whammy: physiological loss keeps nutrients from being absorbed and psychological concerns suppress food intake. This exchange draws attention to the necessity for intersectoral strategies for geriatric nutrition, not just addressing the supply of trace metals but also the social and mental health determinants of food consumption. Social engagement with food, nutrition education on nutrient-rich food, and access to good nutrition interventions enhance intake and quality of life in the elderly (Cristina et al., 2021). By understanding these complicated challenges, caregivers and medical providers can develop more effective nutritional plans that support healthy aging (Figure 6.17).

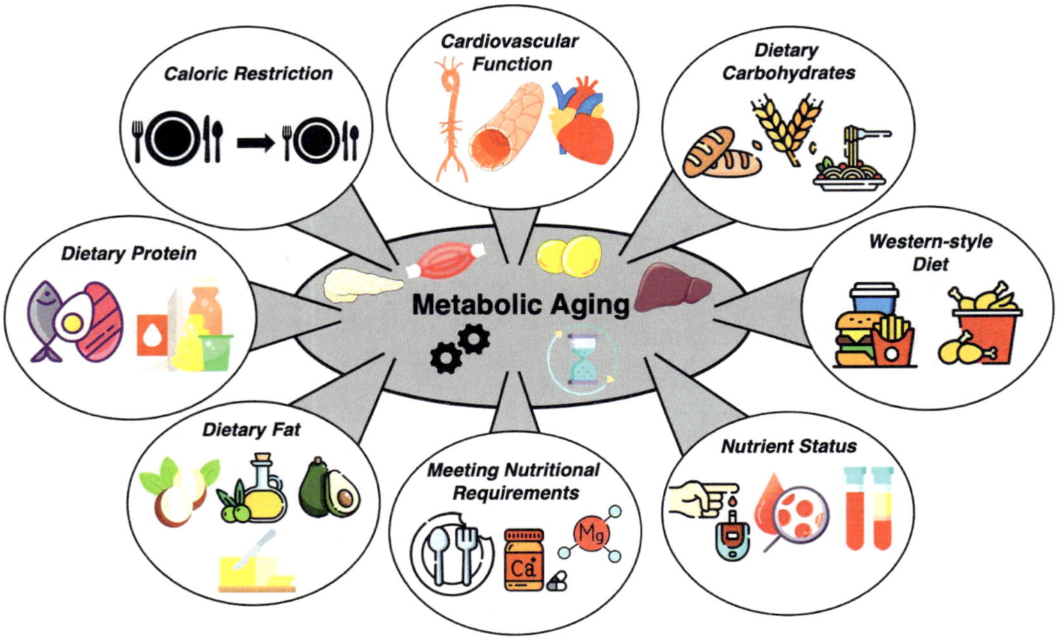

Figure 6.17. Nutrition and metabolic aging.

Source: https://www.frontiersin.org/files/Articles/1191958/fnut-10-1191958-HTML/image_m/fnut-10-1191958-g001.jpg.

6.6.2. Interaction with Medications

Drug interaction is a relevant factor in the nutritional management of the elderly. Older individuals will be taking multiple drug medications to rectify chronic ailments, and thus, the risk of drug interaction with trace metals, which play crucial roles in numerous biochemical reactions, becomes increasingly significant. The metals not only preserve various biochemical processes but also influence the effect and toxicity of drugs. For example, zinc is important for immune response and can affect the pharmacokinetics of certain antibiotics. In accordance with the geriatric consideration, physicians must consider how trace metal insufficiency or excess would alter the absorption, distribution, metabolism, and excretion of drugs and thereby lead to untoward effects or less than optimal therapeutic effectiveness. Furthermore, medications commonly used in elderly patients can have an influence on trace metal status as well. Certain drugs possess a characteristic to increase the elimination of trace metals and thereby develop deficiencies over time. For instance, diuretics, which are frequently employed in treating hypertension and heart failure, might augment the renal elimination of potassium, magnesium, and zinc and thereby increase their deficiency. This is why individualized nutritional assessments in older patients are mandatory, whose aim is not only to enhance ingestion of trace metals but also to identify potential drug interactions. Understanding these conditions can lead to more prudent prescribing, with medications and nutrition weighed in balance to provide total health while diminishing the potential for metal deficiency complications. Lastly, the interface between trace metal needs and medication interactions is established by the applicability of individualized medicine in geriatric nutrition. Tailored treatment regimens according to trace metal status could provide an extended treatment approach for chronic diseases among the elderly. For example, combining dietary modification or trace metal supplementation like copper could render certain drug therapies more effective, e.g., Alzheimer's disease and its associated cognitive impairment (Jadhav et al., 2024). Moreover, novel monitoring techniques, aided by advances in sensor technologies as described by recent studies (Junior et al., 2024), would be capable of facilitating real-time trace metal level monitoring and drug interactions. This combined approach would immensely improve drug effectiveness and the quality of life for the elderly by ultimately resulting in healthy outcomes.

6.6.3. Importance of Personalized Nutrition Plans

Individualized nutrition planning is paramount to addressing the unique nutritional needs of the geriatric population, particularly trace metal requirements. During aging, there is a change in metabolic function and nutrient requirements that impacts their ability to metabolize and absorb nutrients. For instance, aging individuals suffer from trace metal deficiencies such as zinc, selenium, and copper, which have far-reaching implications for overall health and mental well-being. Personalized nutrition regimens can easily correct such deficiencies by formulating individual-specific dietary advice in terms of the health status of the individual, his or her dietary habits, and individual requirements, thereby enhancing their quality of life and lessening the risk of chronic diseases typical of aging. The application of individualized nutrition in the diets of older adults decreases the risk factors for neurodegenerative diseases, such as Alzheimer's disease, which is now very prevalent among older persons. Evidence suggests that trace metals play an important role in the pathophysiology of Alzheimer's and other cognitive impairments. For instance, deficiencies or imbalances of essential metals lead to oxidative stress and inflammation, further exacerbating neurological impairment. By the application of tailored nutrition, the provision of food interventions can include food items rich in protective trace metals and thereby improve cognitive well-being. This tailored approach not only provides older adults with control over their health but also promotes preventive measures that may lead to healthier aging, highlighting the relative importance of individualized nutrition interventions among the elderly. Besides, the application of technology in developing customized nutrition counseling has exhibited promising potential for improving health outcomes among the elderly. Wearable technologies with optical sensors and real-time monitoring features can provide valuable insights into the nutrient intake and overall health status of a person. This innovation is coming in tandem with the emerging paradigms in healthcare, demonstrating how personalized nutrition can be integrated with other innovations such as artificial intelligence and the internet of things, as considered in recent studies (Junior et al., 2024). These types of innovation are capable of leading to dynamic nutrition adaptations based on ongoing data to make sure that aging individuals receive optimal amounts of nutrients needed for health sustenance. Lastly, these personalized nutrition methods, supported by technology, are not only required for the fulfillment of trace metal requirements of the elderly but also for global health management throughout the aging process.

SUMMARY

Trace metal requirements for elderly nutrition are the way through which multidirectional aging-related challenges can be overcome. As aging impairs the capacity of the gastrointestinal tracts to absorb and utilize nutrients, a specialized approach is required. The declining efficiency of nutrient absorption can lead to malnutrition, which exacerbates diseases in various organ systems, including the nervous, musculoskeletal, and cardiovascular. According to the literature, nutritional treatment of the elderly should involve a comprehensive understanding of gastrointestinal changes to limit the risk for malnutrition as well as its complications (Rémond et al., 2015). Besides, some trace metals, such as zinc and copper, also play a major role in maintaining good health among the elderly. Studies have established that despite the availability of adequate zinc status among most elderly populations, a significant proportion of them remain in the deficient category, which makes it crucial to conduct in-depth food evaluation (Paterson, 1982). Consequently, trace metal intake from foods that contain zinc will be added to various functions in the body, thereby promoting long-term health and well-being in the elderly. The current controversy surrounding trace metal requirements also highlights the necessity for constant evaluation of eating habits and food source contributions towards meeting specific nutritional needs. Application of dietary recommendations that assist in concentrating on nutrient-rich foods can significantly improve health status in the geriatric population. With the increasing aging population, the integration of knowledge of the individual nutritional status and functional capacity will be essential in preventing deficiencies and improving quality of life. An effective holistic knowledge of trace metal nutrition is thus an important component in the overall plan for geriatric care (Rémond et al., 2015).

The contribution of trace metals in the geriatric diet cannot be overstated because these micronutrients play a critical role in most of the physiological functions needed to support good health in older individuals. Trace metals, including zinc, copper, and selenium, are crucial trace metals that facilitate vital processes such as immune function, antioxidant defense, and enzyme action. As aging proceeds, the bioavailability of such metals might decline due to changes in gut absorption and diet and cause deficiencies. Thus, an individualized nutritional intervention to maximize the intake of trace metals can provide significant health benefits. Recognition of trace metal requirements in the aged enables clinicians to organize dietary regimes that will yield optimal levels, with resultant prevention of age-associated disease states, such as cognitive dysfunction and compromised immunity. Furthermore, trace metal interaction with food constituents is of crucial significance in geriatric nutrition. A few foods, including phytate- and oxalate-rich foods, are inhibitory to trace metal absorption, and nutritional management is thereby more complicated. For instance, phytates found in whole cereals and legumes can be a barrier to zinc intake. Therefore, the overall strategy in the therapy of the elderly on how to manage their diet should account for such interactions in order to maximize trace metals' bioavailability. In addition, this highlights the importance of health education of elderly people based on food choice to enhance nutrient uptake and minimize inhibitors and thereby enhance well-being. Taking a holistic approach to geriatric nutrition strengthens the argument for increased research into optimizing trace metal availability in this high-risk group. In conclusion, enhancing our understanding of trace metal requirements among elderly individuals is essential for their overall health and well-being. There are indications that poor intake of such nutrients further exacerbates age-related illnesses, such as cognitive impairment and chronic disease. Therefore, nutritional interventions addressing such requirements must take top priority in geriatric healthcare. The use of multidomain approaches, such as dietary modification in combination with physical activity and psychological support, can be synergistic and enhance the multifactorial nature of health in the elderly. Interventions within community settings, educating older adults on trace metal nutrition, can equip them with enhanced compliance with dietary recommendations, hence better health consequences. This integrative approach emphasizes the imperative need for ongoing research and intervention trials to identify successful nutrition regimens for geriatric populations (Journal of Problem Based Learning in Higher Education, 2023; Wu et al., 2023).

A CLOSER LOOK

MALNUTRITION AND DEHYDRATION IN THE GERIATRIC ADULT

Malnutrition and dehydration are emergent and often underdiagnosed with problems in geriatric adults and have considerable effects on their general health and quality of life. With age, many physiological, psychological, and social changes can lead to inadequate food intake and inadequate fluid intake. Reduced appetite, impaired sense of taste or olfactory function, difficulty with chewing or swallowing, and chronic illnesses such as dementia or gastrointestinal disease typically interfere with normal eating habits. Polypharmacy, or the use of many drugs, may even exacerbate loss of appetite or cause side effects like dry mouth or nausea. Besides this, mobility and cognitive impairments may render an older adult incapable of cooking food or accessing fluids, thus risking malnutrition and dehydration. Depression and loneliness may reduce hunger for food or fluid consumption, and economic constraints may limit the availability of affordable, healthy food (Figure 6.18).

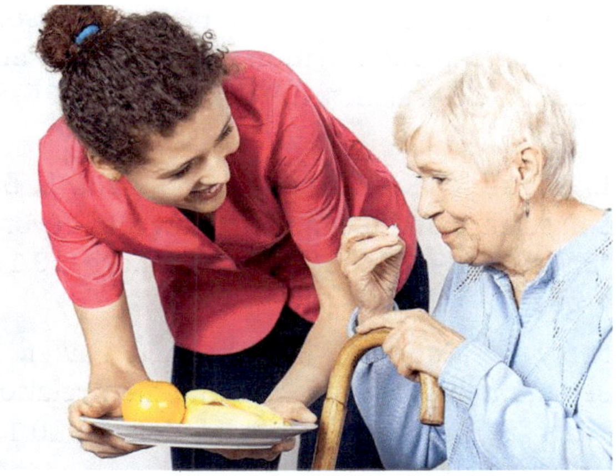

Figure 6.18. Malnutrition in the elderly.

https://external-content.duckduckgo.com/iu/?u=https%3A%2F%2Fimages.onlymyhealth.com%2Fimported%2Fimages%2F2021%2FSeptember%2F23_Sep_2021%2Fbig2.jpg&f=1&nofb=1&ipt=6246e32262dfe54f1f6dd655a91078963f31e3997a849689578a823536fcf75b

Dehydration in the elderly is particularly dangerous due to decreased perception of thirst and compromised kidney function, both of which affect fluid status. The implications of these conditions are increased susceptibility to infection, slowed wound healing, impaired muscle function, and higher hospitalization and mortality rates. Hence, an imperative to implement regular nutritional screening, increase hydration awareness, and provide personalized dietary advice is essential to ensure maximum nourishment and hydration for the elderly. Multidisciplinary approaches involving caregivers, dietitians, and physicians are essential in recognizing high-risk individuals and in managing the complexities of changing interactions leading to geriatric malnutrition and dehydration.

REFERENCES

1. Abreu, A. P., Martins, R., & Nunes, J. (2023). Emerging applications of *Chlorella sp.* and *Spirulina* (*Arthrospira*) sp. *Bioengineering*, *10*, 955–955. https://doi.org/10.3390/bioengineering10080955 (accessed on 12th July 2025).
2. Arnold, M., Buttriss, J., Chiofalo, B., Fox, J., Ghosh, P., Greppi, G., Griessen, D., et al. (2017). Role of proteins and of some bioactive peptides on the nutritional quality of donkey milk and their impact on human health. https://core.ac.uk/download/pdf/154842854.pdf (accessed on 12th July 2025).
3. Dr. Arpita Maitra, Dr. Swagata Gayen, Dr. Divya Pandya, Dr. Anwesha Banerjee, Dr. Rekha Puttannavar (2024). Trace elements in health & disease–A boon in disguise. https://doi.org/10.53555/jaz.v45iS3.4420(accessed on 12th July 2025).
4. Maggio, M., De Vita, F., Lauretani, F., Nouvenne, A., Meschi, T., Ticinesi, A., Dominguez, L. J., Barbagallo, M., Dall'aglio, E., & Ceda, G. P. (2014). The Interplay between Magnesium and Testosterone in Modulating Physical Function in Men. *International journal of endocrinology, 2014*, 525249. https://doi.org/10.1155/2014/525249(accessed on 12th July 2025).
5. Volkert, D., Beck, A. M., Cederholm, T., Cruz-Jentoft, A., Goisser, S., Hooper, L., Kiesswetter, E., Maggio, M., Raynaud-Simon, A., Sieber, C. C., Sobotka, L., van Asselt, D., Wirth, R., & Bischoff, S. C. (2019). ESPEN guideline on clinical nutrition and hydration in geriatrics. *Clinical nutrition (Edinburgh, Scotland)*, *38*(1), 10–47. https://doi.org/10.1016/j.clnu.2018.05.024(accessed on 12th July 2025).
6. Betz, U. A. K., Arora, L., Assal, R. A., Azevedo, H., Baldwin, J., Becker, M., Bostock, S., et al. (2023). Game changers in science and technology–now and beyond. *Technological Forecasting and Social Change*, *193*, 122588–122588. https://doi.org/10.1016/j.techfore.2023.122588 (accessed on 12th July 2025).
7. Ducros, V., Faure, P., Ferry, M., Couzy, F., Biajoux, I., & Favier, A. (1997). The sizes of the exchangeable pools of selenium in elderly women and their relation to institutionalization. *The British journal of nutrition*, *78*(3), 379–396. https://doi.org/10.1079/bjn19970158(accessed on 12th July 2025).
8. Rémond, D., Shahar, D. R., Gille, D., Pinto, P., Kachal, J., Peyron, M. A., Dos Santos, C. N., Walther, B., Bordoni, A., Dupont, D., Tomás-Cobos, L., & Vergères, G. (2015). Understanding the gastrointestinal tract of the elderly to develop dietary solutions that prevent malnutrition. *Oncotarget*, *6*(16), 13858–13898. https://doi.org/10.18632/oncotarget.4030(accessed on 12th July 2025).
9. Elsaadany, A. (2017). The influence of dietary boron supplementation on performance and some physiological parameters in Bandarah chickens 2- laying period. *Egyptian Poultry Science Journal*, *37*, 105–122. https://www.semanticscholar.org/paper/b607cb4e3cc2e43a7954c31f81b8b664d973fcf2 (accessed on 12th July 2025).
10. Full issue. (2023). Entire issue. *Journal of Problem Based Learning in Higher Education*, *11*, 1–156. https://doi.org/10.54337/ojs.jpblhe.v11i3.8226 (accessed on 12th July 2025).
11. Hever, J., & Cronise, R. J. (2017). Plant-based nutrition for healthcare professionals: Implementing diet as a primary modality in the prevention and treatment of chronic disease. *PubMed*, *14*, 355–368. https://doi.org/10.11909/j.issn.1671-5411.2017.05.012 (accessed on 12th July 2025).

12. Hills, R. D., Pontefract, B., Mishcon, H. R., Black, C. A., Sutton, S. C., & Theberge, C. R. (2019). Gut microbiome: Profound implications for diet and disease. *Nutrients, 11*, 1613–1613. https://doi.org/10.3390/nu11071613 (accessed on 12th July 2025).

13. Jadhav, D., Saraswat, N., Vyawahare, N. S., & Shirode, D. S. (2024). Targeting the molecular web of Alzheimer's disease: Unveiling pathways for effective pharmacotherapy. *The Egyptian Journal of Neurology Psychiatry and Neurosurgery, 60*. https://doi.org/10.1186/s41983-023-00775-8 (accessed on 12th July 2025).

14. Kaliniak-Dziura, A., Skałecki, P., Florek, M., Kędzierska-Matysek, M., & Sobczak, P. (2024). Chemical composition and elements concentration of fillet, spine, and bones of common carp (*Cyprinus carpio*) in relation to nutrient requirements for minerals. *Animals: an Open Access Journal from MDPI, 14*. https://www.semanticscholar.org/paper/17538ddb78d575e0361293342cf1762b68ff8785 (accessed on 12th July 2025).

15. Khan, Z., Liu, W., Mubeen, I., Alrefaei, A. F., Alharbi, S. N., Muhammad, F. G., Ejaz, A., et al. (2023). Cobalt availability in the soil plant and animal food chain: A study under a peri-urban environment. *Brazilian Journal of Biology=Revita Brasileira de Biologic, 83*, e270256. https://www.semanticscholar.org/paper/0de1ace867998315ae3fcd99147f795f4bb1b2ee (accessed on 12th July 2025).

16. Leal-Junior, A., da Silva, J. S., Macedo, L., Marchesi, A., Morau, S., Valentino, J., Valentim, F., et al. (2024). The role of optical fiber sensors in the new generation of healthcare devices: A review. *Sensors & Diagnostics, 3*, 1135–1158. https://doi.org/10.1039/d4sd00032c (accessed on 12th July 2025).

17. Lorenzo-López, L., Lema-Arranz, C., Fernández-Bertólez, N., Costa, S., Costa, C., Teixeira, J. P., Pásaro, E., et al. (2022). Relationship between DNA damage measured by the comet-assay and cognitive function. *Mutation Research/Genetic Toxicology and Environmental Mutagenesis, 883, 884*, 503557–503557. https://doi.org/10.1016/j.mrgentox.2022.503557 (accessed on 12th July 2025).

18. Majeed, M., Chavez, M., Nagabhushanam, K., & Mundkur, L. (2021). Zinc supplements in COVID-19 pathogenesis–Current perspectives. *Austin Journal of Nutrition & Metabolism, 8*. https://doi.org/10.26420/austinjnutrmetab.2021.1107 (accessed on 12th July 2025).

19. Millena, C. G., Binaday, J. A. B., Bulawan, C. B., Nipas, E. G. D., Ruivivar, S. S., & Rosales, A. L. (2024). Nutritional composition and mineral bioavailability of selected root and tuber crops in the Bicol Region, Philippines. *Food Research*. https://www.semanticscholar.org/paper/b8ec06947fa81f788d23c385cc5747150b90fffa (accessed on 12th July 2025).

20. Neri, M. C., & d'Alba, L. (2021). Nutrition and healthy aging: Prevention and treatment of gastrointestinal diseases. *Nutrients, 13*, 4337–4337. https://doi.org/10.3390/nu13124337 (accessed on 12th July 2025).

21. Niego, A. G. T., Rapior, S., Thongklang, N., Raspé, O., Jaidee, Lumyong, S., & Hyde, K. D. (2021). Macro fungi as a nutraceutical source: Promising bioactive compounds and market value. *Journal of Fungi, 7*, 397–397. https://doi.org/10.3390/jof7050397 (accessed on 12th July 2025).

22. Oršolić, N., & Jazvinšćak Jembrek, M. (2024). Royal jelly: Biological action and health benefits. *International Journal of Molecular Sciences, 25*, 6023–6023. https://doi.org/10.3390/ijms25116023 (accessed on 12th July 2025).

23. Paterson, P. (1982). Zinc levels of hospitalized elderly. https://core.ac.uk/download/590879860.pdf (accessed on 12th July 2025).

24. Piccoli, G. B., Cupisti, A., Aucella, F., Regolisti, G., Lomonte, C., Ferraresi, M., D'Alessandro, C., et al. (2020). Green nephrology and eco-dialysis: A position statement by the Italian Society of Nephrology. *Journal of Nephrology, 33*, 681–698. https://doi.org/10.1007/s40620-020-00734-z (accessed on 12th July 2025).

25. Sajjadi, S. S., Foshati, S., Haddadian-Khouzani, S., & Rouhani, M. H. (2022). The role of selenium in depression: A systematic review and meta-analysis of human observational and interventional studies. *Scientific Reports, 12*. https://doi.org/10.1038/s41598-022-05078-1 (accessed on 12th July 2025).

26. Saleem, M., Iqbal, J., Shi, Z., Garrett, S., & Shah, M. (2022). Distribution and bioaccumulation of essential and toxic metals in tissues of *Thaila* (*Catla catla*) from a natural lake, Pakistan and its possible health impact on consumers. *Journal of Marine Science and Engineering*. https://www.semanticscholar.org/paper/8290d81d43774bf441c65663e620a349f775cd3e (accessed on 12th July 2025).

27. Sgarbieri, V. C., & Pacheco, M. T. B. (2017). Premature or pathological aging: Longevity. *Brazilian Journal of Food Technology/Brazilian Journal of Food Technology, 20*. https://doi.org/10.1590/1981-6723.19416 (accessed on 12th July 2025).

28. Sharma, R., Martins, N., Kuča, K., Chaudhary, A., Kabra, A., Rao, M. M., & Prajapati, P. K. (2019). Chyawanprash: A traditional Indian bioactive health supplement. *Biomolecules, 9*, 161–161. https://doi.org/10.3390/biom9050161 (accessed on 12th July 2025).

29. Staehelin, H. B. (2017). Micronutrients and Alzheimer's disease. https://core.ac.uk/download/85209142.pdf (accessed on 12th July 2025).

30. Whitmee, S., Haines, A., Beyrer, C., Boltz, F., Capon, A., Ferreira de Souza Dias, B., Ezeh, A., et al. (2015). Safeguarding human health in the Anthropocene epoch: Report of The Rockefeller Foundation–Lancet Commission on planetary health. *The Lancet, 386*, 1973–2028. https://doi.org/10.1016/s0140-6736(15)60901-1 (accessed on 12th July 2025).

31. Wu, X., Zhang, T., Tu, Y., Deng, X., Sigen, A., Li, Y., Jing, X., et al. (2023). Multidomain interventions for non-pharmacological enhancement (MINE) program in Chinese older adults with mild cognitive impairment: A multicenter randomized controlled trial protocol. *BMC Neurology, 23*. https://doi.org/10.1186/s12883-023-03390-5 (accessed on 12th July 2025).

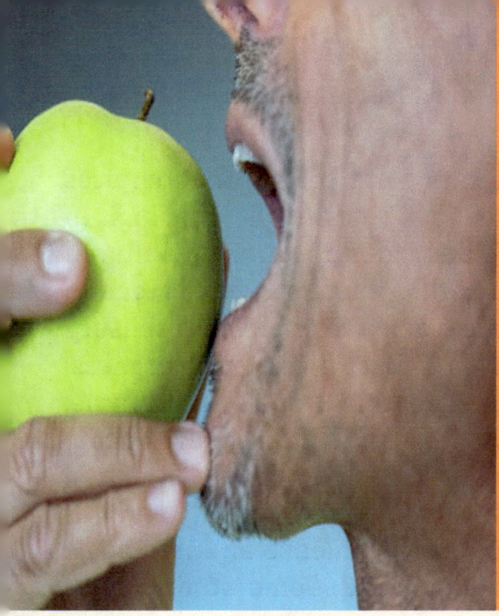

Chapter 7
SMELL, TASTE, AND ORAL SOMATOSENSATION: AGE-RELATED CHANGES AND NUTRITIONAL IMPLICATIONS

Contents

Introduction

The sensory systems of smell, taste, and oral somatosensation play critical roles in shaping human experience and behavior, particularly regarding nutrition and food intake. As these senses provide essential information about food quality and safety, they also enhance the enjoyment of eating. However, age-related changes can significantly affect these sensory modalities, leading to alterations in dietary preferences and nutritional intake. Research has shown that older adults frequently experience declines in olfactory and gustatory perception, which can diminish their ability to enjoy food. These changes in sensory perception are not merely physiological; they can result in profound implications for health and well-being, exacerbating issues like malnutrition and decreased appetite among the elderly. Understanding these sensory shifts is vital for developing appropriate dietary interventions and nutritional guidelines tailored to this population. The intricate relationship between diet, sensory perception, and nutritional outcomes has garnered increasing attention in contemporary research.

Variations in chemosensory abilities are often linked to dietary habits, with certain food choices showing associations with poorer sensory functioning. For instance, a Western-style diet high in saturated fats and refined sugars has been correlated with impaired odor identification and altered taste perception, especially in older adults. Individuals adhering to healthier dietary patterns tend to exhibit more robust sensory capacities, suggesting a reciprocal influence between diet and sensory perception. Such findings indicate that not only do sensory changes impact dietary preferences, but the prevailing diet may also further exacerbate sensory decline, creating a detrimental cycle. Investigating these interactions is paramount for highlighting potential strategies for enhancing sensory function through proper nutrition. Finally, the genetic factors underlying taste perception have also been shown to intersect with swallowing physiology, underscoring the complexity of oral sensory systems. Alterations in genetic taste status can significantly influence an individuals swallowing mechanics, thus affecting how they perceive and consume food. Some studies have suggested that variations in genetic predisposition toward specific tastes may either enhance or inhibit swallowing efficacy, especially in populations experiencing swallowing disorders. While evidence regarding this intersection remains mixed, it encourages further exploration of how genetic factors might contribute to nutritional outcomes. The implications of these research efforts are profound, suggesting that personalized nutritional approaches that consider both sensory and genetic influences may lead to more effective strategies in promoting healthy eating behaviors across different age groups and health statuses.

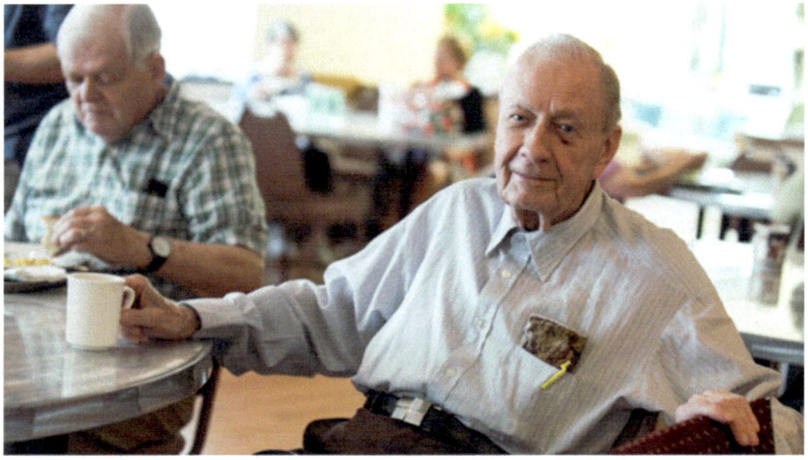

Figure 7.1. Smell and Taste Change as You Age.

Source: https://www.nia.nih.gov/sites/default/files/inline-images/smell-taste-older-people-inline.jpg

Definition of smell, taste, and oral somatosensation

The understanding of smell, taste, and oral somatosensation is pivotal in the context of nutrition and age-related changes. Smell, or olfaction, serves as a critical sensory system enabling individuals to detect and identify odors in their environment, influencing food preferences and choices. This chemosensory experience allows for an assessment of the hedonic value of food, which is crucial for fostering appetite and satisfaction during meal consumption. Research indicates that individual differences in odor sensitivity significantly impact flavor perception and enjoyment of food products. For example, studies conducted across various demographics reveal clustering of subjects into groups based on their sensitivity to specific odors, affecting their overall experience of flavors in food, emphasizing the intricate link between smell and nutritional behavior (Braghieri A et al., 2021). In addition to smell, taste plays a significant role in the overall sensory experience of food. Taste perception is mediated by receptors located on the tongue that respond to five basic taste modalities: sweet, sour, salty, bitter, and umami. These basic tastes convey essential information about the nutritional quality of food, aiding in the identification of safe and nourishing options versus potentially harmful substances. The integration of taste and smell contributes to the overall flavor profile, influencing food preferences that are critical for healthy eating habits. Furthermore, genetic and environmental factors have been shown to affect preferences for certain taste qualities, thereby shaping dietary behaviors throughout life. Understanding these mechanisms is essential for addressing age-related changes in culinary pleasure and acceptance, as preference patterns may shift with maturity (Törnwall et al., 2013). Oral somatosensation encompasses the tactile perceptions experienced within the oral cavity, including temperature, texture, and astringency. These sensations significantly influence the enjoyment of food, complementing the taste and smell. For instance, the perceived texture of a food item can enhance or diminish the overall flavor experience, with certain textures being more appealing to different demographic groups. Moreover, this aspect of sensory perception may also change with age, as individuals experience variations in sensitivity to texture and temperature. The oral sensory response not only contributes to the satisfaction of eating but is also an important factor in determining food choices. Collectively, the interplay of smell, taste, and oral somatosensation serves an evolutionary purpose, guiding individuals toward foods that fulfill their nutritional needs while also providing sensory pleasure, which may become increasingly pivotal as age-related changes occur (Törnwall et al., 2013).

Importance of these senses in daily life

The integration of smell, taste, and oral somatosensation profoundly influences daily life, especially in contexts related to nutrition and overall well-being. These senses not only facilitate the enjoyment of food but also play crucial roles in health and survival. For instance, the ability to taste and smell allows individuals to distinguish between nutritious foods and harmful substances, thereby aiding dietary choices. This sensory interaction is particularly vital for head and neck cancer patients, who experience altered perceptions of food due to their condition. Research shows that changes in food perception involve more than just taste; they encompass texture, temperature, and other oral sensations that affect overall eating experiences and quality of life. Therefore, a comprehensive understanding of these senses can lead to tailored nutritional interventions, significantly improving patient well-being and dietary engagement (R Riantiningtyas et al., 2023). Furthermore, the relationship between sensory perception and eating behaviors underscores the nutritional implications of smell, taste, and oral somatosensation. Aging is associated with notable declines in these senses, which can result in decreased appetite, altered food preferences, and insufficient nutrient intake. The impact is particularly significant among older adults, who may rely heavily on these senses for food enjoyment and social interactions during mealtime. When the sensory experience of eating diminishes, it can lead to not only nutritional deficits but also reduced social cohesion and emotional well-being. As observed in patients recovering from various medical conditions, maintaining these senses plays an integral role in fostering a positive relationship with food and enhancing adherence to necessary dietary recommendations during recovery (Brodbeck A et al., 2022). Additionally, the interplay between sensory health and everyday nutritional practices emphasizes the need for targeted research and interventions. The current literature points to a gap in understanding oral somatosensory changes, especially among vulnerable populations such as the elderly and cancer patients. By prioritizing studies that explore how these alterations affect food perceptions, healthcare providers can develop personalized strategies to improve dietary experiences. For example, those with diminished taste might benefit from enhanced textures or the use of spices to compensate for lost flavor perception. Overall, recognizing and addressing the importance of smell, taste, and oral somatosensation in daily life can lead to better health outcomes and improved quality of life for individuals across the lifespan (R Riantiningtyas et al., 2023).

7.1 The Physiology of Smell

The physiology of smell, or olfaction, is a complex process that begins when volatile molecules enter the nasal cavity and bind to olfactory receptors situated in the olfactory epithelium. These receptors are part of a sophisticated signaling pathway that transmits sensory information to the olfactory bulb in the brain, ultimately informing the perception of scent. Notably, the olfactory system interacts closely with the gustatory system, which is responsible for taste. This multisensory relationship highlights the interconnectedness of smell and taste in the overall eating experience. As age alters the olfactory and gustatory capabilities, this can significantly impact dietary habits and nutritional intake, emphasizing the need to understand these physiological changes as individuals age. Age-related changes in the physiology of smell can lead to a diminished ability to perceive aromas, affecting food preferences and consumption patterns. Studies indicate that the sensitivity of olfactory receptors declines with age, which may lead to alterations in taste perception and an overall reduction in the enjoyment of food ((Dietsch et al., 2024)). This phenomenon is particularly pertinent in understanding nutritional implications for older adults, as diminished sensory experiences can result in decreased appetite and subsequent weight loss or malnutrition. Addressing these issues necessitates a clinical lens that combines an understanding of sensory physiology with nutritional strategies tailored to the specific needs of elderly populations.

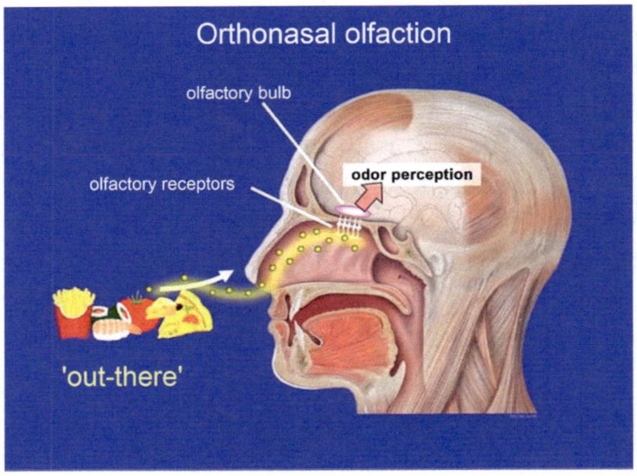

Figure 7.2. Physiology of smell.

Source: https://image.slidesharecdn.com/physiologyofsmell-160426050206/85/physiology-of-smell-10-638.jpg?cb=1666279449

Moreover, the interplay between taste, smell, and swallowing physiology marks a critical area of examination in the context of age-related changes. Research suggests that taste can significantly influence swallowing function, providing an avenue for therapeutic interventions, particularly in individuals with dysphagia, a condition prevalent among the elderly ((Dietsch et al., 2022)). By incorporating taste manipulation strategies into treatment plans, healthcare professionals can foster improved swallowing outcomes and enhance the overall quality of life for older adults. Continued exploration into the physiological mechanisms behind olfaction, taste, and their combined effects on nutrition will yield valuable insights into effective dietary recommendations and interventions for aging populations.

7.1.1 Mechanisms of olfactory perception

The mechanisms of olfactory perception are fundamental to understanding human sensory experiences and their implications for nutrition and health. Olfactory perception begins with the detection of odor molecules, which bind to olfactory receptors located in the nasal epithelium. This process involves a complex neural pathway where the activated receptors send signals to the olfactory bulb, leading to the processing and identification of smells. Age-related changes in olfactory function can significantly affect an individuals perception of flavors and their overall appetite. Studies have demonstrated that declines in olfactory sensitivity are prevalent among older adults, which can diminish food enjoyment and lead to nutritional deficits. Such changes underline the importance of olfactory cues in taste perception, as the integration of these senses is crucial for effective eating behaviors and dietary choices.

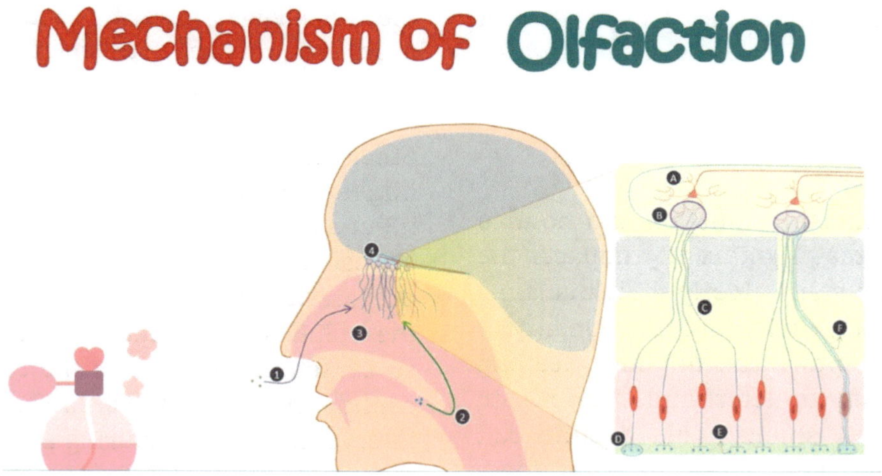

Figure 7.3. Mechanisms of olfactory perception.

Source: https://i.ytimg.com/vi/oYp10Ea9h8c/maxresdefault.jpg

The interplay between olfactory perception and taste is further evidenced in clinical contexts, especially in managing conditions like dysphagia. Here, the manipulation of taste can influence swallowing outcomes, highlighting the multisensory nature of feeding. A narrative review examining the physiology of taste and swallowing indicates that enhancing olfactory input through targeted tastes may improve swallowing efficacy and safety. However, individual factors such as genetic taste status also play a significant role in this complex interaction. While mixed evidence exists regarding the direct correlation between olfactory perception and swallowing success, there is a growing recognition of the need for further research in this area. This gap is particularly notable in studies involving participants with dysphagia, where tailored interventions may yield better outcomes and enhance quality of life (Damra et al., 2023). Future exploration of olfactory mechanisms must consider the individual differences that impact both smell and taste perception. As aging populations confront declining sensory functions, understanding how these changes affect dietary intake becomes paramount. Studies suggest that nutritional interventions that incorporate olfactory stimulation could potentially counteract age-related declines in appetite and food intake. For instance, aroma-enhancing strategies can be employed during meal preparations to make food more appealing to older adults, thereby encouraging consumption. Ultimately, a comprehensive understanding of olfactory mechanisms not only informs clinical practices in nutrition and swallowing therapy but also fosters a holistic approach to enhancing the quality of dietary experiences across different age groups (Dietsch et al., 2024).

7.1.2 Age-related decline in olfactory function

The decline in olfactory function is a notable aspect of aging that significantly impacts the quality of life for many elderly individuals. As people age, the sensitivity and functionality of the olfactory receptors can diminish, leading to a reduced ability to detect and discriminate between different smells. This decline can profoundly affect their ability to enjoy food, as approximately 90% of those with smell loss report a diminished eating experience. The impairment of olfactory function not only alters food perception but can also lead to poorer nutritional choices, resulting in a decrease in overall dietary intake. Without the stimulating aromas that enhance flavor, older adults may struggle to find pleasure in meals, underscoring the importance of maintaining olfactory health as part of a comprehensive approach to nutrition in aging populations (Fjaeldstad et al., 2024). Moreover, the relationship between olfactory decline and nutritional intake warrants further exploration, especially considering the implications for maintaining adequate food consumption among the elderly. Flavor perception, fundamentally reliant on the interplay between taste and smell, often diminishes due to age-related sensory decline. Consequently, older adults may become less inclined to eat, leading to potentially significant nutritional deficits. Although flavor enhancement techniques have been suggested to mitigate these effects, research indicates that this approach lacks consistency in effectiveness for enhancing food intake among older individuals. Specifically, studies have shown that even flavor-enhanced foods do not necessarily improve the appeal or consumption levels in those with impaired olfactory function, highlighting a critical gap in nutritional strategies tailored for aging populations (Essed et al., 2009). In light of these challenges, fostering a multisensory dining experience could be a strategic avenue to enhance the enjoyment and intake of food among older adults suffering from olfactory decline. Engaging other senses, such as texture and visual appeal, might counterbalance the reduced olfactory input and restore some degree of enjoyment in eating. Programs that promote cooking and food preparation can also contribute to improving the culinary experience for older individuals, as evidenced by studies indicating increased confidence and quality of life following cooking interventions. By nurturing a holistic approach that incorporates various sensory elements into food experiences, we can better support the nutritional needs of the aging population while addressing the concurrent decline in olfactory function (Fjaeldstad et al., 2024).

7.1.3 Impact of diminished smell on food preferences

The decline in olfactory function as individuals age significantly affects food preferences and dietary choices. As the sensory capability to detect and identify aromas diminishes, the enjoyment of food may decline, leading to altered eating habits. Reduced olfactory input can result in a lessened perception of flavors, making food less appealing and potentially contributing to inadequate nutrition among older adults. This sensory decline not only influences taste but can also diminish the overall experience of eating, hence impacting long-term dietary adherence and nutritional intake. The implications of these changes can be profound, particularly as they relate to age-related health issues that necessitate a balanced diet for maintenance and prevention of chronic conditions. Furthermore, the relationship between diminished smell and food preferences can be linked to broader nutritional implications for older adults. Research indicates that changes in the gastrointestinal tract, which often occur with aging, further complicate the ability to retain nutrients from food. For instance, alterations in mechanical digestion and nutrient absorption can exacerbate the effects of sensory decline, as the combined challenges may lead to an increased risk of malnutrition among older individuals. Consequently, they may gravitate towards less nutrient-dense foods that are easier to consume yet fail to meet dietary requirements for vitamins and minerals, undermining their overall health. Addressing these nutritional gaps is crucial, particularly in developing dietary guidelines tailored to the unique needs of the aging population to mitigate the consequences of sensory decline. From a practical standpoint, it is essential to adapt food products and meal solutions that cater to the evolving preferences of older consumers experiencing diminished smell and taste. Studies highlight the importance of food texture and flavor enhancement as effective strategies for improving food acceptance among these individuals. Specifically, softer food textures have been found to be more appealing, making them easier to chew and swallow. Additionally, enhancing flavor profiles, particularly through the thoughtful use of salt and fat substitutes, can significantly improve the sensory experience of meals for older adults. By designing food options that consider these factors, such as those explored in recent research on meat products, stakeholders can create nutritionally adequate meals that promote healthy eating and encourage independence in the elderly population, thereby supporting their quality of life ((Bordoni et al., 2015), (Conroy et al., 2018)).

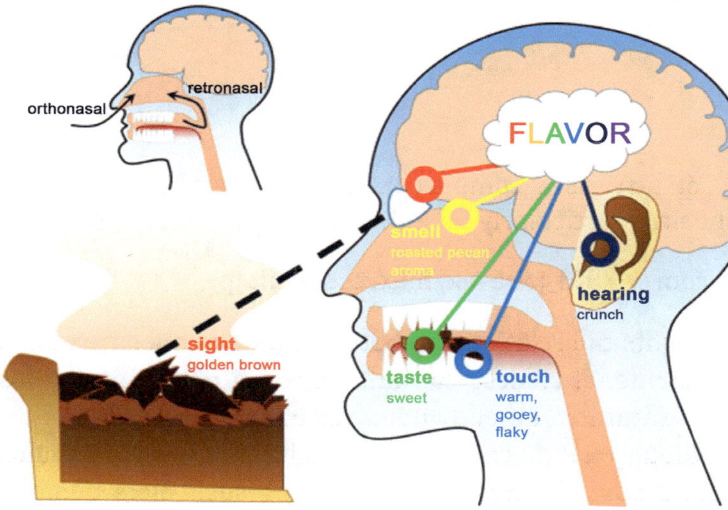

Figure 7.4. Brain tricks to make food taste sweeter.

Source: https://i0.wp.com/sitn.hms.harvard.edu/wp-content/uploads/2016/01/Figure_1v3.png

7.2 The Physiology of Taste

The physiology of taste is a complex interplay of sensory systems that fundamentally impacts nutrition and health, particularly as individuals age. Taste perception is mediated through taste buds located primarily on the tongue, which are responsible for detecting five primary taste modalities: sweet, sour, salty, bitter, and umami. Each of these modalities signals different nutritional information, prompting the intake or avoidance of certain foods. Interestingly, age-related changes in the gustatory system, such as declining taste bud number and neurological alterations, can dramatically affect taste perception, leading to either neglect or overconsumption of specific flavors. This dysregulation in taste sensitivity can result in educational and clinical challenges, particularly among the elderly population, where maintaining adequate nutrition is critical for health and well-being. Hence, understanding the physiological mechanisms underlying taste is vital in addressing dietary needs in aging adults.

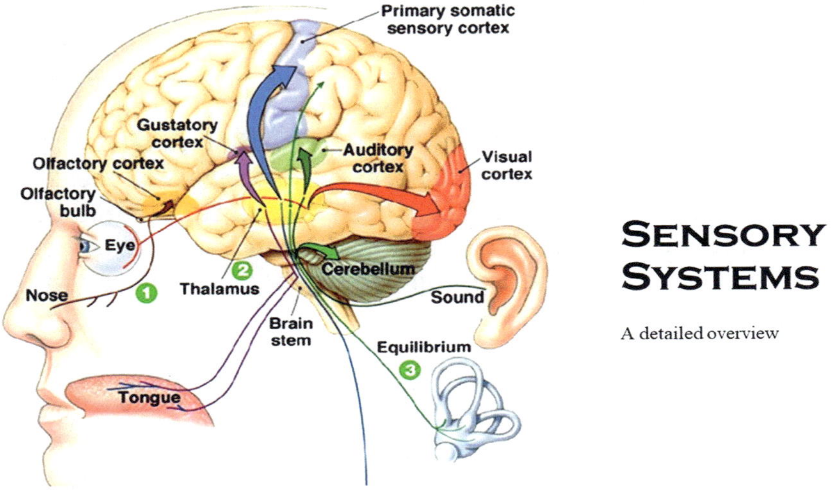

Figure 7.5. Physiology of taste is a complex interplay of sensory systems that fundamentally impacts nutrition and health, particularly as individuals age

Source: https://i.ytimg.com/vi/BRl_jzU5-dk/maxresdefault.jpg

Recent research highlights the relationship between diet composition and sensory perception, shedding light on how nutritional choices can influence the physiology of taste. A Western-style diet, characterized by high saturated fat and added sugar, has been linked to altered chemosensory abilities, suggesting that dietary habits can serve as catalysts for sensory changes rather than mere reflections of existing conditions. Participants consuming such diets demonstrated poorer odor identification ability, greater sensitivity to certain bitter compounds (PROP), and unique patterns in taste enhancement, indicating a shift in gustatory processing. These alterations not only complicate the experience of food but may also lead to poorer dietary choices over time, exacerbating health challenges associated with aging. Therefore, it is crucial to consider how diet-related changes in taste perception might affect nutritional intake and, ultimately, the health of aging individuals (Appel et al., 2016). Furthermore, genetic factors also play a significant role in shaping taste perception and swallowing functions, emphasizing the need for a nuanced understanding of gustatory physiology. Research has indicated that individual genetic variations can lead to significant differences in taste sensitivity, which in turn may influence swallowing mechanics. For instance, individuals with heightened taste sensitivity might exhibit altered swallowing patterns, impacting their ability to consume a balanced diet. While the existing literature on genetic taste status and its interaction with swallowing is somewhat inconsistent, studies suggest that genetic predispositions can affect how individuals experience and respond to different flavors. This interplay between taste perception and physiological function highlights the importance of personalized nutritional strategies, particularly for those with swallowing disorders. By incorporating an understanding of genetic taste status and its effects, healthcare practitioners might better address the unique dietary needs of individuals, promoting healthier eating habits, particularly among the aging population (Damra et al., 2023).

7.2.1 Mechanisms of gustatory perception

Gustatory perception primarily hinges on the intricate mechanisms of taste bud function, which are essential for detecting and processing flavors. These taste buds, located mainly on the tongue, possess specialized cells called taste receptor cells that are responsive to different taste modalities, including sweet, sour, salty, bitter, and umami. Each type of taste receptor is linked to specific signaling pathways that convey sensory information to the brain. For instance, sweet and umami tastes are mediated by GPCRs (G-protein coupled receptors), while bitter tastes primarily involve distinct receptor families. As organisms age, the efficacy of these pathways can decline, leading to altered taste perception. This change highlights the importance of understanding gustatory mechanisms, particularly in the context of nutritional intake among older adults, as diminished taste sensitivity can significantly affect dietary choices, nutritional quality, and overall health. The development and differentiation of gustatory receptor cells provide a framework for understanding how taste perception evolves over a lifetime. Recent advancements in cellular biology have enabled researchers to isolate taste bud cells and develop in vitro models to study their function more closely. For example, studies utilizing TBD cell lines have characterized various receptor expressions, including T1R3 and T2R8, which are crucial for detecting sweet and bitter sensations, respectively (N/A, 2011). These models have revealed important insights into how taste receptors respond to stimuli, such as sour flavors, and how they maintain structural integrity through three-dimensional cultures that mimic natural tissue architecture. This cellular approach illuminates the dynamic nature of gustatory mechanisms and emphasizes the need for ongoing research into how these processes may change with age, affecting older adults' ability to perceive tastes and potentially influencing their nutrition. Age-related changes in gustatory perception can be understood through an exploration of both physiological alterations and the broader implications for nutrition and health. As individuals age, there is often a decrease in the number of functioning taste buds, leading to diminished sensitivity to certain tastes. Additionally, the sensory pathways linking taste receptors to the brain may undergo degeneration, resulting in a reduced ability to discriminate among flavors. This decline can impact food enjoyment and intake, causing older adults to opt for unhealthier, more palatable options to compensate for decreased flavor perception. Thus, it is crucial to examine gustatory perception not only as a standalone sensory mechanism but in relation to other sensory modalities, particularly olfactory and oral somatosensory systems. Understanding these interconnections is key to addressing the nutritional challenges faced by the aging population, fostering healthier dietary practices that support overall well-being (Dumont V et al., 2018).

7.2.2 Changes in taste sensitivity with age

As individuals age, significant changes in taste sensitivity become apparent, primarily due to both physiological and neurological factors. The human gustatory system, which is responsible for the perception of taste, not only undergoes a decline in the number of taste buds but also experiences alterations in the way these buds respond to various stimuli. Research suggests that older adults may demonstrate reduced sensitivity to certain taste qualities, particularly bitter and sweet flavors, which can influence dietary preferences and nutritional intake. The decline in taste perception may consequently lead to a diminished appetite and a reduced interest in eating, potentially compromising overall health and energy levels as people age. Understanding these changes is crucial for developing dietary interventions that cater to the evolving taste profiles of older populations, ultimately promoting better nutritional habits. A critical aspect of aging and taste sensitivity is the role of genetics in individual taste perception. The bitter compound 6-n-propylthiouracil (PROP) has been identified as a marker for distinguishing variations in taste sensitivity among individuals, including older adults. Those who are genetically predisposed to heightened sensitivity to PROP frequently exhibit distinct food preferences, which can be attributed to the different affinities of the TAS2R38 bitter receptor variants. These genetic differences may also influence individuals responses to essential nutrients, particularly as age-related changes affect overall consumption patterns. Furthermore, certain genetic factors could engage in complex interactions with physiological changes related to aging, leading to differences in metabolic processing of food. These insights have vital implications for tailoring dietary recommendations that address the nutritional needs and preferences of older adults, thereby supporting healthier aging. In addition to shifts in taste perception, aging significantly impacts the consumption of high-protein foods, crucial for maintaining muscle mass and overall health. Older adults often face barriers to adequate protein intake due to declining chemosensory and physical abilities, as well as changes in living situations. Many of these high-protein foods, like meat and dairy, may become less appealing or more difficult to consume due to their texture or preparation requirements. As noted in recent research, these factors not only influence dietary choices but also raise concerns about nutrition adequacy among the elderly population. Consequently, it is essential to explore and address the challenges associated with protein consumption in older adults, such as the affordability and accessibility of high-protein options. By doing so, we could foster higher protein intake and subsequently enhance the overall nutritional status and quality of life for the aging demographic, making it a vital area of investigation in nutritional science (Barrett et al., 2013).

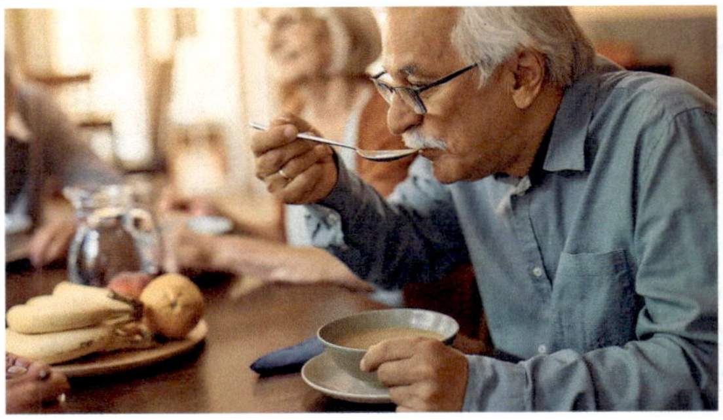

Figure 7.6. Changes in taste sensitivity with age.

Source: https://www.uhhospitals.org/-/media/Images/Social/Senior-Man-Eats-Soup-With-Friends-1413582310-Blog-OpenGraph.jpg

7.2.3 Relationship between taste and dietary choices

The relationship between taste and dietary choices is profoundly influenced by an individual's sensory perceptions, particularly taste, which is modulated by several factors, including age. As individuals grow older, the sensory experience of taste may diminish due to physiological changes in taste receptors and olfactory functions. This decline can lead to altered food preferences and dietary habits, often resulting in a reduced intake of essential nutrients. Additionally, research indicates that as populations experience economic growth, their dietary patterns shift towards higher consumption of ultra-processed foods (UPFs), which are characterized by added sugars, fats, and sodium. The industrialization of food systems and globalization facilitate this transition, leading to concerns over dietary quality and health outcomes ((Baker P et al., 2020)). Thus, understanding how taste perception correlates with dietary choices is crucial in addressing nutritional health, especially among aging populations. Childrens dietary choices also exhibit a significant relationship with taste, strongly influenced by early experiences and familial practices. From a young age, preferences for certain flavors and textures are established, which can persist into adulthood. Parental exposure to various foods during formative years plays a pivotal role; children tend to mirror their parents dietary habits, leading to long-term implications for their nutritional health. Research underlines that when parents model positive eating behaviors while encouraging the exploration of diverse foods, children are more likely to develop healthy eating patterns, thereby preventing nutrition-related issues later in life ((Scaglioni S et al., 2018)). This intergenerational influence underscores the importance of family dynamics in shaping dietary choices, indicating that interventions aimed at enhancing childrens diet should address not only food exposure but also parental behavior and attitudes towards nutrition. Moreover, the interplay between taste preferences and dietary choices has broader implications for public health strategies. Educators and healthcare professionals are increasingly recognizing the necessity of incorporating sensory experiences in nutritional education programs. Such initiatives can facilitate a better understanding of healthy eating habits and establish a foundation for lifelong dietary choices. Given the challenges posed by the prevalence of UPFs in modern diets, particularly in economically advanced regions, focusing on taste-related interventions may effectively promote healthier alternatives ((Baker P et al., 2020)). By fostering an appreciation for natural flavors and whole foods, these programs could counterbalance the negative impacts of industrial food production and encourage a shift towards diets that prioritize healthful nutrients. Ultimately, bridging the gap between taste experiences and dietary choices can play a crucial role in improving public health outcomes and nurturing a culture of nutrition-consciousness across generations.

7.3 Oral Somatosensation

Oral somatosensation plays a critical role in the perception of flavor and the overall gustatory experience, significantly influencing dietary choices and nutritional health. This sensory modality encompasses a range of tactile experiences, such as temperature, texture, and pain, that contribute to how individuals perceive foods and beverages. As individuals age, alterations in oral somatosensation can lead to altered food preferences and a decreased ability to derive pleasure from eating. Age-related changes in sensitivity to different textures and temperatures can lower consumption of essential nutrients, thereby impacting overall health. Given that oral somatosensation is integral to flavor perception, it serves as a bridge connecting taste and smell to the physiological responses associated with food. Enhancing awareness of these changes can benefit dietary recommendations tailored to older adults, promoting improved nutritional intake and quality of life. The association between dietary habits and oral somatosensation warrants attention, particularly when considering the effects of a Western-style diet characterized by high amounts of saturated fats and sugars. Evidence suggests that individuals consuming such diets demonstrate poorer chemosensory functions, which may further exacerbate age-related sensory decline. Research indicates that individuals on a Western-style diet exhibit decreased odor identification ability and altered taste perceptions, particularly regarding sweetness and fat discrimination. These findings are critical because they highlight a bidirectional relationship where diet impacts olfactory and gustatory functions, while these altered perceptions could influence continued adherence to unhealthy eating patterns. Consequently, a cycle is established that may hinder the consumption of nutrient-rich foods, leading to implications for aging populations who are particularly susceptible to both sensory decline and nutritional deficiencies (Appel et al., 2016). Moreover, the interplay between oral somatosensation and airway protection mechanisms emphasizes the complexity of swallowing and cough control, factors that are vital for maintaining health in older adults. Deficits in oral somatosensation may affect one's ability to perform safe swallowing, a necessary action for preventing aspiration and associated health complications. This is particularly relevant for older adults, who may already face challenges in these areas due to age-related neurological changes. Effective airway protection requires a nuanced understanding of both swallowing and cough behaviors, which share overlapping control mechanisms (BRANDIMORE et al., 2014). As deficits arise in oral somatosensation, the risk of swallowing difficulties becomes more pronounced, necessitating targeted interventions to enhance sensory experiences related to food and promote safer eating practices. By recognizing these relationships, healthcare providers can better address nutritional and health outcomes for aging populations.

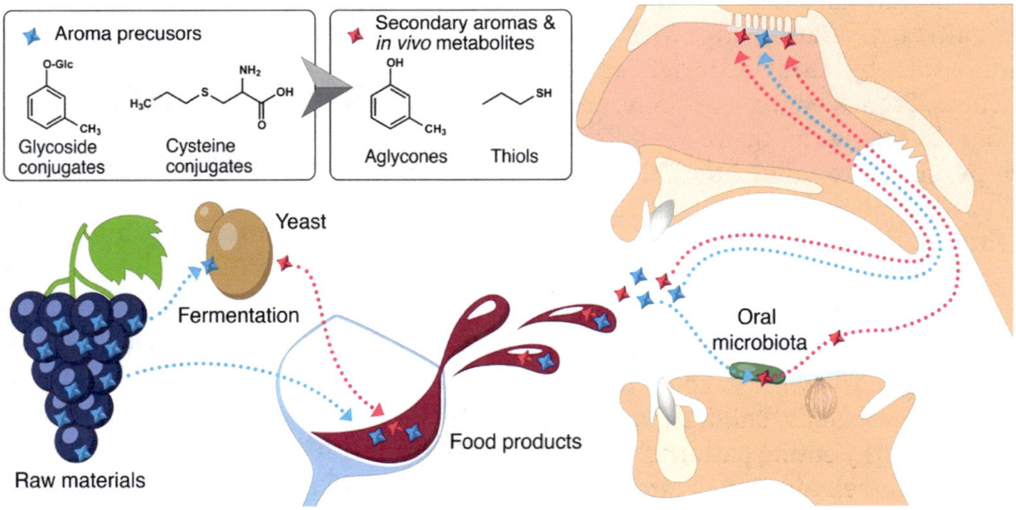

Figure 7.7. Impact of Oral Microbiota on Flavor Perception.

Source: https://www.mdpi.com/foods/foods-10-02006/article_deploy/html/images/foods-10-02006-g001.png

7.3.1 Definition and role in flavor perception

In the context of flavor perception, it is essential to understand the multifaceted components that contribute to this sensory experience. Flavor is not solely determined by taste but is significantly influenced by olfactory signals, oral somatosensation, and even visual aspects. The human mouth contains taste buds that primarily detect basic tastes—sweet, sour, bitter, salty, and umami. However, the complex interplay of these taste signals with olfactory cues, particularly during food consumption, leads to the perception of flavor as a holistic experience. As noted in contemporary research, various factors including aging and dietary habits can alter both taste and smell sensitivity, subsequently impacting flavor perception. Enhanced understanding of these interactions has implications for nutritional behavior, especially as populations age and nutritional dilemmas become increasingly pertinent in promoting health and well-being. The role of olfaction in flavor perception is paramount, as it is the sense most closely tied to the analysis of food aromas. Odor molecules released from food stimulate olfactory receptors in the nasal cavity, which then influence the perception of flavor significantly. This relationship underscores the notion that flavor is a combination of input from both taste and smell, crafted into a singular experience. Recent studies in human olfaction illustrate how factors such as genetic variation can lead to differences in olfactory sensitivity among individuals. (N/A, 2023) highlights that environmental adaptations have allowed humans to navigate sensory preferences, further complicating the flavor experience in diverse contexts. Particularly for older adults, a decline in olfactory function could result in diminished flavor perception, which might unintentionally lead to reduced food intake and nutritional deficiencies over time. Moreover, the aspect of oral somatosensation contributes to the complexity of flavor perception through tactile experiences, influencing how individuals perceive temperature, texture, and spiciness in food. These sensory experiences work in concert with taste and smell, collectively creating a unique flavor profile for each food item. Research has indicated that processed foods tend to alter these sensory connections due to their textural and chemical modifications, thereby impacting overall flavor perception. (Ashley N Gearhardt et al., 2022) presents evidence that highly processed foods may evoke addictive responses, complicating dietary choices and nutrition. As individuals age, understanding the interaction between these sensory modalities becomes vital in addressing potential health risks associated with poorer dietary habits, ensuring that nutritional strategies consider holistic approaches to flavor perception.

7.3.2 Age-related changes in oral somatosensory function

As individuals age, significant changes occur in oral somatosensory function, impacting the overall experience of flavor and texture in food. Sensory receptors in the oral cavity, including those responsible for touch and temperature, deteriorate over time, which can lead to diminished sensitivity. This reduction in sensitivity alters not only the perception of food but also the enjoyment and acceptance of various textures and flavors. The changes in oral somatosensory function are often accompanied by a decline in taste and olfactory sensitivities, culminating in a more muted gastronomic experience. Consequently, older adults may exhibit altered dietary preferences, potentially opting for foods that are stronger in flavor or texture to compensate for these sensory declines, thereby influencing their nutritional intake and health outcomes. Moreover, the interaction between oral somatosensory function and dietary habits becomes increasingly complex with age. Research indicates that individuals consuming a Western-style diet, characterized by high saturated fat and added sugars, experience poorer chemosensory perceptions. Specifically, those adhering to such diets exhibit impaired odor identification abilities and differences in taste sensitivity (Appel et al., 2016). These dietary patterns can compound the effects of age-related changes, further contributing to an overall decline in olfactory and gustatory function. Such findings highlight the imperative for targeted dietary interventions that consider both sensory changes and nutritional needs, ultimately aiming to support healthier eating behaviors in older adults. This underscores the potential for improving somatosensory function through dietary adjustments, which could enhance the quality of life for aging populations. In addition to dietary influences, genetic factors also play a role in oral somatosensory function and swallowing physiology. Studies suggest that genetic taste status may significantly impact how individuals perceive taste and, consequently, how they interact with food (Damra et al., 2023). This interplay between genetics and aging could further complicate the understanding of oral somatosensory function in older adults, as individual differences in perception could lead to diverse eating habits and nutritional outcomes. Additionally, the interdependence of taste and swallowing highlights the importance of considering genetic backgrounds when assessing swallowing difficulties in older individuals. Ultimately, recognizing the multifaceted nature of these influences provides a comprehensive framework for addressing the nutritional challenges faced by the aging population, emphasizing the need for personalized dietary strategies to accommodate sensory changes.

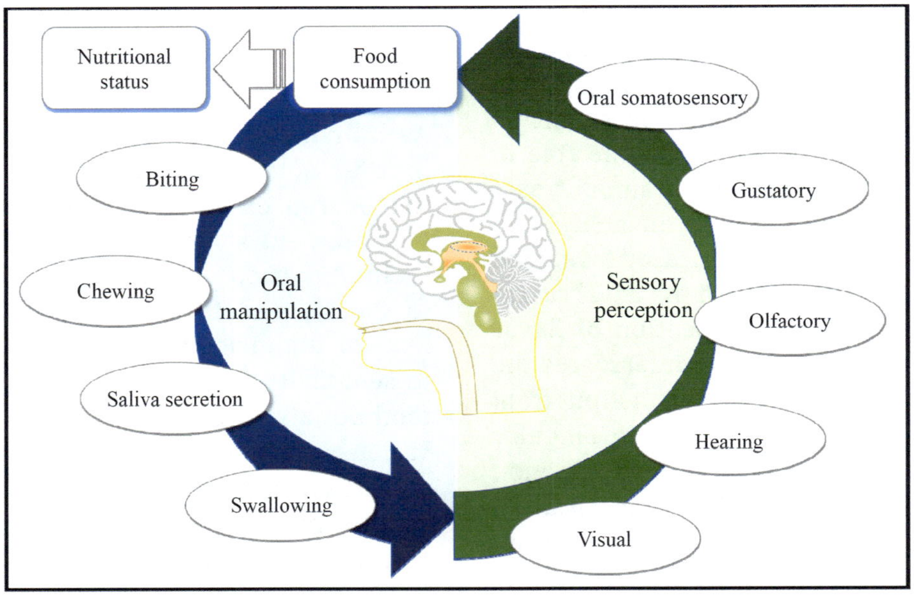

Figure 7.8. Food for the elderly based on sensory perception.

Source: https://ars.els-cdn.com/content/image/1-s2.0-S2665927122001551-gr2.jpg

7.3.3 Effects on eating behavior and food enjoyment

The intricate relationship between sensory perception and eating behavior is deeply influenced by taste, smell, and oral somatosensation, particularly as individuals age. With advancing years, the decline in olfactory and gustatory functions can significantly alter food enjoyment, which in turn impacts dietary habits and nutritional intake. Research indicates that diminished sensory perception often leads to the preference for stronger flavors or the consumption of more nutrient-dense foods to compensate for reduced taste intensity. This shift can result in a paradox where older adults may gravitate toward high-caloric, flavorful foods, thereby increasing the risk of nutritional imbalances. Understanding how these sensory changes influence food preferences is crucial for developing age-appropriate dietary guidelines that promote both enjoyment and nutrition, addressing the unique needs of the aging population. Furthermore, as societal norms evolve, the acceptance of alternative protein sources plays a significant role in shaping eating behaviors. Contemporary trends indicate a growing interest in innovative food options, such as plant-based meat alternatives and insect-based proteins. Nevertheless, the acceptance of these novel foods varies significantly among different populations, influenced largely by taste experiences, personal preferences, and cultural norms. Studies reveal that attitudes toward consuming insects, for instance, are often shaped by perceptions of novelty and sustainability, although resistance due to food neophobia remains prevalent in Western societies (Kr Töger et al., 2022). As consumers contend with both traditional dietary practices and emerging global food trends, the interplay between sensory experience and cultural acceptance becomes a pivotal factor in enhancing food enjoyment and promoting healthier eating choices. Moreover, plant-based meat alternatives (PBMA) represent a burgeoning sector aimed at addressing concerns over sustainability and health. However, the transition from traditional meat to PBMA is often met with motivational barriers, such as social rituals and conflicting eating goals (Steffen Jähn et al., 2021). These hurdles can significantly impede individuals' willingness to embrace PBMA, even when they closely mimic the sensory qualities of animal meats. To effectively encourage dietary shifts, it is essential for marketers and food developers to consider these barriers and implement strategies that enhance the sensory appeal of such alternatives. By fostering positive sensory experiences and addressing consumer concerns, it is possible to facilitate a greater acceptance of diverse food options that not only satisfy but also promote a balanced diet, especially as the population ages and seeks both enjoyment and nutritional adequacy.

7.4 Nutritional Implications of Sensory Changes

The sensory changes associated with aging significantly impact nutritional intake and preferences, creating a complex relationship between diminished sensory perception and dietary adequacy. As individuals age, alterations in the ability to smell and taste can lead to a decline in appetite and food enjoyment, which ultimately affects nutritional status. The diminished acuity of taste and smell can render familiar foods bland and less appealing, thereby discouraging older adults from consuming necessary nutrients. Such changes necessitate careful dietary planning to ensure adequate intake of vital vitamins and minerals, which are crucial for maintaining health and preventing age-related diseases. Moreover, the interplay of these sensory changes can exacerbate feelings of isolation, further compounding the risk of malnutrition as older adults may rely on convenience foods with lower nutrient density for quick meals rather than more balanced options. Furthermore, the nutritional implications of sensory changes can be particularly profound in individuals with developmental or neurogenic disorders, such as Down syndrome, wherein the dynamics of oral somatosensation intersect with dietary habits. These individuals often face challenges related to both taste and texture sensitivity, which can complicate their willingness to explore diverse food options.

Consequently, their dietary intake may lack variety and essential nutrients, as the enjoyment of food is closely linked to sensory experiences. Properly addressing these sensory changes through tailored nutritional interventions can encourage healthier eating patterns and enhance overall well-being. This aligns with findings that show how sensory and motor deficits can alter oral behaviors, highlighting the need for an integrated approach to nutritional care that considers the individuals sensory experiences alongside their dietary requirements (Madhavan A et al., 2023). Finally, understanding the intersection of sensory changes and nutrition underscores the importance of incorporating sensory enhancement strategies into dietary planning for elderly and special populations. Modifications can include flavor enhancement through herbs and spices, as well as the introduction of appealing food textures to stimulate interest in eating. These strategies not only aim to improve palatability but also address the psychological dimensions of eating, aiming to mitigate the social isolation that can accompany age-related sensory declines. Moreover, interventions to improve the environment in which individuals eat—such as making mealtime social or enhancing the visual appeal of the food—can stimulate both taste and smell. Ultimately, recognizing and strategically addressing the nutritional implications of sensory changes can lead to improved dietary intake, thus fostering better health outcomes among aging individuals and those with specific dietary challenges (Farhangdoust M, 2024).

7.4.1 Impact on nutrient intake and dietary quality

The interplay between sensory perception and dietary quality is particularly salient in understanding the impact of age-related changes on nutrient intake. As individuals age, alterations in smell, taste, and oral somatosensation contribute to a decline in meal enjoyment and acceptance, leading to poorer dietary choices. Older adults often experience a diminishment in taste sensitivity, particularly for sweet and salty flavors, which can result in a decreased appetite and reduced food intake. This decline can hinder nutrient diversity, causing a reliance on monotonous, less nutrient-dense foods. Such shifts not only affect caloric intake but potentially lead to deficiencies in essential vitamins and minerals, precipitating a cascade of health issues. Therefore, it is crucial to consider how the aging sensory experience shapes food preferences and dietary habits in older populations (Croxford S, 2023). In addition to sensory changes, the broader context of food systems plays a significant role in nutritional outcomes. Nutritional professionals are increasingly called to navigate complex food environments affected by socio-economic factors that influence accessibility and affordability of healthy foods. For instance, food insecurity can lead to reliance on low-cost, high-calorie options, exacerbating issues related to malnutrition among older adults. Increased understanding of personal biases and cultural backgrounds can enhance dietary recommendations and support better food choices tailored to individual needs. This requires nutritionists to engage in interdisciplinary approaches that foster trust and enhance dietary quality through culturally relevant strategies, ensuring that older adults have access to the variety of foods necessary for optimal health (N/A, 2023). Moreover, sensory experiences aligned with food consumption involve more than taste and aroma; they encapsulate a holistic view of dietary quality influenced by environment and lifestyle. As older individuals encounter sensory declines, creating supportive food environments becomes paramount. Strategies may include improving the palatability of nutritious foods through culinary initiatives that enhance flavor profiles or modifying meal presentations to stimulate visual appeal. Empowering older adults with knowledge about sensory preferences can help align their diets with health goals, inciting a shift in food choices. By emphasizing a sensory-rich eating experience, caregivers and health professionals can facilitate better engagement with food, ultimately striving to improve nutrient intake and overall dietary quality in aging populations (Croxford S, 2023).

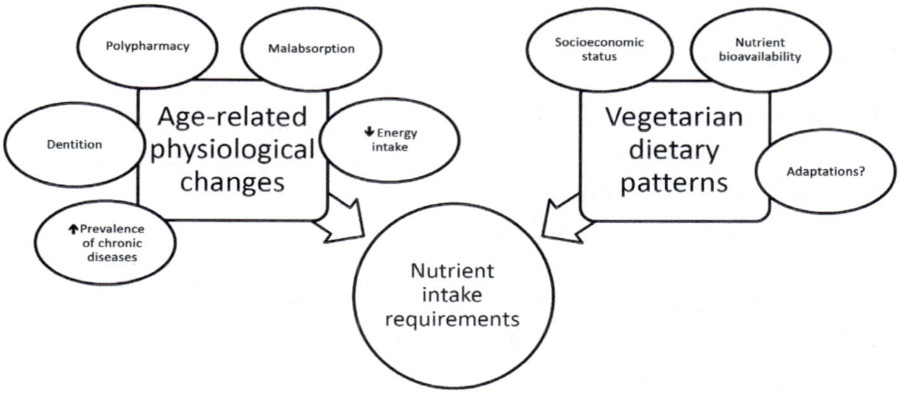

Figure 7.9. Age-related physiologic changes and decreased energy intakes that are commonly observed in older populations can result in reduced nutritional status.

Source: https://www.researchgate.net/publication/316090161/figure/fig1/AS:963429548453927@1606710912755/Factors-determining-the-nutrient-intake-requirements-of-older-and-elderly-vegetarian.gif

7.4.2 Potential for malnutrition in older adults

The potential for malnutrition in older adults is a pressing concern that emerges from the interplay of age-related physiological changes and evolving nutritional needs. As individuals age, their sensory perception, particularly taste and smell, tends to diminish. This decline can lead to a reduced appetite and altered food preferences, which subsequently impact their nutritional intake. With a decreased ability to perceive flavors and scents, older adults may find less enjoyment in eating, leading to decreased food consumption and insufficient nutrient intake. Neurodegenerative changes and dental issues further exacerbate these difficulties, making it crucial to understand how sensory declines influence dietary habits. Addressing these issues is essential for provide older adults with a balanced diet that meets their nutritional requirements and helps prevent malnutrition, which can significantly affect their overall health and quality of life (Agerberg et al., 1996). In addition to sensory declines, older adults often experience physiological and mechanical changes in their gastrointestinal tract (GIT) that can further contribute to malnutrition. The aging process is associated with several alterations in the GIT, including diminished mechanical disintegration of food, compromised gastric motility, and reduced efficiency in nutrient absorption. These factors can hinder the bodys ability to adequately digest and utilize essential nutrients, underpinning the importance of tailored dietary strategies. While older adults may consume what seems to be an adequate amount of food, the quality and bioavailability of nutrients can be significantly impaired. This dysfunctional state of the gastrointestinal system presents a unique intersection with malnutrition, creating a cycle where inadequate nutrient absorption can lead to deteriorating health outcomes and increased vulnerability to conditions such as frailty and chronic disease (Bordoni et al., 2015). Preventing malnutrition in older adults necessitates a multifaceted approach that integrates dietary solutions, nutritional education, and supportive interventions. Awareness of the unique challenges faced by this population is essential for health care providers, caregivers, and family members alike.

Developing dietary guidelines that consider the physiological changes of the aging GIT, while promoting nutrient-dense food choices, can play a pivotal role in combating malnutrition. Moreover, incorporating sensory-enhancing interventions and fortifying foods with essential vitamins and minerals may further encourage older adults to maintain adequate nutritional intake. To effectively address this public health issue, collaborative efforts among nutritionists, geriatricians, and researchers are critical in identifying and validating biomarkers that facilitate the assessment of food intake, nutrient bioavailability, and the overall nutritional status of older adults, ultimately improving health outcomes and quality of life (Bordoni et al., 2015).

7.4.3 Strategies to enhance flavor and nutrition

The enhancement of flavor and nutrition in food preparation is essential for addressing age-related changes in taste and smell, which can significantly impact dietary habits. One effective strategy is the incorporation of various herbs and spices, which not only elevate the sensory experience of meals but also provide numerous health benefits. Research indicates that specific spices, such as turmeric and ginger, possess anti-inflammatory properties and contribute to better overall health, particularly in older adults. By utilizing these flavor enhancers, not only can meal palatability be improved, but nutritional density is also increased, thereby addressing potential deficiencies often seen in aging populations. This dual approach highlights the importance of rethinking how we flavor food, making culinary creativity a key component in promoting healthier eating habits among the elderly. Additionally, the role of food presentation cannot be overlooked when considering strategies to enhance flavor and nutrition. Visual appeal has a profound effect on the perception of taste and can significantly influence appetite, particularly in older adults who may experience diminished sensory acuity.

Techniques such as vibrant plating and contrasting colors can stimulate appetite and entice individuals to consume a wider variety of foods. Furthermore, engaging the sense of touch through varied textures in food can contribute to a more enjoyable eating experience. As sensory environments vary widely across different contexts influenced by socio-economic factors, it is crucial to account for these elements in designing meal options that cater to individuals needs, especially when addressing the discrepancies highlighted in the notion of sensory inequities (N/A, 2023). Finally, educational strategies aimed at enhancing flavor comprehension and nutritional awareness among older adults are vital. Workshops and cooking classes that focus on the medicinal properties of ingredients foster a deeper understanding and appreciation for food choices. Through these programs, participants can be educated on combining flavors in innovative ways that also preserve or enhance nutritional value, such as using healthy fats that promote flavor while aiding in nutrient absorption. Moreover, sharing the cultural significance of diverse culinary practices can motivate individuals to engage with their food, potentially reversing the declines in appetite that may accompany aging. Therefore, a multifaceted educational approach, factoring in the importance of smell, taste, and texture, can profoundly improve nutritional outcomes within this demographic (Velasco C et al., 2018).

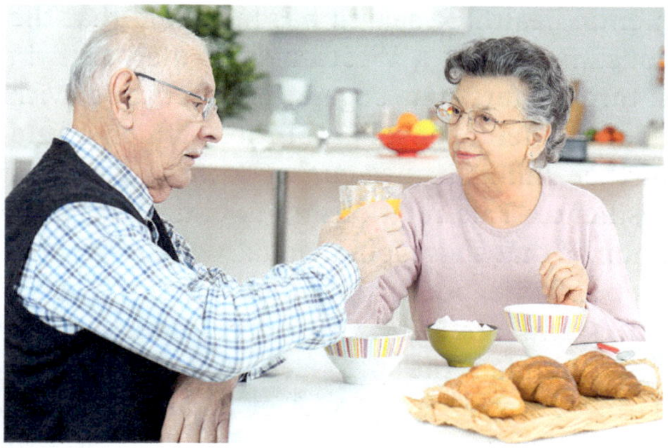

Figure 7.10. Strategies to enhance flavor and nutrition.

Source: https://www.discoveryvillages.com/wp-content/uploads/2022/01/top-tips-to-improve-nutrition-in-the-elderly.jpg

7.5 Psychological and Social Factors

Psychological and social factors significantly influence how individuals experience and perceive taste and smell, especially as they age. An individuals dietary habits are closely tied to their social environment and psychological well-being. Research indicates that people consuming a Western-style diet, which is typically high in saturated fats and sugars, may exhibit impaired olfactory identification and distinct taste preferences. The consumption patterns established within social groups can shape these sensory perceptions, leading to poorer nutritional choices over time. As such, the psychological impact of one's dietary context—often reflective of social norms—can ultimately impede the adoption of healthier eating habits. This dynamic illustrates how social influences can reinforce dietary preferences that may further adversely affect sensory perception and overall health, complicating efforts to modify diet in older populations. In addition to dietary influences, psychological factors such as food neophobia and individual hedonic responses play crucial roles in shaping taste experiences. Studies demonstrate that odor sensitivity correlates with flavor perception, highlighting the psychological dimension of taste. Individuals with high sensitivity to certain flavors tend to have more refined and nuanced experiences with food, while those with lower sensitivity often rate sweeter options more favorably. This variability in psychological response affects nutritional choices, as those less sensitive may gravitate toward sweeter, less nutritious foods. Furthermore, preferences shaped by past experiences and cultural contexts can create significant barriers to trying new foods, impacting both nutritional intake and sensory enjoyment in older adults.

Therefore, understanding these psychological factors can provide valuable insight into potential interventions aimed at improving dietary habits. Social factors, including cultural norms and communal eating practices, further complicate the landscape of taste and smell perception. The shared experience of meals often influences food choices and preferences, especially within familial or communal settings. In many cultures, the collective enjoyment of food is intertwined with social bonding, which can lead to the reinforcement of preferred flavors and textures among group members. This phenomenon is particularly significant for older adults, who may face social isolation that can exacerbate dietary deficiencies by limiting exposure to varied foods. Research supports the notion that communal eating not only enhances enjoyment through shared sensory experiences but also encourages healthier eating patterns. Such insights underscore the importance of considering social dynamics and support systems when addressing nutritional challenges related to age-related changes in smell and taste perception, advocating for more integrative approaches to dietary interventions.

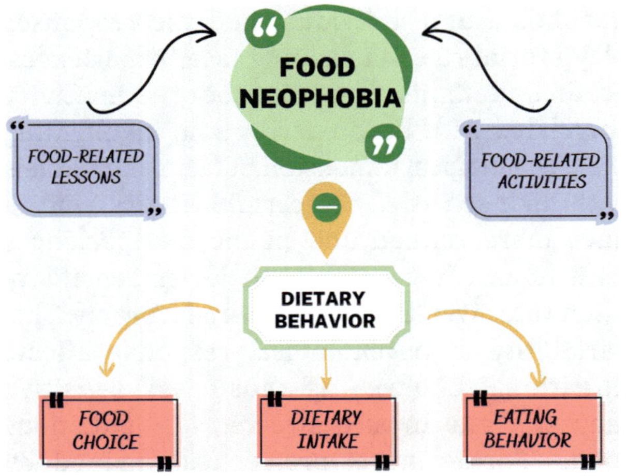

Figure 7.11. A narrative review on food neophobia throughout the lifespan.

Source: https://static.cambridge.org/content/id/urn%3Acambridge.org%3Aid%3Aarticle%3AS0007114522003713/resource/name/S0007114522003713_figAb.png?pub-status=live

7.5.1 Influence of sensory changes on mental health

Sensory changes, particularly in the domains of smell and taste, can have profound implications for mental health, especially as individuals age. The degradation of these senses often correlates with an increased risk for mental health disorders, such as depression and anxiety. The interplay between diminished sensory input and emotional well-being is complex; for example, individuals experiencing a loss of taste may find mealtime less enjoyable, leading to decreased appetite and potential malnutrition. This diminished appetite can further exacerbate feelings of sadness or isolation, creating a cyclical relationship between sensory decline and mental health outcomes. Enhanced understanding of these connections underscores the significance of sensory health as a crucial component of holistic well-being, particularly in older populations who are already at greater risk for psychological conditions. Moreover, dietary choices are intrinsically linked to our sensory perceptions, thereby impacting mental health. Research has indicated that the consumption of a Western-style diet, high in saturated fats and sugars, is associated with poorer chemosensory abilities, which could further diminish ones quality of life and mental resilience. This relationship is underscored by findings that suggest individuals with a Western diet exhibit poorer olfactory identification skills and altered taste perceptions, which can diminish the pleasure associated with eating experiences (Appel et al., 2016). Poor dietary habits not only impair sensory health but also feed into negative emotional states, leading to a downward spiral impacting mental health and nutritional status. Understanding this dynamic can guide interventions aimed at promoting nutritious diets that align with sensory health, thus fostering psychological resilience. Furthermore, the mechanisms through which taste influences swallowing and overall nutritional intake highlight the importance of sensory experiences for mental wellness. Taste sensation is not merely a physical process; it engages complex neural pathways that affect mood and cognitive functions. Impairments in taste perception can disrupt swallowing behaviors and lead to reluctance in consuming nutritionally necessary foods, which can result in adverse health outcomes, including malnutrition (Dietsch et al., 2022). The psychological repercussions of these dietary changes can manifest as declining mental health, emphasizing the need for careful management of sensory health in aging populations. By focusing on the broader implications of sensory changes, healthcare providers can develop strategies to address both nutritional needs and mental well-being through targeted interventions that emphasize the restoration or preservation of sensory functions.

7.5.2 Social implications of altered eating experiences

The experience of eating extends beyond mere sustenance; it encompasses social interactions, cultural practices, and emotional connections that constitute its rich tapestry. Alterations in the sensory dimensions of eating, particularly relating to smell and taste, can disrupt these interpersonal bonds. For instance, individuals with diminished olfactory function often report a significant decline in their enjoyment of food ((Fjaeldstad et al., 2024)). This decline not only affects personal satisfaction but may lead to alienation in social dining environments, where shared meals typically serve as a medium for building relationships. Consequently, the implications of altered eating experiences can extend to social withdrawal, changing the dynamics of interaction within families and peer groups. When individuals opt out of communal eating due to diminished sensory enjoyment, they risk missing out on the fundamental experiences that foster social cohesion. Moreover, the multisensory experience of eating highlights the intricate relationship between taste perception and social settings. Research indicates that taste plays a crucial role in swallowing and overall eating enjoyment, both of which are central to social gatherings ((Dietsch et al., 2024)). When individuals experience changes in their taste perception—whether due to age, health conditions, or altered sensory function—the resulting difficulty can hinder participation in shared meals. As dining often serves as a cultural touchstone, impaired taste not only alters individual experiences but can also shift the cultural significance of food within communities. Family recipes may lose their meaning if one can no longer appreciate their flavors, while traditional food rituals might diminish in importance, reflecting the broader social implications of altered eating experiences. Additionally, the social ramifications of these altered eating experiences underscore the need for innovative interventions. Addressing the decline in sensory enjoyment among those affected can potentially reintegrate individuals into their social circles. Approaches such as enhancing the visual and textural aspects of food, as suggested in a study focusing on patients with smell loss, demonstrate the potential for restoring pleasure in eating ((Fjaeldstad et al., 2024)). These adaptations can revitalize communal dining experiences and affirm the inherent value of food as a social connector. Hence, as we consider the broader nutritional implications of age-related sensory changes, it becomes clear that addressing the social aspects of altered eating experiences is essential for promoting overall well-being and community engagement.

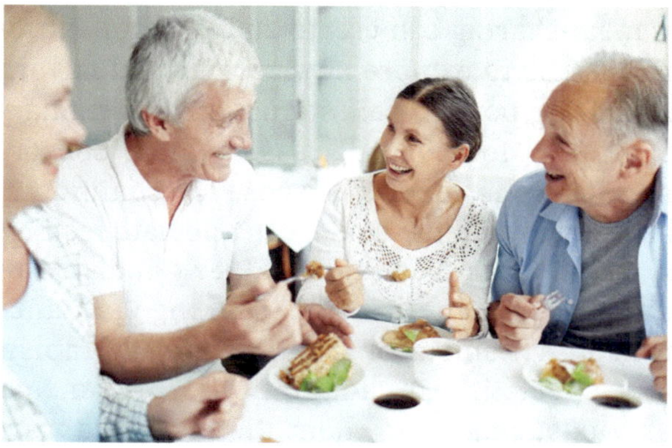

Figure 7.12. Social implications of altered eating experiences.

Source: https://bestlifeonline.com/media-library/older-white-people-eating-together.jpg?id=53254838&quality=82&strip=all

7.5.3 Coping mechanisms for individuals experiencing changes

As individuals age, they often confront significant changes in sensory perception, particularly in the realms of smell and taste. The decline of these senses can lead to a diminished quality of life, including alterations in dietary habits and nutritional intake. To cope with these changes, individuals may benefit from employing various strategies that emphasize adaptation. For instance, utilizing stronger flavors and spices in cooking can compensate for a decreased sensitivity to taste, thereby encouraging a more pleasurable eating experience. Additionally, engaging in mindful eating practices may foster greater appreciation for food textures and aromas, ultimately reinforcing positive associations with meals. Such coping mechanisms not only help maintain nutritional health but also bolster emotional well-being during this challenging transition. Social support plays a significant role in the coping processes of individuals experiencing age-related sensory changes. Connecting with others who share similar experiences can provide an essential network for emotional resilience. Group activities involving cooking or meal-sharing can create an environment for individuals to explore new recipes and flavors, promoting both social interaction and culinary creativity. Moreover, discussing these sensory modifications fosters a sense of community and understanding, which can alleviate feelings of isolation or frustration. Elderly individuals might also benefit from seeking guidance from nutritionists or occupational therapists who specialize in adaptations for sensory loss, ensuring that their dietary needs are met optimally. This comprehensive approach encourages adaptive coping mechanisms that acknowledge both the physical and psychological aspects of aging. Educational interventions are crucial for equipping individuals with the knowledge and skills to navigate sensory changes effectively. Workshops or informational sessions focusing on the implications of altered taste and smell can empower older adults to make informed dietary choices. Additionally, teaching practical strategies for enhancing flavor perception, such as incorporating umami-rich foods or using aroma-enhancing techniques, can significantly mitigate the impact of sensory loss. Research suggests that understanding the scientific basis for these changes can facilitate acceptance and reduce anxiety regarding food-related experiences (N/A, 2022). Ultimately, fostering an informed perspective on sensory adaptation not only enriches the nutritional quality of life for aging individuals but also enhances their overall well-being. With such educational support, older adults can develop robust coping mechanisms that enable them to navigate the complexities of aging with greater confidence (Pande S, 2022).

7.6 Research and Future Directions

The exploration of age-related changes in smell, taste, and oral somatosensation presents numerous avenues for future research, particularly regarding their implications on nutrition and overall health. As individuals age, alterations in sensory perception can significantly impact dietary choices, leading to reduced food intake and subsequent nutritional deficiencies. Investigating these sensory changes could inform interventions aimed at promoting healthier eating habits among older adults. Future studies may focus on the mechanistic pathways linking sensory decline to altered appetite regulation and food preferences. This could include examining how changes in chemesthesis affect nutrient absorption and overall health, specifically in populations with certain medical conditions. With a better understanding of these relationships, it is possible to develop targeted nutritional strategies that accommodate the sensory preferences of older adults, thereby improving both their dietary intake and quality of life. Furthermore, expanding research on oral somatosensation may contribute valuable insights into age-related dysphagia and its nutritional consequences. Given the complexity of swallowing mechanisms and their interconnection with sensory perceptions, future studies could adopt an integrative biophysiological framework similar to that proposed in other areas of research. Such a framework could elucidate how sensory feedback impacts the coordination of swallowing and its associated neural pathways. For example, specific attention could be paid to populations with developmental disorders like Down syndrome, where structural anomalies influence both the oral cavity and sensory feedback mechanisms. Understanding these dynamics will not only pave the way for advanced therapeutic interventions but also highlight the importance of tailoring dietary strategies that mitigate the risk of aspiration and malnutrition in vulnerable groups (Madhavan A et al., 2023). Lastly, the implications of highly processed foods (HPFs) on sensory perception, especially in the context of aging, warrant rigorous investigation. Recent evidence suggests that HPFs may possess addictive qualities, thereby moderating individuals food choices and consumption behaviors as they age (Ashley N Gearhardt et al., 2022). This line of inquiry emphasizes the need to assess how sensory changes influence the propensity for compulsive eating behaviors, further complicating nutritional outcomes.

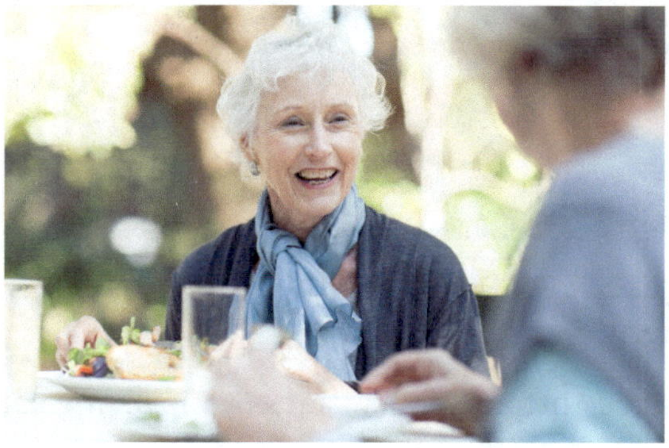

Figure 7.13. Changes in Taste and Smell With Age.

Source: https://fthmb.tqn.com/FJk2usCXCW7qERjzXvpZwGUcXz8=/2000x1333/filters:fill(87E3EF,1)/GettyImages-557920551-56c8e8a75f9b5879cc4545cb.jpg

Future research should aim at establishing criteria for evaluating HPFs addictive potential and its intersections with sensory processing. Identifying nutritional patterns tied to sensory changes could promote public health initiatives that combat unhealthy eating habits prevalent in older adults. By exploring the nexus between sensory perception and dietary preferences, researchers can contribute to the development of comprehensive strategies to enhance the nutritional health of aging populations, ultimately reducing the burden of age-related malnutrition.

7.6.1 Current studies on sensory changes and nutrition

Recent studies examining the interplay between sensory changes and nutrition reveal significant implications for both dietary habits and health outcomes. Research indicates that individual variations in taste perception can considerably influence swallowing physiology and nutrition. While genetic taste status plays a crucial role, findings remain mixed regarding its impact on swallowing outcomes. For instance, a review highlighted that only a subset of studies reported significant effects of genetic taste status on swallowing abilities, suggesting that further exploration is needed to understand these relationships comprehensively. The limited number of studies that incorporate genetic factors indicates a gap in existing literature, which clinicians could address by considering how individual sensory experiences shape dietary choices and swallowing function (Damra et al., 2023). In addition to genetic influences, dietary patterns also affect chemosensory abilities. A notable study investigated the correlations between Western-style diets, characterized by high saturated fat and sugar content, and chemosensory perception. Participants consuming such diets exhibited poorer olfactory identification abilities, variations in taste sensitivity, and distinct flavor processing patterns compared to those maintaining healthier diets. These findings suggest that a diet rich in unhealthy components may not only alter sensory perception but could also reinforce detrimental dietary habits. The small to moderate effect sizes observed in these relationships call for an understanding of whether these dietary-induced sensory changes precede the adoption of unhealthy eating patterns or result from them.

Thus, addressing dietary choices may be pivotal in enhancing sensory functions and overall health (Appel et al., 2016). Together, these studies underscore the complex relationship between sensory perception and nutrition, particularly as individuals age. As sensory abilities such as taste and smell decline, older adults might gravitate towards less nutritious food choices, potentially exacerbating health issues. Addressing this challenge requires an interdisciplinary approach, combining insights from nutrition science, genetics, and sensory psychology to develop comprehensive dietary strategies. By acknowledging the integral role that sensory changes play in nutrition and health, future research can better inform interventions designed to improve dietary quality among aging populations. Ultimately, fostering an understanding of how sensory perception impacts food choices may prove essential in promoting healthier diets and enhancing quality of life for individuals across the lifespan (Damra et al., 2023)(Appel et al., 2016).

7.6.2 Emerging therapies to address sensory decline

As the population ages, sensory decline in smell, taste, and oral somatosensation poses significant challenges not only to individual quality of life but also to nutritional health. Emerging therapies targeting these sensory declines are increasingly at the forefront of geriatric care. For instance, olfactory training has shown promise in enhancing olfactory function in elderly individuals, potentially leading to improved appetite and dietary choices. This approach involves the repetition of exposure to specific scents, activating olfactory receptors and elements of neuroplasticity. Such sensory rehabilitation therapies not only have potential therapeutic benefits but also carry lower risks compared to pharmaceutical interventions, reflecting a shift towards more holistic treatment modalities for sensory impairments associated with aging. In addition to olfactory training, advancements in neurotechnology signify a new frontier in sensory rehabilitation. For example, Brain-Computer Interface (BCI) technologies are being investigated for their ability to assist in cognitive and sensory processing in individuals experiencing prolonged disorders of consciousness. Studies indicate that electroencephalographic (EEG) measures, including the N1 and P3 components of auditory evoked potentials (AEPs), can provide crucial insights into sensory perception and awareness in patients with cognitive-motor dissociation (Coyle et al., 2024).

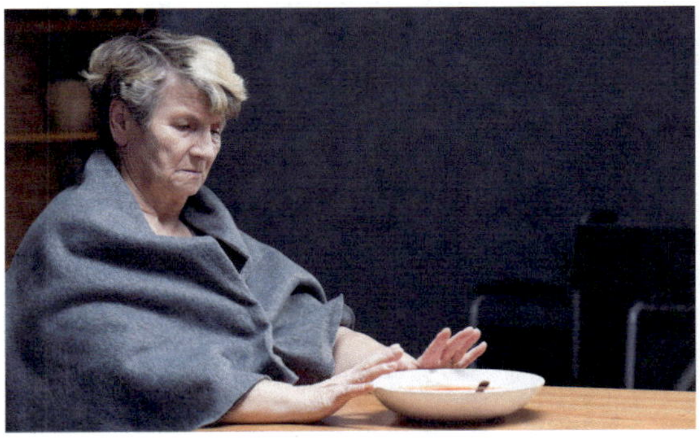

Figure 7.14. Dealing With Loss Of Taste In The Elderly.

Source: https://www.seatonseniorliving.com/wp-content/uploads/2022/08/Dealing-With-Loss-Of-Taste-In-The-Elderly..jpg

As these technologies evolve, they present the possibility of developing more personalized therapies that can address multiple facets of sensory decline, thereby enhancing overall well-being in older adults. Moreover, dietary interventions that augment taste and flavor perception are gaining traction as another avenue for addressing sensory decline. For instance, research has indicated that modifying food textures and enhancing flavor profiles through seasoning can help stimulate engagement with food among older adults experiencing diminished taste sensitivity. As a consequence, nutritional education and collaborative cooking initiatives that promote sensory-rich experiences are gaining recognition as effective strategies (Coyle et al., 2024). These interventions underscore the necessity of integrating sensory training with nutritional practices, fostering not just the maintenance of sensory function but also promoting healthier eating habits, ultimately contributing to better health outcomes in the aging population.

7.6.3 Importance of interdisciplinary approaches in research

The exploration of sensory experiences, particularly in relation to smell, taste, and oral somatosensation, necessitates an interdisciplinary approach that brings together diverse fields such as psychology, nutrition, and sensory science. Each of these disciplines contributes unique insights that enhance the understanding of how age-related changes affect eating behaviors and nutritional implications. For instance, psychology offers valuable frameworks for understanding how emotional and cognitive processing influences taste perception, while nutrition focuses on the physiological aspects of food intake and its impact on health. By fostering collaboration across these fields, researchers can develop comprehensive models that better account for the complexities of human sensory experiences and their implications for dietary habits. Moreover, the integration of different scientific methodologies is crucial for addressing the multifaceted nature of food experiences. As highlighted in the study of food textural acoustics, challenges arise when examining how particular sensory experiences, such as the sound of food, impact the perception of taste and enjoyment, particularly for individuals with swallowing disorders. The findings suggest that existing methods may be inadequate in capturing the richness of these experiences (TF K et al., 2023). An interdisciplinary approach can improve research design by incorporating diverse perspectives and techniques, allowing for a more holistic understanding of food-related phenomena, including how aging alters sensory perceptions. This collaborative effort is essential for developing effective interventions to improve nutritional outcomes for diverse populations. Furthermore, technologies like LeviSense exemplify the potential of interdisciplinary research to enhance our understanding of multisensory integration during eating experiences. By systematically examining how different stimuli, such as visual and olfactory cues, influence taste perception, this innovation highlights the importance of integrating knowledge from sensory research, psychology, and culinary arts (Ablart et al., 2020). The insights gained from such interdisciplinary studies not only further academic discourse but also have practical implications for creating novel culinary experiences that cater to different age groups and enhance the enjoyment of food. Ultimately, embracing interdisciplinary collaboration ensures that research in this area is robust, relevant, and capable of addressing the complex interactions between sensory perception, age-related changes, and nutritional practices.

SUMMARY

The intricate interplay between age-related changes in sensory modalities, particularly smell, taste, and oral somatosensation, and their nutritional implications is a critical area of study. Understanding how aging affects these senses is essential, as diminished sensory function can lead to changes in dietary habits and nutritional intake. As older adults often experience a decline in the ability to perceive flavors and aromas, the result may be a less enjoyable eating experience and, consequently, diminished nutritional status. Furthermore, research suggests that such modifications in sensory perception can form a feedback loop, influencing food choices that prioritize convenience over nutrition, thereby exacerbating health-related issues associated with aging. Moreover, the impact of dietary choices on sensory perception cannot be overlooked. Evidence points to the significance of dietary patterns, particularly those characterized by high saturated fats and sugars, in modulating chemosensory abilities (Appel et al., 2016). The findings from studies underscore a concerning trend: individuals adhering to a Western-style diet exhibited poorer olfactory identification and altered taste perceptions when compared to those consuming a more balanced diet. This relationship highlights the necessity for nutritional interventions aimed at promoting healthier eating habits to support sensory functionality in older populations. By fostering awareness of dietary impacts on the senses, it may be possible to enhance the overall dining experience and nutritional adequacy in aging individuals. Finally, addressing sensory challenges through interventions can have profound implications for improving quality of life among aging populations. The potential for enhancing sensory processing through nutritional modifications suggests a promising avenue for research and practical application. As explored in recent studies, sensory processing affects emotional regulation and behavior, particularly in populations experiencing further complexity, such as autistic children and adolescents (Hatem et al.). By understanding the mechanisms linking sensory perception with dietary habits, effective strategies can be developed to encourage healthier eating practices that not only enhance sensory experiences but also support emotional and behavioral adjustments. Ultimately, promoting the optimization of taste, smell, and somatosensory functions may lead to a more enjoyable and nutritionally rewarding relationship with food among older adults.

The intricate interplay between smell, taste, and oral somatosensation is crucial for understanding how these senses change with age and their subsequent impact on nutrition. As individuals age, sensory perception can decline, leading to a reduced ability to taste and smell, which in turn affects dietary choices and preferences. This sensory decline can result in a decreased appetite and insufficient nutritional intake, heightening the risk of malnutrition in older adults. Moreover, age-related changes in oral somatosensation can modify the eating experience, influencing food texture perception and leading to alterations in food choices. Comprehensive analysis of these sensory attributes indicates a pressing need for tailored nutritional strategies that accommodate the unique sensory experiences of the elderly population. Research has highlighted the role of oral somatosensation, which encompasses not only taste perception but also interrelated sensory modalities such as chemosensation and thermal perception. Enhanced understanding of these oral sensory processes offers valuable insights into how they vary among individuals, particularly with respect to taster status. The discovery of genetic polymorphisms that categorize individuals as hyper-tasters, tasters, or tolerant tasters points to significant differences in sensory perception, particularly in response to flavors and textures in food. These variations have implications for dietary habits, as they can determine individual preferences and tolerances for different food components, such as the pungency of spices, which plays a vital role in enhancing flavor profiles in meals, particularly in older adults whose sensory thresholds may have shifted (Spence et al., 2024). Furthermore, exploring the complex dynamics of oral sensory processing has revealed that individuals experience chemostimulant intensity differently across various regions of the oral cavity. Studies indicate that an interaction between touch type, taster status, and oral location influences the perception of flavors and sensations, suggesting that sensory experiences are not uniform. This nuanced understanding could facilitate the development of interventions aimed at improving eating experiences through flavor enhancement or modification, catering to the specific needs of older adults. As sensory sensitivity diminishes with age, the ability for individuals to personalize their flavor experience through spices and ingredients may be hindered, emphasizing the importance of creating appealing and nutritious meals tailored to their sensory capabilities (Smith et al.).

CLOSER LOOK

TASTE AND SMELL IN THE ELDERLY

Taste and smell in the elderly reveals that these senses often diminish with age, significantly affecting quality of life, nutrition, and safety. The decline in taste and smell—collectively known as chemosensory perception—is typically gradual, beginning around the age of 60. This reduction may stem from a natural decrease in the number and sensitivity of taste buds and olfactory receptors. In addition, age-related changes in the brain's processing of sensory information, dental issues, medications, and chronic conditions such as Alzheimer's or Parkinson's disease can further impair these senses. Taste is generally less affected than smell, with sweet and salty flavors often being the first to weaken.

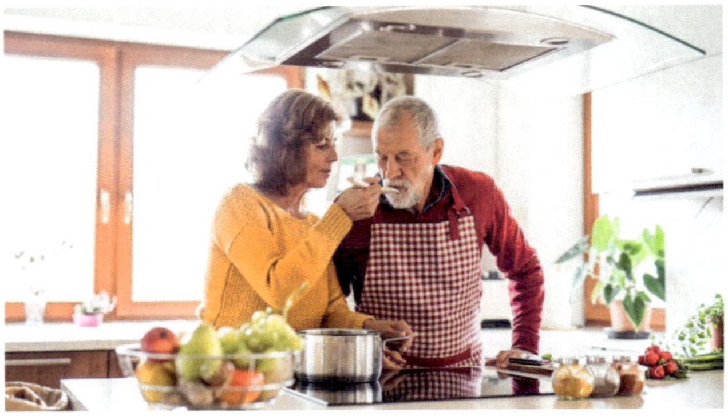

Figure 7.15. Managing Taste and Smell Changes in Older Persons.

Source: https://comfortkeepers.ie/img/asset/aW1hZ2VzL2FnZWluZy1ncmFjZWZ1bGx5LmpwZw/ageing-gracefully.jpg?w=1400&h=788&s=0ff5dbb8c3511babcc04d8fabdfd6a3a

This can lead elderly individuals to overuse salt or sugar to compensate, increasing their risk for hypertension or diabetes. Loss of smell can also compromise the ability to detect spoiled food or gas leaks, posing health hazards. Moreover, the diminished enjoyment of eating may lead to decreased appetite, poor nutrition, weight loss, or even depression. Maintaining oral hygiene, managing medication side effects, and encouraging flavorful yet healthy meals with varied textures and temperatures can help mitigate these sensory losses. Understanding the importance of taste and smell in elderly care is crucial for promoting overall well-being and ensuring that older adults continue to engage positively with their environment and dietary habits.

REFERENCES

1. Aarthi Madhavan, Larissa Lam, Nicole M. Etter, Krista M. Wilkinson (2023) A biophysiological framework exploring factors affecting speech and swallowing in clinical populations: focus on individuals with Down syndrome. Volume(14). Frontiers in Psychology. doi: https://doi.org/10.3389/fpsyg.2023.1085779
2. Abby Brodbeck, Grace Helminak, Emma Jacobson, Dominque Islas, Media S. Esser, Erica M. Phelps, Abby C Streeton, et al. (2022) NANN Research Summit 2022. Volume(22), E78 - E85. Advances in Neonatal Care. doi: https://www.semanticscholar.org/paper/067cac7462808f5dbbac8715ea18c595b53c6b18
3. Ablart, D, Chi, TV, Maggioni, E, Marzo, et al. (2020) LeviSense: A platform for the multisensory integration in levitating food and insights into its effect on flavour perception. doi: https://core.ac.uk/download/336585489.pdf
4. Ada Braghieri, Alessandra Bendini, Corrado Pacelli, Luisa Torri, Maria Piochi, Rossella Di Monaco, Sharon Puleo, et al. (2021) Food neophobia, odor and taste sensitivity, and overall flavor perception in food. doi: https://core.ac.uk/download/551069687.pdf
5. Agerberg, Atkinson, Bartoshuk, Bartoshuk, Baum, Baum, Baum, et al. (1996) Geriatric Oral Health and Its Impact on Eating. doi: https://deepblue.lib.umich.edu/bitstream/2027.42/111258/1/j.1532-5415.1996.tb06419.x.pdf
6. Appel, Bertino, Cicerale, Heather M. Francis, Martin R. Yeomans, Mattes, Megan J. Oaten, et al. (2016) Chemosensory abilities in consumers of a western-style diet. doi: https://core.ac.uk/download/46166611.pdf
7. Ashley N. Gearhardt, Alexandra G. DiFeliceantonio (2022) Highly processed foods can be considered addictive substances based on established scientific criteria. Volume(118), 589-598. Addiction. doi: https://doi.org/10.1111/add.16065
8. Banni S, Crnjar R, Melis M, Tepper BJ, Tomassini Barbarossa I (2014) Genetic sensitivity to the bitter taste of 6-n-propylthiouracil (PROP) and its association with Physiological mechanisms controlling Body Mass Index (BMI). doi: https://core.ac.uk/download/pdf/54598551.pdf
9. Barrett, Becker, Braun, Chernoff, Cowart, Evans, Gollub, et al. (2013) The consumption of protein-rich foods in older adults: An exploratory focus group study. doi: https://core.ac.uk/download/20665247.pdf
10. Bordoni, Alessandra, Dupont, Didier, Gille, Doreen, Kachal, et al. (2015) Understanding the gastrointestinal tract of the elderly to develop dietary solutions that prevent malnutrition. doi: https://core.ac.uk/download/286575279.pdf
11. BRANDIMORE, Alexandra Essman, GODOY, Juliana, HEGLAND, Karen Wheeler, TROCHE, et al. (2014) A framework for understanding shared substrates of airway protection. doi: https://core.ac.uk/download/268274789.pdf
12. Carlos Velasco, Anton Nijholt, Kasun Karunanayaka, Melle Nieling, Qian Janice Wang, Klemens Knoeferle, Charles Spence, et al. (2018) Multisensory Human-Food Interaction. . Frontiers research topics. doi: https://doi.org/10.3389/978-2-88945-518-8
13. Conroy, Paula M. (2018) Development, assessment and optimisation of meat systems for the aging consumer through processing and packaging modification. doi: https://core.ac.uk/download/161818987.pdf

14. Coyle, Damien, Du Bois, Naomi, Hill, N. Jeremy, Korik, et al. (2024) Objective neurophysiologic markers to aid assessment of prolonged disorders of consciousness (PDoC). doi: https://core.ac.uk/download/624084191.pdf

15. Damra, Rana H., Dietsch, Angela M., Lee, Theresa S., Mulheren, et al. (2023) The Effect of Genetic Taste Status on Swallowing: A Literature Review. doi: https://core.ac.uk/download/610527554.pdf

16. Dietsch, Angela M., Mulheren, Rachel W., Westemeyer, Ross M. (2024) Applying the Evidence: Taste Manipulation as a Dysphagia Management Strategy. doi: https://core.ac.uk/download/620961190.pdf

17. Essed, N.H. (2009) Flavor enhancement of food as a stimulant for food intake in elderly people. doi: https://core.ac.uk/download/pdf/29249979.pdf

18. Fjaeldstad, Alexander Wieck (2024) Using Cooking Schools to Improve the Pleasure of Food and Cooking in Patients Experiencing Smell Loss. doi: https://core.ac.uk/download/613712071.pdf

19. Hatem, Samar H., Montoya, Pedro, Riquelme, Inmaculada, Sabater Gárriz, et al. (2025) A multidimensional investigation of the relationship between skin-mediated somatosensory signals, emotion regulation and behavior problems in autistic children. doi: https://core.ac.uk/download/653726945.pdf

20. Karani TF, Pillay M (2023) It's crunch time: Exploring the sensibility of food textural acoustics for individuals with dysphagia. doi: https://core.ac.uk/download/642810832.pdf

21. Manely Farhangdoust (2024) Pictorial Satisfaction: Consuming Food Porn in the Digital Age. doi: https://doi.org/10.32920/26052574.v1

22. Phillip Baker, Priscila Machado, Thiago M. Santos, Katherine Sievert, Kathryn Backholer, Michalis Hadjikakou, Cherie Russell, et al. (2020) Ultra-processed foods and the nutrition transition: Global, regional and national trends, food systems transformations and political economy drivers. Volume(21). Obesity Reviews. doi: https://doi.org/10.1111/obr.13126

23. R. Riantiningtyas, Florence Carrouel, A. Bruyas, W. Bredie, Camille Kwiecien, A. Giboreau, A. Dougkas (2023) Oral Somatosensory Alterations in Head and Neck Cancer Patients—An Overview of the Evidence and Causes. Volume(15). Cancers. doi: https://www.semanticscholar.org/paper/e9f461eee84f154048a73446812b08420b7942ad

24. Shania Pande (2022) Policy Focus: How can our understanding of physiology help us mitigate and adapt to climate change?. Physiology News. doi: https://doi.org/10.36866/pn.127.9

25. Sharon Croxford (2023) Role of food in our teaching and practice. Volume(80), 448-451. Nutrition & Dietetics. doi: https://doi.org/10.1111/1747-0080.12852

26. Silvia Scaglioni, Valentina De Cosmi, Valentina Ciappolino, Fabio Parazzini, Paolo Brambilla, Carlo Agostoni (2018) Factors Influencing Children's Eating Behaviours. Volume(10), 706-706. Nutrients. doi: https://doi.org/10.3390/nu10060706

27. Smith, S (2025) Neural and Psychological Mechanisms of Oral Sensation. doi: https://core.ac.uk/download/169433292.pdf

28. Spence, Charles (2024) The king of spices: on pepper's pungent pleasure. doi: https://core.ac.uk/download/603241292.pdf

29. Steffen Jähn, Pia Furchheim, Anna-Maria Strässner (2021) Plant-Based Meat Alternatives: Motivational Adoption Barriers and Solutions. Volume(13), 13271-13271. Sustainability. doi:

https://doi.org/10.3390/su132313271

30. Tieneke Kröger, Jacqueline Dupont, Lucy Büsing, Florian Fiebelkorn (2022) Acceptance of Insect-Based Food Products in Western Societies: A Systematic Review. Volume(8). Frontiers in Nutrition. doi: https://doi.org/10.3389/fnut.2021.759885

31. Törnwall, Outi (2013) Genetic and Environmental Influences on Chemosensory Perception and Preferences. doi: https://core.ac.uk/download/16390763.pdf

32. Victoria Dumont, Maryse Delaunay-El Allam, Nadège Roche-Labarbe (2018) Psychobiological foundations of early sensory-motor development and implications for neonatal care. Routledge eBooks. doi: https://doi.org/10.4324/9781315642765-33

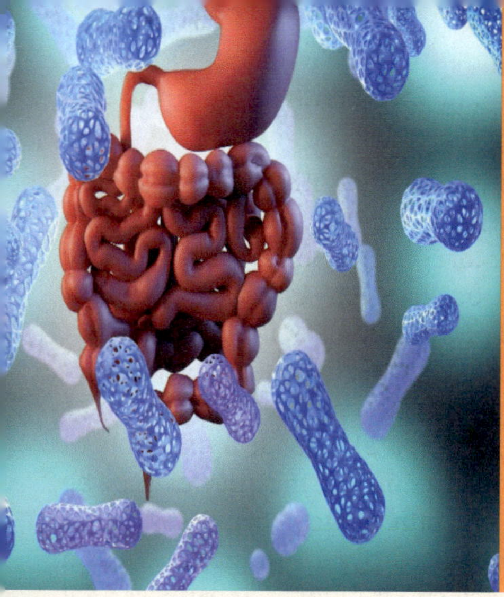

Chapter 8
AGING GUT

Contents

Introduction

The aging gut serves as a significant focus within the field of gerontology, particularly due to its implications for health and quality of life in older adults. As individuals age, various physiological changes take place in the gastrointestinal system, impacting not only digestion but also overall metabolic health. These changes may lead to a decline in gut function, which can exacerbate age-related diseases, increase susceptibility to infections, and influence the absorption of essential nutrients. Notably, studies have shown that the human colonic neuromuscular functions may decline with age, leading to altered motility patterns and increased gastrointestinal disorders. Through a comprehensive examination of how these transformations affect health outcomes, the implications of an aging gut can be better understood, paving the way for targeted interventions aimed at enhancing gut health in older populations (Ahmed et al., 2018). In light of the complexities surrounding gut health, understanding the specific physiological mechanisms in play is crucial. The functionality of the gut is closely tied to its muscular and neuronal properties, which are known to exhibit variations with aging. Research indicates that cholinergic functions, responsible for muscle contractions in the colon, weaken significantly with age, especially in the ascending colon. Furthermore, while the overall density of myenteric neurons remains stable, some specific changes can occur, such as the increase in neurons exhibiting choline acetyltransferase immunoreactivity. This phenomenon suggests that while the quantity of neurons might not decline, their functional efficacy does weaken, resulting in diminished motility and increased gastrointestinal discomfort. Exploring these intricate dynamics becomes imperative for developing strategies to counteract the negative effects of aging on gut function (Ahmed et al., 2018). Moreover, the impact of dietary influences on gut motility cannot be overlooked, especially as glucose intake has been shown to trigger specific motor responses in the gastrointestinal tract. A study examining the motor response of the antro-pyloro-duodenal region to glucose infusions illustrates how nutrient composition and delivery can regulate gastrointestinal activity. As the body ages, the response to such stimuli can alter, resulting in reduced effectiveness in regulating digestion and nutrient absorption. This insight underscores the necessity for tailored dietary recommendations that account for age-related changes within the gut. By investigating the interplay between aging and dietary factors, researchers can contribute to a better understanding of how to promote gut health and overall well-being among older adults .

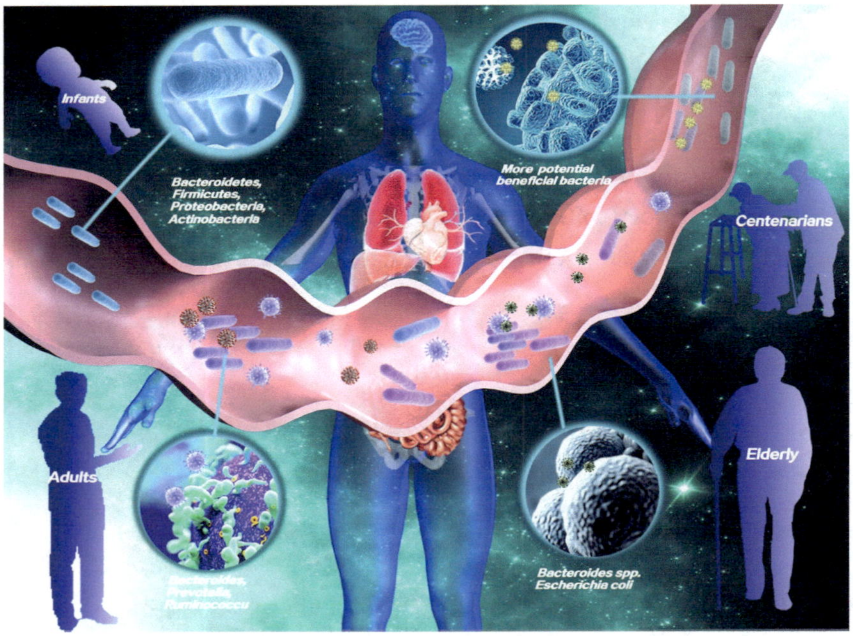

Figure 8.1. Aging Gut Microbiome in Healthy and Unhealthy Aging.

Source: https://www.aginganddisease.org/article/2024/2152-5250/148648/AD-16-2-980-g1.jpg

Definition of the aging gut

The concept of the aging gut encompasses a spectrum of physiological changes that occur within the gastrointestinal (GI) system as individuals advance in age. Notably, this aging process is not merely a byproduct of chronological aging; rather, it is characterized by various alterations, including changes in gut motility, microbial composition, and integrity of the gut barrier. As people age, the diversity and abundance of beneficial gut microbiota typically decline, contributing to a dysbiotic state that can exacerbate gastrointestinal disorders and systemic diseases. This transformation is significant as it not only affects digestion and nutrient absorption but also has broader implications for overall health, influencing metabolic processes and immunity, reflecting the critical role the gut plays in maintaining homeostasis. Thus, understanding the aging guts definition lays the groundwork for exploring interventions and lifestyle adjustments that promote gut health in older adults. Aging gut-related changes also correlate closely with numerous health complications, notably neurodegenerative disorders and chronic diseases. Emerging studies illustrate a compelling connection between gut health and neurological functions, highlighting the role of the microbiome in modulating the brain-gut axis. For instance, altered gut microbiota composition is increasingly being investigated for its involvement in conditions such as Parkinson's disease, where dysbiosis may precede or exacerbate neurological symptoms. Research suggests that an imbalance in gut bacterial populations may instigate inflammatory responses, leading to a cascade of neuroinflammatory changes. Furthermore, the bidirectional communication within the microbiota-gut-brain axis could elucidate how gut health deterioration affects cognitive and emotional well-being, reinforcing the idea that an integrated approach to health must consider gut aging dynamics as critical to preventing neurological decline and promoting longevity (Caputi et al., 2018). In addition to neurological implications, the aging gut presents significant associations with systemic health conditions, such as chronic kidney disease (CKD) and cardiovascular diseases.

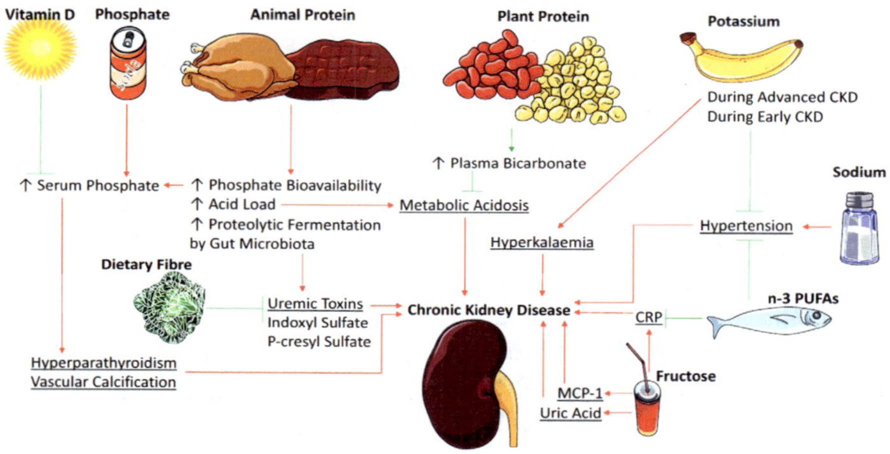

Figure 8.2. Mechanisms of dietary factors impact on chronic kidney disease..

Source: https://www.mdpi.com/nutrients/nutrients-09-00265/article_deploy/html/images/nutrients-09-00265-g001.png

The deterioration of gut health contributes to increased intestinal permeability, often termed leaky gut, which allows for the translocation of bacteria and their components into circulation. Such changes can trigger systemic inflammation, a known risk factor for both CKD and cardiovascular pathologies. Specifically, the dysregulated immune response precipitated by an unhealthy gut microbiome may aggravate renal function decline, establishing a feedback loop of deterioration. Recent research underscores the potential of targeting gut health through diet and probiotics as a means to mitigate such comorbidities. By elucidating the mechanisms linking gut aging to systemic diseases, scholars aim to foster a more nuanced understanding of how the aging gut interplays with various health conditions, opening avenues for preventive strategies tailored to the elderly population (Ekström et al., 2017).

Importance of gut health in aging

The interaction between gut health and aging is increasingly recognized as a pivotal factor in promoting longevity and mitigating age-related diseases. As individuals age, the gut microbiota undergoes significant transformations that can influence overall health. Research indicates that shifts in microbial diversity and composition may correlate with various chronic conditions prevalent among the elderly, such as obesity, diabetes, and cardiovascular disease. A well-balanced gut microbiota is essential for maintaining metabolic homeostasis, which is essential as metabolic processes tend to decline with age. Consequently, fostering a diverse gut microbiome through a healthy diet, prebiotics, and probiotics may not only enhance digestive health but also support immune function, ultimately playing a crucial role in extending healthy lifespan and improving quality of life in older adults. The ecological properties of the gut microbiota are equally vital in the context of aging. Specific microbial strains can produce metabolites beneficial for health, such as short-chain fatty acids, which possess anti-inflammatory and immune-modulating effects. These beneficial metabolites can support cognitive functions and even influence mood, which is particularly relevant given that mental health issues often escalate with age. A detailed analysis of the gut microbiota reveals that biodiversity is linked to better health outcomes in older individuals; higher biodiversity indicates resilience against gastrointestinal disorders and other age-related diseases. Notably, a study highlighted the robust correlation between gut microbiota biodiversity and healthy aging, suggesting that maintaining microbial diversity can serve as an important indicator of age-associated health, affirming the crucial role of gut health in the aging process (Bazzani A et al., 2020)(Bazzani et al., 2020). Moreover, lifestyle factors play a significant role in shaping gut health as individuals age. Nutritional habits, physical activity, and stress levels affect the gut microbiomes composition and functionality. Diets rich in fiber, fermented foods, and polyphenols can enhance gut microbial diversity, while processed foods and high sugar intake tend to diminish it. In addition, regular physical activity has been shown to positively influence gut health, leading to improved metabolic outcomes and decreased inflammation. This suggests that interventions aimed at modifying diet and exercise patterns could be effective in promoting a healthier gut microbiome, ultimately influencing health outcomes in aging individuals. As the global population ages, understanding and emphasizing the importance of gut health will be paramount in addressing the health challenges associated with aging, highlighting the ongoing need for research in this critical area of gerontology.

8.1 The Anatomy of the Gut

The anatomy of the gut plays a crucial role in the overall health and functionality of the gastrointestinal system, especially as individuals age. The gut comprises various components, including the esophagus, stomach, small intestine, and large intestine, each playing unique roles in digestion and nutrient absorption. As individuals progress through the aging process, changes in gut anatomy and physiology can profoundly affect health outcomes. For instance, the epithelial lining of the gut may become thinner, leading to a reduced ability to absorb essential nutrients. Furthermore, aging is associated with alterations in gut motility, which can increase the risk of conditions such as constipation and gastrointestinal discomfort.

Understanding these anatomical changes is vital in developing targeted interventions that can help maintain gut health throughout an individuals lifespan. In addition to structural changes, the aging gut also experiences significant shifts in its microbiome composition. The gut microbiome consists of trillions of microorganisms that contribute to digestion, immune function, and overall metabolic health. Research indicates that the diversity and abundance of beneficial bacterial species decline with age, while pathogenic organisms may proliferate, disrupting the delicate balance necessary for optimal gut function. This dysbiosis can lead to a host of issues, including inflammation, impaired immune responses, and even mental health challenges. The interplay between aging and microbiome health underscores the importance of dietary habits and lifestyle choices in promoting gut health. For example, incorporating a diet rich in prebiotics and probiotics may support microbial diversity and mitigate the adverse effects of aging on the gut. Moreover, stress plays a critical role in how the gut functions and ages. Chronic stress has been found to influence gut permeability and motility, consequently affecting the gut-brain axis. As one ages, the impact of stress on gut health may be exacerbated, leading to increased susceptibility to gastrointestinal diseases. Recent studies suggest that health care providers must bridge the gap between understanding the brains influence and its relationship with gut function. By recognizing the significance of psychosocial factors, health practitioners can better tailor interventions aimed at promoting gut health in older adults. As our comprehension of the guts anatomy and its interactions with stress deepens, it becomes evident that an integrative approach is necessary for maintaining a healthy gut throughout the aging process (Estrine J et al., 2006) (Carmody et al., 2012).

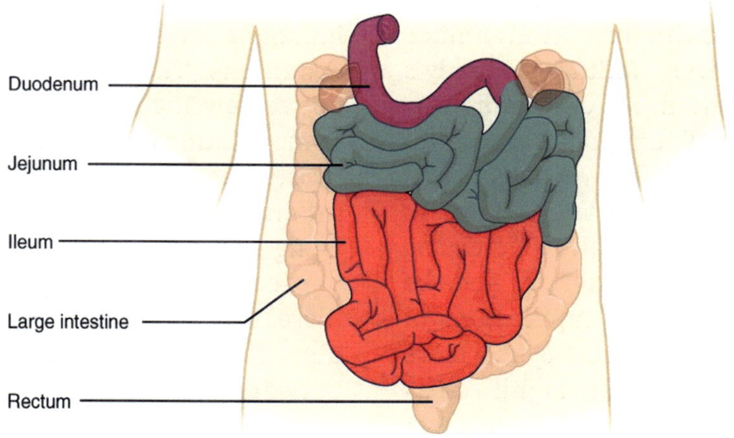

Figure 8.3. The Anatomy of the Gut.

Source: https://s3-us-west-2.amazonaws.com/courses-images-archive-read-only/wp-content/uploads/sites/403/2015/04/21031729/2417_Small_IntestineN.jpg

8.1.1 Overview of the gastrointestinal tract

The gastrointestinal tract (GIT) serves as a complex and vital system responsible for the digestion of food and the absorption of nutrients within the human body. It encompasses a series of organs, including the mouth, esophagus, stomach, small intestine, large intestine, and anus, all of which work in harmony to process ingested materials. The breakdown of food begins in the mouth, where mechanical and chemical processes initiate digestion, followed by the esophagus, which transports food to the stomach. Here, gastric acids further decompose food matter before it progresses to the small intestine, where the majority of nutrient absorption occurs. As individuals age, however, the efficiency of the GIT can wane, leading to various digestive issues that impact overall health and nutrition. As people age, significant physiological changes occur in the GIT, affecting its structural and functional characteristics. These changes may manifest as a decline in gastrointestinal motility, which refers to the coordinated contractions of the digestive tract that facilitate food movement. Additionally, there may be a reduction in the secretion of important digestive enzymes, potentially compromising the digestion and absorption processes. For instance, alterations in the intestinal walls integrity can hinder nutrient uptake, effectively limiting the body's access to essential vitamins and minerals. This deterioration in GIT function is critical to understanding the interplay between aging and nutritional health, particularly as it relates to malnutrition in older adults, a topic of increasing global concern as life expectancy rises and the population ages further. The implications of reduced GIT functionality extend beyond mere digestive discomfort; they can significantly influence the nutritional status of the elderly, thus heightening their vulnerability to various health complications. As noted in research, the aging GIT struggles to meet the nutritional demands of the body effectively, leading to a greater risk of malnutrition and associated health issues that impact multiple organ systems, including the nervous, musculoskeletal, and immune systems. Addressing this multifaceted problem requires a comprehensive commitment to developing dietary guidelines that support the unique challenges faced by the aging population. Proposed solutions must account for the functional decline of the GIT while enhancing nutrient bioavailability and optimizing dietary intake, ensuring that elderly individuals receive adequate nourishment to maintain health and well-being (Bordoni et al., 2015). Moreover, understanding the role of probiotics may play in mitigating these challenges, as they have been linked to improved gut health and reduced antibiotic use in specific populations (Connors et al., 2019).

8.1.2 Changes in gut structure with age

The aging gut undergoes significant structural changes that impact its overall functionality. As individuals age, the composition and diversity of the gut microbiota shift, leading to an imbalance that may contribute to various health issues. Research has indicated that older populations typically exhibit a higher Firmicutes to Bacteroidetes ratio, which is associated with inflammation and could exacerbate age-related conditions. These alterations in gut flora are not merely incidental; they play a pivotal role in modulating immune responses, as evidenced by studies suggesting that low-grade, chronic inflammation can develop throughout the aging process. Such inflammatory states are particularly concerning, as they are linked to increased vulnerability to neurodegenerative disorders, creating a profound connection between gut health and cognitive function in the aging population (Bauer et al., 2017). Moreover, the neuromuscular functionality of the gut diminishes with age, particularly in the ascending colon. Investigations into human colonic neuromuscular responses indicate that older adults experience a decline in cholinergic function, evidenced by the increased likelihood of muscle relaxation rather than contraction in response to electrical stimulation. These changes reflect a complex interplay between the integrity of various neuronal pathways and muscular responsiveness as age progresses. Additionally, while certain types of neurons remain stable in number, an increase in specific cholinergic neuron populations occurs, illustrating that the gut does not simply deteriorate but rather adapts in a manner that may compromise its contractile efficacy (Ahmed et al., 2018). The implications of aging on gut structure are further illustrated by changes in the blood-brain barrier and cerebral blood flow, which are intricately linked to the functionality of the gastrointestinal system. Aging is associated with impaired vascular functions, particularly impacting how the brain communicates with peripheral systems, including the gut. Studies indicate that alterations in gut microbiome diversity correlate with observed declines in cognitive function, suggesting a bi-directional relationship through the brain-gut axis. As individuals age, these interactions may exacerbate cognitive decline and overall wellbeing, emphasizing the need for a holistic understanding of aging that encompasses both gut health and neurological outcomes (Bauer et al., 2017). Enhanced knowledge of these interconnections will be vital in addressing the multifaceted health challenges that arise in older populations.

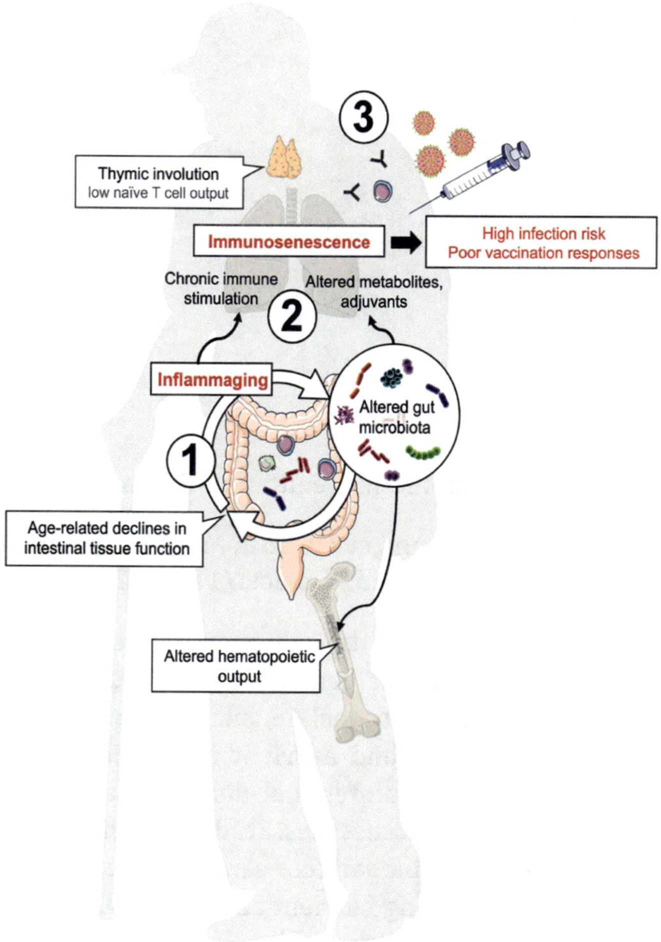

Figure 8.4. The aging gut microbiome and its impact on host immunity.

Source: https://media.springernature.com/full/springer-static/image/art%3A10.1038%2Fs41435-021-00126-8/MediaObjects/41435_2021_126_Fig1_HTML.png

8.1.3 Role of gut microbiota in digestion

The role of gut microbiota in digestion becomes increasingly significant as individuals age, particularly with the structural and functional changes observed in the aging gastrointestinal tract. As one advances in age, the efficiency of the digestive system tends to diminish, leading to a decreased ability to extract vital nutrients from food. These alterations include a decline in gastrointestinal motility and the mechanical disintegration of food. This reduced functionality not only impacts the immediate digestion process but also poses a risk for malnutrition among the elderly population, as essential nutrients may not be adequately absorbed or assimilated. Understanding the symbiotic relationship between gut microbiota and the digestive system is crucial, as these microbial communities assist in the metabolic breakdown of complex carbohydrates and proteins, ultimately enhancing nutrient bioavailability during a time when maintaining nutritional intake is paramount for health and well-being (Bordoni et al., 2015).

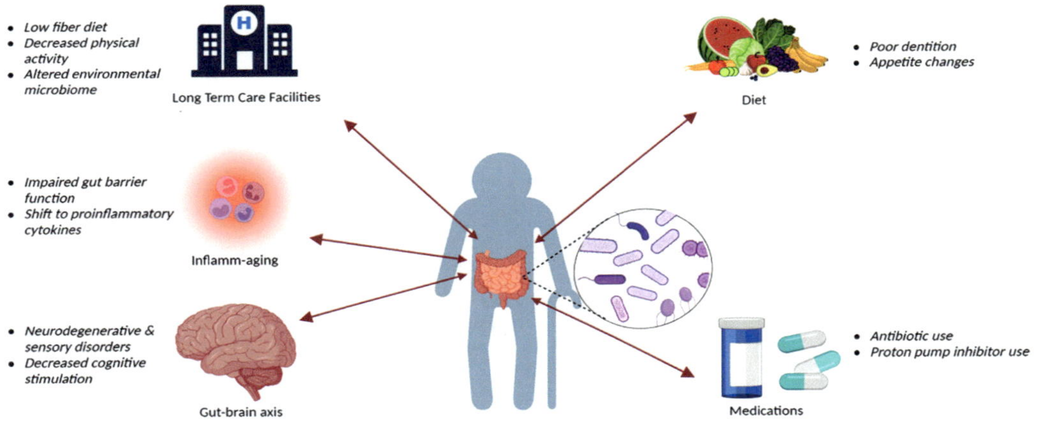

Figure 8.5. The Role of the Gut Microbiome in Health and Disease in the Elderly.

Source: https://media.springernature.com/lw1200/springer-static/image/art%3A10.1007%2Fs11894-024-00932-w/MediaObjects/11894_2024_932_Fig1_HTML.png

In addition to the structural changes in the gastrointestinal tract, the composition of gut microbiota itself is affected by aging, which can further complicate digestive processes. The diversity and abundance of beneficial bacteria tend to decline, such as Lactobacillus and Bifidobacterium species, which are pivotal in fermentation and nutrient absorption. The resultant dysbiosis can lead to an increased susceptibility to gastrointestinal disorders and impaired immune function, consequently heightening the risks of chronic diseases. Studies indicate that certain probiotic strains, like Lactobacillus delbrueckii subspecies bulgaricus, can exert beneficial effects on digestion by improving metabolic pathways and enhancing nutrient absorption. Such strains provide a promising avenue for dietary interventions that may mitigate the adverse effects of aging on gut health and overall nutrient assimilation, illustrating the indispensable role of gut microbiota in supporting digestion in older adults (Devirgiliis et al., 2017). Addressing the interplay between gut microbiota and digestion in the context of aging provides a framework for potentially effective nutritional strategies. Given the complexity of the aging gut, promoting a diverse and balanced gut microbiota through dietary means may simultaneously enhance digestion and overall health. This can include the incorporation of fermented foods that are rich in beneficial probiotic strains, as they can help restore microbial balance, optimize nutrient uptake, and alleviate some digestive dysfunctions prevalent in older adults. Moreover, understanding the unique metabolic capabilities of various probiotics can enhance their application in targeted therapies for age-related digestive issues. Addressing these factors holistically may not only counteract the deleterious effects of physical aging but also significantly improve the quality of life for the elderly population, emphasizing the crucial role that gut microbiota play in the digestive process as individuals age (Bordoni et al., 2015) (Devirgiliis et al., 2017).

8.2 The Aging Process and Gut Function

The intricate relationship between the aging process and gut function has become a focal point in contemporary geriatric research. As individuals age, a marked decline in the diversity and composition of the gut microbiome is often observed, which can significantly influence overall health outcomes. This alteration in microbial diversity is not merely a consequence of aging but rather acts as a catalyst for various physiological changes. For instance, as microbial balance shifts towards dysbiosis, this can induce chronic inflammation and oxidative stress, which are closely linked to neurodegenerative diseases. The implications of these changes extend far beyond digestive health; they are intertwined with cognitive functions and the neural underpinnings of aging. Investigations into the gut microbiomes composition reveal a critical relationship with neurological health, raising important questions about prevention and treatment strategies for age-related cognitive decline (Ru Bíz et al., 2024). Moreover, the declining functionality of the gut during the aging process is accentuated by a variety of external factors such as diet, medication, and lifestyle.

A nutrient-rich, diverse diet can potentially mitigate some of the negative effects associated with gut dysbiosis, while poor dietary choices may exacerbate microbial imbalances, leading to a vicious cycle of decline. In particular, specific phyla within the gut microbiome—such as Firmicutes and Bacteroidetes—have been associated with both healthy aging and cognitive impairments. Recent studies indicate that individuals with age-related cognitive disorders, such as Alzheimer's disease and dementia, exhibit notable differences in the relative abundance of these microbial communities compared to healthy older adults. Therefore, understanding how lifestyle factors influence gut function may provide valuable insights into strategies for promoting health in the elderly (Coradduzza D et al., 2023). The exploration of therapeutic interventions targeting the gut microbiome holds immense potential for enhancing cognitive function in aging populations. A burgeoning area of research is focused on harnessing probiotics, prebiotics, and dietary modifications to restore microbial balance and support gut health. Evidence suggests that such interventions could strengthen the gut-brain axis, thereby improving neurocognitive outcomes. Furthermore, as the role of the gut microbiome becomes increasingly recognized in the context of aging, it may also emerge as a promising biomarker for assessing cognitive decline. The link between gut health and neurodegeneration invites a reevaluation of traditional treatment approaches for age-related cognitive disorders, suggesting that integrated strategies encompassing dietary, microbial, and neurological dimensions could foster healthier aging processes (Ru Bíz et al., 2024)(Coradduzza D et al., 2023).

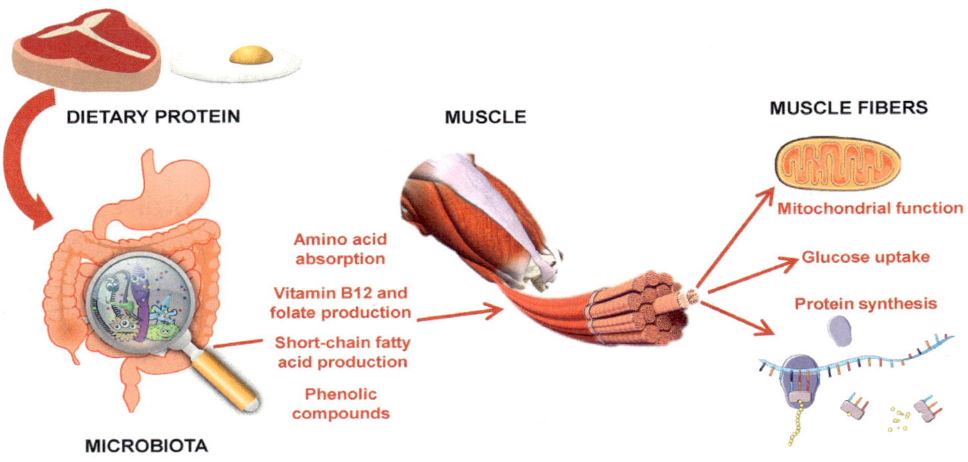

Figure 8.6. Gut Microbiota, Muscle Mass and Function in Aging.

Source: https://www.mdpi.com/nutrients/nutrients-11-01633/article_deploy/html/images/nutrients-11-01633-g001.png

8.2.1 Impact of aging on digestive enzymes

As individuals age, a significant decline in the efficacy of digestive enzymes becomes apparent, directly influencing nutrient absorption and overall gastrointestinal health. Enzymatic activity plays a crucial role in the mechanical and chemical breakdown of food, facilitating the release of essential nutrients into the bloodstream. However, age-related physiological changes in the gastrointestinal tract, such as reduced gastric acid production and altered gut motility, contribute to diminished enzymatic function. This decline can adversely affect the digestion of macronutrients, notably carbohydrates, proteins, and fats, thus impairing the bioavailability of nutrients and exacerbating malnutrition among the elderly population. Despite the critical nature of these changes, comprehensive insights into the dynamics of aging digestive enzymes remain insufficient, highlighting an urgent need for targeted research to fully understand the implications on health outcomes among aging individuals (Bordoni et al., 2015). The interplay between aging and digestive enzyme functionality not only influences nutrient absorption but also holds the potential to exacerbate inflammatory responses within the gut. With the aging process often associated with a state known as inflammaging—characterized by chronic, low-grade inflammation—an inefficient digestive system may further amplify this condition. Altered enzymatic activity can contribute to undigested food particles in the gut, promoting dysbiosis, which is a disruption of the gut microbiome. This imbalance can lead to adverse health outcomes, including increased intestinal permeability and heightened immune responses. Consequently, the elderly may experience a heightened vulnerability to digestive disorders and systemic diseases, underpinning the importance of investigating the relationships between digestive enzymes, gut health, and inflammation (Guantario B et al., 2019). Moreover, understanding the impact of aging on digestive enzymes is critical for formulating dietary interventions aimed at alleviating malnutrition risks in the elderly. Research indicates that strategic dietary changes, including incorporating easily digestible nutrients and probiotics, could enhance digestive function and restore gut homeostasis. Probiotics, in particular, have shown promise in mitigating some age-related digestive issues through mechanisms that bolster mucosal barrier integrity, enhance immunity, and modulate inflammatory responses. By integrating such findings into dietary guidelines and interventions, researchers can aid in the development of personalized nutrition strategies that account for the altered digestive capacities in aging individuals. These interventions stand to improve the quality of life for older adults and mitigate the health risks associated with malnutrition and digestive decline (Bordoni et al., 2015).

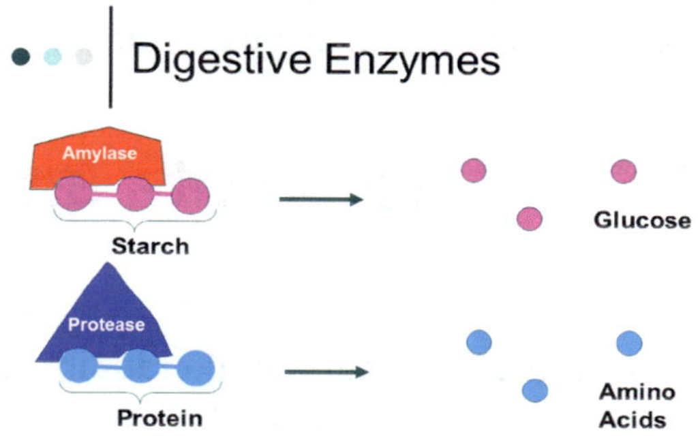

Figure 8.7. Digestive Enzymes.

Source: https://www.sliderbase.com/images/referats/953b/(29).PNG

8.2.2 Changes in gut motility

As the human body ages, the gastrointestinal (GI) system undergoes significant changes that manifest as alterations in gut motility. These changes are integral to the overall function of the gut and play a critical role in digestion and nutrient absorption. In particular, the propulsion of food throughout the digestive tract slows down, leading to an increased risk of gastrointestinal disorders such as constipation and diverticulosis. Research has shown that the frequency of various motor responses in the gut decreases with age. The frequency of pressure waves in the antrum and pylorus, essential components of the digestive process, becomes less frequent, which can compromise the efficiency of food breakdown and transit through the GI tract. Such motor dysfunction not only affects digestion but also reduces the bioavailability of nutrients essential for health in older adults. Moreover, specific changes in gut motility have been linked to the physiological responses triggered by food intake. For instance, studies indicate that glucose infusion can significantly alter gastric motility patterns. Intraduodenal glucose infusions have been shown to increase isolated pyloric pressure waves (IPPWs) and pyloric tone, illustrating these responses dose-dependent nature. However, as people age, the hierarchical motor responses at the pylorus and other regions of the gastrointestinal tract may weaken, leading to inadequate responses to dietary changes. This diminished sensitivity to nutrient stimuli underscores the importance of understanding gut motility in aging, as it directly impacts the aging populations capacity to ingest and process vital nutrients effectively, ultimately influencing their overall health status (Besanko et al., 2013). The implications of these motility changes extend beyond mere digestive efficiency; they are closely entwined with nutritional outcomes and, consequently, health risks. The aging of the gastrointestinal tract contributes to increased susceptibility to malnutrition, which can lead to various comorbidities affecting multiple organ systems, including the skeletal and immune systems. Reduced gut motility diminishes the ability to digest and absorb nutrients, thus compounding the risks associated with age-related malnutrition. Research indicates that the mechanical and biochemical processes of the aging gastrointestinal system progressively lose effectiveness, further complicating nutrient absorption and, ultimately, health. Addressing gut motility in the elderly is increasingly vital, as it entails not only dietary adaptations to meet these biological changes but also the necessity for health systems to implement guidelines catering to the nutritional needs of the aging population (Bordoni et al., 2015).

8.2.3 Effects of aging on nutrient absorption

As individuals age, significant physiological changes occur within the gastrointestinal tract that adversely affect nutrient absorption. The mechanical processes involved in food breakdown, including chewing and swallowing, often decline with age, resulting in less effective digestion. Moreover, alterations in gastrointestinal motility can lead to slower transit times through the digestive system, which may hinder the absorption of essential nutrients. These changes in motility, combined with a decrease in secretory functions of the digestive enzymes, can substantially affect the bodys ability to extract and utilize nutrients from food. Consequently, the aging gut struggles to meet the nutritional needs of the elderly, contributing to poorer overall health and increased susceptibility to malnutrition and related health risks. Additionally, the integrity and function of the intestinal wall play a crucial role in nutrient absorption, and aging can compromise this aspect significantly. Changes in the structure of the intestinal mucosa, such as reduced surface area and altered permeability, contribute to decreased nutrient bioavailability. This degradation of the mucosal barrier not only exacerbates nutrient absorption issues but also increases the risk of inflammation and other gastrointestinal disorders. Furthermore, this compromised barrier function can facilitate the entry of harmful pathogens, increasing the potential for infections and gastrointestinal disturbances. Notably, the consequences of these changes extend beyond the gut itself, as malnutrition in the elderly can lead to a myriad of complications affecting multiple organ systems, further entrenching the cycle of decline associated with aging (Bordoni et al., 2015). Addressing the challenges associated with nutrient absorption in the aging population requires a multifaceted approach. It is essential to consider dietary interventions tailored to the unique needs of older adults, focusing on enhancing nutrient bioavailability and ensuring adequate dietary intake. Furthermore, research initiatives should emphasize identifying biomarkers linked to food intake and nutrient absorption to create effective dietary guidelines. With funding for relevant research, such as the pilot RCT on the management of iron deficiency anemia among older individuals (Donaldson et al., 2018), it becomes increasingly feasible to combat malnutrition through targeted dietary strategies. By understanding the dynamics of the aging gut and its influence on nutrient absorption, healthcare professionals can better support the nutritional health of the elderly, ultimately improving their quality of life.

8.3 Gut Microbiota and Aging

As individuals age, significant alterations occur not only in bodily systems but also in the composition and function of gut microbiota. The decline in microbial diversity is a critical component of these changes, leading to a precarious balance in the gut ecosystem. This imbalance can predispose the elderly to various gastrointestinal disorders, which are notably prevalent in this demographic. Specifically, gastrointestinal disorders, including chronic constipation, faecal impaction and incontinence, are a major cause of morbidity in the elderly (Colyer et al., 2013). The degradation of beneficial bacteria, alongside an increase in pathogenic strains, signifies an urgent need to understand how aging affects gut health. Research into the microbiotas role reveals that maintaining a diverse microbial population is crucial for gastrointestinal health, which directly correlates with overall well-being in older adults. Moreover, the functional alterations in gut microbiota extend beyond digestive implications, significantly influencing metabolic processes and immune responses. As gut bacteria play a vital role in shaping the host's immune system, an aging population often experiences diminished immunity alongside altered microbiota composition. This shift not only heightens the risk of infections but may also exacerbate chronic health conditions prevalent in older adults. Incontinence and sexual dysfunction are often increased in the aged human population. In rats and mice, the pattern of micturition and faecal clearance also changes with ageing and is suggestive of bladder and bowel dysfunction (Black et al., 2013). A better understanding of these interconnected systems highlights the necessity for targeted interventions that could restore microbial balance and improve physiological function, thereby enhancing the quality of life for older individuals. Interventions aimed at modifying gut microbiota are gaining traction as potential solutions to some of the challenges posed by aging. Dietary changes, prebiotics, and probiotics have shown promise in restoring gut health, thus offering a pathway toward improved health outcomes.

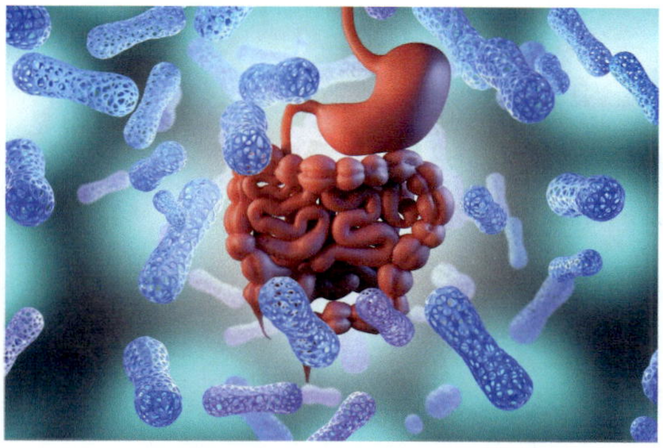

Figure 8.8. Younger gut microbiota age reduces cardiovascular disease risk in older adults.

Source: https://www.news-medical.net/images/news/ImageForNews_782785_1718338614640129.jpg

The adoption of plant-based diets rich in fiber can lead to increased microbial diversity, supporting a more resilient gut ecosystem. Additionally, probiotic supplementation has been indicated as a beneficial strategy to counteract age-related declines in microbial diversity. As research progresses, it emphasizes the significance of personalized nutrition and microbiome-targeted therapies in addressing age-specific health issues. By focusing on the role of gut microbiota in the aging process, we can harness these strategies to mitigate the onset of gastrointestinal disorders, foster better immunity, and ultimately enhance the aging experience.

8.3.1 Composition of gut microbiota in older adults

The composition of gut microbiota in older adults is a subject of growing importance in the realm of health science, as alterations in these microbial communities are intricately linked to the aging process. As individuals age, research indicates a shift toward a less diverse microbiota, often characterized by increased levels of specific pathogenic bacteria and diminished populations of beneficial microbes. This dysbiosis can lead to various health issues, including increased inflammation, metabolic disorders, and cognitive decline. Understanding the unique factors that influence gut microbiota in older adults is crucial for developing strategies to mitigate these changes and promote healthy aging. The possibility of reversing age-related dysbiosis through lifestyle interventions, such as diet and physical activity, shows great promise in restoring balance within the microbiome and enhancing overall health outcomes for the elderly population. Engaging in regular physical activity has emerged as one of the promising strategies to positively influence gut microbiota in older adults. Recent studies have shown that individuals adhering to the World Health Organizations physical activity recommendations exhibit a higher abundance of beneficial bacterial taxa, such as Lactobacillus and F. prausnitzii. These microbes are known to contribute to gut health and overall well-being.

Conversely, those who are sedentary display higher levels of disease-associated bacteria, like D.piger and Enterobacterales. These findings underscore the potent role of physical activity in shaping gut microbiota composition, suggesting that an active lifestyle may indeed serve as a means to promote not only microbial diversity but also the health of older adults. Therefore, encouraging physical activity among aging populations should be a fundamental component of strategies aimed at enhancing microbiome health. The intricate relationship between gut microbiota and sleep quality in older adults is another critical area of research that reveals significant connections impacting health. Aging is frequently associated with sleep disturbances that can exacerbate health problems and contribute to psychological stress. Studies exploring the bidirectional relationship between sleep and gut microbiota have indicated that microbial diversity is linked to sleep quality, with higher gut microbiota richness correlating positively with improved objective sleep measures. Specific bacterial taxa, such as Ruminococcus and Veillonella, have been tentatively associated with healthier sleep patterns. These findings emphasize the need for further investigation into the mechanisms connecting gut health and sleep, particularly as both domains play vital roles in the cognitive and emotional functioning of older adults. Such research could inform clinical interventions aimed at enhancing both sleep quality and microbiome health, ultimately fostering better aging experiences for the elderly population.

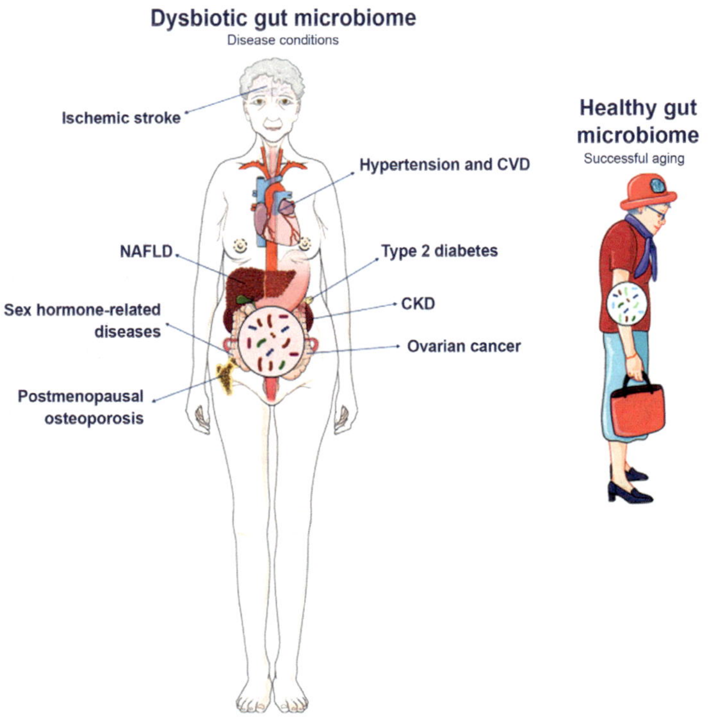

Figure 8.9. Aging and Gut Dysbiosis.

Source: https://media.springernature.com/lw685/springer-static/image/chp%3A10.1007%2F978-3-031-35064-1_16/MediaObjects/484868_1_En_16_Fig1_HTML.png

8.3.2 Effects of diet on gut microbiota diversity

The gut microbiota serves as a critical component of human health, especially as individuals age. The diversity of microbial populations within the gastrointestinal tract is profoundly influenced by dietary choices, which can dictate not only the composition of gut microbiota but also its functionality. Research has established a correlation between dietary patterns and microbiota diversity, indicating that specific diets can promote a flourishing microbial community. In particular, diets rich in fibers—found in fruits, vegetables, and whole grains—support the growth of beneficial bacteria, thus enhancing microbial diversity. Additionally, these dietary fibers serve as prebiotics, fueling the growth of beneficial strains while inhibiting pathogenic species. Consequently, an enriched microbiota diversity is essential in fostering immune health and metabolic balance, particularly important for aging populations in mitigating age-related disorders. The effects of high-fat diets (HFD) on gut microbiota diversity further illuminate the detrimental impacts of diet on microbial health as individuals age. Studies have shown that HFD can lead to a significant reduction in microbial diversity, as evidenced by changes in gut composition due to the dominance of specific bacterial phyla like Firmicutes. For instance, a comparative analysis of mice subjected to HFD indicated not only a decrease in beneficial gut bacteria but also disruptions in bone metabolic markers and increased inflammation (Qiao Y et al., 2025). Such alterations may contribute to the development of conditions like osteoporosis, emphasizing the multifactorial nature of dietary impacts on gut health. Furthermore, the implications extend beyond localized gut effects, suggesting that imbalances in microbial diversity could transform metabolic and inflammatory pathways that influence systemic health in aging individuals. Conversely, low-protein diets (LP) present a fascinating alternative with beneficial implications for gut microbiota and overall health. Research indicates that LP diets can augment species diversity by promoting the growth of taxa such as Verrucomicrobiota, which are associated with improved glucose homeostasis and enhanced immune responses (Vaddi P et al., 2024). The interaction between dietary protein levels and gut microbiota has been scrutinized, revealing that an LP diet can lead to changes in microbiome composition that confer metabolic advantages for aging populations. Notably, the shifts in microbial diversity resulting from LP diets correlate positively with metabolic health outcomes, such as improved glucose tolerance and regulation of inflammatory pathways. Thus, considerations of dietary composition become imperative in the context of aging, advocating for mindful dietary interventions that enhance gut microbiota diversity and promote better health outcomes among the elderly.

8.3.3 Relationship between gut microbiota and immune function

The relationship between gut microbiota and immune function is critical, especially as individuals age. The gut houses trillions of microorganisms, which play a pivotal role in the modulation of immune responses. As the gut microbiota composition shifts due to factors such as diet, lifestyle, and aging itself, there can be significant implications for immune health. Dysbiosis, or an imbalanced gut microbiome, can lead to systemic inflammation and a higher risk of autoimmune diseases and infections in older adults. Moreover, studies suggest that lifestyle modifications, such as increased physical activity and dietary adjustments, can enhance microbial diversity and functionality, thus bolstering immune function. This interplay demonstrates that a proactive approach towards maintaining a healthy gut microbiome can serve as a protective factor against age-related immune decline, emphasizing the importance of tailored interventions in promoting health during aging (Kruger K et al., 2021). Understanding the mechanisms behind gut microbiotas influence on the immune system is essential for developing therapeutic strategies for age-related illnesses. The gut microbiome contributes to immune regulation through interactions with various immune cells and mediators. For instance, gut-derived metabolites like short-chain fatty acids (SCFAs) play a crucial role in maintaining intestinal barrier integrity and modulating systemic inflammation.

These metabolites enhance the production of regulatory T cells, which help prevent exaggerated immune responses. Conversely, dysregulated immune pathways can arise from gut dysbiosis, leading to increased susceptibility to infections and chronic diseases among the elderly. The intricate balance between the microbiota and the host immune system is further complicated by the bi-directional communication between the gut and central nervous system, reinforcing the need for a holistic understanding of this relationship in the context of aging (Caputi et al., 2018). Furthermore, the exploration of dietary influences sheds light on the potential for targeted interventions. Specific nutrients, including dietary fiber, polyphenols, and polyunsaturated fatty acids, have shown promising effects on gut microbiota composition and diversity. This, in turn, can strengthen immune responses and mitigate chronic inflammation that often accompanies aging. Adequate protein and energy intake are also essential to support muscle mass and immune function, highlighting nutritional choices as key players in maintaining health in older adults. Regular exercise has been found to positively affect the gut microbiome, enhancing its biodiversity and functionality, while also promoting immune health. Collectively, these findings suggest that optimizing diet and lifestyle can enhance gut microbiota diversity, fostering a more robust immune system and potentially mitigating some adverse effects of aging (Kruger K et al., 2021).

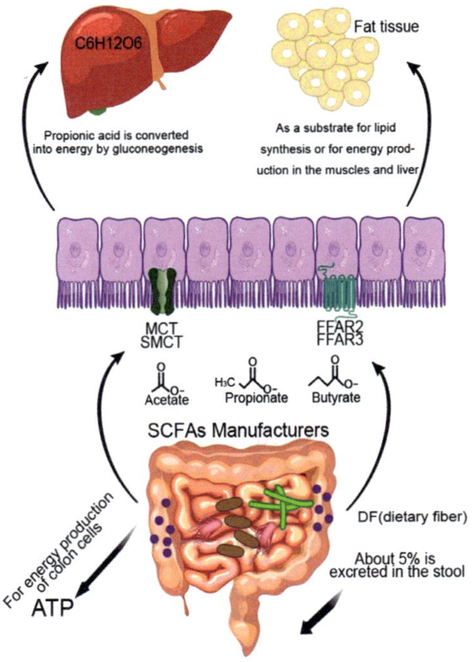

Figure 8.10. Gut microbiota-derived short chain fatty acids act as mediators of the gut-liver-brain axis.

Source: https://media.springernature.com/lw685/springer-static/image/art%3A10.1007%2Fs11011-025-01554-5/MediaObjects/11011_2025_1554_Fig1_HTML.jpg

8.4 Common Gut Disorders in the Elderly

As individuals age, the gastrointestinal system undergoes significant changes that often lead to common gut disorders, notably chronic constipation. This condition emerges as a prevalent issue in the elderly, attributed to various factors, including decreased gastrointestinal motility and dietary changes. The aging guts reduced efficiency in processing food contributes not only to constipation but also elevates the risk of fecal impaction, making it a major cause of morbidity in this population

(Colyer et al., 2013). Additionally, the use of certain medications commonly prescribed for age-related ailments can exacerbate constipation, complicating the health issues many elderly individuals face. Understanding the multifaceted nature of this disorder is critical for developing effective management strategies that can help mitigate its impact on quality of life. Another prevalent issue among the elderly is fecal incontinence, which profoundly affects emotional and physical well-being. The decline in muscle tone and changes in the nervous system can disrupt the complex processes of bowel regulation, leading to involuntary loss of stool. As elderly individuals experience this condition, social stigmas and personal embarrassment can lead to increased isolation and decreased participation in daily activities (Black et al., 2013). Moreover, the impact of fecal incontinence is not solely physical; it often results in psychological distress, emphasizing the need for comprehensive care that addresses both the physical and emotional facets of this disorder. Early identification and intervention remain crucial in managing fecal incontinence effectively, ensuring that affected individuals receive the necessary support and resources. In addition to constipation and fecal incontinence, gastrointestinal disorders such as gastroesophageal reflux disease (GERD) are increasingly common in the elderly population. The aging process may result in changes to the esophageal lining, reduced salivary production, and decreased lower esophageal sphincter function, contributing to the onset and severity of GERD symptoms. This condition can lead to significant discomfort and disrupt the eating habits of older adults, often resulting in a reduced quality of life as they navigate dietary restrictions and seek relief from persistent symptoms. Compounding these issues, the interaction of GERD with existing medications can further complicate treatment regimens. Thus, a holistic approach that encompasses thorough evaluation, dietary changes, and medication management is essential in addressing the complexities of gut disorders in the aging population.

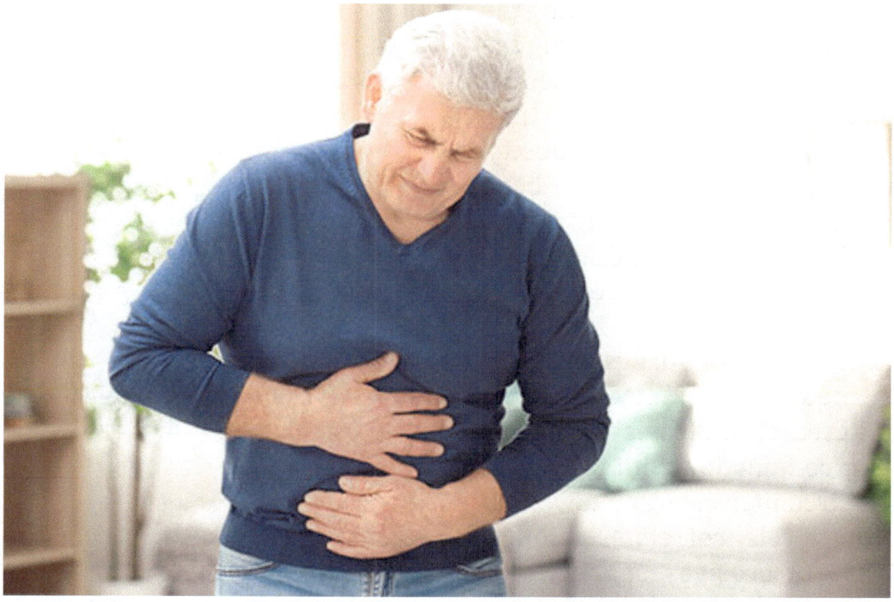

Figure 8.11. Importance of Digestive Health for the Elderly.

Source: https://seniorstridehomecare.com/wp-content/uploads/2018/04/Senior-Male-with-Stomach-Ache.jpg

8.4.1 Gastroesophageal reflux disease (GERD)

As individuals age, various physiological changes can predispose them to gastrointestinal disorders, with gastroesophageal reflux disease (GERD) being a prevalent concern among the elderly population. This condition is characterized by the backward flow of stomach contents into the esophagus, leading to symptoms such as heartburn and regurgitation. The increasing prevalence of GERD among older adults is attributed to several factors, including weakened esophageal sphincter function and changes in esophageal motility. Furthermore, age-related anatomical alterations, such as kyphosis—an exaggerated spinal curvature—can exacerbate GERD symptoms due to altered pressure dynamics in the abdomen. Individuals with spinal deformities may experience changes in posture that affect the alignment of the gastrointestinal tract, thereby influencing reflux episodes (Hirano K et al., 2012). Overall, the interplay between aging and the anatomical changes it brings is critical for understanding the incidence of GERD in the elderly. Identifying the risk factors for GERD in older adults is essential for effective management and intervention. Specific lifestyle habits, such as obesity, smoking, and alcohol consumption, have been documented as significant contributors to the development of GERD symptoms. Additionally, the use of certain medications commonly prescribed in older populations, including nonsteroidal anti-inflammatory drugs (NSAIDs) and other oral medications, may intensify GERDs severity. Research indicates that older age, particularly in conjunction with high body mass index, waist circumference, and low high-density lipoprotein levels, correlates strongly with the incidence of erosive esophagitis, a complication of GERD (Chan et al., 2015). This comprehensive understanding of risk factors is vital for healthcare professionals aiming to mitigate GERD complications in elderly patients who may already be dealing with multiple comorbidities. Lastly, effective management strategies for GERD in the aging population must prioritize a multifaceted approach, incorporating lifestyle modifications, dietary changes, and pharmacological interventions tailored to the individual's health status. Clinicians should encourage patients to adopt behaviors that can mitigate symptoms, such as avoiding lying down immediately after meals, reducing portion sizes, and steering clear of trigger foods known to exacerbate reflux. Additionally, the integration of non-invasive risk assessment models can aid in stratifying patients based on their susceptibility to complications like erosive esophagitis (Chan et al., 2015). By understanding the complex relationship between aging and GERD, healthcare providers can develop more effective therapeutic protocols that improve the quality of life for older adults and address the unique challenges presented by this condition.

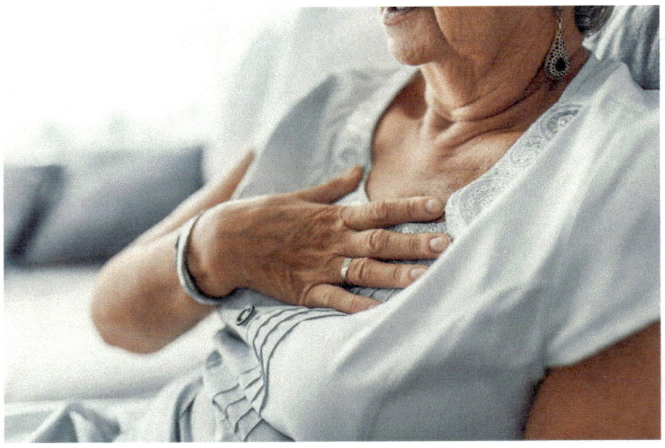

Figure 8.12. GERD and the Elderly Patient.

Source: https://www.gastroenterologyadvisor.com/wp-content/uploads/sites/23/2020/01/chest-pain_SH_1131953909.jpg

8.4.2 Constipation and its prevalence in older adults

Constipation is a prevalent condition among older adults, significantly impacting their quality of life and overall health. The aging process contributes to functional decline within the gastrointestinal tract (GIT), leading to various changes that predispose older individuals to constipation. Reduced gastrointestinal motility, slower transit times, and alterations in the mechanical and chemical digestion of food play crucial roles in this phenomenon. Additionally, the aging gut is often characterized by a diminished capacity to absorb nutrients effectively, further complicating dietary intake and health status—factors that also correlate with the onset of constipation. Understanding these changes in the GIT is vital for addressing the increasing rates of constipation in older adults, as they face not only physical limitations but also psychological and social challenges that can exacerbate their gastrointestinal issues (Bordoni et al., 2015). The relationship between constipation and the aging gut goes beyond mere physical manifestations, encompassing a broader spectrum of health implications. As older adults encounter changes in their neural functions, particularly in the colon, the regulation of bowel movements can become significantly impaired. Studies have shown that with advancing age, the neuromuscular functions in the colon decline, resulting in less effective peristaltic contractions that facilitate bowel evacuation. Specifically, the aging process affects cholinergic functions in the ascending colon, leading to diminished contractile response, which contributes to constipation (Ahmed et al., 2018). This aspect of aging reveals the intricate connection between neurological health and gastrointestinal functionality, highlighting a critical consideration for healthcare providers in managing constipation among elderly patients. Addressing constipation in older adults requires a multifaceted approach that considers their unique physiological and psychological needs. Interventions may include dietary modifications, such as increasing fiber intake and hydration, as well as incorporating regular physical activity tailored to individual capabilities. Additionally, healthcare professionals must prioritize education about the importance of bowel health and the potential complications of untreated constipation, such as fecal impaction or hospitalization. Moreover, screening for underlying medical conditions or medication side effects that could exacerbate constipation is essential for effective management. By adopting a comprehensive strategy that acknowledges the complexities of the aging gut, healthcare systems can significantly enhance the quality of life for older adults grappling with constipation while reducing the associated healthcare burdens (Bordoni et al., 2015).

8.4.3 Inflammatory bowel diseases (IBD) and aging

As individuals age, the risk of developing various health conditions increases, particularly inflammatory bowel diseases (IBD) such as Crohns disease and ulcerative colitis. The interplay between aging and gut health is complex, especially given the aging populations distinctive microbial composition changes. Research indicates that elderly individuals commonly exhibit dysbiosis, a microbial imbalance in the gut, leading to impaired immune function when compared to their younger counterparts. This dysbiosis not only heightens the susceptibility to gastrointestinal disorders but also complicates existing conditions like IBD, exacerbating symptoms and disease severity. With the World Health Organization projecting a significant increase in the global elderly population, a deeper understanding of age-related changes in gut microbiota is essential for managing IBD within this demographic (Agrawal et al., 2016). In addition to alterations in microbial composition, the effects of aging on the immune system contribute significantly to the pathophysiology of IBD. Increased cellular senescence—a hallmark of the aging process—leads to chronic low-grade inflammation, further complicating the clinical picture of IBD. The inflammatory status of the elderly can be exacerbated by lifestyle factors, including dietary habits that promote inflammation, such as high-fat diets. Notably, evidence suggests that elevated fat intakes not only exert negative influences on microbial ecosystems but also compromise immune responses. As the prevalence of IBD rises among aged individuals, identifying dietary patterns that exacerbate or alleviate inflammation is crucial for developing effective management strategies tailored to this population (Leite JSM et al., 2016). Addressing the challenges of IBD in the elderly necessitates a multifaceted approach, incorporating both lifestyle modifications and innovative therapeutic interventions. Probiotics and prebiotics have emerged as potential adjunct therapies, demonstrating a capacity to positively influence gut microbiota composition and enhance immune function in older adults. The utilization of these dietary supplements can help mitigate the detrimental effects of dysbiosis and provide an avenue for managing IBD-associated symptoms. Furthermore, promoting physical activity plays a crucial role in modulating inflammatory responses through the upregulation of heat shock proteins that foster gut health. As research into the aging gut continues to evolve, a comprehensive understanding of IBDs mechanisms in the context of aging will undoubtedly inform future clinical practices aimed at improving health outcomes for the elderly (Agrawal et al., 2016).

8.5 Lifestyle Factors Affecting Gut Health

Lifestyle factors play a pivotal role in maintaining gut health, particularly as individuals age. Diet is arguably the most influential aspect; a diet rich in fiber, fruits, and vegetables promotes a diverse gut microbiome, which is essential for optimal digestive function. Conversely, the consumption of processed foods, high sugar, and unhealthy fats can disrupt microbial balance, contributing to conditions such as dysbiosis, which has been linked to inflammation and a range of chronic diseases. Understanding the impact of dietary choices can help older adults make informed decisions that support their gut health. As the aging process progresses, the guts capacity to adapt to dietary changes may diminish, emphasizing the importance of early intervention in diet-related gut health maintenance and prevention of associated disorders. Physical activity is another crucial lifestyle factor influencing gut health in the aging population. Regular exercise not only improves overall physical health but also positively impacts gut motility and microbiota composition. Studies indicate that engaging in moderate levels of physical activity can enhance microbial diversity and reduce the risk of gastrointestinal disorders.

This is particularly important for older adults, who often experience decreased mobility and changes in gut function. Encouraging regular exercise can mitigate some age-related declines in gut health by promoting better circulation and nutrient absorption. Furthermore, the psychological benefits of physical activity, such as improved mood and reduced anxiety, can contribute to a healthier gut-brain axis, further enhancing gut health in the aging demographic. Additionally, psychosocial factors such as stress and social engagement significantly affect gut health in older adults. Chronic stress can lead to gastrointestinal disturbances, including altered gut permeability and changes in microbial populations, which may exacerbate conditions like irritable bowel syndrome. Cultivating social connections and participating in community activities can buffer against stress, fostering a healthier gut environment. Moreover, mental health considerations linked to lifestyle choices underscore the need for a holistic approach to gut health in the aging population. By emphasizing a lifestyle that incorporates diet, physical activity, and social engagement, interventions can be tailored to improve gut health and overall well-being as individuals age. The intersection of these factors reflects a comprehensive understanding necessary for promoting gut health longevity in older adults.

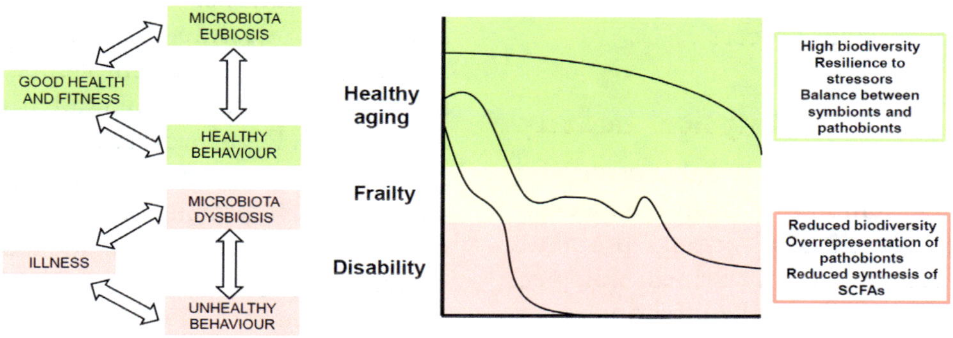

Figure 8.13. The Effects of Lifestyle and Diet on Gut Microbiota Composition.

Source: https://www.mdpi.com/nutrients/nutrients-13-02045/article_deploy/html/images/nutrients-13-02045-g001.png

8.5.1 The role of diet in maintaining gut health

The relationship between diet and gut health is pivotal, especially for aging populations seeking to maintain their well-being. A well-balanced diet directly influences the composition and diversity of gut microbiota, which are crucial for digestive health. For older adults, incorporating dietary strategies such as the Mediterranean Diet may provide substantial benefits. This diet, rich in fruits, vegetables, whole grains, and healthy fats, has garnered attention for its potential to support cardiovascular health and longevity. Many older individuals perceive the Mediterranean Diet as a pleasant way to enjoy food while simultaneously adapting to nutritional needs that can mitigate the impact of aging. However, challenges related to accessibility and cultural acceptance often arise, emphasizing the need for tailored dietary recommendations that resonate with older adults lifestyles, preferences, and sociocultural backgrounds (Tierney A et al., 2023). Moreover, the significance of probiotics and fiber in maintaining gut health cannot be overstated, particularly for the elderly. In qualitative studies, older adults have expressed their belief that live yogurt and probiotics play essential roles in fostering a healthy gut environment, linking gut health to broader aspects like cognitive function and digestive wellness. This understanding showcases an emerging awareness of the guts integral connection to overall health, as well as the potential for probiotics to support a balanced microbiome. Despite considerable advancements in scientific communication about the gut microbiotas effects on health, many older adults remain unaware of specific links between dietary choices and microbiome maintenance. Therefore, educating this demographic about the importance of fiber and probiotic-rich foods as part of their daily diet is paramount for promoting better gut health and, consequently, a healthier aging process (Tierney A et al., 2023). Additionally, it is essential to recognize that stress can adversely impact gut health, which is particularly relevant for older individuals facing various life challenges. Research has shown that the brain and gut communicate extensively, and stress can disrupt this relationship, leading to adverse health outcomes. The concept of a gut-brain axis suggests that mental health can influence physical health, underscoring the importance of a holistic approach to diet and well-being. With evidence indicating that dietary choices can mitigate stress-related gut issues, it becomes clear that mental and emotional well-being cannot be separated from physical health. Encouraging older adults to pursue nutrient-rich diets can foster resilience not only in their physical health but also in their psychological well-being, ultimately contributing to a more robust aging process .

8.5.2 Importance of physical activity

Engaging in regular physical activity is paramount for maintaining health, especially as individuals age. Physical activity promotes the efficient functioning of various biological systems, including the gastrointestinal tract (GIT). Research indicates that exercise can enhance gut motility, thereby facilitating digestion and nutrient absorption. This enhancement is particularly crucial for older adults, whose digestive systems may become less efficient due to aging and related physiological changes. By promoting a more dynamic GIT environment, physical activity can address some of the declines associated with aging, ensuring that nutrients are effectively processed. Consequently, maintaining an active lifestyle serves as a protective factor against malnutrition, which has been increasingly recognized as a pressing issue in geriatric health. Moreover, physical activity exerts a profound influence on mental health, which is intrinsically linked to physical well-being. Aging individuals often face psychological stress that can adversely affect their overall health, including their digestive health. While stress is known to affect bodily functions, including the GIT, regular exercise has been shown to mitigate these adverse effects by promoting mood stabilization and reducing anxiety. This interplay between mental and physical health underscores the holistic benefits of physical activity. By effectively managing stress and anxiety, older adults can promote better gut health, thereby tackling the interconnected dilemmas presented by aging, psychological factors, and nutritional intake. An active lifestyle consequently supports the brain-gut axis, facilitating optimal functioning across systems vital for older individuals. Finally, the relationship between physical activity and nutrition underscores the necessity for comprehensive wellness approaches in aging populations. As the GIT experiences age-related decline, the ability to digest and absorb essential nutrients diminishes, increasing the risk of malnutrition (Bordoni et al., 2015). Regular exercise can play a crucial role in alleviating these issues by stimulating appetite and improving the metabolic processes required for nutrient assimilation. Consequently, structured physical activity programs should be integrated into dietary guidelines aimed at older adults, reinforced by the understanding of their GIT functionality (Bordoni et al., 2015). By emphasizing the synergistic effects of nutrition and exercise, healthcare providers can offer more tailored, effective strategies that promote lasting health benefits, ultimately mitigating the risks associated with aging populations. Such integrated approaches are vital in fostering a healthier future for older adults, addressing both physical and nutritional needs in tandem.

8.5.3 Impact of stress and mental health on gut function

The intricate relationship between stress, mental health, and gut function is increasingly recognized as a critical area of study, particularly in the context of an aging gut. Stress activates the hypothalamic-pituitary-adrenal (HPA) axis, leading to increased cortisol production, which can disrupt the gut microbiomes delicate balance. This dysbiosis may result in gastrointestinal disturbances, including altered motility and increased intestinal permeability. Consequently, such changes can exacerbate feelings of anxiety and depression, creating a vicious cycle where mental health issues lead to further gut dysfunction and vice versa. As individuals age, their resilience to stress often decreases, making them more susceptible to these adverse effects on gut health. Understanding this dynamic interaction emphasizes the need for holistic health approaches that consider both psychological and gastrointestinal factors to promote better health outcomes for the aging population (Estrine J et al., 2006). Moreover, the gut-brain axis serves as the communication pathway between mental health and gut function, highlighting the bidirectional influence between these systems. Stress-induced alterations in the gut microbiota can produce metabolites that influence neurochemical signaling and inflammation, thus affecting mood and cognitive performance. This interaction is particularly significant in older adults, as the aging population frequently experiences heightened levels of stress—be it from physical health declines, loss of independence, or social isolation. Such stressors can exacerbate or potentially lead to the emergence of neurodegenerative conditions, including Parkinsons disease (PD), where gastrointestinal symptoms frequently appear before neurological deficits manifest. Evidence suggests that disturbances in the gut microbiota may initiate or contribute to the progression of PD by influencing inflammation and immune responses within the gut (Caputi et al., 2018). Considering the substantial implications of stress and mental health on gut function, it becomes essential to implement comprehensive management strategies that address both components. Interventions should incorporate stress-reduction techniques, such as mindfulness and cognitive-behavioral therapy, alongside dietary and lifestyle modifications aimed at nurturing a healthy gut microbiome. For instance, promoting the intake of probiotic-rich foods can enhance gut health, while stress-reduction practices can improve overall mental well-being. As research continues to explore the nuanced interactions between stress, mental health, and the aging gut, it is crucial for healthcare practitioners to adopt a more integrated approach in care, recognizing that the mind and gut function collectively influence health outcomes. This highlights the importance of a multi-faceted perspective in addressing the health challenges faced by an aging population (Estrine J et al., 2006).

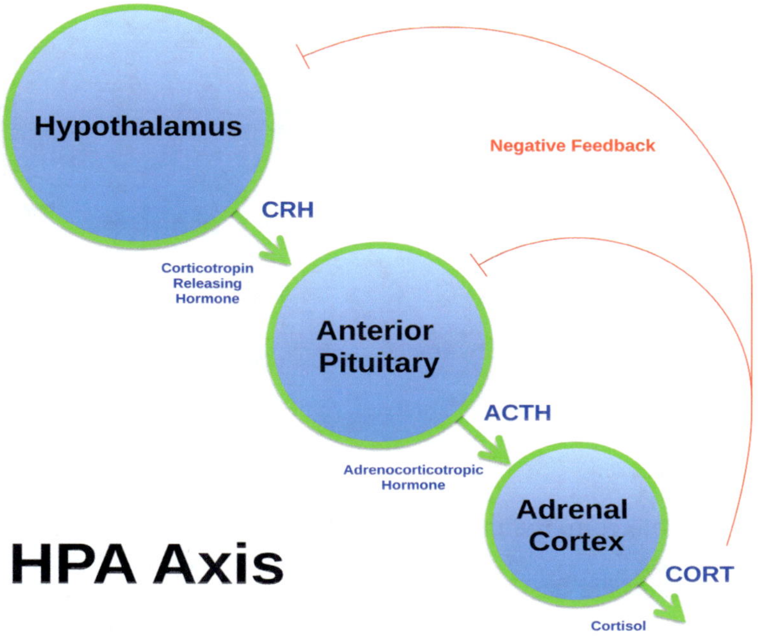

Figure 8.14. Hypothalamic pituitary adrenal axis.

Source: https://upload.wikimedia.org/wikipedia/commons/e/ee/HPA_Axis_Diagram_%28Brian_M_Sweis_2012%29.svg

8.6 Interventions for a Healthy Aging Gut

In the context of interventions aimed at maintaining a healthy aging gut, dietary modifications play a pivotal role. As individuals age, changes in gut microbiota composition can lead to gastrointestinal disturbances and a reduction in overall health. Nutritional strategies focused on incorporating high-fiber foods, probiotics, and prebiotics have demonstrated favorable outcomes. High-fiber diets promote the growth of beneficial gut bacteria, enhancing gut motility and potentially reducing the risk of gastrointestinal diseases. Furthermore, the introduction of probiotics can help restore microbial balance, which is particularly crucial as dysbiosis—an imbalance in the gut microbiome—has been linked to various age-related conditions. As such, these dietary interventions offer a proactive approach to combating the effects of aging on gut health, thereby improving the quality of life for older adults. Additionally, managing stress through various interventions is critical to maintaining a healthy gut in the aging population. Chronic stress has been shown to impact gut health by altering gut microbiota composition and impairing gut barrier function, leading to a range of health issues. Stress management techniques, such as mindfulness meditation, yoga, and regular physical activity, can significantly alleviate stress levels and improve gut health. Evidence suggests that these approaches not only enhance psychological well-being but also foster a healthier gut environment.

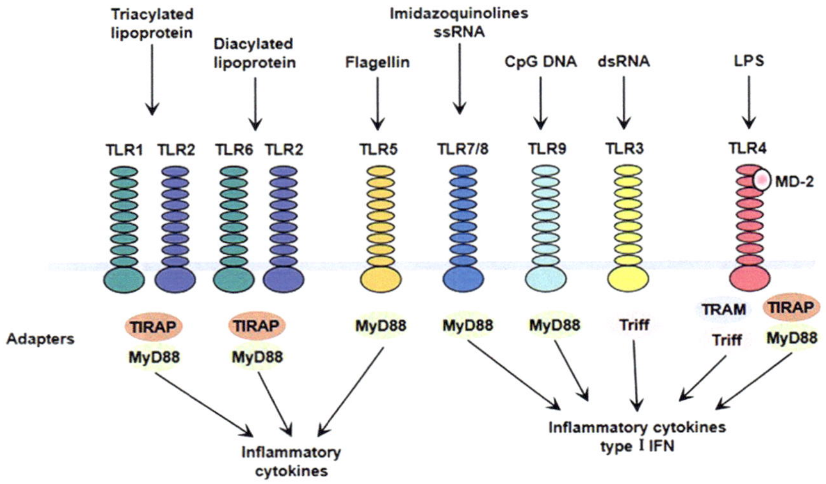

Figure 8.15. Toll-like receptors.

Source: https://www.cusabio.com/manage/upload/201905/Tollike-ligands.jpg

For example, regular exercise has been associated with increased microbial diversity, which is a marker of gut health and resilience. Consequently, integrating stress-reducing practices into daily routines is essential for promoting a healthy gut and, by extension, overall health as individuals transition into later stages of life (Estrine J et al., 2006). Moreover, the interplay between the gut microbiome and neurodegenerative diseases, such as Parkinsons disease, underscores the importance of gut health interventions in the aging population. Research has revealed a bidirectional communication between the gut and the brain, highlighting the guts influence on neurological conditions.

Dysbiosis can exacerbate inflammation and neurodegeneration, creating a vicious cycle that negatively impacts health. Interventions aimed at modulating the gut microbiota through dietary adjustments, including the incorporation of foods rich in antioxidants and omega-3 fatty acids, may mitigate these effects. Furthermore, understanding the role of toll-like receptors (TLRs) in the immune response could pave the way for therapeutic measures that enhance gut health. Hence, addressing the gut-brain axis through targeted interventions not only fosters gut health but may also provide a compelling avenue for supporting neurological health in aging populations (Caputi et al., 2018).

8.6.1 Probiotics and their benefits

The exploration of probiotics and their benefits reveals an essential connection to the aging gut and overall health. Probiotics, live microorganisms that confer health benefits when consumed in adequate amounts, play a pivotal role in maintaining gut health by enhancing the mucosal barrier, regulating inflammation, and modulating immune responses. As individuals age, the composition and diversity of gut microbiota tend to decline, leading to a state known as inflammageing, which is characterized by low-grade chronic inflammation. Research demonstrates that probiotics can counteract these age-related changes by restoring microbial balance and reducing inflammatory markers, ultimately contributing to improved gastrointestinal health and enhanced immune function. These benefits underscore probiotics potential as a valuable intervention for the aging population, addressing both gut health and systemic inflammation in this vulnerable demographic. The scientific literature indicates that probiotics not only aid in gut health but may also possess anti-aging properties. Specific probiotic strains have been shown to impact longevity and healthspan, particularly through mechanisms involving the insulin/insulin-like growth factor signaling pathway. In studies conducted on model organisms like Caenorhabditis elegans, certain probiotics exhibited observable effects on lifespan extension, oxidative stress reduction, and enhanced immune function, thus suggesting that probiotics can mitigate some aging-related physiological declines. The relationship between gut microbiota diversity and healthy aging illustrates that a properly curated microbiome can serve as a buffer against age-associated maladies. Consequently, integrating probiotics into diets could significantly influence aging outcomes by supporting microbial health and reducing the prevalence of age-related diseases, directly linking dietary interventions to improved health in older adults. Furthermore, the relevance of probiotics in the context of aging extends beyond gastrointestinal benefits to encompass broader implications for cognitive and immune health. Research indicates that the gut-brain axis is a critical framework through which probiotics can influence mental health and cognitive function. As aging is often accompanied by neurodegeneration and cognitive decline, maintaining a healthy gut microbiota through probiotics may enhance neuroprotective mechanisms and mitigate risks of conditions such as dementia. Moreover, probiotics can contribute to the modulation of systemic inflammation, aligning with findings that suggest reduced inflammation is crucial for maintaining cognitive health in the elderly. Collectively, these insights highlight the multifaceted benefits of probiotics in the aging process, suggesting that fostering gut health through dietary strategies can have profound implications for enhancing both longevity and quality of life in older adults, as outlined in current research (Guantario B et al., 2019) and (Chaiyasut et al., 2018).

8.6.2 Dietary modifications for gut health

As individuals age, the gastrointestinal tract undergoes significant physiological changes that can impact nutrient absorption and overall gut health. These modifications arise from alterations in digestive motility, mechanical breakdown of food, and the integrity of the intestinal wall. Consequently, the elderly may experience diminished nutrient intake, leading to a higher risk of malnutrition, which in turn exacerbates age-related health conditions. To address these issues, dietary modifications become instrumental in promoting gut health. Implementing diets rich in fiber can enhance gut motility and facilitate effective digestion, thereby countering some of the detrimental effects associated with an aging gastrointestinal system. Additionally, incorporating nutrient-dense foods that are easy to digest can help ensure that older adults receive the essential vitamins and minerals needed to support their overall health and well-being, as outlined in the findings of (Bordoni et al., 2015). Another critical aspect of dietary modifications for maintaining gut health in aging populations lies in the role of gut microbiota. Research has illuminated how specific dietary habits can impact the composition and activity of gut microbial communities, which are pivotal in gastrointestinal processes and immune function. For instance, diets abundant in prebiotics from fruits, vegetables, and whole grains can stimulate the growth of beneficial gut bacteria that produce short-chain fatty acids (SCFAs) crucial for maintaining gut health. These metabolites are not only involved in regulating inflammation but also have implications for metabolic functioning and overall health status in the elderly. The strategic adoption of such high-fiber diets serves to enhance the production of SCFAs, thereby establishing a more favorable gut environment, further supporting the need for systemic dietary interventions within aging populations, as corroborated by (Cadenhead et al., 2017). In addition to fiber-rich diets, the integration of other dietary modifications, such as the Mediterranean-style diet, showcases significant potential in promoting gut health among older adults. This dietary pattern emphasizes healthy fats, lean proteins, and a variety of fruits and vegetables, providing essential nutrients that can bolster gut microbiome diversity. This diversity is pivotal as it relates to improved digestive health and a reduced risk of age-related diseases. Furthermore, these dietary changes can counteract systemic inflammation, which is often exacerbated in aging individuals, reinforcing the interconnectedness of nutrition and gut health. Employing a comprehensive approach to dietary modifications that includes both macronutrients and micronutrients can pave the way for a healthier aging process, significantly affecting the quality of life as individuals navigate the challenges associated with aging, highlighted by the underlying concepts in (Bordoni et al., 2015).

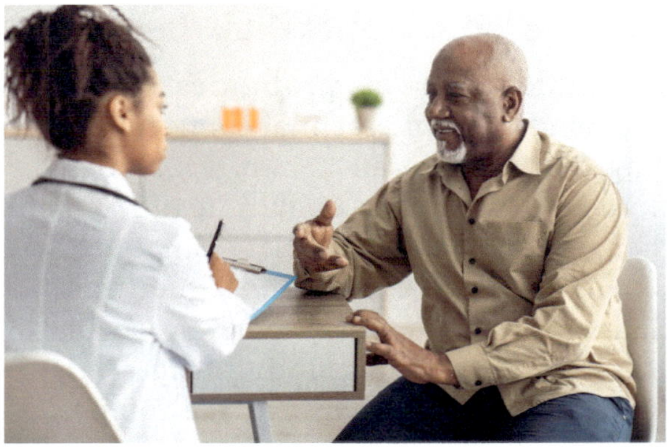

Figure 8.16. Dietary modifications for gut health.

Source: https://assets-global.website-files.com/5e066fbd0d37a10ebf1f4139/659f090c3a70f9a11357de53_shutterstock_2159141583.jpg

8.6.3 Importance of regular medical check-ups

As individuals age, the significance of regular medical check-ups becomes increasingly apparent, particularly with respect to maintaining gut health and overall well-being. Regular examinations serve as a proactive measure for early detection of potential health issues, including gastrointestinal disorders that may arise from age-related changes in gut physiology.

This is especially crucial as the gut microbiome, which significantly influences immune function and metabolic processes, can be adversely affected by aging. Healthcare providers often recommend routine screenings and assessments to monitor gut health, thus enabling timely interventions that may prevent the progression of chronic conditions associated with aging. Regular check-ups also facilitate personalized healthcare strategies, tailored to the unique experiences and health profiles of older adults, ensuring that interventions are optimized for their specific needs. Moreover, routine medical evaluations can help manage and mitigate the effects of chronic illnesses that often coincide with aging. For instance, conditions such as diverticulitis or colorectal cancer are more prevalent in older adults, making screening and early diagnosis vital for effective treatment outcomes. The ability to monitor chronic diseases through regular check-ups allows for adjustments in medication, dietary recommendations, and lifestyle interventions that are essential for maintaining gut health. Health care professionals are also better equipped to provide advice on lifestyle factors that influence gut microbiota, such as diet and exercise. Incorporating holistic approaches into patient care during these check-ups can support enhanced health outcomes and quality of life as patients age. This encompasses addressing both physical symptoms and psychological factors that may impact gut health, underlining the interconnectedness of bodily systems that age together. In addition to the physical benefits, regular medical check-ups contribute to psychological well-being, which in turn can influence gastrointestinal health. The relationship between mental health and gut function is well-documented, with stress and anxiety often leading to dysregulated digestive processes. Consequently, psychiatric disorders among older adults, which can be exacerbated by untreated health conditions, may present additional challenges. Regular consultations provide an opportunity for health care providers to discuss mental health concerns and recommend appropriate interventions. Furthermore, proactive engagement during these visits can help combat feelings of isolation and anxiety prevalent among aging populations. By promoting open communication about gut health and its holistic implications on overall health, regular check-ups foster a supportive environment that encourages adherence to medical advice and a healthier lifestyle, ultimately benefiting the aging gut.

Summary

The examination of the aging gut, it becomes evident that the interplay between gut microbiota composition and overall health is critical as one ages. The gut microbiome undergoes significant changes over time, experiencing a decline in diversity and richness, which has been associated with various age-related diseases. This gradual deterioration impacts not only gastrointestinal function but also plays a role in systemic inflammation and metabolic health. The importance of understanding these transformations cannot be overstated, as they signal a need for interventions that can potentially mitigate the negative effects associated with an aging digestive system. By exploring strategies that target gut health, such as dietary modifications and the use of personalized nutrition programs, we can begin to devise solutions to improve wellness among the elderly population. Furthermore, research has indicated that modern interventions, including AI-based personalized nutrition programs, can have profound effects on gut microbiome dynamics. In studies, participants exhibited significant improvements in both the richness and diversity of their gut microbiota following tailored dietary recommendations designed through advanced technological tools. Notably, the introduction of food elements associated with cardiovascular health, along with a decrease in inflammation-associated microbiota, emphasizes the ability of nutrition to substantially influence gut health. This relationship is particularly relevant given the aging population's susceptibility to conditions such as atherosclerosis and metabolic syndrome, which are intrinsically linked to gut microbiota composition. Thus, the emerging field of personalized nutrition, aided by technology, offers promising avenues for enhancing gut health in aging individuals (K Rouskas et al., 2025). Lastly, addressing the multifaceted nature of gut health in the context of aging necessitates a holistic approach that includes understanding the systemic interactions of biological factors. As highlighted in contemporary reviews on vascular aging and the gut microbiome, the mechanisms influencing cardiovascular health and aging are indeed interconnected. Strategies targeting inflammation, genomic stability, and the gut microbiome itself provide a framework for developing effective health interventions. To combat prevalent age-related diseases, a multifactorial approach is essential, merging insights from nutrition, microbiology, and broader health sciences. As we move toward a comprehensive understanding of aging and its effects on the gut, future research will be instrumental in establishing effective therapies that can enhance healthspan and combat age-related pathologies, ultimately contributing to improved quality of life (Wankumbu SC et al., 2024).

The concept of the aging gut has become increasingly significant in understanding overall health and longevity. One of the key points is the deterioration of gut microbiota diversity as individuals age, which can lead to various health complications. Research suggests that an imbalance in gut microbiota, characterized by a reduction in beneficial bacteria, directly correlates with age-related diseases, including inflammatory disorders and metabolic syndromes. As the gut microbiome plays a crucial role in nutrient absorption, immune function, and inflammation regulation, maintaining its diversity becomes essential. Interventions such as dietary modifications and probiotics are being explored to enhance gut health in the elderly, emphasizing the importance of a multidimensional approach to aging that incorporates both microbiological and nutrition-based strategies. Another relevant aspect of the aging gut discusses the influence of stress on gastrointestinal health. Throughout the life course, stress emerges as a critical factor that can aggravate gut health, manifesting in conditions like irritable bowel syndrome and inflammatory bowel disease. Notably, a gap persists between conventional medical practices that focus on specific ailments and the broader understanding of how stress impacts gut function. Addressing this disconnect necessitates a comprehensive strategy that integrates psychological well-being with gastrointestinal health, advocating for holistic treatment approaches. Moreover, as gut-brain interactions become increasingly acknowledged, exploring the bidirectional relationship opens new avenues for understanding how psychological stressors might exacerbate age-related gut conditions, as indicated in research around both mental and physical health. Finally, emerging epigenetic research highlights a complex relationship between aging, gut health, and chronic diseases. Chronic kidney disease (CKD), for instance, is posited to share links with age-induced changes in the gut microbiome. Emerging evidence suggests that epigenetic modifications may play a role in the susceptibility of older adults to various diseases, including CKD, thereby emphasizing the need for targeted research into the underlying mechanisms. Understanding these relationships is essential for developing new diagnostics and therapeutic strategies tailored to the aging population. Holistic approaches, which consider various influencing factors—including lifestyle, diet, and psychological well-being—will be critical in combating the repercussions of an aging gut and promoting healthier aging processes across demographics (Estrine J et al., 2006)(Ekström et al., 2017).

CLOSER LOOK

GUT MICROBIOME AS A MODULATOR OF HEALTHY AGEING

Gut microbiome as a modulator of healthy ageing highlights its crucial role in maintaining physiological balance and resilience in older adults. The gut microbiome, a complex community of trillions of microorganisms, contributes to digestion, immune system regulation, and even cognitive function. As people age, the diversity and stability of the gut microbiota often decline due to factors such as dietary changes, reduced mobility, chronic illness, and increased use of medications like antibiotics. This microbial imbalance, or dysbiosis, is linked to inflammation, weakened immunity, metabolic disorders, and age-associated diseases such as diabetes, cardiovascular issues, and neurodegenerative conditions.

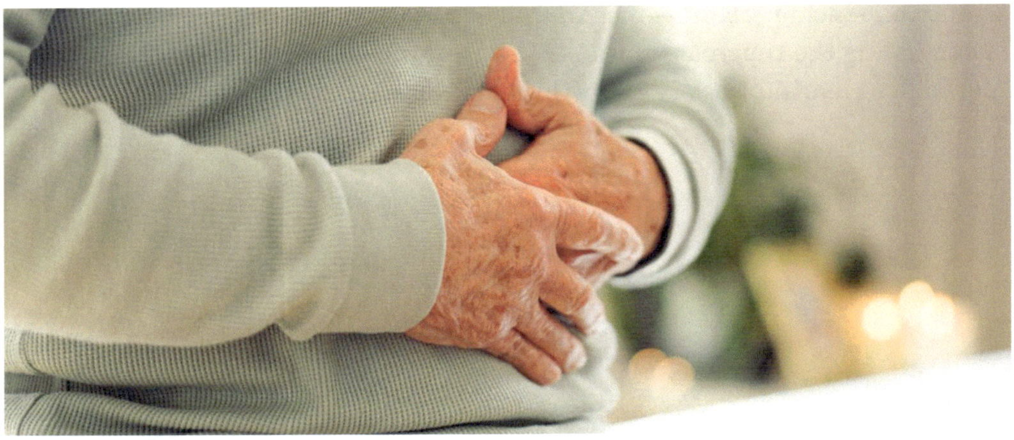

Figure 8.17. Gut Microbiome as a Modulator of Healthy Ageing.

Source: https://external-content.duckduckgo.com/iu/?u=https%3A%2F%2Fbrightcare.co.uk%2Fwp-content%2Fuploads%2F2024%2F07%2FAgeing-Well-Gut-Microbiome.jpg&f=1&nofb=1&ipt=70cbeb8a15fb99d60f14662627043b2f30ff9d8a1fc3710a524a4cfc43a51d2d

Conversely, a diverse and balanced gut microbiota promotes "inflammaging" control—a term describing low-grade chronic inflammation associated with ageing—by producing short-chain fatty acids (SCFAs) that support gut barrier integrity and anti-inflammatory immune responses. Emerging research also shows that the gut-brain axis, the bidirectional communication between the gut and central nervous system, may influence mood, cognition, and mental health in older adults. Diets rich in fiber, fermented foods, and polyphenols, as well as the use of targeted probiotics and prebiotics, show promise in restoring microbiome health. Therefore, nurturing the gut microbiome is increasingly viewed as a key strategy for extending healthspan, reducing disease burden, and promoting vitality in older populations.

REFERENCES

1. Agrawal, Ahmed, Alpers, Anderson, Armougom, Arunachalam, Avonts, et al. (2016) Impact of high fat diets, prebiotics and probiotics on gut microbiota and immune function, with relevance to elderly populations. doi: https://core.ac.uk/download/42155174.pdf
2. Ahmed, Shafi, Broad, John, Carroll, Rebecca, Chin-Aleong, et al. (2018) Changes in neuromuscular structure and functions of human colon during ageing are region-dependent. doi: https://core.ac.uk/download/161396574.pdf
3. Amorim, Fabiano, Ani, Julianne K, Arap, Wadih, Blair, et al. (2019) Biobehavioral effects of Tai Chi Qigong in men with prostate cancer: Study design of a three-arm randomized clinical trial.. doi: https://core.ac.uk/download/323077768.pdf
4. Audrey Tierney, Audrey Tierney, Eibhlís M. O'Connor, Eibhlís M. O'Connor, Eibhlís M. O'Connor, Elke Arendt, Emma O'Shea, et al. (2023) Older adults and healthcare professionals have limited awareness of the link between the Mediterranean diet and the gut microbiome for healthy aging. doi: https://core.ac.uk/download/554220972.pdf
5. Barbara Guantario, Chiara Devirgiliis, Daniela Uccelletti, Marianna Roselli, Paola Zinno, SCHIFANO, EMILY (2019) Caenorhabditis elegans and probiotics interactions from a prolongevity perspective. doi: https://core.ac.uk/download/231749445.pdf
6. Bauer, Bjoern, Chlipala, George, Green, Stefan J., Hartz, et al. (2017) Age Drives Distortion of Brain Metabolic, Vascular and Cognitive Functions, and the Gut Microbiome. doi: https://core.ac.uk/download/232598789.pdf
7. Bazzani A., Castellani G.C., Franceschi C., Garagnani P., Giampieri E., Remondini D., Sala C., et al. (2020) Gut microbiota ecology: Biodiversity estimated from hybrid neutral-niche model increases with health status and aging. doi: https://core.ac.uk/download/385954530.pdf
8. Besanko, L., Burgstad, C., Chapman, M., Deane, et al. (2013) Modulation of individual components of gastric motor response to duodenal glucose. doi: https://core.ac.uk/download/18333704.pdf
9. Black, G., Ranson, R. N, Saffrey, M. J., Tsang, et al. (2013) Age-related changes to lumbosacral spinal cord motoneurons that modulate bladder and bowel functions in male C57BL/6 mice. doi: https://core.ac.uk/download/82978019.pdf
10. Bordoni, Alessandra, Dupont, Didier, Gille, Doreen, Kachal, et al. (2015) Understanding the gastrointestinal tract of the elderly to develop dietary solutions that prevent malnutrition. doi: https://core.ac.uk/download/286575279.pdf
11. Borrego Ruíz, Alejandro, Borrego-García, Juan José (2024) Influence of human gut microbiome on the healthy and the neurodegenerative aging. doi: https://core.ac.uk/download/614635684.pdf
12. Cadenhead, Kristen S, Depp, Colin, Joseph, Jamie, Schmid-Schönbein, et al. (2017) Modified Mediterranean Diet for Enrichment of Short Chain Fatty Acids: Potential Adjunctive Therapeutic to Target Immune and Metabolic Dysfunction in Schizophrenia?. doi: https://core.ac.uk/download/287622216.pdf
13. Caputi, Valentina, Giron, Maria Cecilia (2018) Microbiome-gut-brain axis and toll-like receptors in parkinson\u2019s disease. doi: https://core.ac.uk/download/168404181.pdf

14. Carmody, Rachel Naomi, Wrangham, Richard W. (2012) Human Adaptation to the Control of Fire. doi: https://core.ac.uk/download/28939778.pdf
15. Catarina Ramos, Daniele Magistro, Gemma E Walton, Anya Whitham, Nicola Camp, C. Poveda, Glenn R Gibson, et al. (2025) Assessing the gut microbiota composition in older adults: connections to physical activity and healthy ageing.. GeroScience. doi: https://www.semanticscholar.org/paper/c85dae8b7e66a3bb545aea93b06b59d25d23a2bb
16. Chaiyasut, Chaiyavat, Kesika, Periyanaina, Sivamaruthi, Bhagavathi Sundaram (2018) A REVIEW ON ANTI-AGING PROPERTIES OF PROBIOTICS. doi: https://core.ac.uk/download/482242908.pdf
17. Chan, Wan-Leong, Chang, Full-Young, Chen, Tseng-Shing, Hou, et al. (2015) Establishing a risk scoring system for predicting erosive esophagitis . doi: https://core.ac.uk/download/pdf/82754221.pdf
18. Colyer, Frances, Davies, Heather, Gamage, Prasanna, Ranson, et al. (2013) Ultrastructural analysis of changes in neurons of the mouse internal anal sphincter during ageing. doi: https://core.ac.uk/download/82978021.pdf
19. Connors, Grant, Gould, Kelsie, King, Sarah, Lenoir-Wijnkoop, et al. (2019) Does probiotic consumption reduce antibiotic utilization for common acute infections? A systematic review and meta-analysis.. doi: https://core.ac.uk/download/323070509.pdf
20. Coradduzza D., Cruciani S., De Miglio M. R., Maioli M., Nivoli A., Sedda S., Ventura C. (2023) Age-Related Cognitive Decline, Focus on Microbiome: A Systematic Review and Meta-Analysis. doi: https://core.ac.uk/download/611937490.pdf
21. Devirgiliis, Chiara, Mauri, Pierluigi, Miccheli, Alfredo, Motta, et al. (2017) Combination of metabolomic and proteomic analysis revealed different features among Lactobacillus delbrueckii subspecies bulgaricus and lactis strains while in vivo testing in the model organism Caenorhabditis elegans highlighted probiotic properties. doi: https://core.ac.uk/download/98348104.pdf
22. Donaldson, Alison I C, Myint, Phyo K, Soiza, Roy L (2018) The pale evidence for treatment of iron-deficiency anaemia in older people. doi: https://core.ac.uk/download/153364926.pdf
23. Ekström, Tomas J., Nordfors, Louise, Shiels, Paul G., Stenvinkel, et al. (2017) Current epigenetic aspects the clinical kidney researcher should embrace. doi: https://core.ac.uk/download/84340482.pdf
24. Jaqueline Santos Moreira Leite, Mauricio Krause, Paulo Ivo Homem de Bittencourt, Vinicius Fernandes Cruzat (2016) Physiological regulation of the heat shock response by glutamine: implications for chronic low-grade inflammatory diseases in age-related conditions. doi: https://core.ac.uk/download/pdf/81762055.pdf
25. Judith Estrine, Lisa DeLisle (2006) Stress: Putting the Brain Back Into Medicine. doi: https://core.ac.uk/download/71356692.pdf
26. K. Rouskas, Mary Guela, Marianna Pantoura, I. Pagkalos, M. Hassapidou, E. Lalama, A. Pfeiffer, et al. (2025) The Influence of an AI-Driven Personalized Nutrition Program on the Human Gut Microbiome and Its Health Implications. Volume(17). Nutrients. doi: https://www.semanticscholar.org/paper/6eed13d2f4899e4697c7ef902675ed841441df4f

27. Kenichi Hirano, Naoki Ishiguro, Nobuyuki Hamajima, Norimitsu Wakao, Shiro Imagama, Yukiharu Hasegawa (2012) Influence of lumbar kyphosis and back muscle strength on the symptoms of gastroesophageal reflux disease in middle-aged and elderly people. doi: https://core.ac.uk/download/pdf/81895761.pdf

28. Kruger K., Strasser B., Ticinesi A., Weyh C., Wolters M. (2021) The effects of lifestyle and diet on gut microbiota composition, inflammation and muscle performance in our aging society. doi: https://core.ac.uk/download/521226044.pdf

29. Maria Teresa Wijaya, Ji-Tseng Fang, Geng-Hao Liu, Yuan-Ming Yeh, Ning-Hung Chen, Chih-Ming Lin, Kuain-Yi Wu, et al. (2025) Better objective sleep quality is associated with higher gut microbiota richness in older adults. Volume(47), 4121 - 4137. GeroScience. doi: https://www.semanticscholar.org/paper/e08ea302d01cbe7a4d76b11a86b42c60aaf3ec42

30. Prerana Vaddi, Khristina Young, Molly Easter, Cristal Hill (2024) IMPACT OF LOW PROTEIN DIETS ON GUT HEALTH. Volume(8), 1143 - 1143. Innovation in Aging. doi: https://www.semanticscholar.org/paper/00d236fa6cfe04572438e4bb83da2a95f71b9157

31. San Jose State University, School of Journalism and Mass Communications (1989) Spartan Daily, April 3, 1989. doi: https://core.ac.uk/download/70418816.pdf

32. Silumbwe Ceaser Wankumbu, Xiao-Man Ji, Ming Xu (2024) Decoding vascular aging: implications for atherosclerosis progression and clinical intervention. Exploration of Drug Science. doi: https://www.semanticscholar.org/paper/50994eea967aa98e80add5e151b2a51656ede4de

33. Yajun Qiao, Huimin Zheng, Ruiying Cheng, Juan Guo, Li Ji, Zhibin Liu, Lixin Wei, et al. (2025) High-fat diet-induced osteoporosis in mice under hypoxic conditions. Volume(26). BMC Musculoskeletal Disorders. doi: https://www.semanticscholar.org/paper/f9d000d86ca98dd8b1debc2073347752d7db3064

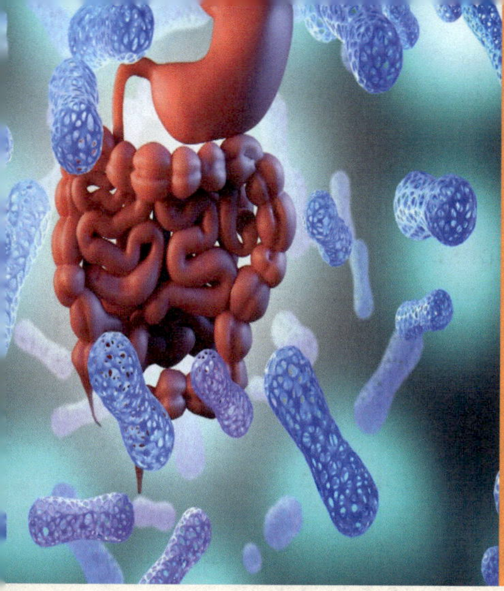

Chapter 9

MACRONUTRIENT AND MICRONUTRIENT NEEDS DEFICIENCIES OF GERIATRIC NUTRIENTS

Contents

Introduction

The increasing age of the world population has thrown a spotlight upon the nutrition of older individuals, particularly macronutrients and micronutrients. As one ages, physiological adaptations like altered metabolism and compromised absorption efficiency give unique nutritional requirements. Meeting these requirements is important for maintaining health, enhancing functionality, and ensuring quality of life in old age. Also, the prevalence of malnutrition in elderly individuals poses a significant health risk, e.g., increased vulnerability to chronic disease, frailty, and mortality. For health practitioners to design targeted dietary interventions that can effectively enhance the health of geriatric populations, a description of the evidence-based deficiencies in nutrients is needed. Therefore, deciphering the complex relationships between diet, intake of nutrients, and overall health outcomes in the elderly population is crucial. The need for an adequate diet in the prevention or minimizing of age-related health disorders cannot be adequately emphasized. Research has demonstrated that both macronutrient and micronutrient deficiencies have been well documented to exacerbate common geriatric conditions, such as cognitive decline and loss of mobility. Specifically, elderly individuals who have poor nutritional status are more vulnerable to the onset of chronic diseases, e.g., cardiovascular and neurodegenerative diseases. Moreover, poor dietary intake can further affect oral health in a vicious cycle of low dietary intake and worse health outcomes. As highlighted in recent literature, oral health is important to maintain good nutrient intake in older people, and therefore, an integrated healthcare model should be followed to improve longevity and quality of life among the elderly (Chan et al., 2023). In order to better appreciate the contribution of dietary patterns to health outcomes in older people, specific dietary interventions that have shown the potential to improve health outcomes must be examined. Foods that are rich in antioxidants and anti-inflammatory activities, for instance, like the Mediterranean diet, have been implicated in improved longevity and retardation of diseases with age. The anti-aging protection provided by such diets is regulated by their wholesome macronutrient and micronutrient composition that contributes to processes of cellular and molecular aging (Fekete et al., 2022). As dietary needs change with aging, personalized dietary counseling that incorporates these healthy eating habits represents an encouraging method to redress nutritional deprivation among the elderly. Upcoming studies should strive to develop combined dietary guidelines that take the unique needs of older individuals in order to establish an environment for successful aging (Figure 9.1).

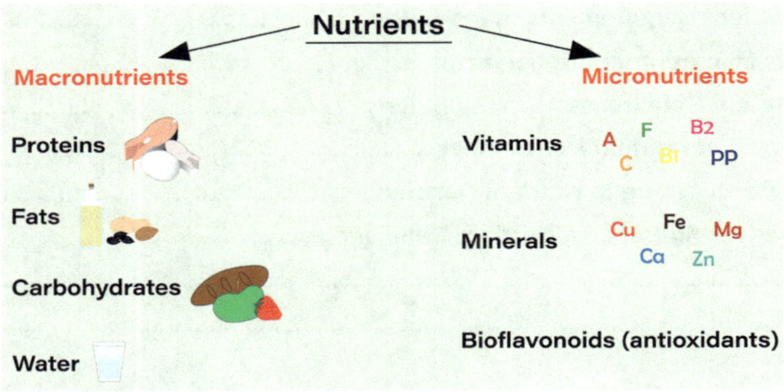

Figure 9.1. Macronutrient and micronutrient needs and deficiencies of geriatric nutrients.

Source: https://www.healthwebmagazine.com/wp-content/uploads/2022/09/macronutrients-and-micronut.jpg.

Definition of Macronutrients and Micronutrients

Macronutrients and micronutrients have significant roles in nutrition to ensure health, especially among the elderly. Macronutrients such as carbohydrates, proteins, and fats are needed in order to supply energy and sustain the functions of the body. Carbohydrates serve as the major fuel, and proteins are necessary for repairing tissues, maintaining muscles, and synthesizing important enzymes. Then there are the fats, though frequently condemned, which play a basic role in helping the absorption of fat-soluble vitamins and maintaining cellular structure. Sufficient macronutrient intake is of extreme significance in elderly people since deficiencies lead to frailty, loss of muscle mass, and impaired physiological function, highlighting the need for balanced nutrition throughout the entire aging process. In contrast, micronutrients, made up of vitamins and minerals, are required in lower quantities but play essential roles in metabolism, immune function, and general well-being. There are often higher chances of micronutrient deficiency associated with growing older due to numerous factors, such as altered digestion, decreased food variety, and others. Certain micronutrients, such as calcium and Vitamin D, play a significant role in bone health, whereas B vitamins perform vital functions in energy metabolism and the functioning of the brain. Systematic review demonstrates that inadequate intake of some micronutrients is associated with frailty in older age and highlights the intricate association of nutrition status with age-related health (Lorenzo-López et al., 2017). The disparity necessitates specific dietary interventions to ensure the nutritional demands of this population are met. One needs to appreciate the complex interaction between a senescent GI tract and nutrient absorption in the management of the elderly's nutrition (Rémond et al., 2015). When the digestive system goes through natural changes, one is less capable of absorbing nutrients, digesting them, and absorbing them, which can contribute to additional malnutrition. This rise in malnutrition not only increases the susceptibility to various health conditions but also deteriorates the organ system functions like the musculoskeletal and cardiovascular systems. Therefore, it becomes crucial to develop dietary guidelines addressing the very specific needs of the elderly, emphasizing nutrient-rich and easily digestible foods. Meeting these nutritional challenges with successful dietary strategies can have a profound effect on improving health outcomes and quality of life in the geriatric population.

Importance of Nutrition in Geriatric Populations

Growth, old or aging creates a plethora of physiological changes that have considerable effects upon nutritional requirements, thus increasing the significance of proper nutrition in geriatric populations. As older individuals experience changes in metabolism, digestion, and absorption, their needs for macronutrients—particularly proteins, carbohydrates, and fats—are different from those of their younger peers. Increased protein intake has been linked with decreased frailty among the population, which is prevalent among the older population. If the body is denied adequate protein, aged individuals are prone to muscle wasting as well as physical disability. Besides, carbohydrates and fats remain essential to maintain energy levels as well as overall health. Therefore, the identification and fulfillment of these macronutrient needs can prove to be invaluable in maintaining healthy aging in geriatric patients. Micronutrients, though lesser thought about, also have their own roles to play in maintaining the health of elderly individuals. Vitamins as well as minerals ensure smooth immune function, bone mineral density, and brain function, all of which assume extreme significance as an individual ages. There have been recent studies to indicate that low intake of specific micronutrients has been observed to be associated with frailty syndrome, hence the need for a well-balanced diet with high levels of such essential nutrients. For example, vitamin D and calcium deficiency have been associated with osteoporosis and fracture risk, while vitamins B12 and E deficiency have been associated with cognitive impairment. Therefore, enhancement of awareness among the elderly towards micronutrient needs is a part of meal planning as it can be a protective factor for most age-related illnesses and also improve the quality of life. The intricate relationship between nutrition and frailty also illustrates the significance of comprehensive diet evaluation in geriatric medicine. As noted in recent reviews, malnutrition is increasingly identified as a syndrome of complexity associated with aging, where nutritional status has a direct role in causing frailty syndrome. Intervention strategies, including the utilization of the Mini Nutritional Assessment (MNA), can help identify people at risk and deliver personalized dietary counseling. These findings underscore the role of both qualitative and quantitative factors in nutrition and indicate that an integrated view of dietary habits is central to supporting healthy aging. To this end, the integration of nutrition-centered interventions into models of geriatric care is central to preventing and managing frailty and keeping older adults more active and functional (Lorenzo-López et al., 2017).

Overview of Nutrient Deficiencies in Older Adults

The prevalence of malnutrition among the elderly is one of the main public health concerns since it can profoundly impact their overall health and well-being. The majority of older adults are short of their nutritional requirements due to some causes, such as decreased appetite, changes in metabolism, and economic limitations. Malnutrition is responsible for numerous health disorders, including frailty, cognitive dysfunction, and immunosuppression. Moreover, the elderly also often possess complex nutritional needs that must be met because they are more prone to developing conditions like osteoporosis and heart disease. Therefore, an understanding of the nutritional requirements and identification of deficiency among this population is crucial in order to optimize their health and lifespan. The association of improved nutritional status and reduced frailty is an indication of the necessity of targeted interventions and policies to promote the correct consumption of nutrients among the elderly, particularly those in nursing homes (Mashfufa et al., 2025). In addition to the physiological changes brought about by the aging process, the multisystem involvement of medical disorders among older patients complicates the management of their nutritional needs. For example, heart failure patients commonly develop malnutrition, mostly as a result of elevated metabolic needs and reduced appetite, resulting in excessive unintended weight loss and continued worsening of health. Research indicates that close to 50% of the patient population is malnourished, which shows the immediate necessity for uniform diagnostic criteria to allow for early detection and intervention (Johnson, 2016). By correcting the nutritional deficiencies among elderly populations, health care systems are able to advance patient outcomes and the quality of life for this high-risk group. Successful interventions in the form of personalized nutrition plans and nutrition counseling are crucial in preventing the severity of malnutrition and enabling healthy aging. Lastly, it is important to highlight the contribution of micronutrients to healthy aging. Vitamins and minerals such as vitamin D, calcium, and B vitamins are often consumed inadequately, significantly affecting bone strength, muscle function, and cognitive function. These deficiencies in micronutrients will inevitably exacerbate pre-existing health issues and cause frailty and therefore it is important that medical professionals review the dietary intake of older patients regularly.

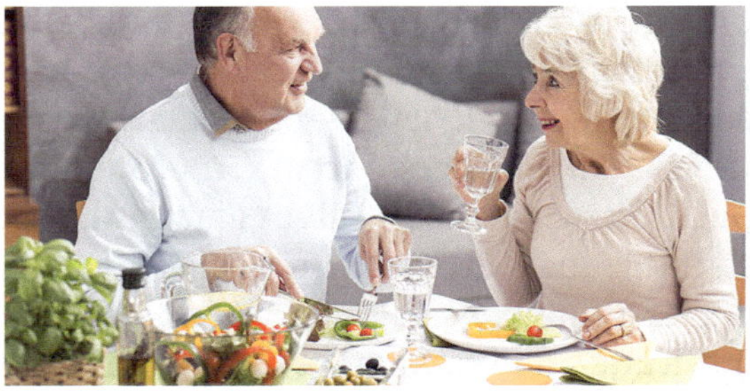

Figure 9.2. Senior nutrition: Special nutrient needs of older adults.

Source: https://www.blueparasol.com/wp-content/uploads/2019/08/Senior-Nutrition-Special-Nutrient-Needs-of-Older-Adults.jpg.

Nutritional interventions should prioritize whole foods, fortified foods, and perhaps supplements if necessary to deliver sufficient quantities of such vital nutrients to the population of older adults. The addition of rigorous nutritional testing and education will enable the identification of deficiencies early enough, ultimately leading to improved health outcomes for the population of older adults as they cope with the complex interaction of aging and diet (Johnson, 2016; Mashfufa et al., 2025) (Figure 9.2).

9.1. Macronutrient Requirements in the Elderly

With advancing age, the needs for macronutrients are significantly altered to accommodate changing physiology, such as a reduction in basal metabolic rate and muscle mass. Proper intake of carbohydrates, proteins, and fat via adequate food intake through a well-planned diet is essential for ensuring the health and functional status of older people. For instance, carbohydrates need to be the bulk of calorie intake in the form of whole grains, vegetables, and fruits for adequate energy and gut health. While protein needs become essential with age, the recommendations suggest 1.0–1.2 grams of protein per kilogram of body weight per day to preserve muscle and prevent sarcopenia. Although fat remains a significant source of energy from food, a concentration on unsaturated fats will contribute to cardiovascular well-being, increasingly significant with older persons who have greater risk factors for heart disease. Older people's deficiency in essential macronutrients is a pressing concern since their deficiency can exacerbate diseases of aging and influence well-being. Evidence indicates that many old people struggle to obtain adequate protein due to poor appetite or nutrient restrictions because of chronic diseases. For instance, a study illustrates that diet disturbance, reflecting that in individuals with celiac disease, suggests broader nutritional deficiencies across the entire population, including the elderly. In addition, the process whereby older adults become accustomed to consuming fewer calories may inadvertently lead to inadequate macronutrient intake, which in turn releases a cascade of negative health effects. There is a need to encourage education and personalized dietary interventions for enhanced awareness and optimal macronutrient intakes through optimal adequacy. Also, note that the individual nutritional needs of older people can be very different based on health status, physical activity level, and food culture. The cross-link between macronutrient intake and health status emphasizes the significance of an equilibrium approach with consideration for the unique needs of older adults. For instance, the elderly may experience difficulties in digesting certain foods, and that necessitates an effective choice of macronutrient sources. A lean protein diet, healthy fats, and fiber can contribute to easy digestion and overall health. In addition, the utilization of nutrient-rich food could even reduce the risk of chronic diseases caused by deficiency and enhance the quality of life in aged populations. Achieving these dietary demands is vital to maintaining optimum health and longevity in older individuals, who increasingly comprise a significant percentage of modern society (Figure 9.3).

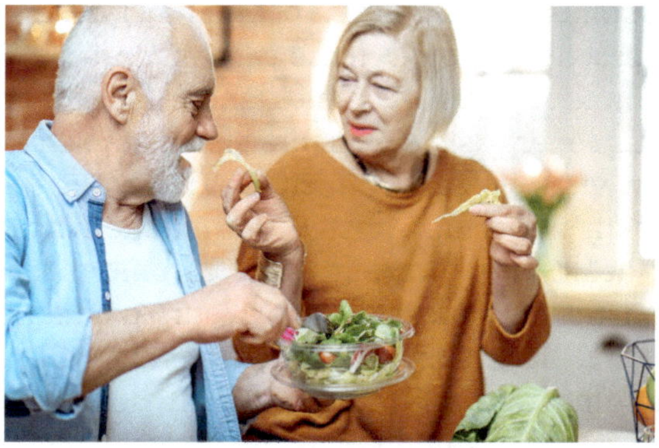

Figure 9.3. Macronutrient requirements in the elderly.

Source: https://bodsupport.com/cdn/shop/articles/rsz_senior-couple-with-healthy-food-at-home-2022-01-19-00-03-37-utc_1200x1200.jpg?v=1699536823.

9.1.1. Role of Carbohydrates in Energy Provision

The role of carbohydrates in energy provision is a matter of particular significance to the aging population, whose dietary needs are particularly diverse from those of more youthful populations. As age increases, basal metabolic rates fall, and thus a redirection of dietary focus towards energy provision and maintenance of general well-being is needed. Carbohydrates are the energy source of excellence, providing valuable fuels for physical and other pursuits. In older adults, inadequate carbohydrate intake may lead to unintentional loss of weight and muscle wasting, which can further encourage worsening of frailty and susceptibility to illness. Hence, a balanced, adequate intake of carbohydrates becomes essential while creating a nutrition regimen for energy balance and prevention of health-related disorders commonly associated with aging, proving the need for age-specific nutritional recommendations for the elderly. Apart from serving as a major source of energy, carbohydrates also contribute to the nutritional profile through an influence on dietary quality and stimulating the intake of other nutrients that are essential. Slow-release carbohydrates, such as whole cereals, vegetables, and fruits, not only release energy slowly but are also rich in dietary fiber, vitamins, and minerals. These nutrients play an important role in the maintenance of gut health and prevention of chronic disease, of particular concern to the ageing population. Recent literature has demonstrated that macronutrient and micronutrient deficiencies are prevalent among older people, particularly in high-risk groups such as women and the elderly. Thus, the addition of high-quality sources of carbohydrates can support maximum nutrient intake, addressing energy needs as well as micronutrient deficiency that is common in aging populations (Rippin et al., 2017). Carbohydrates also have certain interactions with the metabolism of protein and fat, which call for an optimal supply of balanced energy. In instances of inadequate carbohydrate intake, the body may resort to the breakdown of protein for energy through gluconeogenesis, which drains muscle tissue as well as overall health. This is particularly unfortunate in elderly individuals, who already suffer from the inability to maintain muscle as a result of age-related sarcopenia. The supply of sufficient carbohydrates can preserve lean body mass by preventing the utilization of protein stores to produce energy (Demling, 2011). Hence, the prioritization of carbohydrate foods, particularly high-fiber and high-quality foods, can create a synergy that not just encourages energy levels but also musculature health, thereby advocating for a holistic form of geriatric nutrition targeting both macronutrient and micronutrient needs (Figure 9.4).

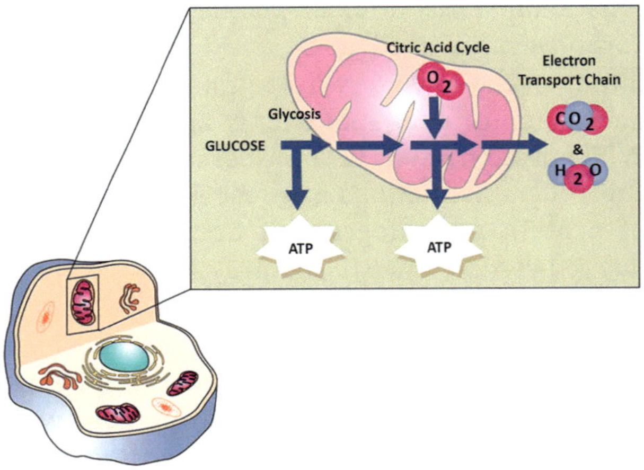

Figure 9.4. The functions of carbohydrates in the body.

Source: https://pressbooks.bccampus.ca/sciencehumannutrition/wp-content/uploads/sites/880/2019/12/image7-1.jpg.

9.1.2. Importance of Protein for Muscle Maintenance

With age, the role of protein in maintaining muscle and overall health becomes increasingly significant. This macronutrient is virtually essential in repairing and building muscle tissue, which is very relevant to the elderly since they are prone to sarcopenia, or muscle mass and strength loss with aging. Protein intake directly influences muscle protein synthesis, a process needed to maintain muscle. In elderly groups, poor protein intake not only worsens muscle loss but also increases susceptibility to injury and other illnesses. Maintaining an adequate supply of protein intake is thus a wise step to enhance muscle conservation and enable independence among the elderly, thereby ensuring an enhanced quality of life and functional status. Moreover, the increased energy requirement and changed metabolism ensuing from aging highlight the necessity for proper protein intake. The aged are likely to suffer from nutritional challenges through inadequate diet consumption, due as loss of appetite, dental problems, or gastrointestinal distress, which can lead to negative protein losses and malnutrition. These have been linked with weakened immune function and heightened susceptibility to many diseases, particularly among those affected by chronic illnesses such as HIV/AIDS. Evidence has shown that proper nutrition, in the form of protein, may have positive impacts on immune status and general health outcomes among older adults, especially those confronted with complex health problems (Miller et al., 2010). Since protein consumption is highly linked with muscle maintenance as well as the immune system, addressing these nutritional needs should continue to be a major concern for health practitioners serving older patients. Protein-fortified foods in frequent meals may play a major role in reversing muscle waste and enhancing the well-being of older people. Lean meat, dairy products, legumes, and nuts not only provide the minimal amino acids necessary for repairing muscle but can also provide other micronutrients for overall better health as well. Furthermore, careful application of nutritional supplements has been advocated when food intake is found to be inadequate. Research indicates that supplementation can lead to improvement in haematological and immune status, ultimately aiding in neutralizing the risks of malnutrition and energy deficiency in this vulnerable population (Vermaak, 2013). Thus, addressing protein intake in the context of other nutritional needs is essential in maintaining muscle conservation and optimizing longevity in the elderly, serving as the foundation of effective geriatric management.

9.1.3. Fats and Their Role in Cognitive Health

In cognitive health, dietary fats play a very crucial role, particularly with increasing age. Omega-3 and omega-6 are essential fatty acids that are components of neuron membranes, which make a proper communication system among brain cells feasible. The fats not only facilitate maintaining the structural integrity of cell membranes but also synaptic plasticity, which is critical for learning and memory. Deterioration in cognitive ability, commonly seen among older persons, can be attributed to poor consumption of such healthy fats. Studies have shown that foods high in omega-3 fatty acids could be associated with a reduced risk of cognitive impairment, thus emphasizing the importance of adding these fats to the older population's diets to ensure that their cognitive abilities remain intact with age. In addition, fats facilitate the absorption of fat-soluble vitamins A, D, E, and K, which are essential for neuroprotection and world brain health. Their deficiency can exacerbate cognitive impairment in old age and impede brain function. For example, vitamin D, which is traditionally associated with cognition, has been identified as having possible neuroprotective benefits against neurodegenerative ailments. The interaction between fats and these micronutrients highlights the balanced consumption of healthy fats to ensure the best utilization of nutrients. Since elderly populations can have challenges accessing necessary nutrients, healthcare providers should highlight personalized nutrition prescriptions that include sources of healthy fats to complement their cognitive health interventions while reducing deficiencies resulting from inadequate diets. Finally, consumption of high levels of unhealthy fats, i.e., trans fats and saturated fats, is a significant contributing factor to cognitive health. Investigations have found that such diets have been associated with an increased risk of Alzheimer's disease and other dementias.

Inflammatory responses triggered by the fats are likely to trigger oxidative stress, and in turn, intensify harm to the neuronal cells and contribute to further speeding up cognitive decline. In addition, poor fat consumption is often accompanied by poor eating habits that may lack brain-nourishing foods needed for cognitive purposes. It follows that education on what constitutes fat in one's diet is crucial, especially for the elderly, who may need to learn how to consume brain-healthy fat rather than unhealthy fat. Emphasizing the benefit of balanced fat intake with other nutrients can ultimately be utilized in supporting cognitive health in geriatric populations, consistent with general dietary recommendations for enhancing mental and psychological well-being (Figure 9.5).

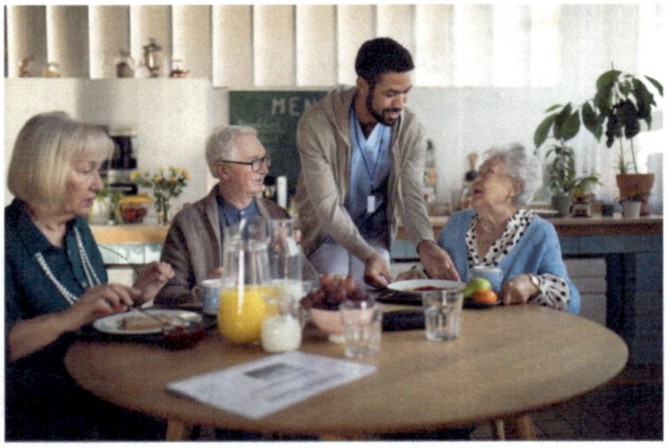

Figure 9.5. The role of nutrition in cognitive health.

Source: https://www.innovatix.com/wp-content/uploads/2025/06/group-of-cheerful-seniors-enjoying-breakfast-in-nu-2024-10-18-09-20-20-utc-1536x1024.jpg.

9.2. Common Macronutrient Deficiencies

The elderly are particularly vulnerable to macronutrient deficiencies due to several reasons, like altered food patterns, physiological changes, and diseases. A common deficiency is protein deficiency, leading to breakdown of muscle and loss of mobility, ultimately impairing functional status. As individuals age, protein needs might increase due to metabolic alterations and greater susceptibility to sarcopenia, a condition characterized by loss of muscle strength and mass. Reduced protein intake not only undermines physical health but might also weaken the immune system, rendering aged individuals susceptible to illness and infection. As noted by evidence in favor of adequate nutritional consumption, correction of protein deficiency through dietary modification or supplementation is critical in the establishment of positive health results among elderly populations (Reckow, 2012). An additional common macronutrient deficiency among the elderly is an inadequate intake of carbohydrates, which serve as a major source of energy. Elderly individuals have diets that lack complex carbohydrates, hence lead to energy deprivation and will lead to exhaustion and poor mental functions. The decrease in the consumption of carbohydrates can be attributed to reasons such as low hunger, toothache, or the perception that low-carbohydrate diets are more beneficial. Complex carbohydrates not only provide energy but also contribute to the health of the intestinal system because they promote healthy digestion through fiber. When elderly diets lack these important carbohydrates, there exists a cycle of side effects, exacerbation of pre-existing conditions, and risk to patients for such illnesses as constipation and dysglycemia (Berger et al., 2019). Lack of fat is another critical issue in the elderly, since important fats are crucial for numerous functions in the body, such as hormone production, nutrient absorption, and cell membrane structure. Despite the widely reported benefits of omega-3 and omega-6 fatty acids to cardiovascular and cognitive health, many elderly individuals do not get their fat requirements from foods. The majority of such deficiencies stems from dietary limitations, weight phobia, or ignorance of the necessity of incorporating healthy fats into their diets. Low-fat consumption compromises nutrient absorption and causes secondary deficiencies of micronutrients. Thus, an increase in dietary consumption to include appropriate sources of healthy fats, such as fatty fish, nuts, and oils is a significant factor in improving the quality and health of the diet in older adults (Reckow, 2012) (Figure 9.6).

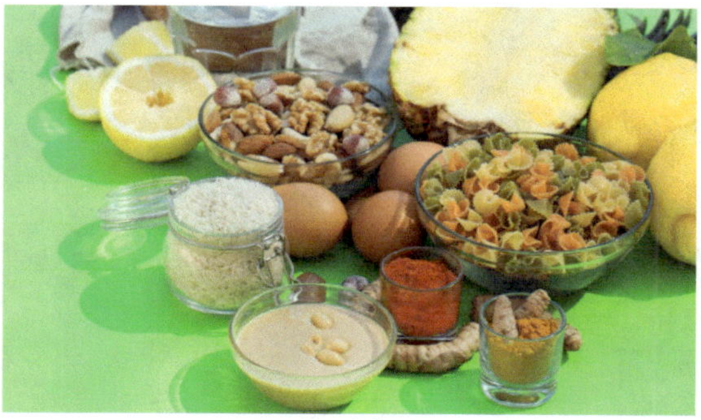

Figure 9.6. Macronutrient deficiencies and excesses.

Source: https://orthofoodie.app/wp-content/uploads/2023/07/low-purine-ingredients-for-dieting-to-stop-gout-2023-11-27-04-50-26-utc-scaled-e1707384770780-1024x541.jpg.

9.2.1. Insufficient Protein Intake and Its Consequences

In the context of geriatric nutrition, insufficient protein intake emerges as a fundamental concern, strongly compromising functional status and overall health among older adults. Proteins play a central role in maintaining muscle strength, muscle mass, and body function, which diminishes with age, due to factors such as hormonal changes and reduced physical mobility. The consequence of inadequate protein consumption may be seen as sarcopenia, or chronic loss of muscle mass and weakness, thereby increasing the risk of falls, injury, and disability. Therefore, the importance of overcoming protein malnutrition is ever more significant to enhance the quality of life and life expectancy among the aged population, who are more susceptible to the myriad of health complications associated with the ageing process and nutrient deficiencies. In addition to its effect on strength and muscle, poor protein intake may adversely affect immune function in elderly people. In the aging process, the immune system undergoes functional decline, and subnormal protein levels exacerbate this effect by rendering the elderly more susceptible to infection and illness. Immune cell and antibody production are dependent on an adequate supply of protein; therefore, caloric restriction undermines the body's ability to effectively respond to pathogens. Furthermore, studies indicate that protein deficiency has the potential to exacerbate the clinical presentation of prevalent chronic diseases among older individuals, such as heart failure and kidney disease. By appreciating the implications of insufficient protein intake, medical professionals can enhance the efficacy of dietary interventions to prevent these adverse effects and enhance the overall condition of general health among older individuals (Choi et al., 2021). Apart from this, research has shown that low protein consumption may impair recovery activities among hospitalized older patients, making proper nutritional care very crucial. Interestingly, the majority of older inpatients were found to end up consuming less than the calculated caloric requirements, which is rather dangerous given that it is linked to a greater rate of malnutrition and insufficient nutrient intake, such as proteins. Low protein intake, often in the setting of micronutrient deficiencies, can significantly increase surgery recovery time, promote postoperative complication rates, and eventually lower survival. In the hospital setting, where hospitals aim to provide holistic care, the significance of fulfilling protein needs with dietary planning and supplementation cannot be overemphasized. Interventions such as providing high-protein diets and assessing individual nutritional needs can go a long way in lowering the dangers of protein deficiency, paving the way for enhanced health outcomes in geriatric patients (Berger et al., 2019).

9.2.2. Low Carbohydrate Consumption and Energy Levels

Low carbohydrate consumption and energy levels have been a nutraceutical concern of research, especially among geriatric patients. Carbohydrates are long-established as a significant source of energy, necessary to provide physical and mental well-being in older adults. When very low carbohydrate intake occurs, the subject becomes tired and has low energy, and age-related decreases in activity and health-related quality of life may be amplified. Although certain proponents of low-carbohydrate diets argue that such restrictions can encourage weight loss and metabolic benefits, the practice can be restrictive in ensuring sufficient energy availability, particularly in the elderly, who can have inherently lower energy needs but still require sufficient calories to meet their daily functional demands.

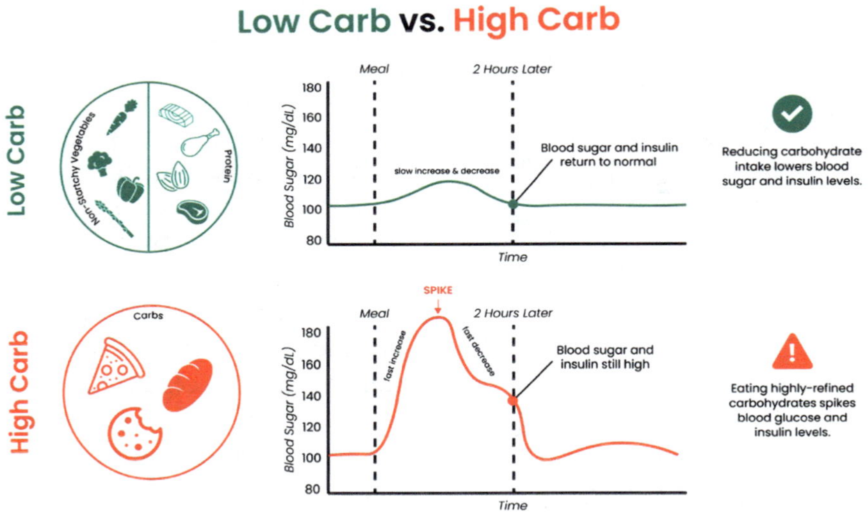

Figure 9.7. Low-carb eating.

Source: https://mylevel2.com/wp-content/uploads/2022/12/Low-vs.-High-Carb-Graphic-1024x627.png.

As described in literature, the short-term efficacy of low-carbohydrate diets may importantly differ in long-term impact on health and youthfulness during aging (Crowe, 2005). Furthermore, studies indicate that imbalanced nutrient intake, particularly in the context of low low-carbohydrate diet, results in deficiencies in essential micronutrients. For older people, maintenance of a wide variety of nutrients is essential since deficiencies compromise immune function, cognitive function, and overall health. Evidence suggests that dietary restriction, such as that occurring with low-carbohydrate diets, can interfere with the consumption of critical vitamins and minerals necessary for older populations (Deriemaeker et al., 2011). For instance, inadequate carbohydrate consumption can result in inadequate dietary fiber consumption, which is paramount for the gastrointestinal tract's health. Consequently, if carbohydrates are replaced by fats or proteins without careful planning, older adults risk denying themselves the cardiovascular safeguard implied by adequate fiber and good nutrient balance, thus the need for a balanced feeding strategy to meet their special requirements. While it is true that there can be short-term weight loss or management on low-carbohydrate diets in certain circumstances, there is debate as to whether such a diet is maintainable and healthy in the longer term for older people. The majority of studies indicate that such dietary habits are adverse, particularly among older people who might require more balanced, energy-providing diets in order to maintain optimal health (Crowe, 2005). Apart from weight issues, older individuals need to be given sufficient carbohydrates to help sustain their metabolic processes. Insufficient energy derived from carbohydrates can lead to adverse effects on muscle and overall systemic metabolic health, both of which are critical to mobility and autonomy in the elderly. Thus, an even protocol with adequate carbohydrate intake, along with other macronutrients, appears essential for the optimal energy levels and nutritional demands in the elderly population (Figure 9.7).

9.2.3. Imbalance of Healthy Fats and Cardiovascular Health

The imbalance of healthy fats has a significant impact on cardiovascular health, particularly among the elderly population, where nutritional demands and metabolic response are different from younger adults. Healthy fats, primarily mono- and polyunsaturated fats, are thought to be crucial to heart health due to their potential to reduce LDL cholesterol and reduce inflammation. Disproportionately high intakes of saturated and trans fats, which increase cholesterol levels and cardiovascular disease, are common among older adults. Lack of proper consumption of healthy oils, for example, olive oil that is high in omega-3 and omega-6 fatty acids, worsens this imbalance, resulting in negative health consequences. Increasing heart disease prevalence among this group highlights the gravity of necessitating dietary interventions that involve the addition of balanced healthy fats to their regular diet (Banda-Nyirenda et al., 2009). Apart from the cardiovascular aspects, there is evidence of a deficiency of essential fatty acids in most elderly people, which are crucial for several physiological processes, including heart rhythm and blood pressure control. The link between low-fat diets and cardiovascular disease is also established by research focusing on the detrimental effects of lipid imbalance in the elderly. Specifically, the lack of consumption of omega-3 fatty acids—contained in fish, walnuts, and flaxseeds—can lead to increased exposure to heart-related illnesses. In addition, global dietary guidelines support placing these essential fatty acids on the priority list to avoid cardiovascular conditions related to aging. Interestingly, the European Food Safety Authority promotes the idea that dietary changes emphasizing healthy fats can foster improved public health outcomes (Agostoni et al., 2010). To address the imbalance of fats and encourage cardiovascular health in the elderly population, policymakers and practitioners are obligated to advocate for holistic nutritional education with an emphasis on healthy intake of fats. This entails creating food-based dietary guidance for specific populations that emphasizes the importance of balanced fat intake. Community-based interventions need to educate older adults regarding the types of fats healthy for the heart and how to include them in their diet. Further, there is a critical need to monitor and analyze food habits on a frequent basis to recommend an individual's health profile. As public health interventions increasingly develop, an appreciation of fat intake and cardiovascular disease can be the driving force for tremendous modifications in the dietary pattern of elderly individuals, thereby reducing cardiovascular morbidity and mortality (Banda-Nyirenda et al., 2009).

9.3. Micronutrient Requirements in the Elderly

Aging has a profound influence on micronutrient requirements, which necessitates an appropriate appreciation of the nutritional requirements among the elderly. With physiological changes occurring, such as decreased digestive efficiency and changed metabolism, the capacity for absorbing and utilizing important vitamins and minerals is impaired. This often leads to deficits in substances crucial for maintaining the individual health, such as vitamin B12, vitamin D, calcium, and iron. All in all, particularly older individuals are at risk of inappropriate nutritional intake due to a variety of symptoms including decreased appetite, impaired mobility, and disease, ultimately placing them at risk of micronutrient deficiency. It is necessary to rectify such deficiencies in order to prevent adverse effects on health like frailty, cognitive impairment, and bone disease, making individualized nutritional therapy a necessity. Moreover, research underscores the value of an even greater diet with a vast richness of micronutrient diversity to promote general geriatric well-being. For instance, interventions that focus on increasing dietary antioxidants such as vitamins C and E have proved to strengthen immune processes and combat oxidative stress typical of the elderly. Further, studies have determined that the elderly population will demonstrate lower levels of adherence to Dietary Reference Intakes for micronutrients compared to other age groups, primarily due to varied diets and dietary limitations.

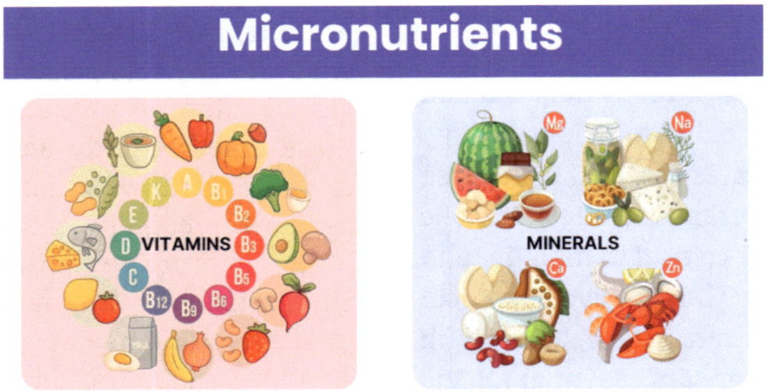

Figure 9.8. Micronutrient requirements in the elderly.

Source: https://images.examples.com/wp-content/uploads/2024/04/Micronutrients-1.png.

The resultant deficiencies in major nutrients have the potential to affect significantly, as seen in studies with celiac populations, wherein micronutrient deficiencies are common regardless of strict dietary adherence, highlighting the need for comprehensive nutrition counseling and monitoring in exposed communities (Castaño González et al., 2018). For resolving these problems, it is essential to create awareness regarding the food strategy that can adequately fulfill the needs of micronutrients in elderly people. Nutritional education must involve the delivery of guidelines not just for selecting foods rich in nutrients but also for incorporating them into the diet daily. A well-balanced diet consisting of fruits, vegetables, whole grains, and lean proteins may prove to be a good defense against the most prevalent nutritional deficiencies among older adults. Further, more recent evidence suggests that supplementation may be beneficial in certain circumstances, especially where dietary modifications alone are ineffective in achieving maximal micronutrient status. As the literature states, less than optimal levels of micronutrients not only undermine physical well-being but can also adversely affect overall quality of life, warranting continued research and targeted public health interventions on this priority area (Banda-Nyirenda et al., 2009) (Figure 9.8).

9.3.1. Essential Vitamins for Immune Function

The effectiveness of the immune response is directly associated with a range of critical vitamins and is a factor that contributes to health, particularly among older individuals. Vitamins A, C, D, and E are each potent regulators of immune response that play a role in cell signaling and fighting pathogens. For instance, vitamin D is a crucial factor in the activation of T-cells, which are tasked with identifying and killing dangerous pathogens. On another note, vitamin C is an antioxidant that protects immune cells from oxidative stress, thereby enhancing their function. Older adults often develop vitamin deficiencies due to decreased dietary intake, compromised absorption, or altered metabolism, leading to their vulnerability to infection and diseases as well. Thus, adequate consumption of these vitamins is important to help promote immune status among the elderly. The function of vitamins extends beyond overall immune function; they are also essential for recovery from infection as well as general control of inflammation. Vitamins A and E, specifically, have a particular function in preserving mucosal integrity that is the body's first line of defense against infection. Furthermore, vitamin E can boost the development of immune cells, and this results in a better response to infection. In individuals suffering from chronic diseases, such as heart disease or diabetes, these vitamins play a particularly important role because they can neutralize inflammatory responses that exacerbate these diseases. It is the appreciation of the complex interplay between vitamins and overall health that underscores the importance of nutrition intervention for the improvement of geriatric patients' vitamin status, especially in patients with specific health issues or malnutrition. Each of these key vitamins' deficiency requires an interdisciplinary approach consisting of dietary modification and supplementation. Screening for vitamin deficiency must be part of a comprehensive geriatric assessment, particularly because it can lead to a vast array of complications in the form of increased susceptibility to infection and wound failure to heal. Vitamin B12 and folate, for instance, are crucial in immune function because they are necessary for cell division and DNA synthesis. Given malnutrition's potential to influence a meaningful level of health outcome among the elderly, there is a need for targeted nutrition therapy to be incorporated as part of routine care. This proactive measure has the ability to mute the negative impacts of micronutrient deficiencies, as suggested by Berger et al. (2019) and validated by the pivotal role played by proper nutrition therapy in recuperation, as noted in Demling (2011).

9.3.2. Importance of Minerals for Bone Health

Bone health is highly dependent on sufficient intake of certain minerals, primarily calcium and phosphorus, that form the basis of bone structure. Of these, calcium is of utmost importance as it constitutes approximately 99% of the body's mineral content in the bones and teeth and plays a primary role in their development and in the bone remodeling process. Poor intake of calcium can lead to decreasing bone density, ultimately bringing about an increased susceptibility to osteoporosis, particularly in aging populations, who by nature lose bone density as they age. Phosphorus also enhances calcium function through the formation of hydroxyapatite, the mineral complex that gives bones their strength. As the aged population has lower dietary calcium and phosphorus levels, it is significant to understand their role in formulating diet recommendations for care of the elderly to optimize bone health and reduce potential fractures (Vermaak, 2013). Apart from calcium and phosphorus, magnesium and vitamin D are significant minerals impacting bone health. Magnesium is also essential in the activation of vitamin D, enabling the absorption of calcium in the intestines. The synergistic action of magnesium, calcium, and vitamin D is most vital in geriatric nutrition since a deficiency in any of these minerals can affect overall bone quality. Research has shown that elderly people are likely to have low levels of magnesium intake, which can increase the risk of bone fragility. Also, the deficiency of vitamin D, common among the elderly due to inadequate exposure to sunlight and nutritional acquisition, can lead to enhanced malabsorption of calcium, thereby aggravating maintenance of bone health. Therefore, a complete nutrition strategy for the elderly must ensure the delivery of sufficient levels of these minerals to build up healthy bones (Alharbi, 2012). The contemporary diet of the majority of elderly individuals tends not to reach the suggested daily intake levels of these essential minerals, leading to serious health complications. It has been reported in a study that a high incidence of nutrient deficiency was common among the elderly who were living in retirement communities, particularly concerning essential micronutrients that are crucial for bone function. Such deficiency verifies the need for more nutritional interventions and education concerning mineral consumption. Through proper dietary regulation and targeted supplementation, mineral consumptions of the elderly may be increased, thereby lessening the occurrence of osteoporosis and fractures. Through these corrections, health can be greatly improved, making quality of life better for geriatric individuals and minimizing the economic burden of age-related bone diseases (Vermaak, 2013) (Figure 9.9).

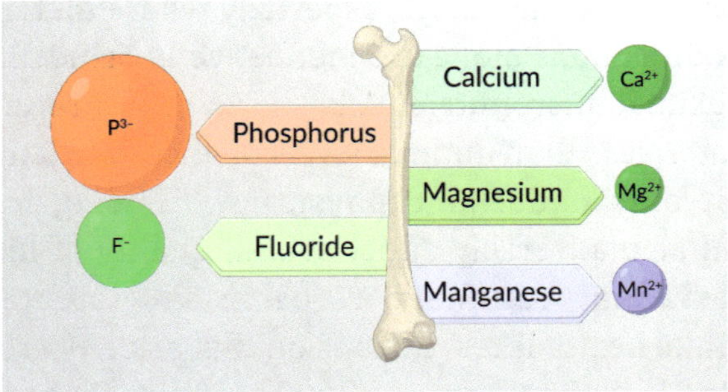

Figure 9.9. Essential minerals for bone health.

Source: https://www.jove.com/files/media/science-education/science-education-thumbs/14021.jpg.

9.3.3. Role Of Antioxidants in Preventing Chronic Diseases

Antioxidant function in the prevention of chronic diseases has gained universal attention, particularly in cases of geriatric nutrition. Chronic diseases such as cardiovascular disease, diabetes, and neurodegenerative diseases disproportionately affect a high number of older people, extensively changing their quality of life. Antioxidants, which are molecules that decrease oxidative stress through the neutralization of free radicals, have been proposed to be one of the important components of preventing the onset and progression of these diseases. A systematic review indicates that increased dietary antioxidant capacity is associated with lower risk of developing frailty, which is typically complicit with chronic disease expression among older individuals. Supplying older people with adequate intake of antioxidant foods, such as fruits, vegetables, nuts, and whole grains, may be an essential strategy in combatting the ill effects of aging on health and well-being (Lorenzo-López et al., 2017). Furthermore, antioxidants play a role not only in the prevention of chronic diseases but also in the treatment of these conditions. Research has depicted how certain antioxidants can play a role in slowing down the inflammatory mechanisms of chronic diseases. Vitamins C and E, as well as carotenoids, for instance, have been observed to promote cognitive performance and decelerate neurodegeneration among elderly subjects.

This is particularly relevant within Alzheimer's disease, where oxidative stress is a significant contributory factor. Therefore, the inclusion of antioxidants in dietary treatments not only aids in the prevention of chronic ailments but also facilitates control of the progression of the diseases, hence improving the overall quality of life among the elderly (Staehelin, 2017). The effect of antioxidant intake highlights the importance of proper nutrition with a sufficient intake of micronutrients among the elderly groups. Deficiencies in vitamins and minerals relative to foods high in antioxidants may enhance susceptibility to chronic diseases. Nutritional assessment and interventions favoring the consumption of antioxidants are therefore of utmost significance for healthcare professionals. A diet with a focus on the significance of fruits and vegetables and responsiveness towards the synergistic function of macronutrients has the potential to develop a protective nutritional setting, as indicated by numerous studies. Through prevention and control of chronic disease by ensuring adequate intake of antioxidants, not only can the disease burden in the elderly be reduced, but also longevity and quality of life among the elderly may be improved. Antioxidant addition to dietary counseling is thus a key component of geriatric practice (Lorenzo-López et al., 2017).

9.4. Common Micronutrient Deficiencies

In the ageing population, common micronutrient deficiencies create a gigantic challenge to overall health and well-being. Vitamin D, vitamin B12, iron, and calcium are just a few nutrients whose deficiency in the diet of the elderly results in a variety of health ailments. For instance, insufficiency of vitamin D results in osteoporosis and cardiovascular disorders, and insufficient vitamin B12 results in cognitive impairment and anemia. The combination of physiological changes with age, i.e., decreased absorption potential and metabolic changes, makes an individual more susceptible to these deficiencies. Therefore, the treatment of these nutrition deficiencies is a must to enhance the quality of life in older adults, as well-nourished older people are in a better position to stay on the move, remain independent, and mentally alert during their later years. Research identifies that some groups of the elderly are especially vulnerable to micronutrient deficiency, typically depending on food habits and illnesses. For individuals with celiac disease, for instance, they characteristically possess malabsorption issues which may lead to iron, iodine, and magnesium deficiencies. In a study on the dietary habit of celiac men, compliance to micronutrients in them was much less than necessary, which resulted in severe health risks due to compromised nutrition status (González et al., 2018). This could be aggravated by wrong food selection, i.e., excessive intake of processed food items that often lack substantial micronutrients. Therefore, personalized nutritional interventions, including supplementation and counseling on health food choice, are part and parcel to avoid such deficiencies and improve the nutritional environment for old people. The role of micronutrients extends beyond individuals' health, influencing public health issues on a broader scale. In settings with chronic diseases like HIV/AIDS, such deficiencies can have a negative effect on therapy outcomes and overall health condition management. Evidence indicates that diet supplemented with fish can greatly enhance health outcomes for ART individuals by improving micronutrient status, which is critical in combating the effects of debilitating disease (Banda-Nyirenda et al., 2009). The awareness of interaction between good nutrition and effectiveness of medical treatments signifies the potential of diet treatments to prevent micronutrient deficiency. Overall, the elderly will fare well from overall nutritional strategies that consider ubiquitous deficiencies, eventually resulting in better health, robustness, and wellbeing (Figure 9.10).

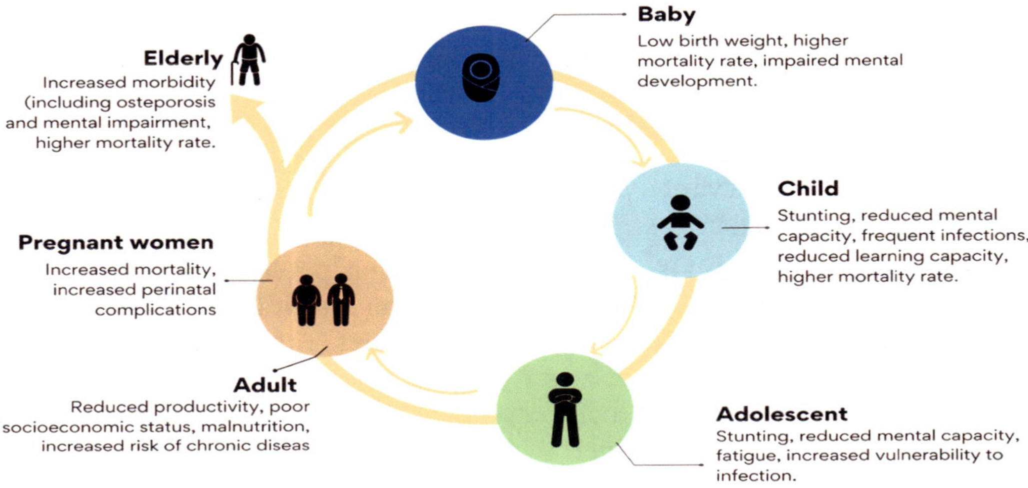

Figure 9.10. Consequences of micronutrient deficiency through the life cycle.

Source: https://www.researchgate.net/publication/366172703/figure/fig2/AS:11431281239060644@1714170148742/Consequences-of-micronutrient-deficiency-through-the-life-cycle-Modified-from-56.tif.

9.4.1. Vitamin D Deficiency and Its Impact on Bone Density

Vitamin D deficiency is a prevalent condition in the geriatric population and has a great deal to do with diminishing bone density. Deficiency inhibits the ability of the body to absorb calcium, which is a necessary mineral in maintaining bone strength and integrity. Age tends to induce a natural decrease in the vitamin D-producing capability of the skin from the sun, and this only contributes to the deficit in older patients who could already be limiting outside activity due to mobility or safety considerations. The consequent decrease in calcium intake can lead to increased resorption of bone and decreased bone mineral density, eventually posing an increased risk of fractures and osteoporosis. Because these conditions are found in over 30% of individuals above the age of 65, vitamin D consumption as food or as a supplement becomes a necessary intervention to enhance bone health among this group. Furthermore, vitamin D deficiency affects more than just bone health and can have impacts on the general health of older individuals. Low vitamin D levels have been linked to higher inflammation and oxidative stress, which can exacerbate age-related disease. Current evidence shows that adequate intake of vitamin D will provide assurance against immunity, which is crucial during health crises such as the COVID-19 pandemic, where socially isolated older citizens are not only suffering from deficiency but also increased risk of infection. Keeping the immune system intact is key to the prevention of infection-related complications and the promotion of recovery. Thus, possessing adequate levels of vitamin D can go a long way in enhancing not only bone integrity but also overall resilience of older adults in the context of broader public health concerns, such as those presented in Iddir et al. (2020) and Mattioli et al. (2020). To combat vitamin D deficiency, some dietary modifications and lifestyle adjustments recommended for elderly patients become the priority. Augmentation of the food intake of foods rich in vitamin D, such as fatty fish, fortified milk products, and egg yolks, becomes essential for patients who are not exposed to sufficient sunlight. Moreover, considering probable impediments to adequate nutrition, particularly via extended seclusion, highlights the necessity for health care professionals to prioritize nutritional assessments as a first priority in geriatric practice. Besides dietetic changes, safe solar exposure whenever feasible is necessary in rehabilitation treatment aimed at increasing bone density and overall well-being outcomes. The integration of these tactics into a total strategy of ensuring macronutrient and micronutrient needs has the potential to significantly lower the undesirable effects of vitamin D deficiency, as manifested in the arguments around geriatric nutrition deficiency generally.

9.4.2. Iron Deficiency and Its Effects on Energy Levels

Iron deficiency remains a matter of utmost concern, particularly in the geriatric case where providing adequate nutritional services must form part of health and well-being existence. The elderly tend to have a higher prevalence of iron deficiency due to multiple reasons, including decreased dietary consumption and absorption, chronic illness, and drug side effects. Iron being an essential factor in hemoglobin synthesis, its deficiency leads to anemia, which presents as weakness and fatigue. Geriatric patients may struggle to carry out regular day-to-day functioning as the lack of hemoglobin impacts oxygenation all over the body and diminishes stamina and overall functional ability. It may also affect a vicious cycle in which decreased energy levels allow more sedentary behavior, which further aggravates the health of geriatric patients. The manifestations of iron deficiency are not restricted to bodily fatigue only; they encompass cognitive and social domains of living that could severely affect quality of life. It has been studied that patients with iron deficiency anemia can be afflicted by derangements in cognitive function, and this can manifest as confusion, irritability, or loss of concentration, impacting their relationship with caregivers, families, and society in general. This state of low energy can not only worsen physical health but also lead to greater feelings of depression and isolation in older people. Iron deficiency treatment, therefore, is not merely a matter of attending to physical symptoms but also determining the total needs of the geriatric patient. Supplementation and dietary therapy programs must take these factors into consideration in order to enhance physical energy as well as mental status in this high-risk group. Effective intervention strategies must be employed to reverse the effects of iron deficiency on energy in the elderly. Healthcare professionals, nutritionists, and carers must act in concert to assess dietary intake accurately and identify vulnerable subjects. Enhancing nutrition education will allow older patients to make informed choices about their diet, which should emphasize foods high in iron and vitamin C, which improve absorption. Besides, health policy will have to construct enabling environments to easily reach healthy food to older adults. Regular screening of iron deficiency along with complementary education interventions will be an important feature for improvement of energy levels as well as health outcome. Through the treatment of both the physical and psychosocial aspects of iron deficiency, we can produce a more resilient geriatric population, enhancing their quality of life and independence (Kinabo et al., 2008; Banda-Nyirenda et al., 2009).

9.4.3. Calcium Deficiency and Risks of Osteoporosis

Calcium deficiency is a significant issue in the elderly, as it plays a major role in maintaining bone health. As age advances, the body is more likely to experience reduced calcium absorption following several physiological changes within the gut. These could be compounded by poor dietary calcium supply, and with that, greater vulnerability to osteoporosis, a condition whereby bones lose their density and become susceptible to fractures. Osteoporosis is also referred to as a silent disease because it occurs with a delayed onset and lacks symptomatic expression until fracture, which illustrates the importance of early dietary interventions to prevent calcium deficiency and the resulting hazard. By encouraging adequate intake of calcium through diet or foods supplemented with it, it is possible to counteract the adverse effects of aging on bone density and general skeletal status, which is particularly crucial in maintaining quality of life among older adults (Rémond et al., 2015). The effects of calcium deficiency extend beyond skeletal integrity because it is directly related to other physiological functions like muscle contraction and nerve impulse. This interconnectivity highlights the necessity for considering not only calcium intake but also the entire eating pattern of elderly groups. Malnutrition, often seen in older individuals, is a twofold burden by limiting both macronutrient and micronutrient intake, like calcium. Reduced appetite, pharmacological influences on nutrient absorption, and socioeconomic factors add further to nutritional deficiencies, thus promoting susceptibility to osteoporosis. These multifaceted problems are solvable only by adopting a multi-component approach that focuses on individualized nutritional care and interventions in the context of complexity embedded in geriatric health (Sandra et al., 2014). To induce awareness regarding food containing calcium and its regular intake can ensure better health outcomes in elderly individuals. In order to combat the rising prevalence of osteoporosis due to calcium deficiency, public health initiatives must aim towards better nutritional education and supply among the aged. With the current population trends shifting towards an aging population, there is an urgent need to develop strategies that encompass nutritional advice specifically designed for geriatric individuals. Dietary maintenance of calcium levels by advocating frequent intake of dairy products, leafy green vegetables, and fortified foods will go a long way in preventing osteoporosis risks. This public health priority should also emphasize recommending regular screening and assessment of bone condition among the elderly. In promoting an integrated approach that includes nutrition, physical activity, and frequent health checks, we can allow aging populations to achieve improved health status levels and live longer in life free from the disabling effects of osteoporosis (Rémond et al., 2015; Sandra et al., 2014) (Figure 9.11).

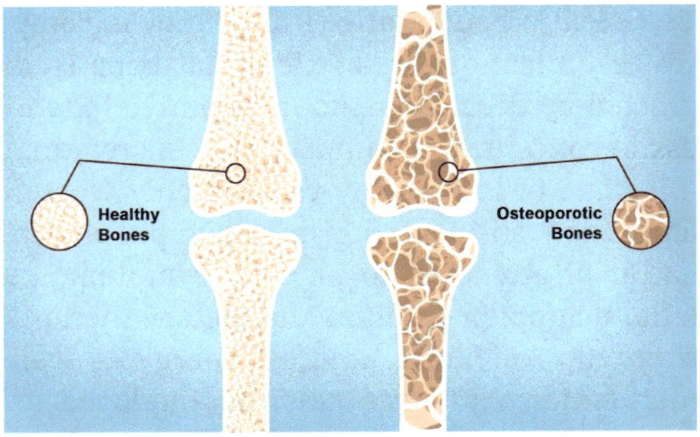

Figure 9.11. Osteoporosis in older adults.

Source: https://cdn.prod.website-files.com/63e3b52a84906f20447ea2e8/676f58c2b93a44d389f2aa58_676f5875b82e956f013d6fff_osteoporosis.png.

9.5. Factors Contributing to Nutrient Deficiencies

An essential cause of nutritional deficiencies among the elderly is the interaction between physiological changes with age and nutrition. With increasing age, individuals lose their appetite, taste perception becomes altered, and smell decreases, which can reduce their food consumption and compromise the quality of diet. Also, cognitive impairments such as dementia or other neurodegenerative disorders can cause meal preparation and food choice issues, further adding to the risk of failing to consume adequate nutrients. These factors in combination would lead to insufficient intake of major macronutrients and micronutrients, thus resulting in increased risk of deficiency leading to further effects on health status among the elderly. These conditions may be addressed by specific nutritional measures that could enhance such deficiencies and provide better health for this group. A significant contributing factor to the nutritional deficiencies of elderly people is the side effects of the administration of drugs and the condition of polypharmacy. The majority of elderly patients are prescribed multiple drugs for chronic conditions, which can adversely affect nutrient metabolism and absorption. Some drugs, such as proton pump inhibitors and other gastric acid suppressants, can compromise the bioavailability of certain key nutrients, such as vitamin B12 and folate. Research has shown that their use has correlated with decreased serum concentrations of key nutrients, implying the need for education among healthcare providers regarding potential impairment in nutrient status in patients. As age advances and medication become complex, these interactions can further complicate their nutritional condition, with a strong demand for holistic care approaches that consider the pharmacological as well as nutritional factors in the elderly (Rue et al., 2005). Lastly, socioeconomic factors such as affordability and accessibility of healthy food have a pivotal position in the nutrient deficiencies of the older population. Most older adults have fixed incomes that do not allow them to buy fresh, high-density foods. As a result, dependence on low-cost processed foods results in the consumption of nutrient-deficient diets. Furthermore, social isolation can discourage cooking, and convenience foods that are also nutritionally deficient become the preferred choice. Recent studies demonstrate that a high percentage of elderly patients are deficient in dietary reference values for certain nutrients, with negative implications for cognitive performance and overall health. This reflects the necessity of broad community support services for improved access to nutritional food for elderly individuals, in addition to educational programs for awareness about nutritional health (Mendonça, 2018) (Figure 9.12).

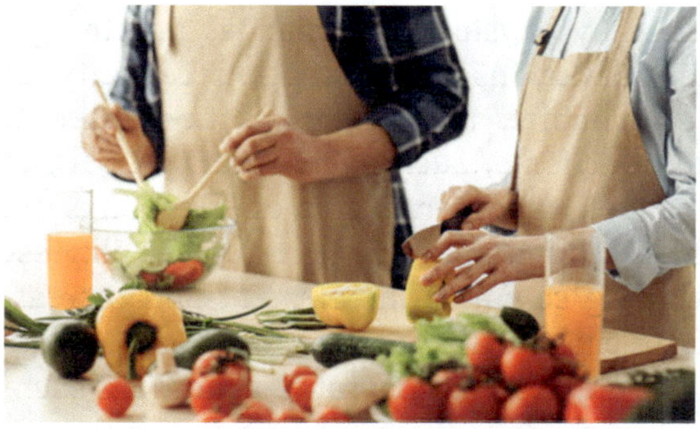

Figure 9.12. Factors contributing to nutrient deficiencies.

Source: https://www.hydratis.co/cdn/shop/articles/225_a096a145-7a15-47f8-8fb0-995342ff10c0.png?v=1743513160&width=500.

9.5.1. Changes in Metabolism with Aging

As one ages, there is a gradual loss in metabolic rate, which significantly affects the nutritional requirements of the subject. Aging is marked by body changes with the reduction of lean muscle tissue but an increase in fat tissue. This transformation can lower the basal metabolic rate (BMR), or the number of calories required to maintain the physiological functions of the individual when at rest. As a result, older individuals struggle to retain macronutrient intake. For the physically active that may be compensating for some of these losses in metabolism, inactivity intensifies the slowing of metabolism. Exercise is crucial, as not only does it help to preserve muscle mass but also stimulates metabolic processes that are vital to health. This is particularly relevant due to the potential for heightened oxidative stress with aging, which can further influence energy metabolism and the utilization of nutrients, requiring proper dietary intake to counteract such difficulties. The influence of aging on metabolism goes beyond macronutrient requirements to include micronutrient needs as well. Based on studies, some micronutrient deficiencies have been determined to be caused by physiological changes due to aging, e.g., reductions in absorption capacity and eating habits. Deficiency in these essential micronutrients, such as vitamins B12, D, and C, as well as minerals zinc and iron, has been linked to a number of age-related illnesses, including cognitive impairment and increased risk of chronic diseases. For instance, oxidative stress and neurodegenerative conditions such as Alzheimer's disease have meaningful implications for the function of antioxidant micronutrients in diet (Staehelin, 2017). A proper dietary balance containing high levels of fruits, vegetables, lean proteins, and whole grains is necessary to ensure that older adults are provided with sufficient levels of these micronutrients to support metabolism and overall well-being. Besides, hospitalization in elderly individuals presents a higher risk for the development of nutritional deficiencies that play an important role in their recovery and future health condition. Under hospital conditions, the majority of patients usually present with inadequate caloric intake through various factors including diminished appetite and restrictive diets, whereas others are given less than the needed 1500 kcal/day (Beger et al., 2019). This caloric deficit can lead to reduced reservoirs of vital micronutrients, further exacerbating the problems of aging. A thiamine deficiency, for instance, can impair energy metabolism and even cognitive function, emphasizing the need for system-wide screening for micronutrient deficiency on hospitalization. Proactive measures, such as enrichment of hospital food with micronutrient packs and supply of caloric needs, are essential to address these deficiencies in an appropriate manner and improve outcomes in patients. These reflect growing awareness of the importance of customized nutritional measures in the elderly to maximize recovery and quality of life (Figure 9.13).

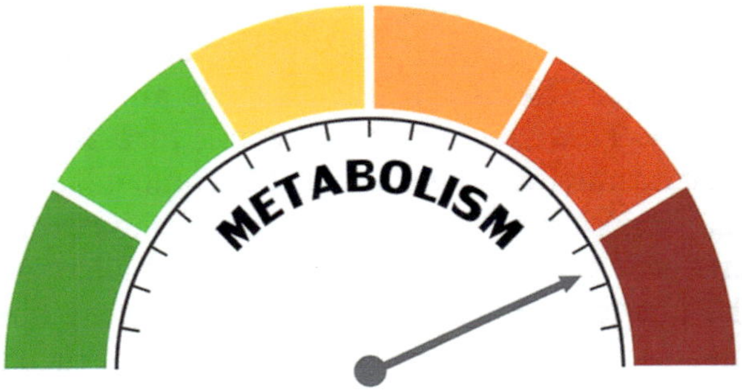

Figure 9.13. Surprising findings about metabolism and age.

Source: https://content.health.harvard.edu/wp-content/uploads/2023/04/223480bb-1ca3-4de4-88ba-b2fa11b11636.jpg.

9.5.2. Dietary Restrictions and Preferences

Dietary preferences and restrictions play a significant role in influencing the nutritional status of the elderly, particularly in deficiency of macronutrient and micronutrient. Over time, dietary patterns may be determined by an individual's condition of health, religion, or ethnicity. These dietary options have a powerful impact on nutrient intake, with many elderly individuals selecting low-sodium or low-fat diets in an attempt to manage chronic illness, such as hypertension and cardiovascular disease. However, these restrictive diets can have the side effect of leading to deficiencies in important nutrients. As an example, while a low-fat diet can be great for the cardiovascular system, it minimizes the intake of necessary fats, such as omega-3 fatty acids, that support brain activity and overall health in older adults. Consideration of these dietary patterns is integral to the development of effective interventions that will optimize nutrient intake and improve health outcomes in this population (Nnanna, 2025). Moreover, nutritional knowledge of the elderly person also exerts a significant influence on their food habits and operations. A hard-hitting study had reported that a large percentage of elderly participants were adequately knowledgeable concerning basic nutrition, with reference to their food choices. However, nutritional knowledge alone is not sufficient to guarantee avoidance of nutritional deficiencies. The study highlighted that the majority of individuals still suffered severe micronutrient deficiencies, such as vitamin B12, vitamin C, iron, and zinc. Consequently, the interface between food knowledge and actual eating habits requires targeted education programs that enhance awareness in conjunction with enabling older populations to make healthy and informed diet choices. Inscribing educational interventions to meet individual dietary constraints and the dangers that go with them is necessary in overcoming such prevalent deficiencies and promoting a better quality of life among seniors (Nnanna, 2025). Socioeconomic status may also further complicate the nutritional status of older people. Lower economic resources may restrict access to nutrient-dense foods, while cultural factors may define food choices less conducive from a nutritional angle. The dilemma continues to be in reconciling personal taste and limitations with the requirement for an adequately balanced diet that satisfies the macronutrient and micronutrient requirements of the elderly. In addition, one needs to acknowledge the fact that some dietary restrictions, although potentially useful in the management of particular health conditions, might not suit the integral nutritional demands required for health and vigor with advancing age. Addressing these relevant sociodemographic determinants is critical in understanding how to properly counter micronutrient deficiency, as studies reveal that inadequate intake of nutrition can lead to various other health complications, including cognitive impairment and weakened immunity, further justifying the deployment of optimal nutritional interventions specifically for elderly populations.

9.5.3. Socioeconomic Factors Affecting Food Access

Socioeconomic status greatly influences food access, and more importantly, in the geriatric population who are apt to have certain problems in relation to their nutritional needs. Economic constraints such as lower incomes and higher prices for foods can restrict access to nutrient-dense foods necessary for the maintenance of health in the elderly. Furthermore, the majority of elderly may be living on fixed wages that limit their purchasing capacity and lead them to choose quantity instead of quality when they purchase food. Therefore, micronutrient and macronutrient deficiencies are prevalent, leading to conditions such as malnutrition, dementia, and increased mortality. Socioeconomic dynamics extends beyond economics; they involve education, which affects nutritional knowledge and the ability to make fully informed dietary choices and therefore overall health in older adults. Transportation problems and food deserts further complicate the issue of food access for low-income older populations. The majority of older adults may not have reliable access to alternative means of transportation and therefore cannot access grocery stores or food markets with improved alternative food choices. This restriction leads to an excessive reliance on convenience stores or fast-food chains, which typically have highly processed low-nutrient foods. In addition, access to healthier food stores is typically determined by socioeconomic status; more affluent communities are more likely to have a larger selection of grocery store chains, whereas low-income neighborhoods suffer from a lack of these outlets. The combined effect of such barriers to influence tends to be articulated in below-optimal eating habits, as shown in research showing the correlation between access to quality sources of food and nutritional status among the elderly, reaffirming the imperative for systemic reform in the rectification of these inequalities and maximization of dietary intake. Incorporation of knowledge of such socioeconomic influences into nutritional assessments is valuable in averting malnutrition among geriatric populations.

Appropriate nutrition assessment, as emphasized in contemporary healthcare interventions, must consider not only food consumption, but also socioeconomic factors resulting in food-related challenges. Food security through interventions such as community nutritional interventions and improved transportation options can significantly impact the nutritional health of older adults. This concords with findings which demonstrate that careful nutritional evaluation should include socioeconomic data and the employment of nutritional screening as a part of clinical assessment, thereby allowing interventions to be appropriately targeted. By tackling the intricate interconnections between food availability and socioeconomic factors, healthcare professionals can more effectively combat the shortages that threaten the health of this vulnerable population, ultimately leading to better overall health outcomes among older adults suffering from nutritional deficiencies.

9.6. Strategies for Addressing Nutrient Deficiencies

Interdisciplinary treatment of nutrient deficiencies among geriatric populations involves dietary maximization, monitoring, and education. One of the primary strategies is screening for older adults' nutritional well-being to identify the deficiencies. This can be done by performing regular screening processes with dietary screening and biochemical analysis of the levels of nutrients. Besides that, personalized diet treatment based on needs, predilections, and comorbidities are the secret to overall improved well-being. For instance, type 1 diabetes patients may need special care for their diet; however, recent research indicates a lack of specific guidelines that are able to offer optimal support to the population (Sarteau et al., 2024). Thus, developing tailor-made nutrition programs that consider medical history along with current health status is able to maximize dietary outcome and subsequently enhance health. Another key aspect in nutritional management of deficiencies is attention to protein intake, particularly for older adults. Current revisions of protein needs for diet suggest that older individuals can gain benefits from increased protein intake, with recommended levels higher than the previously recommended 0.8g·kg·-1day-1, up to 1.0g·kg·-1day-1 (Morgan et al., 2023). This adaptation is an acknowledgment of the requirement for protein not just for muscle preservation but for general metabolic wellness in aging individuals. The inclusion of varied protein sources, both vegetable and animal, will help provide a balanced amino acid profile, which plays an important role in remodeling certain muscles and avoiding sarcopenia. Furthermore, training in protein timing and quality can also optimize the muscle health of older populations by enabling more effective nutrient utilization and maintaining an active lifestyle. Finally, the application of community programs can greatly minimize nutrient deficiency among the elderly population. Programs may involve nutrition seminars, cooking instruction, and counseling focused on improving dietary knowledge and enabling the consumption of healthier foods. Particularly, making healthy foods accessible and affordable is essential, as money and mobility issues can significantly hamper elderly individuals' capacity for gaining enough nutrients. Collaborations with food banks, meal delivery services, and health agencies are excellent means of providing nutrient-dense foods, particularly in rural areas. By fostering a community environment that is conducive and supports nutrition education and access, there is the possibility of significantly improving nutritional outcomes and bridging gaps among the geriatric population (Figure 9.14).

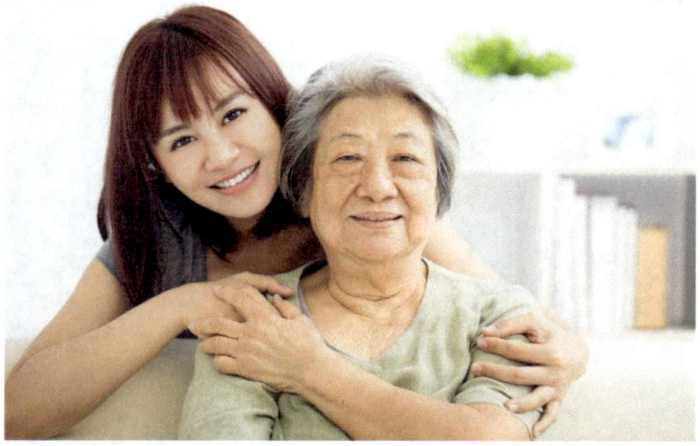

Figure 9.14. Nutritional deficiencies in older adults.

Source: https://sa1s3optim.patientpop.com/assets/images/provider/photos/2638004.jpg.

9.6.1. Nutritional Education and Awareness Programs

Nutritional awareness and education programs are fundamental to address the unique dietary needs of the geriatric population, particularly in the case of macronutrient and micronutrient deficiencies. These interventions provide older individuals with relevant information about their nutritional requirements so that they can make informed decisions about their diet. Tailor-made education programs can significantly influence older people's nutrition knowledge, especially within the context of increasing prevalence of chronic diseases in this age group. By attending to the distinct nutritional concerns of the elderly, such programs can bridge the gap between dietary advice and food consumption, thereby improving overall wellness outcomes and quality of life. Targeted nutritional education can also counteract the intricacies caused by polypharmacy, which is prevalent among elderly populations. As noted in some studies, the majority of older adults experience nutrient deficiency due to the interaction between medications and foods (Alharbi, 2012). Awareness of nutrition programs provides guidelines in the best way one can manage to prevent such interactions, which ensure proper nutrition for older individuals while on medication. Furthermore, the inclusion of interactive elements, such as meal planning and culinary demonstrations, may enhance the involvement and first-hand nutrition knowledge of participants. This approach provides a platform upon which older adults are actually able to seek out their food choices and learn about meal preparation for healthy diets. Furthermore, incorporation of nutritional education within community programs, such as retirement communities, has proven to be effective in dietary adequacy promotion among older adults. Research indicates that the majority of patients in such settings will likely suffer from poor nutrient intake, hence necessitating certain intervention strategies (Sarteau et al., 2024). Through monitoring of macronutrient and micronutrient needs, these interventions can potentially combat prevalent deficiencies in low dietary fiber and vitamin intake. Assembly of elderly in group meetings and peer-organized activities can also create a feeling of community and eventually re-emphasize the importance of healthy eating. Appropriate educational materials help elderly not only meet their nutritional needs but also gain increased social benefits that support healthy eating habits.

9.6.2. Importance of Regular Health Screenings

Routine screening is an important role in early diagnosis and management of nutritional deficiency conditions in elderly populations. As aging patients are likely to undergo physiological changes that affect their nutritional status, routine screening will be able to identify individuals who are at risk for deficiencies in major macronutrients and micronutrients. It is possible to early intervene through personalized nutritional guidance that not only can enhance overall health but also decrease the incidence of chronic disease since malnutrition is highly correlated with disease states such as sarcopenia and osteoporosis. It is worth mentioning that food and nutritional intake form the foundations of health, as witnessed in current studies on chronic and degenerative diseases interactive with nutrition, the significance of the inclusion of routine health screenings in preventive healthcare plans. Moreover, health screening measures of nutritional status provide vital information that guides healthcare providers towards effective nutrition interventions. For instance, the DETERMINE checklist, which is used to measure nutritional risk, has been shown to identify at-risk individuals across various age groups. While limited in scope, the evidence indicates that regular screening is able to recognize high and moderate nutritional risk, particularly among the oldest, old, who are likely to have a higher proportion with poor nutrient intake. Early detection and correction of these gaps can have a beneficial impact on energy and protein status, which are essential to maintain muscle mass and overall functional well-being in older adults. Therefore, the inclusion of health screenings in routine geriatric practice promotes an active approach to the management of nutrition-related health risks (Brunt et al., 1999). Even more important, regular health screenings not only facilitate clinical interventions but also allow older adults greater control over nutritional status. Encouraging screening participation encourages awareness and informs people about the importance of consuming well-balanced food with essential nutrients. Because most older adults can have difficulty in preparing balanced meals or accessing healthful food, timely health screenings can result in personalized education programs that encourage better diets. This future-directed approach is particularly relevant given the strong frequency of association between poor dietary behaviors and health outcomes for older adults, including weight change and chronic disease presence. As such, health screenings serve as a bridge, bridging geriatric populations to optimal interventions and support systems, effectively enhancing their nutrition status and quality of life (Brunt et al., 1999) (Figure 9.15).

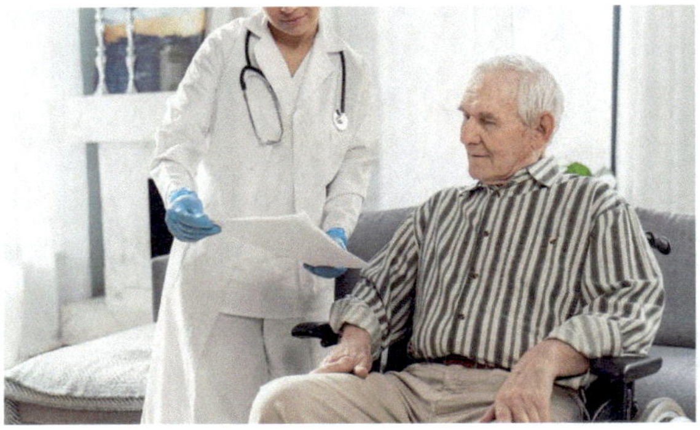

Figure 9.15. Regular health screenings in elderly.

Source: https://nycdocs.com/assets/images/blog/20241021073735.jpg.

9.6.3. Role of Dietary Supplements in Geriatric Nutrition

The practice of using dietary supplements in geriatric care has gained increasing significance in the context of the unique macronutrient and micronutrient deficiencies encountered in the elderly. Because of physiological changes with increasing body age, the body's capacity to utilize nutrients decreases, thus increasing the likelihood of nutritional deficiency. Dietary supplements, which can comprise vitamins and minerals, play a pivotal role in the avoidance of such deficiencies. A balanced diet of the required nutrients, particularly by supplements when diet is inadequate, has been established to play a crucial role in maintaining cognitive abilities and overall health among the elderly. Of significance is the prevention of neurodegenerative conditions, such as Alzheimer's, by the protective elements of micronutrients that illustrate how nutritional deficiencies are to be corrected with supplementation as one age, ultimately resulting in healthier and independent life later in years. In addition to cognition, supplements also contribute significantly to the management of other common geriatric deficiencies. Some micronutrients like Vitamin B12, iron, and zinc are often low in older adults, leading to adverse health consequences like anemia and compromised immunity. Therefore, the supplementation of targeted supplements—as suggested by newer studies—must be a part of the nutrition planning of geriatrics. For example, Berger et al., (2019) identifies that elderly hospital malnutrition has consequences on critical micronutrient deficits, where systematic supplementation regimens come into play. In incorporating multi-micronutrient administrations with hospital admission or as routine dietary practice, clinicians can ensure that older patients attain their basic nutritional needs, thereby averting resulting complications attributable to deficiencies. Furthermore, the demand for diet supplements during geriatric care should consider interaction and equilibrium in micronutrients. For all that supplementation can successfully correct specific deficiencies, imbalance or excess can be an issue. This comes into play particularly for older patients with existing illness since certain micronutrients will exacerbate or interact with medications. For instance, the relationship between amyloid protein accumulation in Alzheimer's disease and specific metal micronutrients illustrates the delicate interaction between dietary requirements and health outcomes (Staehelin, 2017). Hence, it is essential that nutritional supplement schemes for the elderly be well planned individually, considering not just the prevailing deficiencies but also the overall scenario of their lifestyle and health. This should lead to supplementation which will do them good in total and not worsen their condition.

SUMMARY

Correction of macronutrient and micronutrient deficiency prevalent among the geriatric population is necessary for overall improvement in their health and wellbeing. Aging is likely to lead to physiological changes that complicate nutrient intake and metabolism, and therefore, there is a necessity for a considerate nutritional plan that is attuned to the particular requirements of older adults. Studies have determined that malnutrition not only has consequences on physical health but also oral health, with a vicious cycle that may significantly reduce quality of life. Therefore, healthcare providers must prioritize nutrition as the core component of care for older adults, embracing interventions that ensure adequate intake of nutrients to avert frailty and other diseases of aging (Chan et al., 2023).

Furthermore, a detailed exploration of the relationship between food intake, oral health, and geriatric nutrition can significantly enhance the quality of life among older people. Poor oral health can lead to impaired ability to consume a balanced diet, which further leads to nutritional deficiencies. The substitutability of oral health and diet explains the need for holistic approaches that integrate both into elderly health care systems. By paying attention to these associations, medical professionals can strive to reduce the prevalence of malnutrition and promote overall better health outcomes among seniors (Chan et al., 2023). Finally, an emphasis on the gut microbiotas contribution to our health as we age is paramount. Studies have shown that optimal gut microbiome is linked with improved metabolic and cognitive functioning, facets often impaired in the elderly population as a whole due to lack of nutrition. The inclusion of dietary interventions that promote an increase in microbiota diversity, along with probiotics and prebiotics, represents a hopeful area of research for enhancing geriatric health. By making a commitment to a holistic model that incorporates nutrition and microbiome health, we can enhance the elderly population's potential to not only live longer, but to enjoy an enhanced quality of life into their elderly years.

Understanding the nutritional needs of the elderly is essential in the preservation of their health and functionality. Older adults go through unique physiological changes that influence their dietary needs, necessitating focus on both macronutrients and micronutrients. Macronutrients, i.e., proteins, fats, and carbohydrates, play important roles in the delivery of energy, preservation of muscle mass, and overall body function. As people get older, maintenance of lean body mass is more critical in order to avoid frailty, so proper protein consumption is crucial. In addition, dietary fats must be mostly unsaturated for the health of the cardiovascular system, and carbohydrates must be chosen based on their high fiber content for proper digestion and general metabolic well-being. Thus, macronutrient intake is a significant aspect of older adult diet planning since it has a significant impact on their physical well-being and quality of life. In addition to macronutrients, special attention should also be provided to the micronutrient needs of older adults since deficiency will result in serious health consequences. Micronutrients like vitamins and minerals play a crucial role in maintaining an array of biochemical processes and prevents chronic diseases. For instance, deficiencies of vitamins D and B12 are highly common among elderly people and may result in impaired cognitive performance and bone architecture. Studies reveal that low dietary intakes of certain micronutrients are related to frailty syndrome, which underscores the importance of a diet with an adequate supply of nutrients. Older people are also likely to have impaired absorption of some minerals, further complicating their nutritional status. A well-balanced strategy involving a variety of whole foods has been found to cut down these risks by ensuring adequate uptake of micronutrients, thereby leading to maximum health benefits in this susceptible group (Lorenzo-López et al., 2017). The effectiveness of nutritional intervention in reversing deficiency among the aged population emphasizes the need for individualized training modules for nutrition. Studies revealed that most nutrition and dietetics professionals report unmet educational needs in the areas of geriatric care, particularly among nutrition, healthcare, and community health fields (James et al., 2019). This means there is a need for ongoing professional development and research into the dietary needs of older people. Additionally, creating awareness of the dietary options in community settings can allow older people to make more suitable nutritional decisions. Furthermore, the implementation of nutritional screening tools, such as the Mini Nutritional Assessment, can help determine at-risk individuals for malnutrition. These practices collectively are directed toward promotion of nutrient consumption and overall health and functioning in older adults, with focal point on an active geriatric nutrition approach.

A CLOSER LOOK

MICRONUTRIENT NEEDS OF THE ELDERLY

Micronutrient needs of the elderly mean that advancing age carries with it both increasing vulnerability to deficiency as well as altered nutrient absorption. As metabolism slows and calorie intake often decreases, older adults must meet their nutritional needs with fewer calories, making micronutrient density crucial. Common deficiencies include vitamin D, vitamin B12, calcium, magnesium, and iron. Vitamin D is essential for bone health and immune function, yet synthesis through sunlight declines with age, necessitating dietary or supplemental sources. Calcium needs increase with age-related bone loss and osteoporosis risk (Figure 9.16).

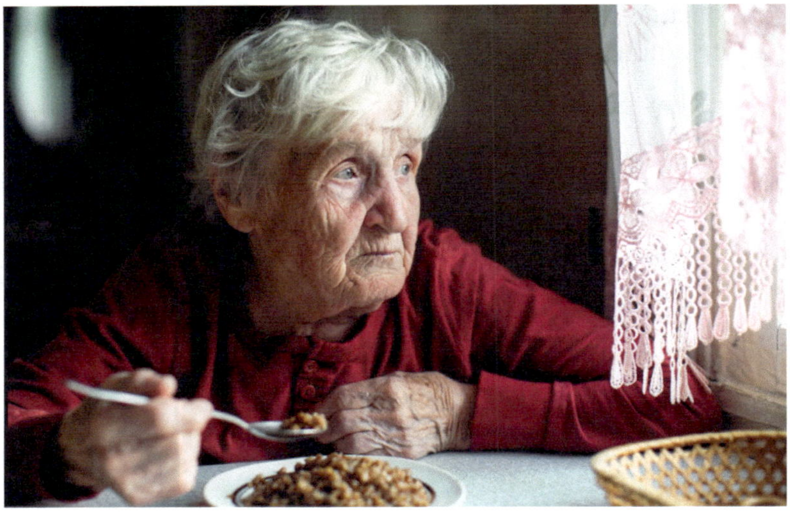

Figure 9.16. Impact of loneliness on micronutrient intake in aging adults.

Source: https://www.news-medical.net/images/news/ImageForNews_793586_17295187538424618.jpg.

Vitamin B12 utilization can be impaired by reduced stomach acid or drug-nutrient interactions, leading to dementia or anemia if left uncorrected. Magnesium supports cardiovascular and neuromuscular function, yet its intake is frequently suboptimal. Iron requirements vary by gender and health condition, but although menopausal women need less iron, older people with chronic illness can be at risk for iron-deficiency anemia. Zinc, folate, and vitamin A are also necessary for protection against infection, vision, and cell repair. A diverse diet that contains a good number of fruits, vegetables, whole grains, lean meats, and fortified foods can satisfy these needs. In some cases, supplementation is needed, especially when diet, absorption, or appetite limits consumption. Care of micronutrient status is an integral component of geriatric nutritional management, keeping energy intact, disease at bay, and healthy ageing in place.

REFERENCES

1. Deriemaeker, P., Aerenhouts, D., De Ridder, D., Hebbelinck, M., & Clarys, P. (2011). Health aspects, nutrition and physical characteristics in matched samples of institutionalized vegetarian and non-vegetarian elderly (> 65yrs). *Nutrition & metabolism*, *8*(1), 37. https://doi.org/10.1186/1743-7075-8-37(accessed on 12th July 2025).
2. Alharbi, O. M. (2012). Residents living in a retirement community are at risk for numerous nutrient inadequacies. https://core.ac.uk/download/61634083.pdf (accessed on 12th July 2025).
3. Rippin, H. L., Hutchinson, J., Jewell, J., Breda, J. J., & Cade, J. E. (2017). Adult Nutrient Intakes from Current National Dietary Surveys of European Populations. *Nutrients*, *9*(12), 1288. https://doi.org/10.3390/nu9121288(accessed on 12th July 2025).
4. Crowe T. C. (2005). Safety of low-carbohydrate diets. *Obesity reviews : an official journal of the International Association for the Study of Obesity*, *6*(3), 235–245. https://doi.org/10.1111/j.1467-789X.2005.00196.x(accessed on 12th July 2025).
5. Kinabo, J., Bader, E., & Palma, G. (2008). Nutrition country profile United Republic of Tanzania. https://core.ac.uk/download/pdf/11307195.pdf (accessed on 12th July 2025).
6. Banda-Nyirenda, D., Hâsken, S. M. C., & Kaunda, W. (2009). Impact of nutrition and fish supplementation on the response to antiretroviral therapy, Zambia: A literature review. Reducing poverty and hunger by improving fisheries and aquaculture www.worldfishcenter.org. https://core.ac.uk/download/pdf/6514806.pdf (accessed on 12th July 2025).
7. Beccari, T., Bertelli, M., Caruso, P., & Ceccarini, et al. (2022). Clinical assessment for diet prescription. https://core.ac.uk/download/539311437.pdf (accessed on 12th July 2025).
8. Berger, M. M., Pantet, O., Schneider, A., & Ben-Hamouda, N. (2019). Micronutrient Deficiencies in Medical and Surgical Inpatients. *Journal of clinical medicine*, *8*(7), 931. https://doi.org/10.3390/jcm8070931(accessed on 12th July 2025).
9. Rémond, D., Shahar, D. R., Gille, D., Pinto, P., Kachal, J., Peyron, M. A., Dos Santos, C. N., Walther, B., Bordoni, A., Dupont, D., Tomás-Cobos, L., & Vergères, G. (2015). Understanding the gastrointestinal tract of the elderly to develop dietary solutions that prevent malnutrition. *Oncotarget*, *6*(16), 13858–13898. https://doi.org/10.18632/oncotarget.4030(accessed on 12th July 2025).
10. Morgan, P. T., Witard, O. C., Højfeldt, G., Church, D. D., & Breen, L. (2025). Dietary protein recommendations to support healthy muscle ageing in the 21st century and beyond: considerations and future directions. *The Proceedings of the Nutrition Society*, *84*(3), 245–258. https://doi.org/10.1017/S0029665123003750(accessed on 12th July 2025).
11. Brunt, A. R. (1999). The relationship between the DETERMINE checklist, social factors, and nutritional risk in rural, community-dwelling, elderly women. https://core.ac.uk/download/38905182.pdf (accessed on 12th July 2025).
12. Mak T, Louro Caldeira S. The Role of Nutrition in Active and Healthy Ageing: For prevention and treatment of age-related diseases: evidence so far. EUR 26666. Luxembourg (Luxembourg): Publications Office of the European Union; 2014. JRC90454(accessed on 12th July 2025).
13. Castaño González, L. A., Churruca Ortega, I., González, T., et al. (2018). Celiac male's gluten-free diet profile: Comparison to that of the control population and celiac women. https://core.ac.uk/download/185553616.pdf (accessed on 12th July 2025).

14. Chan, A. K. Y., Tsang, Y. C., Jiang, M., Leung, K. C. M., Lo, E. C. M., & Chu, C. H. (2023). Diet, nutrition, and oral health in older adults: A review of the literature. *Dentistry Journal, 11*, 222–222. https://doi.org/10.3390/dj11090222 (accessed on 12th July 2025).

15. Choi, J. T., Hatch, G. F., Jalali, O., et al. (2021). Malnutrition in orthopedic sports medicine: A review of the current literature. https://core.ac.uk/download/643776758.pdf (accessed on 12th July 2025).

16. Demling, R. H. (2011). Nutrition, anabolism, and the wound healing process: An overview. https://core.ac.uk/download/28936579.pdf (accessed on 12th July 2025).

17. Eldeib, S. (2025). The role of early-life nutrition in preventing micronutrient deficiencies: Focus on vitamin D, omega-3, and iron during the first 1000 days & role of gum versus cow milk in toddlers' nutrition. *International Journal of Clinical Studies and Medical Case Reports*. https://www.semanticscholar.org/paper/37644517aa5cf1fa5cc0d526f950ea15cbc2c58e (accessed on 12th July 2025).

18. Fekete, M., Szarvas, Z., Fazekas-Pongor, V., Fehér, Á., Csípő, T., Forrai, J., Dósa, N., et al. (2022). Nutrition strategies promoting healthy aging: From improvement of cardiovascular and brain health to prevention of age-associated diseases. *Nutrients, 15*, 47–47. https://doi.org/10.3390/nu15010047 (accessed on 12th July 2025).

19. Carlo Agostoni, Jean-Louis Bresson, Susan Fairweather-Tait, Albert Flynn, Ines Golly, Hannu Korhonen, Pagona Lagiou, Martinus Løvik, Rosangela Marchelli, Ambroise Martin, Bevan Moseley, Monika Neuhäuser-Berthold, Hildegard Przyrembel, Seppo Salminen, Yolanda Sanz, Sean (J.J.) Strain, Stephan Strobel, Inge Tetens, Daniel Tomé, Hendrik van Loveren and Hans Verhagen (2010). EFSA Panel on Dietetic Products, Nutrition, and Allergies (NDA); Scientific Opinion on establishing Food-Based Dietary Guidelines. https://core.ac.uk/download/13781037.pdf (accessed on 12th July 2025).

20. Iddir, M., Brito, A., Dingeo, G., Sosa, S., Samouda, H., La Frano, M. R., & Bohn, T. (2020). Strengthening the immune system and reducing inflammation and oxidative stress through diet and nutrition: Considerations during the COVID-19 crisis. *Nutrients, 12*, 1562–1562. https://doi.org/10.3390/nu12061562 (accessed on 12th July 2025).

21. James, G. E. (2019). Professional development needs in nutrition and dietetics. https://core.ac.uk/download/227521177.pdf (accessed on 12th July 2025).

22. Johnson, S. L. (2016). Proportion of heart failure patients who meet criteria for malnutrition upon hospital admission based on ASPEN guidelines. https://core.ac.uk/download/268250816.pdf (accessed on 12th July 2025).

23. La Rue, A., McCaddon, A., Kant, A. K., Termanini, B., Greenwood, C. E., Fu, C. S., Rose, C. S., et al. (2005). Vitamin status and cognitive function in a long-term care population. https://core.ac.uk/download/pdf/3840573.pdf (accessed on 12th July 2025).

24. Lorenzo-López, L., Maseda, A., de Labra, C., Regueiro-Folgueira, L., Rodríguez-Villamil, J. L., & Millán-Calenti, J. C. (2017). Nutritional determinants of frailty in older adults: A systematic review. *BMC geriatrics, 17*(1), 108. https://doi.org/10.1186/s12877-017-0496-2(accessed on 12th July 2025).

25. Mattioli, A. V., Sciomer, S., Cocchi, C., Maffei, S., & Gallina, S. (2020). Quarantine during COVID-19 outbreak: Changes in diet and physical activity increase the risk of cardiovascular disease.

Nutrition Metabolism and Cardiovascular Diseases, *30*, 1409–1417. https://doi.org/10.1016/j.numecd.2020.05.020 (accessed on 12th July 2025).

26. Mendonça, N. M. P. (2018). Dietary intake, B vitamins, and health outcomes in the very old: Analysis of the Newcastle 85+ study. https://core.ac.uk/download/188733721.pdf (accessed on 12th July 2025).
27. Miller, T. L., Neri, D., Schaefer, N., et al. (2010). The effect of aging, nutrition, and exercise during HIV infection. https://core.ac.uk/download/pdf/8645052.pdf (accessed on 12th July 2025).
28. Nnanna, O. A. (2025). Dietary pattern, nutritional status, and micronutrient levels in an elderly population in Arochukwu local government area of Abia State, Nigeria. *International Journal of Science and Research Archive*. https://www.semanticscholar.org/paper/65e6db5b0f18cd3723c4930dbeed4f27449c8574 (accessed on 12th July 2025).
29. Reckow, J. (2012). The impact of time of day, sleep, and nutrition on age-related changes in cognitive performance. https://core.ac.uk/download/235077053.pdf (accessed on 12th July 2025).
30. Sarteau, C. A., Ercolino, G., Fruik, A., et al. (2024). Nutritional status, dietary intake, and nutrition-related interventions among older adults with type 1 diabetes: A systematic review and call for more evidence toward clinical guidelines. https://core.ac.uk/download/619687422.pdf (accessed on 12th July 2025).
31. Staehelin, H. B. (2017). Micronutrients and Alzheimer's disease. https://core.ac.uk/download/85209142.pdf (accessed on 12th July 2025).
32. Tardy, A. L., Pouteau, E., Márquez, D., Yilmaz, C., & Scholey, A. (2020). Vitamins and minerals for energy, fatigue, and cognition: A narrative review of the biochemical and clinical evidence. *Nutrients*, *12*, 228–228. https://doi.org/10.3390/nu12010228 (accessed on 12th July 2025).
33. Vermaak, E. (2013). The influence of a nutritional supplement on lung function and immune status of HIV-positive patients in the Mangaung metropolitan. https://core.ac.uk/download/222966441.pdf (accessed on 12th July 2025).
34. Wahyu, E., & Sari, Y. K. (2025). Nutritional status correlated with frailty among elderly. https://core.ac.uk/download/651466228.pdf (accessed on 12th July 2025).
35. Zeppa, S. D., Agostini, D., Ferrini, F., Gervasi, M., Barbieri, E., Bartolacci, A., Piccoli, G., et al. (2022). Interventions on gut microbiota for healthy aging. *Cells*, *12*, 34–34. https://doi.org/10.3390/cells12010034 (accessed on 12th July 2025).

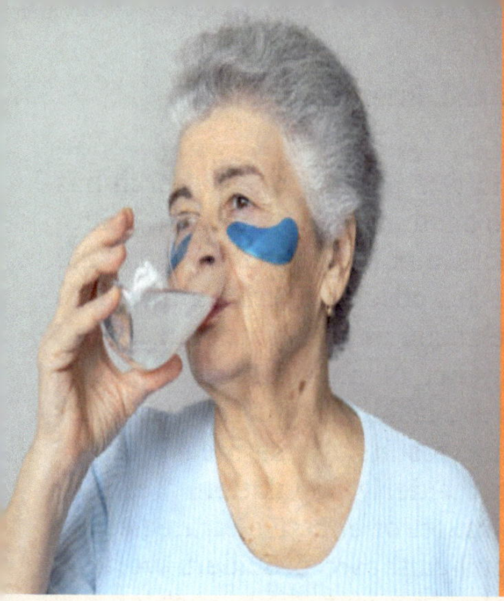

Chapter 10
HYDRATION AND FLUID BALANCE IN THE ELDERLY

Contents

Introduction

As the population ages in modern society, older adults are becoming the main focus of healthcare debates, particularly in the context of fluid balance and hydration. Age-related physiological changes accompany aging and have a significant impact on the body's ability to maintain proper hydration efficiently. Muscle waste, impaired kidney function, and altered thirst perception add to the older adult's susceptibility to dehydration. This is compounded by the prevalence of chronic disease and polypharmacy, not only demanding more fluid consumption but also impeding assessment of hydration status. Awareness of older individuals' vulnerability to dehydration is important as poor hydration has been linked with increased rates of morbidity and mortality within this population. It is important to study effective approaches aimed at enhancing fluid intake and addressing the barriers precluding older individuals from maintaining peak levels of hydration. Findings indicate that the prevalence of dehydration in older individuals has been approximated at 20%–30%, presenting an urgent need for a comprehensive assessment and management approach tailored to this population. Research has indicated that water-loss dehydration has been found to be linked to a laundry list of adverse health consequences, such as increased morbidity, disability, and mortality. It is important to comprehend the complex nuances of dehydration in older adults because these obstacles pose distinctive hindrances that physicians need to overcome. One of the main barriers is the social and institutional factors that may discourage alcohol consumption, such as fear of incontinence or physical limitations to accessing drinking sources. Overcoming such barriers in an integrative fashion might lead to better drinking habits, which might have an eventual impact on healthier results. These measures are particularly urgent given the projected demographic increase of the elderly population, a call for action for productive measures to prevent dehydration. The recognition of effective strategies for the assessment and avoidance of dehydration risk is important for healthcare providers working with older adults. Recent research emphasizes the utility of clinical presentations, such as dry tongue, as an accurate screening tool for dehydration among older people. The effectiveness of such assessment can guide timely interventions to reverse dehydration and ensure fluid balance, which is a critical component in sustaining health and enhancing quality of life among older adults. Empirical evidence indicates that if trained adequately, healthcare personnel can successfully apply these screening tools to screen for hydration status among older adults to provide an active management of fluid maintenance. With the advancement of knowledge in the area of hydration dynamics of older adults, more studies are required to enhance these tools and develop multi-faceted interventions aimed at this vulnerable population, thereby ushering in healthier aging in various settings (Vivanti et al., 2010; Cook et al., 2019) (Figure 10.1).

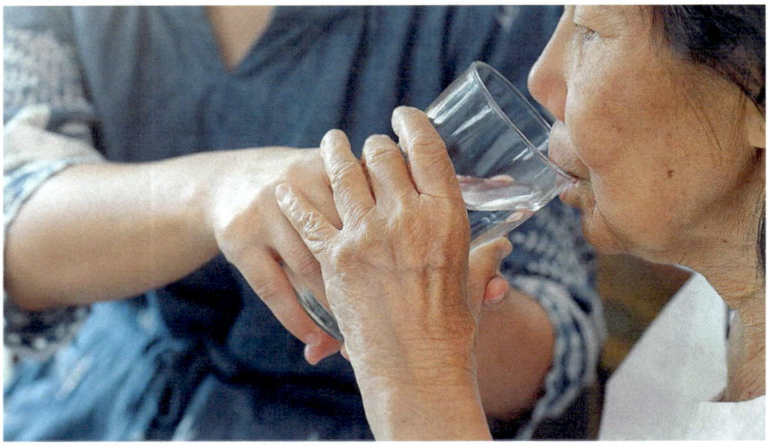

Figure 10.1. An elderly woman gets glass of water from a caregiver for hydration.

Source: https://cura.systems/wp-content/uploads/elderly-woman-gets-glass-water-from-caregiver-for-hydration.jpg.

Importance of Hydration in Overall Health

Incorporating regular fluid consumption, particularly water, into daily habits is the cornerstone of maintaining optimal hydration levels. Offering advice on individual fluid consumption may significantly empower older people to make good choices that enhance their hydration level based on dietary advice in a bid to enhance their quality of life. Furthermore, the link between chronic disease prevention and hydration cannot be overstated. Adequate fluid replacement ensures renal function by assisting in the efficient elimination of waste products as well as the conservation of electrolyte balance. As outlined in the current dietary guidelines, hydration has a role to play in the prevention of disease conditions like osteoporosis, which is still a major health concern among the elderly. Proper hydration aids the effective functioning of bone formation mechanisms and may avoid fractures due to osteoporosis (LeBoff et al., 2022). Hydration is also essential for maintaining blood pressure, thereby avoiding cardiovascular-related conditions. Proper hydration can allow the body's metabolism of fats and carbohydrates so that energy requirements are adequately met. Hydration enables digestion and absorption of nutrients, which is of extreme significance for the elderly who may have compromised digestive function. Fluid intake, in particular, can avert constipation, which is common in the elderly, thus providing total gastrointestinal health. Therefore, promoting water consumption and informing older individuals about the need for proper hydration can establish an environment of active health promotion. The contribution of hydration to health cannot be overstressed, particularly in the elderly population, which is faced with unique challenges to fluid equilibrium. With advancing age, physiological changes such as impaired sensation of thirst, reduced kidney function, and alterations in body composition enhance susceptibility to dehydration. Thus, older people can have an episode of water-loss dehydration ranging between 20% and 30%, associated with severe health outcomes, including increased mortality and morbidity. These must be treated with a proactive intervention to encourage fluid intake and reverse barriers to hydration in its quest (Cook et al., 2019). Through the encouragement of an appreciation of hydration's crucial role, caregivers and healthcare providers can help older adults better maximize health through improved fluid balance, critical to their well-being and health. Another area of hydration to consider is how it influences mood and cognitive status, especially in older adults. Research has shown that even mild dehydration affects the condition of mood so that there would be less vigor and increased sensations of fatigue or irritability (Vidal, 2015). This is particularly pertinent because cognitive impairment is already present in aging populations. Maintaining proper hydration would go a long way in supporting mental acuity and emotional stability, which are important determinants of the quality of life in the older adult population. Also, since emotions are intricately intertwined with physical health, promoting a positive mood through hydration can have a deep impact on cognition and social competency among the elderly. Thus, understanding the emotional aspect of hydration can be an integral part of devising overall care plans for the elderly. To be capable of fighting off the risk of dehydration, specific interventions must be employed that account for the unique needs of the elderly. Interventions can include identification of individual barriers to adequate fluid intake, such as mobility impairment, cognitive impairment, or social isolation, that lead to decreased drinking behavior (Cook et al., 2019). Care home initiatives, for instance, can include offering timed reminders to drink and convenient access to fluids. Encouraging social drinking sessions, where socializing is merged with hydration, is also a way of enhancing fluid intake and has the added benefit of promoting psychological health. Thus, the development of a stronger idea about the dualistic need for hydration in the elderly can contribute to improving their physical and mental health, finally leading to improved quality of life and lower health-related complications.

Overview of Fluid Balance in the Elderly

Fluid balance among the elderly is a significant concern due to changes with age in physiology.

As individuals get older, body composition changes, which in turn normally reduces the proportion of total body water. This change has the potential to cause dehydration to be more probable, and frequently, it will go unnoticed. The elderly will not react with normal responses of thirst and thus will be unaware of the necessity to consume fluids. Moreover, age-related alterations in kidney function may interfere with urine concentration by the body, thus complicating fluid retention and excretion. The outcome of such changes is heightened susceptibility to dehydration, which is apt to exacerbate health conditions such as urinary tract infection, confusion, and impaired physical functioning. Hence, the need for proper hydration becomes all the more crucial in order to promote overall well-being and prevent adverse outcomes in this population. The dietary recommendations for fluid intake are also essential because they guide older adults to better hydration practices. A study reveals that older adults drink water in amounts comparable to those of young adults and would equal 2.0 liters/day for women and 2.5 liters/day for men (Alexy et al., 2010). However, most elderly people fail to attain these suggested levels due to several factors, like reduced appetite, mobility, and intellectual impairment. This fluid underconsumption can generate many complications, like kidney stones and compromised heat regulation. Facilitating access to fluids, increasing fluid-containing food options, and promoting regular hydration habits are central strategies that caregivers and healthcare providers should embrace to enhance fluid intake in older people. Furthermore, the interplay between malnutrition and hydration is a central issue in older people. Malnutrition among older people is common, often augmented by changes in intestinal physiology and nutrient absorption precipitated by aging (Rémond et al., 2015). This malnutrition may compromise the body's ability to retain fluids, making dehydration more likely. In addition, declining sensory abilities such as taste and smell are likely to lead to reduced levels of thirst, further complicating hydration. The effects of inadequate hydration combined with malnutrition have the potential to introduce drastic health problems such as frailty and increased susceptibility to illness. Integrative dietary guidelines that recognize these complexities and address the unique nutritional needs of older people are required in order to produce successful strategies for fluid balance and overall health (Figure 10.2).

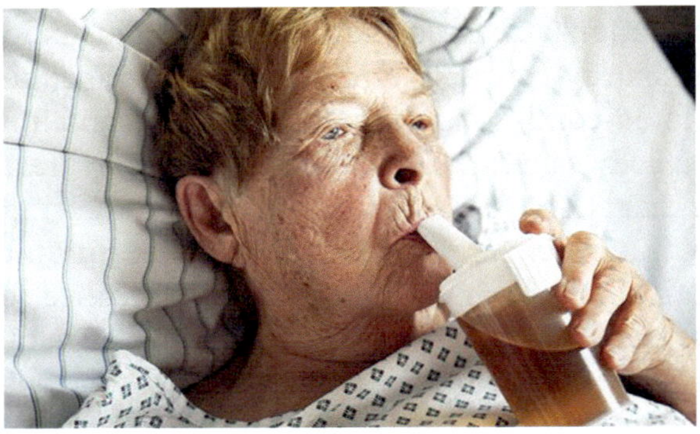

Figure 10.2. Fluid balance.

Source: https://dm1zcrsul8wju.cloudfront.net/sites/rcn_nspace/files/styles/tile_image/public/Assessing_and_documenting_fluid_balance_tile-iStock.jpg?itok=IBxTKAfY.

10.1. Physiological Changes in Aging

Physiological changes that occur with aging decrease the sense of thirst and reduce the body's ability to maintain water. As a result, elderly individuals are often unable to recognize their fluid needs, which will increase the risk of dehydration. This is augmented by other conditions such as chronic illness, drugs, and mobility impairment that will further impede fluid intake. Several physiological changes occur with aging that have a significant impact on fluid balance and hydration. Surprisingly, the aging kidney has a low glomerular filtration rate, reducing its ability to concentrate urine effectively and manage fluid balance. This impairment in renal function is likely to trigger alterations in fluid retention and increase susceptibility to dehydration, particularly in the elderly. Also contributing to the vulnerability are hormonal changes of aging, such as reduced secretion of antidiuretic hormone (ADH), which disables the body's capacity for water retention during fluid deficits. Older adults can be dehydrated subconsciously without the ability to compensate, increasing the health risks of fluid imbalance. Joined with the hydration issues of aging are alterations in gastrointestinal function. As the elderly gastrointestinal tract goes through chemical and mechanical changes, nutrient and fluid absorption can decrease, increasing the risk for malnutrition and dehydration. These changes include decelerated gastric emptying, decreased intestinal motility, and reduced digestion, compromising the optimization of nutrient and fluid intake. The consequences of inappropriate hydration are particularly challenging for the elderly, as it may lead to serious complications such as urinary tract infections, kidney stones, and even cognitive impairment. Data related to these physiological changes highlight the absolute need for personalized hydration practices, considering both fluid intake and absorbency capacity among the elderly, ultimately enhancing their well-being and health. Moreover, the causality of poor hydration and its physiological impact can further be explicated in terms of the risk of malnutrition. Research demonstrates that the elderly consume less fluid than recommended, particularly in the face of difficulty with swallowing that is common in conditions such as dysphagia secondary to stroke. Patients with dysphagia had a daily average of 781 ml of thickened liquids prescribed by their doctors, falling below recommended levels of fluid intake in hospitalized adults, according to a retrospective review. Not only does this deficiency exacerbate hydration deficits, but it also perpetuates a malnutrition cycle affecting more than one organ system. The resolution of these connected conditions through holistic hydration and dietary programs is important; this encompasses the provision of liquid intake monitoring methods, as well as individualized nutritional methods for the specific requirements of the aging gastrointestinal system, as previously mentioned (Murray et al., 2014; Rémond et al., 2015) (Figure 10.3).

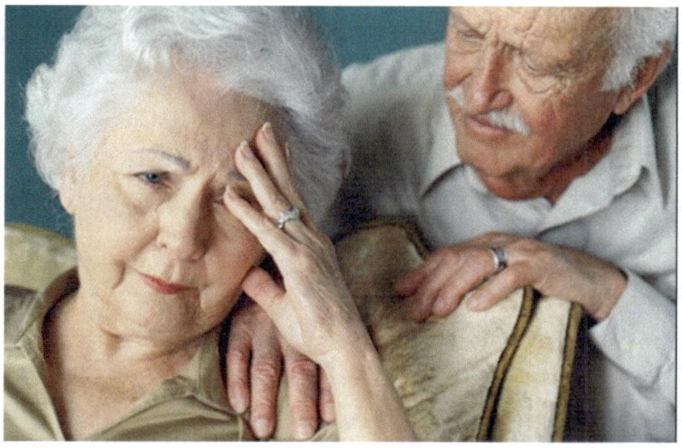

Figure 10.3. Psychological changes of aging.

Source: https://www.avensonline.org/blog/wp-content/uploads/2016/05/Psychological-aging.jpg.

10.1.1. Decreased Thirst Sensation

A reduced sense of thirst among the elderly is a significant challenge in the maintenance of adequate hydration and fluid balance. As age progresses, physiological alterations occur that lead to impairment of the body's thirst mechanism, rendering older people less responsive to the messages of the need for fluid ingestion. Decreased sensitivity of osmoreceptors is specifically known to contribute to this decreased sense of thirst, endangering low intake of fluid. This is of particular note in light of the crucial role that proper hydration plays in a variety of the body's processes, such as temperature regulation and cardiovascular homeostasis. Consequently, the interplay of these alterations with aging renders the older population vulnerable to dehydration, and there is a call for increased caregiver monitoring and anticipatory intervention to increase fluid intake in care regimes (Bak et al., 2016). The impact of reduced perception of thirst is extensive, considering the dehydration risk among successive generations. Evidence indicates that approximately 20%–30% of the elderly may experience water-loss dehydration, a situation readily overlooked due to the insidious presentation of early symptoms (Cook et al., 2019). Dehydration can have disastrous outcomes, including increased morbidity, mortality, and overall reduction in quality of life. Furthermore, common factors related to aging, including decreased muscle mass, decreased kidney function, and decreased cognitive function, also contribute to the susceptibility to poor hydration. These complications underscore the need for interventions that take into consideration the unique challenges of aging populations in having adequate fluid status, hence preventing improved health status among this vulnerable group (Cook et al., 2019).

To be able to challenge the threats of decreased sensation of thirst, specially implemented measures must be adopted in care settings. Detection of limitations on adequate fluid intake is most important; these are mostly physical disability, social isolation, and fear of incontinence that can discourage older individuals from drinking adequate amounts of water. It is important that caregivers take on a facilitative approach that not only identifies such barriers but also promotes a setting for hydration, such as ensuring that fluids are readily accessible and encouraging social drinking habits. These efforts can make a significant contribution to enhancing fluid intake and avoiding dehydration among the elderly. Directed studies research, such as that being fostered by the FP7-funded NU-AGE trial, aim to enhance effective nutrition approaches that address such problems and ultimately lead to healthier aging (Bak et al., 2016).

10.1.2. Changes in Kidney Function

Kidneys play an important role in fluid and electrolyte balance, particularly in the elderly, who predominantly endure changes in kidney function. With increasing age, renal mass is lost concomitant with a decline in glomerular filtration rate (GFR) and affects the body's ability to excrete excess water and maintain electrolyte balance. Decreased renal blood flow and altered renal tubular function are aggravated by age and cause this loss. Consequently, older people can be put at increased risk of both fluid overload and dehydration since their kidneys are unable to respond properly to changes in fluid intake. Furthermore, the impact of such physiological adaptation demands careful monitoring of hydration status, especially since an optimal hydration regimen can vary considerably in older people due to such renal adaptations. Also, the hydration status of older people is inversely related to kidney function and health. For instance, normal hydration facilitates a number of renal processes, including solute dilution in urine. Under normal hydration, individuals tend to have elevated urinary output and low concentration of urine when the body is properly hydrated, which reflects optimal kidney function. Research has indicated void number to be a simple yet effective biomarker of hydration status; increased urination frequency is generally found to correlate with maximum levels of hydration, leading in turn to enhanced kidney function (Burchfield, 2015). Familiarity with the intrinsic correlation between hydration and renal function within elderly populations is thus central to the development of effective health strategies to combat both dehydration and subsequent stresses upon renal function. Moreover, hydration status measurement with methods such as bioelectrical impedance is able to provide valuable information regarding kidney function in the elderly. Bioelectrical impedance analysis offers a noninvasive technique to measure body composition and the distribution of water, which can explain hydration dynamics

(Siervo et al., 2015). The use of this technique, particularly in older subjects, points towards the importance of accurate measurements of hydration. Because fluid balance impacts various body functions, including renal filtration and excretion, assessment of hydration status using the new technologies would complement the quality of overall health. Routine assessment of kidney function alongside hydration status assessment is an integral component for the promotion of fluid balance and avoidance of kidney-related complications among the elderly (Figure 10.4).

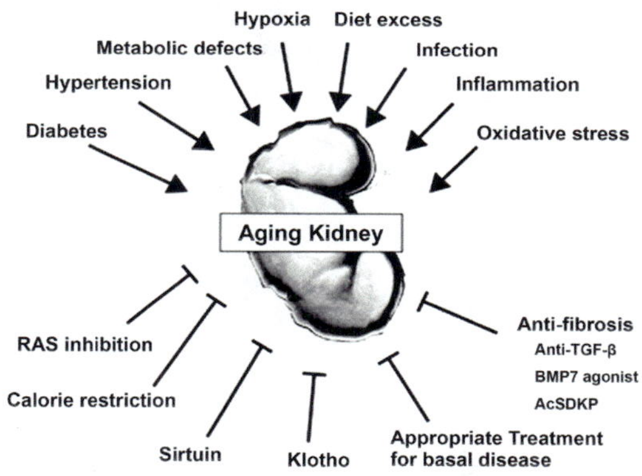

Figure 10.4. Pathophysiology of the aging kidney and therapeutic interventions.

Source: https://media.springernature.com/full/springer-static/image/art%3A10.1038%2Fhr.2012.159/MediaObjects/41440_2012_Article_BFhr2012159_Fig1_HTML.jpg.

10.1.3. Altered Body Composition

Aging results in incredible changes in the body composition that have a significant effect on hydration and fluid balance. The most dramatic change is the loss of lean body mass with simultaneous gain in fat mass. This remodeling decreases the total water content of the body, and this happens primarily in lean tissues. Consequently, the elderly person may acquire a relative insufficiency of body water reserves, and it is therefore necessary to monitor their hydration closely. Moreover, aging also brings along with it some physiological changes, such as decreased muscle mass and altered metabolism, and these can compromise the body's ability to hold and distribute water and make it more susceptible to dehydration (Bak et al., 2016). Recognizing these shifts in composition can assist caregivers and healthcare professionals with creating effective hydration plans specific to the needs of the aging population. Further, hormonal changes related to age greatly impact fluid balance in older adults. As one ages, there is a reduction in the release of anti-diuretic hormone (ADH) and other regulatory hormones, which disrupts the processes responsible for maintaining homeostasis. This disruption can lead to a blunted perception of thirst, resulting in failure among older adults to sense their own level of hydration. Aging has been found to reduce the sensitivity of osmo- and baro-receptors, the sensors for fluid shifts within the body (Bak et al., 2016). Aging reduces sensitivity, increasing susceptibility to dehydration and overhydration and making fluid management among the elderly difficult (Bak et al., 2016). As a result, physiological changes in hydration status ensue, and it is important to highlight hydration education and practice among the caregivers of the elderly to promote optimal hydration and prevent adverse effects of compromised body composition on health. In advanced stages of other illnesses, like cancer, the consequences of compromised hydration and fluid balance are all the more severe. Bioelectrical impedance vector analysis (BIVA) is a recently emerging technique in development as a promising tool to assess the hydration status of patients with advanced illness. There is evidence that hydration levels are proportionate to the severity of symptoms, associated physical findings, and survival. In other words, inadequate hydration can aggravate the symptoms and complicate the course of treatment, thereby creating a disease-dehydration vicious cycle. This highlights the necessity of ongoing monitoring of hydration status in elderly patients with varied health problems. With the application of the latest assessment methods, medical practitioners are able to manage fluid balance more effectively, optimize treatment modalities, and enhance the quality of life of older people with complex medical conditions.

10.2. Risks of Dehydration

Risks of dehydration in the elderly population are multifaceted and can significantly affect general well-being and health. As the physiological aging process continues, decreased sensation of thirst and alterations in the function of the kidneys can contribute to a great risk of poor fluid intake. This situation is compounded further in assisted living or nursing home settings, in which the individuals tend to be dependent on others for hydration. Evidence indicates that none of the health care environments exhibit frequent assessment of fluid intake by residents, where only 17% routinely utilize thickened fluid intake measures in patients with dysphagia, consequently leading to glaring hydration management deficiencies (Murray et al., 2014). Thus, this absence of monitoring can raise the risk for dehydration, leading to such complications as urinary tract infections, confusion, and even hospitalization, all of which pose additional dilemmas for health care professionals. Moreover, cognitive impairment that is typical with aging, particularly in illnesses such as dementia, can further complicate fluid balance. Numerous older people may not be aware of their fluid needs or clearly articulate their thirst and therefore attain seriously low fluid intakes. In others, staff caring for them may not know that they need to provide interventions. An actual case study illustrates how one family member observed the care staff properly implement hydration protocols despite the challenges posed by residents who do not want to drink or have challenges with drinking (Cook et al., 2017). This points to the necessity for tailored hydration strategies toward achieving fluid balance and averting the risk of dehydration.

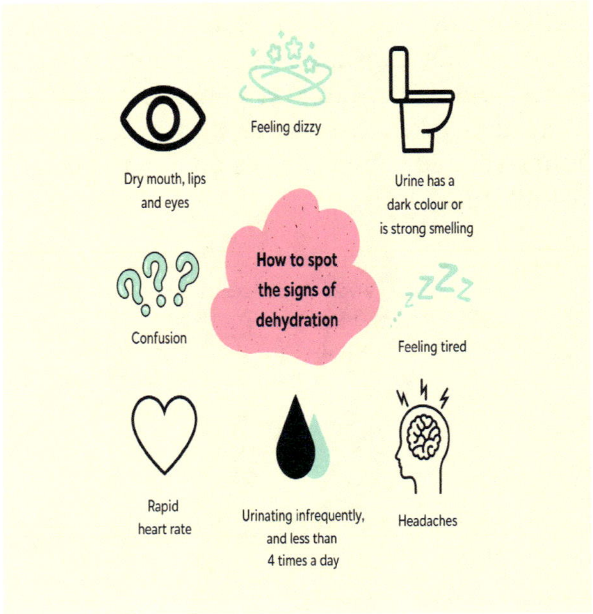

Figure 10.5. Symptoms of dehydration in the elderly.

Source: https://lottie.org/_next/image/?url=https%3A%2F%2Fapi.prd.lottie.org%2Fimages%2FSigns_and_symptoms_of_dehydration_9dde739a02.png&w=3840&q=75.

The implementation of evidence-based daily fluid goals is vital in ensuring vulnerable patients stay hydrated to preserve their health and quality of life. Psychological factors also play a significant role in fluid intake in the elderly, as well as physical dehydration complications. The desire to drink is influenced by social interaction, mealtime settings, and the palatability of fluids. In the majority of elderly people, the act of eating and drinking is done in groups, where socialization is able to either negatively or positively affect fluid intake. Organizations that take a special interest in being hydrated as part of the care, as noted in some research, are likely to experience better compliance among residents (Murray et al., 2014). Involving residents' discussion of fluid choice is likely to raise their acceptability to drink and enhance their hydration status. Lastly, it is necessary to overcome not only the physiological but the psychological barriers to being hydrated by reducing the risks of dehydration as well as improving health outcomes among the older population (Figure 10.5).

10.2.1. Common Causes of Dehydration in the Elderly

Familiarity with the common causes of dehydration in the elderly is crucial to avert the risks of the condition. The most significant among these is the physiological alterations that come with aging. The more they age, the less muscle mass and kidney function they have, making their capacity for water retention useless. Furthermore, the elderly tend to have a diminished sense of thirst, which leads to insufficient intake of fluids. These physiological changes lay the groundwork for susceptibility to dehydration, particularly when heat or illness strikes. Adequate Intakes (AI) of water by the European Food Safety Authority suggest 2.0 liters for women and 2.5 liters for men, applying the same values for the elderly category as well. These findings are found on urinary osmolarity and hydration status findings in various groups of people, ensuring an optimal intake to prevent dehydration (Alexy et al., 2010). However, it ought to be noted that these can vary considerably on an individual basis regarding activity levels, climate, and dietary habits. Differences need to be understood to develop specific hydration regimens that meet the unique needs of older populations to achieve the best health outcomes as they age Results have indicated that an incidence of water-loss dehydration in the elderly can be between 20% and 30%, and thus there is a need to utilize active management strategies to provide adequate hydration in this population (Cook et al., 2019). Another causative agent of dehydration in elderly patients is the status of chronic diseases and the associated polypharmacy that their therapy entails. Diabetes, heart failure, and renal insufficiency directly contribute to a person's fluid requirement and loss. Drug therapy, particularly diuretics and other fluid shift causes, predisposes to dehydration through enhancement of fluid loss. Moreover, the side effects of certain medications result in symptoms such as dry mouth or nausea, which hinder fluid intake. Awareness about these risks is important for health care workers and caregivers, as it is easy to overcome such challenges by individualized interventions and encourage fluid intake while combating intrinsic illness (Vivanti et al., 2010). Environmental factors are also a determining factor in dehydration among older adults. Inadequate environmental access to fluids or physical constraints can significantly elevate the risk of dehydration. Social constraints in the form of isolation or diminished motivation to drink are responsible for decreased fluid intake. Fear of incontinence can also lead some older adults to restrict fluid intake intentionally. Management of these multifactorial causes requires a multidisciplinary approach, for example, the creation of hydration-promoting environments and social interactions encouraging drinking. Through the application of specific interventions, like accessible fluids and frequent encouragement for older individuals to drink, the risk of dehydration can be greatly reduced, ultimately optimizing quality of life and health outcomes (Cook et al., 2019).

10.2.2. Symptoms and Signs of Dehydration

In older individuals, detection of signs and symptoms of dehydration is critical since their body's response to loss of fluids is very different from that of younger individuals. Older individuals have a blunted sense of thirst, which can lead to them not replacing lost fluids appropriately and being more prone to dehydration. Early indications can be slight fatigue, dryness of the mouth, and decreased urine output. As the illness progresses, more severe symptoms, such as confusion or dizziness, take center stage, and it is necessary for caregivers and medical staff to closely monitor these symptoms. These indicators are easily overlooked, particularly among elderly patients who may not be able to perceive their signals of thirst or complaints of distress. Failure to treat dehydration not only aggravates pre-existing health conditions but also can lead to disastrous consequences, including urinary tract infections and kidney problems, hence rendering the management of chronic diseases prevalent among the aged infeasible (Fusch et al., 2009). For instance, dehydration may lead to disturbances in electrolytes, resulting in weakness of the muscles and impairment of mental status. In the elderly, the signs may either simulate or worsen dementia or depression and lead to misdiagnosis and inappropriate management strategies. Furthermore, dehydration has also been linked to the risk of falls, which is a high-priority concern in the geriatric patient population because weakened muscles and cognitive alterations can compromise balance and coordination.

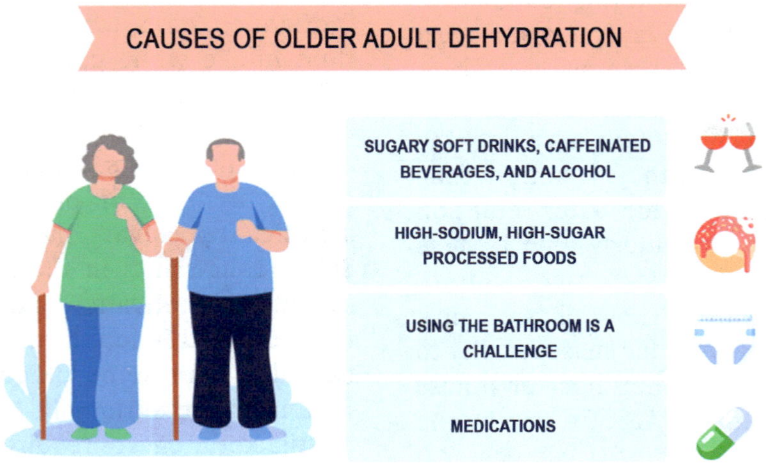

Figure 10.6. The link between dehydration and dementia in older adults.

Source: https://invitacryonyc.com/wp-content/uploads/2022/06/link-between-image-04.png.

The onset of dryness or sunken eyes may also be utilized as a visual cue that fluids are of the highest priority, reinforcing the need for regular monitoring in this high-risk age group. To better understand the physiological effects of dehydration in older adults, one must better understand how overall fluid balance is controlled in healthy subjects. When dehydrated, the body will typically employ compensatory mechanisms to hold onto water and electrolytes, like the augmented secretion of antidiuretic hormone (ADH). These control mechanisms may, however, be impaired by older individuals. A complete evaluation for hydration status will typically include monitoring of biochemical markers as well as clinical indicators. For instance, an increase in serum sodium level indicates a deficiency in body water and can be utilized by clinicians during diagnosis for dehydration. These values are significant since signs of dehydration will sometimes overlap with the symptoms of the common underlying medical diseases among elderly patients, making precise diagnosis difficult, but needed intervention unavoidable. Apart from hydration status detection, preventive measures must be considered to guarantee proper fluid consumption in the elderly. Education on the significance of hydration aimed at both patients and carers is critical in prevention. Encouragement of routine fluid intake without having to feel thirsty must be included in routine care processes among the elderly. Interventions such as the addition of hydrating foods, reminders to drink, and drinking variety can help to alleviate the risk of dehydration. Further, awareness of the relationship between dehydration, cognitive function, and physical functioning instills a sense of urgency into these prevention techniques. Although hydration plays a key role in overall health, fluid status in the older individual must be a priority of their care plan because they may be less capable of recognizing or stating their need for hydration (Figure 10.6).

10.2.3. Consequences of Severe Dehydration

Severe dehydration may have severe implications, particularly for the elderly, whose physiological compensation for fluid imbalance can be compromised. With advancing aging, processes such as deteriorating kidney function, compromised thirst perception, and cachexia can serve to enhance the risk of dehydration, leading to severe health complications. Research has shown that an impairment in hydration status is not only physically apparent but also psychologically apparent, as demonstrated by research that describes the effects of hydration on mood and cognitive performance. More specifically, acute dehydration has been shown to produce disturbance in mood, and this disturbance may contribute to exacerbating feelings of confusion and irritability, particularly in older persons already with some cognitive impairment or emotional instability. Hence, the effects of acute dehydration are far-reaching and extend beyond physical health, touching overall quality of life in the elderly. Physiological effects of acute dehydration in the elderly are wide-ranging and usually occur as elevated morbidity and mortality rates. Dehydration due to water loss, seen in cross-sectional studies, occurs in 20%–30% of the elderly, a figure that gives serious concern. It is also characterized by a rise in serum osmolality, a diagnostic value that also indicates the body's harmful effects of fluid loss. As dehydration worsens, the body becomes susceptible to such issues as urinary tract infection, kidney stones, and even acute kidney injury, which can instantly snowball into more severe health crises.

The intense stress placed on body systems, along with the intrinsic vulnerabilities of aging, underscores the need for tight monitoring of hydration status in the older population. Prophylactic measures are therefore paramount in reducing the prevalence and consequences of dehydration in the elderly group. Intervention against the multifaceted issues of dehydration in the elderly requires an integrative approach that recognizes individual and systemic barriers to proper hydration. Most older adults in care environments are confronted with challenges like the lack of access to fluids, anxiety about incontinence, and reduced social interaction that can lower the pleasure in drinking. Fluids can be increased by specific strategies that involve the care providers as well as the residents. For instance, interventions designed to create a conducive environment toward hydration are able to eradicate risks from low fluid intake because individuals will take more fluids when they are comfortable and when they feel their needs are being met and satisfied. Also, research operations, such as those covered in the FP7-funded NU-AGE trial, are aimed at investigating ideal dietary measures among older adults, with the aim of prioritizing hydration and fluid balance within elderly care, thus reducing the frequency of dehydration-related complications (Cook et al., 2019).

10.3. Importance of Hydration

Hydration is critical to general health, particularly among older individuals who are at a higher risk of dehydration. As people get older, the body also experiences physiological changes such as a decrease in the amount of total body water and a reduced thirst response, which predispose it to dehydration. It is not just a minor inconvenience; it can bring about significant discomfort to physical and psychological well-being and result in more significant health outcomes. Literature indicates that water-loss dehydration has been approximated to affect the elderly to the value of 20%–30%, and this emphasizes the importance of preventive hydration practice. Instilling these can include standardized hydration reminders and creating a fluid-conducive environment to facilitate fluid intake, which can be preventive in minimizing the risk of dehydration in the elderly (Cook et al., 2019). Furthermore, hydration status is highly correlated with emotional state, and this gives another strong justification for its importance in older adults. Research has shown that even mild dehydration could cause mood alterations, influencing such qualities as vigor, acuity, and sociability. Most especially, the effect of hydration on mood was highly visible in women since higher urine concentration was associated with undesirable changes in emotional states. It would seem from such research that adequate hydration has a significant part to play in ensuring mental health, particularly in older women who may see their mood changed by hormonal fluctuations or transitions in life. Thus, as a bodily need, hydration is likewise necessary for the intention of maintaining healthy-mindedness and high quality of life in the elderly (Vidal, 2015). It is crucial to recognize barriers to healthy hydration among the elderly and implement good solutions. Common obstacles include restricted mobility, loss of cognition, and physical limitations that make fluid access harder. Additionally, cultural factors can discourage frequent fluid intake, such as concerns about incontinence or discomfort when going outside. It is required to overcome these challenges via an integrated strategy, like training staff in residential care homes and enhancing social settings that are favorable for drinking. By persistence and clearing these obstacles, it is possible to enhance the intake of fluids, thereby reducing dehydration and its associated clinical complications. These prevention programs can result in improved health outcomes as well as greater independence among older people (Cook et al., 2019) (Figure 10.7).

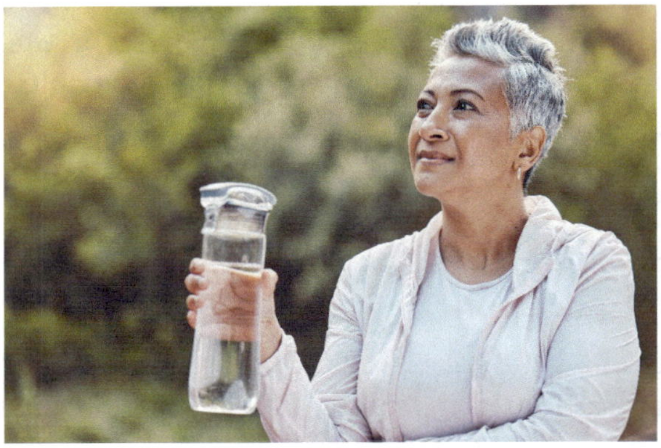

Figure 10.7. Hydration for seniors.

Source: https://www.humangood.org/hs-fs/hubfs/AdobeStock_559073243-1.jpeg?width=2000&height=1334&name=AdobeStock_559073243-1.jpeg.

10.3.1. Role of Water in Bodily Functions

Water plays a crucial role in various body processes that are essential in maintaining one's health, particularly for the older generation. Being a constituent element of cells, tissues, and organs, water facilitates biochemical reactions and medium for metabolic processes. They involve digestion, nutrient absorption, and waste elimination, all of which are highly crucial in sustaining life. In the older adult, physiological changes, such as decreased perception of thirst and impaired renal function, can compromise hydration status. These changes can damage the body's ability to regulate temperature, as well as its ability to balance electrolytes, thus leading to a predisposition to heat illnesses and other problems. By understanding the intricate dynamics between water and bodily processes, medical practitioners can further emphasize the importance of adequate hydration in this group, ensuring their overall health and well-being. Beyond its role in metabolism, water is critical for fluid balance, which is central to organ function and overall homeostasis. The body requires an optimal balance of fluids to support sufficient blood volume, and this, in turn, is important for transporting oxygen and nutrients to tissues. In older people, risk from dehydration is increased due to factors such as impaired skin turgor, diminished capacity of the kidneys to concentrate, and chronic disease that may influence fluid retention. Evidence shows that poor hydration can lead to severe complications like urinary tract infection and kidney stone formation (Hadley, 2017). Hydration thus becomes essential for the elderly as it not only minimizes health risks but also optimizes physical and cognitive functioning and provides a better quality of life. Additionally, hydration affects wound healing and recovery from disease, and thus it is especially significant among older people with medical issues. For example, proper tissue hydration is critical for optimal functioning of the wound healing processes, like granulation and re-epithelialization. Proper hydration levels enable an environment conducive to a moist wound, which helps in optimizing healing time and reducing healing complications (e.g., infection) (Rippon et al., 2016). Furthermore, older people have lower recovery rates, and impaired hydration status will exacerbate these lags and can lead to negative health consequences. Thus, a more effective strategy for hydration in health care settings can be a double benefit: greater overall hydration status and supporting healing processes in older people, which will ultimately be of long-term benefit to their health and recovery.

Through educating older people and their caregivers about body changes that impact the perception of thirst and fluid status, it is easier to emphasize the need for proactive hydration practices in care facilities. Repeated workshops and training sessions through community centers or residential care facilities can be a vital part of this educational process, instilling awareness that leads to a hydration culture among older populations. Thus, the education of the elderly can lead to increased fluid consumption and the reduction of problems with dehydration. Another effective method for enhancing the hydration of elderly individuals is through the intake of hydrated foods as part of their diets. Foods that have a lot of water, such as fruits and vegetables, make a significant contribution to overall fluid intake. The inclusion of foods like watermelon, cucumber, and oranges in meals can provide fluids in a palatable way. Moreover, soup and broth can be nourishing, hydrating meals, particularly for dysphagia patients. Making meals pleasing to the palate and properly colorful will stimulate appetite, with the bonus effect of spurring more fluid intake. Under these circumstances, caregivers and medical professionals must try to craft meal plans that meet nutritional requirements but focus equally on hydration. Through balancing the nutritional choice with the need for hydration, overall health outcomes among older adults can be improved, resulting in a richer and healthier life for these individuals. The virtue of repetition and the convenience of access in facilitating older adult hydration cannot be overstated. Developing a habitual pattern of drinking fluids helps to encourage the practice of drinking fluids at fixed intervals throughout the day. Health care providers can suggest certain times for fluid consumption, like before each meal or during some specific activity, in such a way that this becomes a part of their habit in the long term. Also, provision for readily available fluid is significant; provision of water stations and placement of liquids within reachable ranges will be able to bridge the gaps towards hydration. Assistive drinking aids and cups for those with mobility constraints can also help in attempts towards hydration. By the implementation of strategic means of integrating fluid intake into the patient's daily routine, caregivers can effectively enhance the likelihood of proper hydration, translating to enhanced general health and minimizing the dangers of dehydration among the elderly.

10.3.2. Impact on Cognitive Function

The link between cognitive performance and dehydration is particularly critical for the elderly. Cognitive impairments as mild as reduced attention span and reduced short-term memory, up to more severe changes in executive function and processing speed, have been linked to dehydration. Because older adults may have a diminished sense of thirst, they are unaware of their level of hydration, leading to unjustified reductions in cognitive performance. Not only is dehydration harmful to synaptic operations needed for thought, but it can also cause increased anxiety and mood disturbances, aggravating cognitive decline. Actually, a prevalence of 20%–30% of older adults could be experiencing water-loss dehydration, which suggests an urgent need for interventions to promote adequate fluid intake to maintain cognitive function in this population, since other factors such as polypharmacy and reduced renal function complicate the hydration problem further (Cook et al., 2019). In addition, acute adverse effects extend beyond transient cognitive function to long-term mental health and quality of life outcomes. Research has shown that even slight levels of dehydration can affect mood states, as supported by mood report variability in relation to hydration status. The Profile of Mood States (POMS) assessment proved that changes in hydration—indicated by urine osmolality and specific gravity—statistically significantly predicted cognitive acuity and vigor, especially in women (Vidal, 2015).

These findings emphasize the extremely significant interaction between hydration and cognitive performance, particularly in vulnerable groups like older adults. Interestingly, having adequate hydration may not only enable cognitive performance but also enhance the overall quality of life, which emphasizes education campaigns for fluid intake enhancement. Preventing dehydration-induced decreased cognitive function among the aged requires more sophisticated measures. Identifying individual and architectural barriers to underhydration can promote healthier behaviors. Simple solutions may involve altering care environments, using assistive technologies, or providing social drinking opportunities to promote consistent fluid consumption. Health professionals should strive to proactively evaluate hydration status and promote interventions according to individual need, especially in patients with cognitive impairment. These interventions have the potential to improve dehydration risk and may improve some of the cognitive impairments of poor fluid balance. With the demographic shift toward an aging population, researchers and clinicians need to conduct targeted studies and interventions to achieve cognitive resilience despite the presence of hydration impairments (Cook et al., 2019) (Figure 10.8).

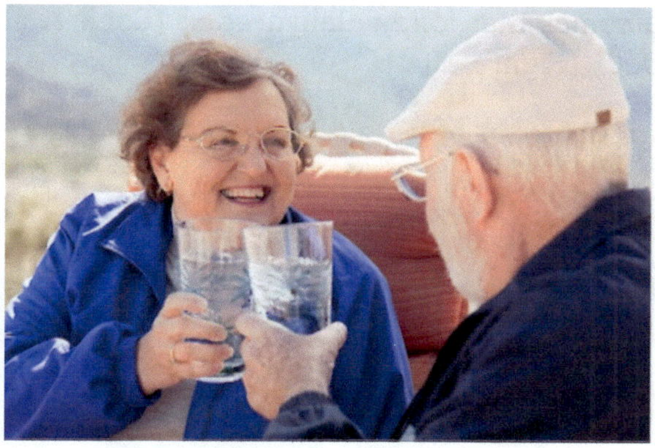

Figure 10.8. Hydration affects cognitive function in seniors.

Source: https://www.seniorhelpers.com/site/assets/files/445476/a_senior_couple_clinking_glasses_of_water.480x0.webp.

10.3.3. Effects on Physical Health and Mobility

The interplay of hydration and physiological health among the aging population is central to maintaining overall health and mobility. It may have a range of undesirable health effects like cognitive impairment, fatigue, and physical endurance loss, all leading to impaired mobility. For the elderly, who may already experience natural declines in physical function, superimposing the issue of dehydration on top can further elicit or exacerbate illness. Quoted in research, dehydration has also been associated with increased morbidity and mortality among the elderly, specifically due to exacerbation of chronic illness and reduced disease immunity (Vivanti et al., 2010). This connection emphasizes the importance of ongoing monitoring of fluid intake to protect against dehydration risks, thus promoting healthy aging and greater physical functioning. Other than its effect on general health, hydration plays a significant part in mobility among older people. As it maintains good hydration, the body can maintain the best muscle function and joint lubrication for effective movement and balance. Conversely, inadequate intake of fluids can lead to physical decline, such as weakening of the muscles, increased risk of falls, and limited independence—concerns that are vital to maintaining a high quality of life. Literature has established that elderly individuals are put at greater risk of dehydration during protracted heat, thus decreasing mobility further and leaving them susceptible to falls (Black et al., 2013). Therefore, adequate hydration is a key component in the preservation of mobility and the promotion of functional independence among the elderly population. Dehydration in the elderly also improves physical health, in addition to enhancing emotional and psychological state. It is the cause of confusion, irritability, and social withdrawal, which may discourage the elderly from participating in mobility-enhancing activities. The merit of hydration extends beyond the ability to survive; it is holistic in its approach to health, incorporating emotional fulfillment and social interaction. Facilities that treat older patients must have integral hydration policies that include education on the necessity for the intake of fluids, particularly in warmer months when hydration becomes an even more significant consideration (Black et al., 2013). By establishing conditions that prioritize hydration, caregivers can efficiently maximize the physical mobility and emotional well-being of their older residents and promote a healthier, more active way of life.

10.4. Recommended Fluid Intake

Guidelines for recommended fluid intake in older individuals are crucial to health preservation and prevention of dehydration, which may have critical implications among this age group. As the body gets older, physiological changes like decreased muscle mass and impaired kidney function predispose older adults to dehydration and fluid loss. Such changes can lead to an impaired response to thirst, often rendering geriatric patients unaware of their fluid requirements. Consequently, periodic assessment and promotion of adequate fluid intake have become cornerstones of geriatric practice, placing hydration at the cornerstone of healthy aging. Laying down dehydrations prevalence as purportedly standing at 20%-30% among the elderly lays emphasis on specific measures of fluid intake to counter probable complications such as morbidity and mortality (Cook et al., 2019). Environmental as well as individual water barriers have to be overcome by measures aimed at delivering the recommended fluid consumption among the elderly. For instance, the ability to access water sources physically can be limited by mobility issues, while cognitive impairments may hinder the experience of thirst. It has been proven that groundbreaking approaches, such as caregiver support in domestic settings, can optimize fluid consumption in older populations. The existence of resources like the Drinks Diary has been promising to measure fluid intake carefully so that interventions can be tailored to precise needs and tendencies (Jimoh et al., 2015). By enhancing hydration-conducive culture, health professionals can bridge barriers to consumption and encourage older patients to take a proactive approach towards fluid balance. Furthermore, varying guidelines dictate amounts of fluid intake required to maintain optimal hydration. The European Food Safety Authority and US recommendations advise 1.5–2 liters per day of water consumption in the elderly. These quantities, however, are based on the patient's health condition, food supply, and drugs that may affect fluid needs. Therefore, adopting an individualized method for assessment and recommendation of fluid needs in the elderly is critical. Constant monitoring, combined with teaching about fluid-containing foods and liquids, can maximize compliance with these recommendations. Lastly, keeping older adults in good hydration status can maximize quality of life in general, enable cognitive functioning, and reduce the risk of degenerative health outcomes that follow dehydration (Cook et al., 2019) (Figure 10.9).

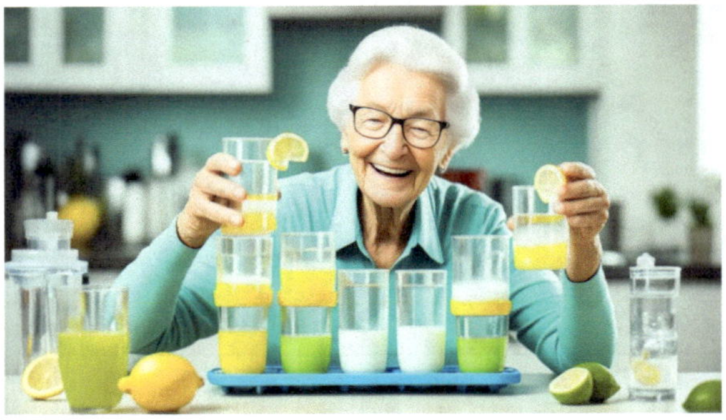

Figure 10.9. Recommended-fluid-intake-for-elderly-individuals.

Source: https://greatsenioryears.com/wp-content/uploads/2024/01/recommended-fluid-intake-for-elderly-individuals-1024x585.jpg.

10.4.1. Daily Fluid Intake Guidelines for the Elderly

It is impossible to overestimate the importance of adherence to guidelines for daily fluid intake in older people, considering that hydration plays a role in overall health and well-being. Older people have peculiar difficulties with fluid intake, including altered physiology to decrease the sensation of thirst and potential cognitive impairment that can interfere with their ability to perceive the need for fluid replacement. As per the European Food Safety Authority and U.S. National Institutes of Health recommendations, older persons should consume between 1.5 and 2.0 liters of fluid daily, though certain considerations like activity level, climate, and personal medical conditions should be considered when setting specific requirements. Adherence to these guidelines can easily minimize the risk of dehydration, prevalent in this age group and leading to severe health conditions, indicating the need for specific hydration strategies. To effectively monitor fluid intake among older age groups, novel methods are being explored to accommodate the daily needs of hydration efficiently. Research highlights the reliability of the self-completed Drinks Diary as a reliable method for assessing fluid consumption in older people living in care homes. The method was found to be highly reliable against direct observation and can accurately classify individuals into either consuming adequate amounts of fluids or not, based on established guidelines (Jimoh et al., 2015). Including simple assessment tools may assist in optimizing hydration care in the elderly. Furthermore, creating an awareness among caregivers and health professionals on the possibility of underreporting fluid intake using traditional monitoring methods is important since it directly affects the well-being of elderly individuals. Combined with monitoring fluid intake, education is an equally important factor in improving hydration among the elderly. Education of older adults on signs of dehydration, such as dry mouth or less urine output, can empower them to become more active participants in managing their fluid intake. Small interventions, such as facilitation of regular fluid breaks at social occasions or mealtimes, can have significant effects on intake levels throughout the day, particularly in the care environment. Notably, studies also indicate that higher levels of knowledge concerning hydration status are directly correlated with improved overall health and cognitive function in older adults (Burchfield, 2015). Consequently, the prevention of fluid intake advice on a day-to-day basis through education and targeted intervention can not only prevent dehydration but also improve the quality of life for an older adult.

10.4.2. Factors Influencing Individual Fluid Needs

The assessment of an individual's fluid needs in the older person is highly influenced by many physiological as well as environmental factors. First, physiological alterations that accompany progressive aging can lead to reduced perception of thirst and reduced renal function, both of which complicate fluid status. Older adults may not even sense their fluid requirements, and therefore, there is an increased risk of dehydration. Environmental conditions, such as temperature and humidity, also come into play, particularly in those with warmer climates, where water loss through sweating can be colossal. Also, the individual's level of physical activity will influence fluid requirements. People leading inactive lifestyles will likely need lower fluid intake than those with more dynamic lifestyles, implying intake needs to be tailored to the individual's lifestyle and surroundings. In addition to environmental and physiological factors, dietary intake also plays a major role in determining the amount of fluid needed in older people. Older people tend to experience problems of malnutrition, which affect their hydration status. As has been observed in the literature, alterations in the aging gastrointestinal tract can slow down the ability to absorb nutrients and fluid, compromising patients for both malnutrition and dehydration (Rémond et al., 2015). Furthermore, dietary practices can limit the consumption of fluids; for example, individuals prone to eating low-fluid foods or those who consume caffeinated drinks may suffer from overall dehydration. Therefore, the health practitioners must assess the dietary patterns of the elderly in a bid to create guidelines to promote efficient fluid consumption, thereby enhancing overall health outcomes and eliminating malnutrition and dehydration consequences. Also, medications and individual health status influence fluid intake among the elderly. Chronic diseases such as diabetes and heart failure might require individual fluid management. For instance, those with cardiac disease may be required to limit fluids for fear of edema as well as overload, while those with diabetes may find that their needs vary based on glycemic control and related hydration status. Furthermore, drugs can exacerbate dehydration through an increase in urine output or shifting of electrolytes. This complex interdependence of pharmacotherapeutic interventions and health conditions necessitates an individualized approach to hydration management, emphasizing the importance of ongoing assessment and adjustment of fluid intake in accordance with evolving health conditions and medications. Comprehension of these elements thus emerges as a critical determinant for ensuring optimal fluid balance and hydration in older adults (Figure 10.10).

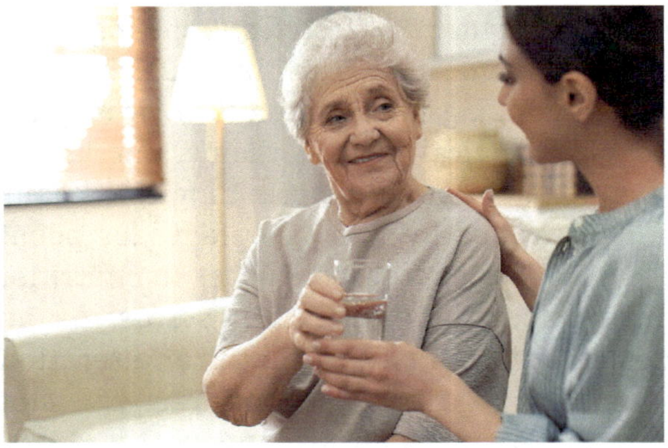

Figure 10.10. Factors influencing individual fluid needs.

Source: https://www.hugheshomecare.net/wp-content/uploads/2021/09/LARGE-bigstock-Young-Woman-Giving-Water-To-El-351487985-1.jpg.

10.4.3. Sources of Hydration Beyond Water

The worth of being well-hydrated in the elderly is not merely drinking water. Numerous foods carry high hydration value that can be included in a fluid intake regimen. Fruits and vegetables that are water-dense, such as cucumbers, watermelon, and oranges, provide hydration as well as vitamins and minerals essential for good health. In the elderly, who may have trouble with appetite or gastrointestinal function, the inclusion of these foods as part of normal meals can serve as a source of both nutrition and hydration. Pairing foods for hydration can stimulate consumption, alleviating dehydration problems, a particular concern in later years, as the body's physiological response to thirst will diminish effectiveness with increasing age. Other than fruits and vegetables, beverages can also play a big role in meeting the need for hydration. Non-caffeinated herbal teas, flavored water, and broths are great alternatives that can provide liquid intake without the ill effects commonly associated with caffeine or sugary beverages. Drinking high-electrolyte fluids, such as sports drinks or coconut water, may be beneficial as well, particularly in active elderly patients or those with diseases that put them at risk for fluid loss. These alternative sources of hydration can be tailored based on the individual's preference and medical needs, thus creating a more enjoyable hydration regimen that need not rely solely on pure water. In the identification and utilization of these alternatives, caregivers and healthcare providers can enhance care for fluid balance for the elderly. In addition, the relationship of nutrition to hydration identifies the necessity for intensified health intervention for the aging population. Malnutrition and dehydration have been evidenced to be common among older populations, more often accompanied by cognitive impairment and sociocultural factors that deteriorate their ability to receive adequate nutrition and fluid balance. The setting of guidelines to prevent dehydration supports the strength of individualized care plans that incorporate both nutrition as well as hydration needs, as noted in the ESPEN study by Volkert et al. (2019). Support of the intake of fluid-containing foods and beverages as part of the daily diet can significantly contribute to the condition of hydration, which affects the overall quality of life and enhances health outcomes in the elderly. Thus, medical practitioners need to embrace a multidimensional approach to hydration, incorporating source diversity as an essential part of their care plan.

10.5. Strategies for Promoting Hydration

Encouraging proper hydration in older people calls for a multidimensional approach specifically geared toward addressing the distinctive challenges characteristic of this group. Part of an effective strategy is boosting awareness among caregivers and physicians about the indicators of dehydration as well as the significance of regular fluid consumption. Effective training interventions can potentially equip residential care workers with the knowledge to identify at-risk individuals for dehydration and hence enhance their ability to provide effective intervention on time. Apart from that, using observational measures to monitor fluid intake can establish standards and alert early to potential issues. By establishing a culture that supports hydration, care workers are able to significantly decrease the risk of dehydration, which affects about 20%–30% of older people and is associated with increased morbidity and mortality rates (Cook et al., 2019). Apart from staff training, the use of individualized fluid plants in older residents can be a main method to increase fluid balance. Such plans should consider personal preferences, nutritional requirements, and such physical or mental impairment that may hamper fluid consumption. For instance, offering residents options for their preferred beverages, such as smoothies or flavored water, can stimulate interest in fluid consumption (Cook et al., 2019). Having realistic daily fluid intake goals, such as the ones applied in successful care homes, can motivate staff members and residents together to monitor hydration. Such personalized approaches not only respect autonomy but also foster an enabling environment where drinking is a shared activity, thereby rendering the experience interactive for all participants. Social interaction also plays an important role in encouraging fluid intake among the elderly. Older individuals living alone can have low enthusiasm for drinking independently, particularly those who live in residential care facilities where they witness minimal or no social engagement. In order to combat this, organizing group activity that includes hydration breaks can actually increase fluid intake while offering social interaction. Forms of communal hydration efforts can be in the form of social tea times or scheduled hydration-focused social events, where residents can enjoy a drink together. Engaging family members in planning hydration also helps in an empowering support system, which is experienced in care settings where families are part of giving hydration advice based on residents' personal choices (Cook et al., 2019). Through these social strategies, caregivers can render the environment more facilitative in ensuring elderly individuals reach an optimal state of hydration (Figure 10.11).

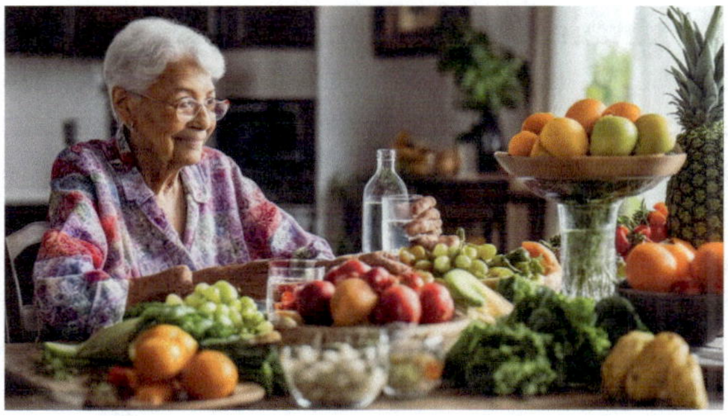

Figure 10.11. Strategies for promoting hydration.

Source: https://greatsenioryears.com/wp-content/uploads/2024/01/promoting-hydration-in-elderly-individuals-1024x585.jpg.

10.5.1. Encouraging Regular Fluid Consumption

Encouraging regular fluid intake in older adults is critical in providing proper hydration and overall health. With increasing age, physiological changes reduce their body water content, and they become less able to perceive thirst, placing them at greater risk of dehydration complications. Compounding these are other causative factors such as confusion, cognitive impairment, and the occurrence of other clinical states so that frequent hydration becomes a necessity in care settings to create proper hydration habits. The inclusion of structured hydration interventions in the older adult population has the potential to positively contribute to fluid intake and mitigate adverse consequences of suboptimal hydration. This will need to be done through an integrated approach with education of the health care professionals, placing significance on the pivotal role they play in promoting fluid intake among the residents, particularly those with cognitive and mobility impairments (Almeda et al., 2024). To encourage effective regular fluid consumption, habits of hydration must be integrated into daily activities in care homes. Evidence supports that interventions delivering fluids at a set time and consistently can have a substantial impact on an older individual's fluid intake. This can be supplemented by other complementary measures, including using verbal reminders and incorporating social interaction to provoke more engaging drinking episodes. A drinking-friendly setting, with hydration stations at hand and the offering of requested beverages, can also encourage residents' increased consumption levels. Further, continuous evaluation and monitoring of each patient's hydration requirements enables the identification of and reaction to fluid intake barriers, thereby meeting each resident's unique needs and limitations in terms of hydration (Cook et al., 2019). The full use of hydration support in care homes is at the heart of ensuring adequate fluid intake in older people. Care staff must ensure this through making hydration an integral part of daily health care and developing useful practices that ensure a balance between the preferences and needs of residents. These practices may include daily fluid therapy, innovative assistive devices that facilitate easier drinking for mobility-impaired residents, and exposing residents to hydration activities centered on wellness. By incorporating residents into such activities, staff can build a hydration culture that not only increases fluid intake but also increases socialization and quality of life. Bridging the particular barriers to fluid intake prevalent in older people will enable care homes to encourage an enabling environment, ultimately yielding enhanced health results and well-being for their residents (Cook et al., 2019; Almeda et al., 2024).

10.5.2. Utilizing Hydration Aids and Reminders

By recognizing the unique hydration challenges that older individuals face, including those residing in nursing homes, the application of hydration reminders and aids is a vital strategy. Cognitive impairment, such as diminished thirst perception and memory loss, typically also increases the risk of dehydration in this population. Organized hydration interventions, therefore, such as timed fluid delivery and reminders, become essential to the assurance of adequate fluid intake. By using visual cues, like purposefully positioned signs reminding residents to take fluids, awareness and encouragement can be greatly increased. In addition, given that numerous older adults might struggle with mobility impairment, aids to help them stay hydrated, like adaptive drinking cups and easy-to-handle water bottles, gain significance. By addressing both physical and cognitive barriers, these interventions have the potential to instill a culture of hydration to support the general well-being of nursing home residents (Almeda et al., 2024). The role of healthcare personnel in promoting hydration cannot be overstated as they play a pivotal role in initiating and maintaining such hydration interventions. Educational programs for staff that focus on hydration and offer education and support to motivate residents to drink in a timely fashion can have significant impacts on outcomes related to fluid balance. Further, it has been demonstrated that the integration of behaviorally based educational programs is effective, evidenced through a change in rates of urinary tract infections among older adults using multi-component interventions, such as education, audits, and feedback (Bath et al., 2019). Continued collection of feedback by working staff on residents' fluid intake behaviors can also promote a more reflexive mode of hydration care, thereby facilitating early intervention. This staff-management interface can make processes robust and robust in addressing the specific needs of the individuals, thereby enhancing the older residents' care environment. Lastly, resilience to the employment of technology can significantly contribute to building strength in the programs designed to promote hydration among the elderly. Platforms such as mobile phone applications that serve also as reminders for fluids or sensors on the wrist that monitor intake of fluids have the promise of creating personalized solutions that address unique requirements. Such technology not only assists alert caregivers but also enables family members and caregivers to track hydration levels in real-time. In addition, the combination of hydration monitoring with the present care management systems has the capability to develop an integrated approach to managing hydration and other health parameters, thus minimizing dehydration complications. As the healthcare systems continue evolving, utilization of such technology in elderly homes would complement traditional practices, leading to an integrative approach to elderly care based on the best fluid balance and hydration (Almeda et al., 2024).

10.5.3. Incorporating Hydrating Foods into the Diet

Incorporating hydrating foods into the diet is an essential strategy for maintaining optimal hydration and fluid balance, particularly among the elderly. As physiological changes, such as decreased thirst sensation and less efficient renal functioning, make older adults more vulnerable to dehydration, there is a crucial need to explore food sources that contribute to fluid intake. Foods with high water content—such as cucumbers, tomatoes, and watermelons—can significantly augment hydration levels. Moreover, these hydrating foods often offer additional health benefits, including vital vitamins and minerals that are essential for overall well-being. Therefore, incorporating these foods not only addresses hydration but also supports nutritional adequacy in older adults, fostering a holistic approach to maintaining health in this population. The method of integrating hydrating foods into daily meals can be both practical and enjoyable, thereby encouraging increased fluid consumption among the elderly. For instance, preparing soups, salads, and smoothies that highlight water-rich ingredients can serve as delicious alternatives to standard hydration practices. As hydration can frequently be neglected in older adults, making hydrating foods more accessible and appealing could influence their dietary choices positively. Moreover, educational programs highlighting the importance of these foods can empower older adults to make informed nutrition choices, thereby improving their overall health outcomes. The role of caregivers and family members is also pivotal in creating an environment that promotes healthy eating behaviors focused on hydration, making the process a collaborative effort that benefits the individual's quality of life. While the value of hydrating foods is clear, it is equally important to consider the overall dietary patterns in which these foods are situated. Research suggests that maintaining a balanced diet encompassing sufficient hydrating foods can enhance not only hydration levels but also mitigate risks associated with chronic diseases common in the elderly population. Adequate hydration promotes better cognitive function, immune response, and physical health, contributing to improved quality of life. Thus, when designing dietary interventions, healthcare professionals should aim to incorporate a variety of water-rich foods along with other nutrient-dense components to foster a well-rounded nutritional approach. This multifaceted strategy will not only support hydration but will also address the broader challenges of ensuring adequate nutrition among older adults, ultimately promoting longevity and enhancing daily living (Killer, 2014; Pock, 2019) (Figure 10.12).

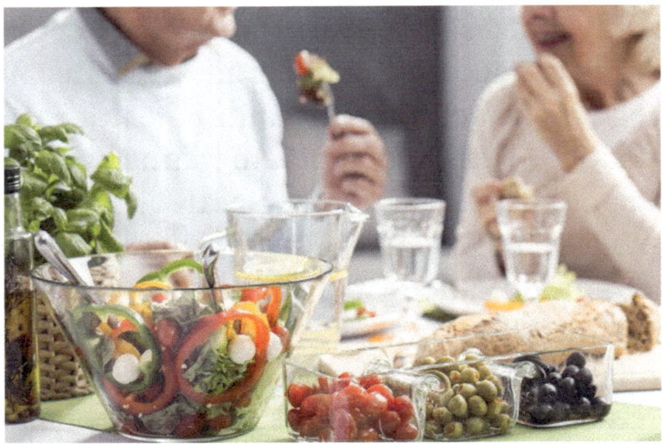

Figure 10.12. Hydrating foods in the diet.

Source: https://abbamt.com/wp-content/uploads/2019/06/shutterstock_426092389.jpg.

10.6. Role of Caregivers and Healthcare Providers

The caregiver and healthcare provider roles are important to the care of hydration and fluid balance in older adults. As individuals age, they will experience physiological changes that may hamper their ability to maintain proper hydration. All family members and paid caregivers play a part in monitoring fluid intake and spotting dehydration. Not only do they need to offer seniors access to water, but they should also encourage regular use at set intervals during the course of a day. In addition, healthcare providers should prioritize educational collaboration with caregivers in creating hydration regimens tailored to individual requirements. Integration of caregivers into care plans can potentially generate better outcomes, considering that they function as key liaison agents between the elderly and professional health care, indicating that overall hydration approaches must be optimized towards improved care. Beyond health-oriented approaches, psychological and emotional aspects of hydration are largely overlooked. Caregivers and health professionals must be made aware that older patients may resist the consumption of liquids due to mobility problems, mental impairment, or lack of motivation. The role of a caregiver extends beyond physical treatment and into motivation, where reassurance and support can be highly influential in an elderly individual's willingness to consume liquids. Apart from that, care providers need to engage caregivers in counseling them on the importance of hydration in order to better comprehend and guide the elderly in a proper manner. By ensuring proper communication and regular support, caregivers can create a positive atmosphere for hydration practices, which in turn promotes the overall fluid balance and wellness of the elderly. The high prevalence of diseases such as dementia complicates the duties of caregivers and care providers in terms of handling hydration. Patients with dementia typically have difficulty perceiving thirst and communicating the necessity for fluids, hence being at a high risk of dehydration (Mole et al., 2018). This calls for caregivers to be vigilant and in touch with monitoring fluid intake while engaging in developing tailored plans to promote hydration. Consultation with healthcare practitioners can aid in the development of customized nutrition and hydration protocols in addressing the unique complications resulting from dementia. Aside from this, the necessity of informing all stakeholders about the key indicators of inadequate fluid intake to provide interventions promptly cannot be overstressed. Through the partnership of the patient's family members, caregivers, and healthcare workers, such risks of dehydration can be mitigated, hence the quality of life among elderly patients with such challenges can be enhanced (Figure 10.13).

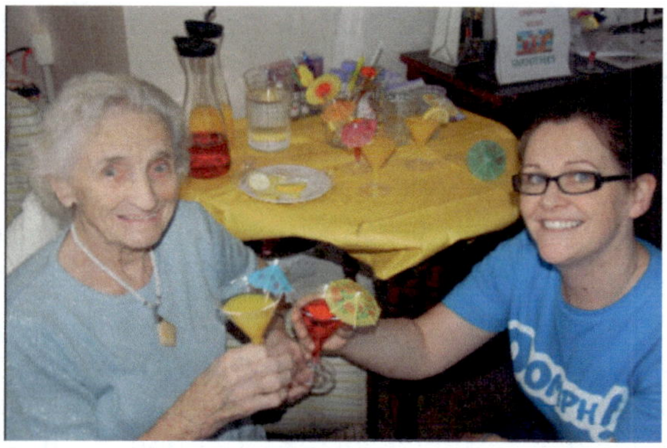

Figure 10.13. The role of caregivers and healthcare providers is crucial in managing hydration and fluid balance.

Source: https://external-content.duckduckgo.com/iu/?u=https%3A%2F%2Flookaside.fbsbx.com%2Flookaside%2Fcrawler%2Fmedia%2F%3Fmedia_id%3D1242153542563405&f=1&nofb=1&ipt=a91bffbbf97c00912e33f7166ac7f33aa0d9b644cf13886071297baa641b7ab6.

10.6.1. Monitoring Hydration Status

Appropriate monitoring of hydration status in older people is important due to the higher risk of dehydration in this age group. With advancing age, physiological alterations such as decreased awareness of thirst and alterations in fluid metabolism make it more difficult to evaluate hydration status. Traditional methods, such as body mass cannot accurately detect changes in hydration because they may be affected by a variety of factors that have no relation to fluid balance. This indicates the necessity for more reliable assessment tools that are able to detect dehydration both quickly and accurately. Current literature does show there are limited established methods of determining hydration status consistently in everyday environments. As recent studies have noted, no single gold standard for evaluating hydration has been widely used, so harmonizing effective monitoring practice between clinical and community contexts has been challenging (Bak et al., 2017). In a clinical environment, the identification of risk for dehydration can be an important factor in determining the health of older patients. New technologies have emerged that emphasize creating realistic and usable tools for monitoring hydration. For instance, recent evidence has suggested that markers such as dry tongue have high sensitivity and specificity for predicting dehydration in older patients. Particularly, data indicate tongue dryness is significantly related to impaired hydration status, detecting 64% sensitivity and 62% specificity in the study population. Such a straightforward screening instrument could allow healthcare workers to rapidly detect individuals at risk and implement early interventions, reducing consequent morbidity and mortality due to dehydration (Vivanti et al., 2010). However, their utility needs further evaluation in diverse populations before widespread use can be considered. Furthermore, the sophistication of hydration monitoring underscores the necessity of developing a multi-modal strategy that synthesizes various methods of evaluation. Although basic observational skills can be helpful to identify hydration status, clinicians must also deal with subjective patient complaints, in addition to objective measurements. Interdisciplinary collaboration may improve monitoring of hydration, allowing a comprehensive, multifaceted grasp of an individual's status. Integration of findings from present research may improve screening protocols by providing pertinent information that does not require significant resources. However, despite improvement, there is the issue of properly preparing staff to maximize the use of these tools. Training sessions on measurements of hydration and what they mean can promote a culture for closer monitoring in care settings. At some point, a greater understanding of geriatric hydration status can equate to improved health management and quality of life, and that hydration is a key priority in geriatric care (Figure 10.14).

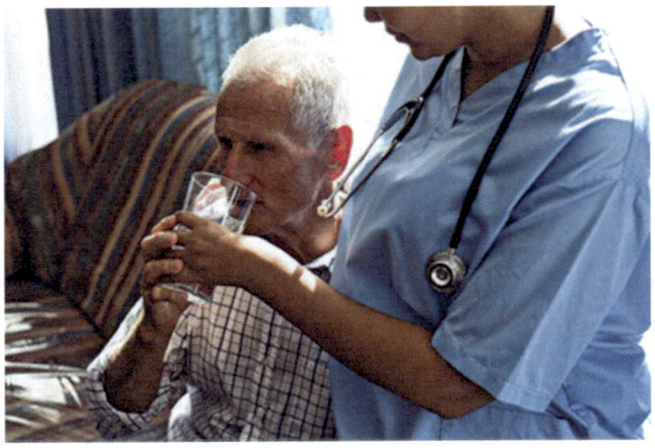

Figure 10.14. Hydration for the elderly in long-term care.

Source: https://hospitalnews.com/wp-content/uploads/2018/08/iStock-830315146.jpg.

10.6.2. Educating Patients and Families

Education of families and patients around hydration and fluid balance is extremely important in maintaining health and well-being, particularly in the elderly. Since the elderly also often experience changes in thirst perception and fluid overload, it becomes the responsibility of the healthcare providers to make them understand the importance of drinking fluids frequently. That kind of education is very important in avoiding dehydration, which can generate some serious health conditions, such as urinary tract infections, confusion, and hospitalization. To this aim, targeted education interventions are to be used to familiarize patients and families with the signs of dehydration and effective hydration interventions. Utilization of visual aids, educational pamphlets, and interactive questioning can aid in learning and retention of such important information, complementing the added value of care provided to this vulnerable population. Secondly, holistic education must address individual conditions and medications that could influence hydration among the elderly. For instance, certain diuretics and antihypertensives might heighten fluid loss or impair fluid absorption, causing the elderly to become reliant on healthcare services. Patients and their families must know about the synergistic interaction of drug regimens and hydration to facilitate their being able to monitor fluid more effectively. In addition, family members can be helped with the maintenance of open lines of communication with the healthcare provider, inviting them to be included in the decision-making process for hydrated care. This collaborative effort not only enhances knowledge but also fosters a support climate wherein family members become empowered to play an active role in the health of their loved ones, ultimately resulting in optimal outcomes and enhanced quality of life. In addition, climatic factors affecting hydration, such as temperature and humidity levels, also require appropriate attention in education. Older people residing in aged care are particularly vulnerable during weather extremes, the claim established by a study that highlighted cooling, hydration, monitoring, and emergency planning during heat waves as important (Black et al., 2013). This necessitates tailored educational programs that accustom patients and families to seasonal changes in order to enable anticipatory measures to control hydration needs better. Through such awareness of the environmental demands, older patients and their families can recognize when supplemental hydration becomes necessary, and thus the value of constant education as an essential component in promoting fluid balance and general well-being in the elderly. In addition, the evidence gathered from community nursing perspectives indicates that teamworking within interdisciplinary teams can be equally significant in care provision, illustrating the wider impact of educating carers and families (Gray et al., 2010).

10.6.3. Implementing Hydration Plans in Care Settings

Hydration plans within care settings are necessary to promote the health and well-being of older adults. Because the rates of hydration have strong effects on general health, the application of systematic procedures to ensure adequate intake of fluids is indispensable. Monitoring hydration must be given priority by care facilities through educating the caregivers about how to recognize the early signs of dehydration and monitor residents' fluid intakes regularly. As a result of increasing reports of heat stroke, particularly among the elderly, the incorporation of hydration strategies into emergency preparedness plans becomes necessary. For instance, facilities operating in regions that are prone to high temperatures must put in place extensive hydration programs characterized by frequent checks and customized hydration programs that are tailored depending on individual needs, which is corroborated by the study that identifies cooling and hydration as the major components of elderly individuals' care during poor weather conditions (Black et al., 2013). Staff participation is essential to the success of hydration programs in care settings. Structured training sessions must be created to highlight the necessity of hydration, knowledge of dehydration signs, and effective communication of hydration needs to residents and families. Interdisciplinary teamwork in the implementation phase will solidify the process so that dietary personnel, nursing personnel, and caregivers all work together to improve hydration. Furthermore, volunteers can assist with these tasks by offering additional help with monitoring fluids and encouraging water intake by residents. But this needs to overcome existing barriers, such as existing arrangements of volunteer support that will keep them from becoming actively involved in hydration programs. Involving all levels of care staff and volunteers allows for multiple means of hydration that can reduce the risk of dehydration among older residents significantly (Godfrey et al., 2013). Monitoring the success of hydration plans is required to ensure that they are sustained and flexible in care settings. Continuity monitoring should be done to assess the implementation of hydration practice, such as residents' health results and feedback from the staff and families. Homes can utilize tools like fluid intake charts or hydration diaries to track advancement and adjust. Moreover, continuous education and reminders of the optimum practices in hydration could increase staff sensitivity and compliance with these plans. Research has suggested that enacting formal hydration procedures can lead to a tremendous reduction in dehydration complications in older adults, thereby highlighting the significance of a precise and formalistic approach to hydration in geriatric care (Black et al., 2013). Adding these elements will not only improve compliance but ultimately contribute to an enhanced standard of care extended to this frail population.

SUMMARY

Healthy hydration and fluid status in the elderly person are paramount to support overall well-being and health. With the aging population undergoing typical physiological changes, they have a compromised ability to detect the sensation of thirst and thus poor fluid intake with consequent dehydration. A good understanding of factors responsible for hydration issues in the elderly person, including medication, mental impairment, and mobility limitation, can aid caregivers and health professionals in creating realistic solutions. These interventions can lower the risk of dehydration, hence improving the quality of life for the older population. The value of hydration is more than a move to respond to physical well-being; it spans through emotional and cognitive well-being to the interconnectedness of the workings of the body. Moreover, new research also shows the link between the level of hydration and mood in the elderly. Acute dehydration was determined to induce adverse mood changes and has significant implications for mental health, particularly in older females. For example, it was discovered that urine specific gravity and osmolality were predictors of changes in vigor and feelings in this group and that hydration status has a significant impact on emotional well-being. Through the use of fluid intake monitoring devices, such as self-report Drinks Diaries, staff can more easily gauge hydration levels and act more effectively in a timely fashion. These actions can prove highly effective in residential care, where proper monitoring is essential to preventing dehydration and sustaining residents' emotional, as well as physical, well-being (Vidal, 2015). Implications of proper hydration extend beyond clinical care to everyday care for older people. Interventions must be used to not only encourage proper fluid consumption but also to educate older individuals with information necessary to recognize the reasons hydration is essential. How effective new approaches, such as the Drinks Diary, demonstrate how successful tools can provide caregivers with accurate information regarding fluid intake and avoid dehydration complications stands as a result. Through prioritizing hydration as a core aspect of care, families and healthcare professionals alike can foster environments of physical and emotional wellness. Ultimately, addressing hydration and fluid balance through a comprehensive perspective is essential, underscoring the need for continued research and responsive actions created specifically for the unique requirements of the elderly (Jimoh et al., 2015).

Fluid balance interaction with overall health in older adults is of first priority since older age groups are particularly vulnerable to fluid imbalance. Dehydration, as physiological reserves get smaller, is extremely dangerous with complications such as decreased cognition, urinary tract infection, and increased morbidity. Effective monitoring and handling of fluid balance are vital for safeguarding the health of this group. Notably, planning for extreme weather event emergencies is a significant element in safeguarding the health of older adults. As outlined in new studies, centers are encouraged to implement total hydration protocols alongside cooling interventions during heatwaves, highlighting the extreme need for interventions especially created for the elderly population (Black et al., 2013). Furthermore, nutrition support comes along with hydration protocols, as adequate fluid consumption is generally correlated with total food consumption. A focus on nutrient-dense foods has the potential to optimize hydration, with greater importance being placed upon achieving dietary needs specific to later life. Specifically, identification of substitutive foods in vulnerable individuals to undernutrition and adequate meal planning becomes paramount (Coxall et al., 2008). With appropriate food intake, older people can successfully avoid the health implications of dehydration and enable better fluid balance. Finally, providing educational programs for caregivers and staff of aged care facilities is essential in the effective battle against these challenges. Spread of information regarding the dehydration signs and symptoms, accompanied by the implementation of proactive hydration measures, will be instrumental in enhancing the health status of older adults to an impressive extent. Facilitating frequent checks, fostering a water-use supportive environment, and employing strategic hydration techniques may lead to improved morbidity in elderly individuals. Focus on the inclusion of hydration in day-to-day care practice thus becomes an integral aspect in promoting longevity and well-being among this at-risk population (Black et al., 2013).

A CLOSER LOOK

CHALLENGE WITH HYDRATION FOR THE ELDERLY

Dehydration in older adults is multifactorial and complex, typically due to a combination of age-related physiological changes, comorbid medical conditions, and environmental or behavioral factors. The body composition of older adults also varies as they age—lean body mass and body water content decrease, reducing their fluid buffers. Concurrently, the sensitivity of the drive for thirst diminishes so that older adults are unaware of the sensation of thirst even when their bodies require fluids. Compounding this issue, renal function worsens with age, impairing urine concentration and water retention ability, thus making older adults prone to dehydration (Figure 10.15).

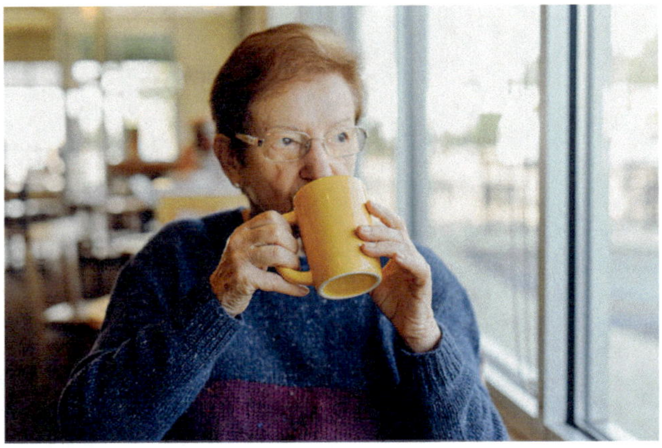

Figure 10.15. Challenge with hydration for the elderly.

Source: https://www.bda.uk.com/static/f2529a4d-ee41-40e3-a0c7e5827edaa0da/Older-Woman-Sipping-Hot-Drink-Tea-Coffee.jpg.

Underlying conditions such as diabetes, congestive heart failure, or cognitive impairment, such as dementia, can also undermine fluid balance and fluid-seeking tendencies. Moreover, some of the drugs consumed by older adults, including diuretics, antihypertensives, and laxatives, enhance fluid loss. Restricted mobility, fear of incontinence, and reliance on other people to deliver fluids also restrict fluids, especially in the nursing home or hospital setting. Elderly patients' dehydration is also associated with serious consequences such as confusion, urinary tract infection, kidney stones, constipation, impaired wound healing, falls and hospitalization. The identification of these risks underlines the urgency of early intervention and detection. Some of the interventions can be daily monitoring of hydration, administering fluids on a regular basis, and advocating for water-rich diets such as vegetables, fruits, and soups. Health workers and caregivers should be trained in recognizing early signs of dehydration, such as dry mouth, sunken eyes, or sudden drowsiness, in a bid to initiate early intervention. Hydration plans must be individualized, culturally sensitive, and adaptive to accommodate varying degrees of independence and cognitive function. Fluid balance throughout life is not merely important for physical health but also for maintaining cognition, emotional status, and quality of life in very old age.

REFERENCES

1. Mole, L., Kent, B., Abbott, R., Wood, C., & Hickson, M. (2018). The nutritional care of people living with dementia at home: A scoping review. Health & social care in the community, 26(4), e485–e496. https://doi.org/10.1111/hsc.12540(accessed on 12th July 2025).
2. Alexy, A., Armstrong, A., Ashraf, A., Aufderheide, B., Badaloo, A., Bagnasco, S., et al. (2010). EFSA Panel on Dietetic Products, Nutrition, and Allergies (NDA); Scientific Opinion on dietary reference values for water. https://core.ac.uk/download/13780775.pdf (accessed on 12th July 2025).
3. Almeda, E., Bandojo, M. B., & Diga, M. C. (2024). Effective hydration interventions for older people living in nursing homes. https://core.ac.uk/download/646458883.pdf (accessed on 12th July 2025).
4. Vivanti, A., Harvey, K., & Ash, S. (2010). Developing a quick and practical screen to improve the identification of poor hydration in geriatric and rehabilitative care. Archives of gerontology and geriatrics, 50(2), 156–164. https://doi.org/10.1016/j.archger.2009.03.003(accessed on 12th July 2025).
5. Rippon, M. G., Ousey, K., & Cutting, K. F. (2016). Wound healing and hyper-hydration: a counterintuitive model. Journal of wound care, 25(2), 68–75. https://doi.org/10.12968/jowc.2016.25.2.68 (accessed on 12th July 2025).
6. Bak, A., Greene, C., & Tsiami, A. (2017). Methods of assessment of hydration status and their usefulness in detecting dehydration in the elderly. https://core.ac.uk/download/84342531.pdf (accessed on 12th July 2025).
7. Bath, J., Dunham, O., Jones, L., et al. (2019). Effectiveness of behavioral interventions to reduce urinary tract infections and Escherichia coli bacteremia for older adults across all care settings: A systematic review. https://core.ac.uk/download/323892311.pdf (accessed on 12th July 2025).
8. Volkert, D., Beck, A. M., Cederholm, T., Cruz-Jentoft, A., Goisser, S., Hooper, L., Kiesswetter, E., Maggio, M., Raynaud-Simon, A., Sieber, C. C., Sobotka, L., van Asselt, D., Wirth, R., & Bischoff, S. C. (2019). ESPEN guideline on clinical nutrition and hydration in geriatrics. Clinical nutrition (Edinburgh, Scotland), 38(1), 10–47. https://doi.org/10.1016/j.clnu.2018.05.024(accessed on 12th July 2025).
9. Rémond, D., Shahar, D. R., Gille, D., Pinto, P., Kachal, J., Peyron, M. A., Dos Santos, C. N., Walther, B., Bordoni, A., Dupont, D., Tomás-Cobos, L., & Vergères, G. (2015). Understanding the gastrointestinal tract of the elderly to develop dietary solutions that prevent malnutrition. Oncotarget, 6(16), 13858–13898. https://doi.org/10.18632/oncotarget.4030(accessed on 12th July 2025).
10. Burchfield, J. (2015). Hydration biomarkers: Creating a user-friendly hydration assessment technique. https://core.ac.uk/download/72840632.pdf (accessed on 12th July 2025).
11. Siervo, M., Prado, C., Hooper, L., Munro, A., Collerton, J., Davies, K., Kingston, A., Mathers, J. C., Kirkwood, T. B., & Jagger, C. (2015). Serum osmolarity and haematocrit do not modify the association between the impedance index (Ht(2)/Z) and total body water in the very old: the Newcastle 85+ study. Archives of gerontology and geriatrics, 60(1), 227–232. https://doi.org/10.1016/j.archger.2014.09.004 (accessed on 12th July 2025).

12. Cook, G., Hodgson, P., Hope, C., Thompson, J., & Shaw, L. (2019). Hydration practices in residential and nursing care homes for older people. Journal of clinical nursing, 28(7-8), 1205–1215. https://doi.org/10.1111/jocn.14727(accessed on 12th July 2025).

13. Coxall, K., Dawes, E., Forsyth, E., et al. (2008). Applying the key principles of nutrition to nursing practice. https://core.ac.uk/download/4145815.pdf (accessed on 12th July 2025).

14. Murray, J., Doeltgen, S., Miller, M., & Scholten, I. (2014). A survey of thickened fluid prescribing and monitoring practices of Australian health professionals. Journal of evaluation in clinical practice, 20(5), 596–600. https://doi.org/10.1111/jep.12154 (accessed on 12th July 2025).

15. Godfrey, M., Smith, J., Green, J., Cheater, F., Inouye, S. K., & Young, J. B. (2013). Developing and implementing an integrated delirium prevention system of care: a theory driven, participatory research study. BMC health services research, 13, 341. https://doi.org/10.1186/1472-6963-13-341(accessed on 12th July 2025).

16. Gray, C. M., James, B., Lauder, W., et al. (2010). Developing community nursing practice: Promoting case management and skill enhancement to support shifting the balance of care. https://core.ac.uk/download/110605.pdf (accessed on 12th July 2025).

17. Hadley, M. C. (2017). Validity of 24-h void duration as an indicator of hydration status. https://core.ac.uk/download/127621296.pdf (accessed on 12th July 2025).

18. Killer, S. C. (2014). Nutrition and hydration implications for trained athletes. https://core.ac.uk/download/288377678.pdf (accessed on 12th July 2025).

19. Koszyczarek, K., Marańska, D., Różańska-Smuszkiewicz, G., et al. (2024). The way to a man's heart is through his stomach—Recommendations after heart surgery (cardiac surgical). https://core.ac.uk/download/620863106.pdf (accessed on 12th July 2025).

20. Périard, J. D., Eijsvogels, T. M. H., & Daanen, H. A. M. (2021). Exercise under heat stress: Thermoregulation, hydration, performance implications, and mitigation strategies. Physiological Reviews, 101, 1873–1979. https://doi.org/10.1152/physrev.00038.2020 (accessed on 12th July 2025).

21. Nwosu, A. C., Mayland, C. R., Mason, S., Cox, T. F., Varro, A., & Ellershaw, J. (2016). The Association of Hydration Status with Physical Signs, Symptoms and Survival in Advanced Cancer-The Use of Bioelectrical Impedance Vector Analysis (BIVA) Technology to Evaluate Fluid Volume in Palliative Care: An Observational Study. PloS one, 11(9), e0163114. https://doi.org/10.1371/journal.pone.0163114(accessed on 12th July 2025).

22. Pock, M. (2019). Lifestyle management for vestibular disorders. https://core.ac.uk/download/287121480.pdf (accessed on 12th July 2025).

23. Shane, A. L., Mody, R. K., Crump, J. A., Tarr, P. I., Steiner, T. S., Kotloff, K. L., Langley, J. M., et al. (2017). 2017 Infectious Diseases Society of America Clinical Practice Guidelines for the Diagnosis and Management of Infectious Diarrhea. Clinical Infectious Diseases, 65, 1963–1973. https://doi.org/10.1093/cid/cix959 (accessed on 12th July 2025).

24. Jimoh, F. O., Bunn, D., & Hooper, L. (2015). Assessment of a Self-Reported Drinks Diary for the Estimation of Drinks Intake by Care Home Residents: Fluid Intake Study in the Elderly (FISE). The journal of nutrition, health & aging, 19(5), 491–496. https://doi.org/10.1007/s12603-015-0458-3(accessed on 12th July 2025).

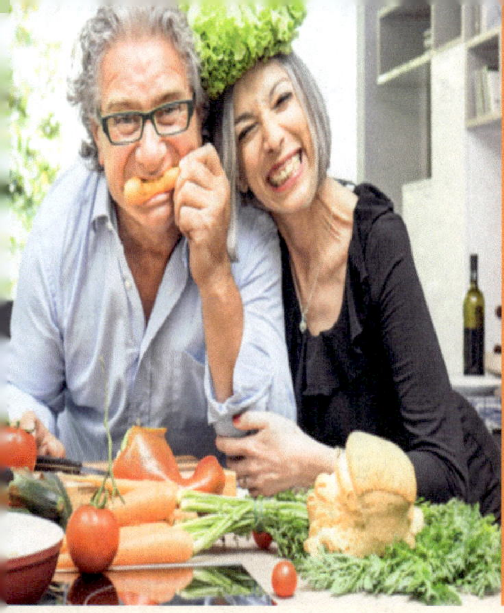

Chapter 11
DIETARY GUIDELINES FOR THE ELDERLY

Contents

Introduction

The elderly population is a matter of growing concern for health care systems throughout the globe, with nutritional needs increasingly significant in the overall maintenance of health. With increasing age, nutritional demands change owing to the metabolic alterations, decreased physical activity, and the development of chronic diseases that may have an impact on diet and nutrition. Therefore, developing a comprehensive framework of dietary guidance for the elderly population is crucial in order to increase their health and well-being. The guidance must include unique health problems prevalent in the geriatric population, such as the risk of cancer that has grown with time. The International Agency for Research on Cancer has put the incidence of approximately one in every five individuals developing cancer in a lifetime, stressing the critical role of nutrition as a preventive option for ageing populations (Bray et al., 2024). Besides, with increasing conditions of ageing like cognitive impairment with dementia, nutrition plays a role in prevention as well as treatment. Care planning for older adults requires consideration of the interactions of nutrition and diseases prevalent in the aging population. Careful auditory and visual stimulation should be part of effective care strategies to preserve cognitive function and reduce the occurrence of delirium in the elderly. Research indicates that malnutrition, often a product of inadequate dietary consumption, can bring about deteriorated physical and mental well-being among the elderly, and as such, it is important that such guidelines contain aspects that assure both physical health and mental capacity (Livingston et al., 2020). In crafting these nutrition guidelines, it is essential to prioritize foods that are not only nutrient-dense but also easy to cook and consume, given the potential limitations that some of the older individuals may have due to mobility or dental problems. Prioritizing whole foods that are dense in important vitamins and minerals while restricting highly processed foods can enable nutrition guidelines to champion healthier results among the older population. Regular assessment of individual dietary habits and needs is essential to make interventions suitably optimized. Ultimately, a well-formulated diet can enhance longevity and quality of life in the elderly, appropriately highlighting that optimal nutrition is responsible for successful aging (Figure 11.1).

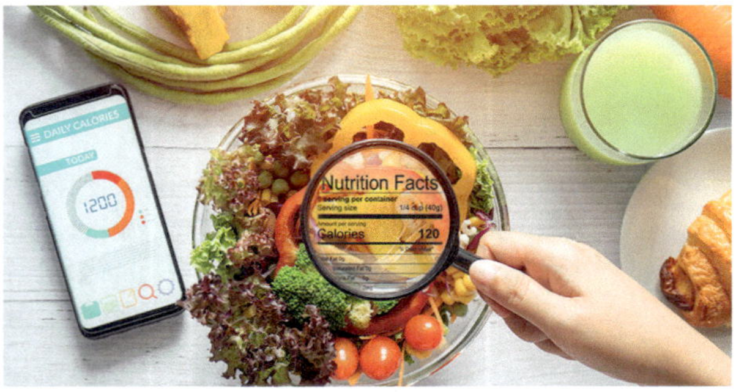

Figure 11.1. Dietary guidelines for the elderly.

Source: https://www.nmamilife.com/wp-content/uploads/2020/10/1-oct-blog-.png.

Importance of Nutrition in Elderly Health

Nutrition has a critical function in preserving health and quality of life among the elderly, considering it has a profound effect on many physiological and psychological processes involved in aging. Elderly individuals have distinctive dietary requirements that are different from younger people because of the altered metabolism, loss of appetite, and possible long-term disease states. Adequate consumption of nutrients, both macronutrients such as carbohydrates, proteins, and fats, and micronutrients such as vitamins and minerals, particularly calcium and vitamin D, plays a critical role in sustaining the energy level, maintaining muscle mass, as well as brain functioning. Moreover, osteoporosis prevention and maintenance of bone health also rely on these micronutrients. A better understanding of these nutritional requirements promotes self-care of health and increases the quality of life of the older population, thus reducing the risk of malnutrition-related morbidity. The importance of nutrition in preventing as well as treating chronic illnesses cannot be overemphasized, particularly among older adults who are likely to have multiple health conditions. Older adults are susceptible to chronic illnesses, including cardiovascular disease, diabetes, and obesity, which can be initiated or exacerbated by a bad diet. Adherence to dietary guidelines for the elderly would assist in preventing the onset and progression of these conditions. For instance, a diet rich in fruits, vegetables, whole grains, and lean protein supports heart health as well as manages blood glucose levels. Additionally, healthier eating favors weight control, which is a salient factor in preventing complications of obesity. This relationship between nutrition and chronic illness underlines the necessity of individualized dietary advice in maintaining the health and well-being of the elderly. Moreover, nutrition is not just crucial for physical well-being but also for emotional and mental well-being. Proper nutrition has been linked with improved cognitive functioning and mental health status, something which is of very great importance when one advances in years. Some nutrients, such as omega-3 fatty acids, antioxidants, and B vitamins, have been shown to be involved in reducing the risk of dementia and age-related cognitive decline in older adults. In addition, nutrition can influence states of mind, and insufficiency of proper vitamins can likely lead to increased instances of depression or anxiety. The inclusion of older adults in planning and preparing meals can also play a part in social contact, which is essential for mental well-being. Lastly, the focus on nutrition through detailed dietary guidelines not only promotes physical health but also overall quality of life among older adults, complementing the mutual dependency of nutritional status and mental health (Livingston et al., 2020; Bray et al., 2024) (Figure 11.2).

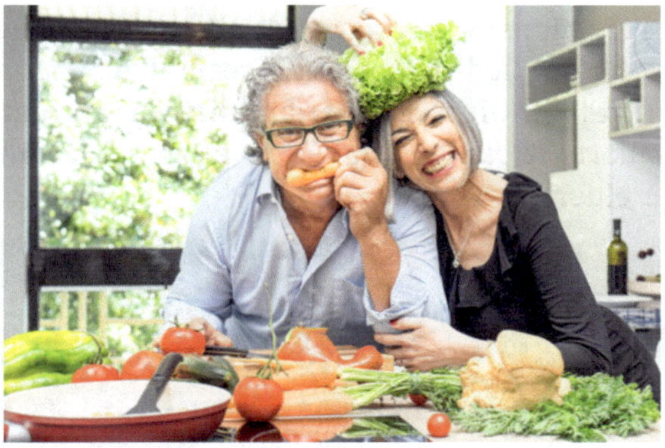

Figure 11.2. Nutrition in elderly health.

Source: https://www.gracebarkerhealth.com/files/2019/03/GettyImages-538650446-1_web.jpg.

Overview of Dietary Guidelines

Dietary guidance is a useful instrument of public health promotion in setting recommended food choices, nutrient consumption, and overall dietary styles to encourage healthier lifestyles. Dietary guidance finds support with scientific evidence of high merit and aims at lowering the risk of chronic disease, improving nutritional well-being, and helping people make better food choices. Particularly for the elderly, who typically face specific health problems such as malnutrition, osteoporosis, and cardiovascular disease, there are now specific dietary suggestions. Recognizing the fact that nutritional needs change with age, these suggestions provide specific advice for the elderly in order to ensure their health, provide the highest possible levels of energy, and promote well-being as a consequence. But it is essential that such guidelines are not only scientifically sound but also available and comprehensible to the target population. An important key to effective dietary guidelines is a triadic awareness-understanding-use among the target public. It has been discovered that while more awareness of consumers regarding dietary guidelines exists, actual consumption is generally lagging behind such awareness (Brown et al., 2011). This means that mere dissemination of the information will not be done, but individuals must also comprehend and apply these guidelines in reality. For older people, how the guidelines are delivered, for instance, through visual diagrams or a presentation at a simple level, can determine whether they will accept nutritional information or not. Thus, stress on the enhancement of comprehension and application of diet guidelines is imperative. There exists an urgent need for additional studies aimed at investigating how these guidelines can contribute to optimal promotion of behavior change in the elderly and optimal improvement of health outcomes among this population. It has also been established through research that the process of developing food-based dietary guidelines (FBDG) requires constant review to guarantee their relevance and effectiveness in the evolving public health environment. For instance, studying the applicability of FBDG to the elderly's needs, food likes and dislikes, and cultural context may provide the necessary data for their best use. Results from studies funded by public health illustrate the role of community sampling and dietary assessment techniques when implementing such guidelines (Madeira et al., 2016). Through continuous observation of consumer behavior and diet, public health authorities can improve guidelines in such a way that the elderly are better served, ultimately offering healthier dieting habits. Thus, an iterative process of guideline development and evaluation ensures enhancement in public health programs to ensure healthy aging and reduce the prevalence of diet-related diseases.

11.1. Nutritional Needs of the Elderly

The dietary needs of the elderly have come under increasing attention regarding their unique physiological and metabolic changes. As a person ages, his/her body undergoes a sequence of changes in the process of digestion, absorption, and use of nutrients and demands accordingly adjusted diets. For example, older people may experience loss of appetite and alteration in the perception of taste and therefore obstruct adequate nutrient intake. So, it is worth going out of your way to eat nutrient-dense foods that are rich in important vitamins and minerals, such as fruits, vegetables, whole grains, lean proteins, and healthy fats. Proper nutritional intervention can bring about the best possible health outcomes, enhance quality of life, and even encourage longevity, and prevent common age-related complications such as osteoporosis and muscle wasting. With the growing prevalence of chronic disease among older age groups, strategic meal planning is a priority. The findings of one recent study were that assisted living communities frequently failed to meet the 2015–2020 Dietary Guidelines for Americans, particularly in the variety of foods in major food groups. Of note, the gaps were largest in fruit and dairy foods, key in providing essential vitamins, calcium, and fluid. Additionally, the majority of menus had excessive saturated fat, sugars, and sodium—ingredients which are likely to aggravate such conditions as hypertension and diabetes. By making an in-depth examination of the nutritional content within such residential centers, the stakeholders are able to identify areas of improvement and regrade diets according to the dietary standards, thereby offering high-quality nutrients to the elderly residents that are consistent with their unique health needs (Schmir, 2018). Moreover, attention needs to be given to individualized dietary interventions that are compatible with individual choices and medical needs. Central to the framing of such interventions is the realization that social factors, such as the presence of companions during meals and cultural food choices, significantly determine eating behavior among the elderly. Integration of the social factors can help to propose a more holistic approach towards the elderly's nutritional demands. Moreover, as written in observations of pet aging, the same principles can be applied on a human scale, where good control of diet can extend life in animals, similarly it can be applied to extend health in the elderly.

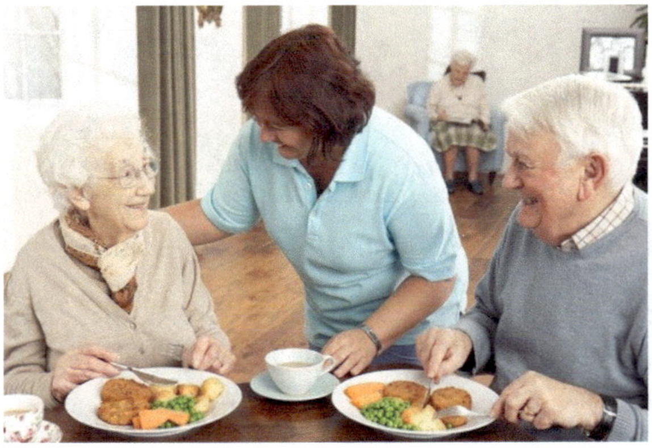

Figure 11.3. Importance of nutrition for aging adults.

Source: https://www.homecareassistanceedmonton.ca/wp-content/uploads/2018/12/Senior-Couple-with-a-Caregiver.jpg.

Thus, nutritionally evidence-based recommendations for older people should not only cover the composition of macronutrients but also create a stimulating and sociable dining atmosphere to maximize health benefits (Lumbis, 2018) (Figure 11.3).

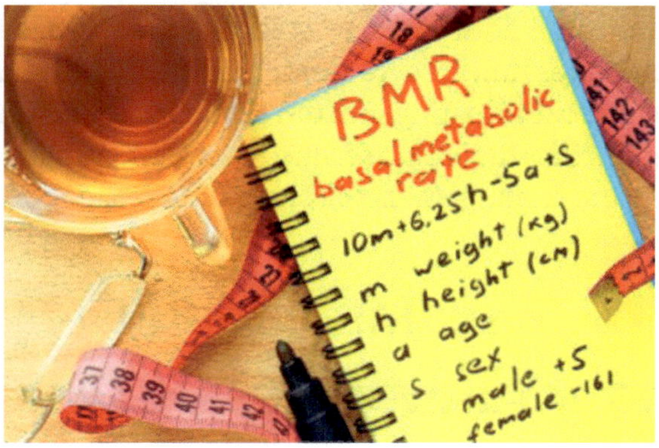

Figure 11.4. Basal metabolic rate (BMR) in nutrition.

Source: https://miro.medium.com/v2/resize:fit:360/0*HbdawLJBbcVNskeX.jpg.

11.1.1. Essential Nutrients for Older Adults

The need for key nutrients increases and becomes increasingly important as one gets older to maintain overall health and well-being. Elderly individuals often experience physiological alterations that may compromise the ingestion, digestion, and absorption of nutrients, thereby increasing their susceptibility to malnutrition. Not only does a functional impairment in the gastrointestinal tract influence the mechanical digestion of food but also the effectiveness of digestion, which may lead to deficiency of valuable nutrients such as protein, vitamins, and minerals. These limitations can be resolved through individualized dietary advice that would have a significant impact on the nutritional status of this group, thereby enhancing the quality of life. Dietary strategies need to be developed based on the unique needs of the elderly to suit their nutritional requirements, ensuring they receive the necessary nutrient intake to sustain aging-related physiological changes and minimize risks of complications (Rémond et al., 2015). The contribution of some nutrients, such as calcium and vitamin D, cannot be overemphasized in the elderly. Both lie at the heart of bone integrity maintenance, which is paramount with the enhanced risk of osteoporosis and fracture in this age group. Bone density is maintained by calcium, while vitamin D aids in calcium absorption, with resulting benefits to skeletal integrity. Research identifies a concerning trend where older adults frequently fall short of recommended dietary allowances for such crucial nutrients, exposing them to bone-related illness (Schmir, 2018).

Top-up with fortified foods or supplements in addition to nutrient-rich whole foods can help mitigate such insufficiencies. Information regarding the significance of well-planned meals that include these critical nutrients is critical to empowering older adults towards better food choices. Additionally, the role of hydration cannot be overlooked in the nutritional requirements for the elderly. Changes in the sensation of thirst will tend to lead to decreased fluid intake and result in dehydration and the ensuing health effects, including cognitive decline and renal function diminishment. They should be encouraged to drink sufficient fluids during the day, and they should concentrate on water and nutrient-rich drinks since they tend to have to make up for reduced kidney activity. In addition, adding moisture to meals through foods that contain lots of moisture—fruits, vegetables, and soups—will also help keep them hydrated. Overall, a comprehensive nutrition plan that addresses the importance of proper hydration, as well as the intake of required vitamins and minerals, can be essential in supporting a healthier aging process and enhancing general quality of life in older adults (Rémond et al., 2015).

11.1.2. Common Deficiencies in Elderly Diets

As people age, the nutritional needs of a person are likely to change as a consequence of physiological as well as psychological factors that are likely to influence nutrient intake. Common protein, vitamin, and mineral deficiencies in the diets of older people are a consequence of diminished appetite, taste loss, and illness, among many others. Protein is essential for maintaining muscle and general health, but elderly people tend to intake below the daily recommended amount, leading to muscle loss and additional frailty. Further, improper intake of vitamins such as B12, D, and folate can result in mental decline and sluggish metabolic activities, contributing to illness. Paying attention to these deficiencies is crucial while assisting in achieving the nutritional needs of the aged and catering to their well-being. It has been suggested that malnutrition among elderly people is not only a matter of inappropriate nutrition but is also subject to the gastrointestinal tract, which, with advancing age, gets less efficient in nutrient absorption. As the studies have elaborated, the chemical and mechanical digestion are compromised, leading to impaired bioavailability of the nutrients and thereby exacerbating deficiency (Rémond et al., 2015). This decline affects the general health of the elderly and makes them more vulnerable to other diseases and reduces their ability to recover from ailments. In addition, nutrition deficiencies have an impact on several organ systems, such as the nervous, musculoskeletal, and cardiovascular systems, promoting a vicious cycle of deteriorating health. Therefore, identifying the interconnection between digestion and nutrition changes with age is important for producing healthy dietary recommendations for the elderly. The Dietary Reference Intakes (DRIs) give a model of healthy nutrition in healthy individuals, but for application in the elderly is particularly challenging with their increased prevalence of chronic diseases and special nutritional needs (Ard et al., 2016). Though DRIs are commonly based on consideration of nutrient deficiencies, consideration must also be given to the prevention and control of chronic diseases, requiring a more sophisticated strategy. Challenges of chronic disease endpoints need to be addressed to create evidence-based guidelines tailored for older adults. This may include reevaluating intake-response models and enhancing the relationship between nutrition and the management of chronic disease.

11.2. Recommended Dietary Allowances (RDAs)

With age, the nutritional needs of people shift significantly, and dietary recommendations, particularly the RDAs, must be reconsidered. The RDAs serve as valuable points of reference, ensuring that elderly citizens obtain adequate amounts of necessary nutrients such as protein, vitamins, and minerals. RDAs owe their origin to a history of scientific effort in optimizing nutritional practices through directional recommendations based on nutrients, much of which has transformed since the earlier period. By understanding the evolution of RDAs, health professionals can more fully appreciate their use in assisting with maintaining health and preventing chronic disease in older people, as the revisions have responded both to advances in the science of nutrition and to shifts in population demographics. This highlights the necessity for specially adapted nutritional advice that specifically meets the physiological and lifestyle variables affecting the elderly. Beyond the consumption of single nutrients, the impact of RDAs extends to influencing total health and well-being. Time and again, studies have demonstrated that adherence to these food guidelines translates into improved nutrition status, reduced incidence of diet-related illness, and improved food security among older adults. Policies and programs to disseminate these guidelines, including federally funded nutrition assistance programs, have been shown to enhance older people's access to healthy food. For instance, a review of food programs indicates that participation in programs can significantly contribute to dietary intake and health outcomes among the elderly (Fox et al., 2004). Thus, aligning food selection with RDAs encourages not just personal health but also public health objectives, underscoring the importance of nutrition among the elderly. Since RDAs play a big role, dissemination of these guidelines to older individuals and their caregivers is important. Misinterpretation of nutritional needs can lead to inadequate nutrient consumption, exacerbation of familiar issues in older age. Interventions that highlight the significance of RDAs in achieving an everyday diet rich in important nutrients can enable older adults to create healthier food choices. As noted, the nutritional context has shifted with cultural and technological advances in food consumption and intake trends; thus, continuous RDAs' growth and communication are instrumental. Based on previous experience on development of such guidelines, experts and decision-makers may construct interactive learning material that effectively targets the geriatric population and promotes lifelong healthy nutrition habits (Carlson, 1991) (Figure 11.5).

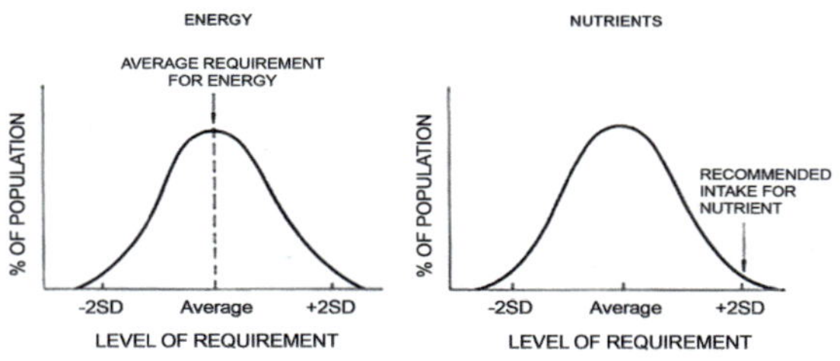

Figure 11.5. Recommended dietary allowances (RDAs).

Source: https://nap.nationalacademies.org/openbook/0309046335/xhtml/img00000.gif.

11.2.1. Overview of Recommended Dietary Allowances (RDAs) for Seniors

RDAs are the major guidelines for giving older persons adequate nutrition in a bid to maintain their health and wellness. The requirements for nutrition change with age due to physiological changes, including alteration of metabolism, structure of the body, and absorptive efficiency. RDAs take these concerns into account, assigning great importance to specific vitamins and minerals required by aging adults, such as calcium, vitamin D, and B vitamins. This targeted strategy meets the heightened vulnerability to deficiencies and imbalance with age, thereby helping in preventing chronic diseases and attaining maximum health longevity. In this regard, adherence to RDAs facilitates an integrated nutritional model and helps health professionals in advising older patients on improving their nutritional status, thereby increasing overall quality of life. Consciousness about the historical development of nutrient-based dietary recommendations also substantiates prevailing policies, particularly among the aging population. Since nutritional standards have been in the United States since Atwater's suggestions for energy and protein in 1894, there has been a huge development in recommendations on nutrients since then. The development and incremental improvements to the RDAs, revised by the National Research Council in 1989, illustrate the ongoing attempt to keep the scientific rigor in making recommendations for diets appropriate to the special circumstances of populations, including the elderly. This historical background not only provides an explanation of the rationale behind the use of individual nutrient targets but also recognizes the importance of continued research in food science. Such research is crucial in formulating effective food guide models that ensure maximal nutritional health among the elderly population in accordance with contemporary dietary standards (Carlson, 1991).

Also, strict compliance with RDAs in the elderly is critical to outweigh the respective health risks of old age. Evidence indicates that diet has a tremendous role in determining the wide variety of health outcomes among older adults, including immune function, cognitive status, and mobility. For instance, poor consumption of necessary nutrients and low caloric intake can lead to adverse effects such as increased frailty, falls, and complications of chronic disease. USDA-initiated aid programs, including food assistance programs, are essential to promoting greater food security and quality of intake among the aged, with broader implications for better overall health outcomes (Fox et al., 2004). These programs demonstrate the core linkage between informed diet culture and supportive systems that allow older adults to pursue their nutritional needs, with a view to stability and promoting healthier aging in populations.

11.2.2. Specific Recommended Dietary Allowances (RDAs) for Key Nutrients

As a person ages, his/her nutrient needs increase, and special RDAs are necessary to maintain them in good health and free from age-related diseases. Key nutrients such as calcium, vitamin D, and vitamin B12 require special attention for the elderly. Calcium is necessary to ensure good bone health because bone loss related to aging increases the chances of fractures. The RDA for calcium in individuals older than age 70 is set at 1,200 mg per day, either from food or supplements. Similarly, adequate vitamin D intake is also important for the absorption of calcium, such that the RDA increases to 800 IU in older people. Importantly, these modifications emphasize the importance of addressing nutrient needs directly related to aging, eventually providing a foundation for overall better health in the aging adult. In addition to calcium and vitamin D, older adults must emphasize an adequate dietary supply of vitamin B12, essential to neurological functioning and red blood cell production. With age, the vitamin B12 absorption may be lower due to reduced stomach acid secretion, for which an RDA of 2.4 micrograms per day is required to reverse any deficiency. In addition, a well-balanced macronutrient intake of proteins and fats is still required to preserve muscle strength and energy levels. The RDA for protein is approximately 1.0–1.2 grams per kilogram of body weight, and this indicates the importance of tailoring diets based on individual needs. Thus, ensuring the elderly get these specific nutrient recommendations can significantly enhance their lives by improving physical health and mental function. To assist further in the health of older individuals, understanding the role of nutrition assistance programs in providing access to necessary nutrients is of utmost significance.

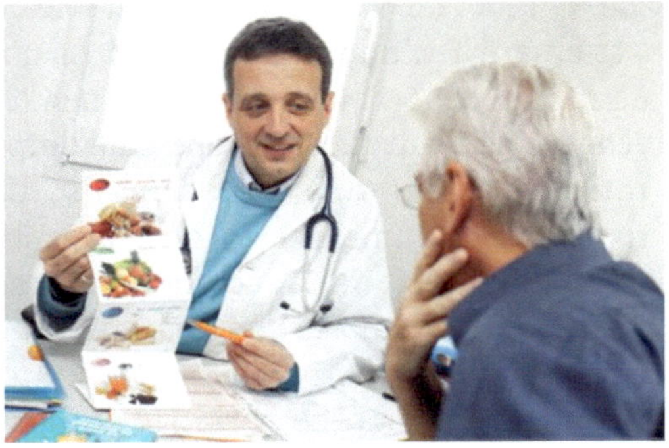

Figure 11.6. Specific recommended dietary allowances (RDAs) for key nutrients.

Source: https://external-content.duckduckgo.com/iu/?u=https%3A%2F%2Ftse1.mm.bing.net%2Fth%2Fid%2FOIP.AuQV3Q2IPpDPt8RbgdqGIwHaE7 %3Fr%3D0 %26pid%3DApi&f=1&ipt=0b4ea593de87eba1b55d286ac182d7d32f7e74001e6ab6ad35fdef4fb8ff41c6.

Programs offered by the USDA offer vital inputs that allow low-income older adults to meet their nutritional needs, thus impacting their nutritional status and overall health outcomes. For instance, food assistance programs prefer to utilize foods rich in nutrients that satisfy the RDAs of important vitamins and minerals outlined in dietary guidelines, like calcium and vitamin D. As noted in Fox et al. (2004), these programs not only ensure food security but also mirror substantial effects on the health of program participants, especially among the most at-risk populations. Thus, if such awareness is developed to a greater extent and individuals become involved in such programs more actively, the nutritional intake gap is narrowed, and the elderly reach and maintain the recommended dietary level (Figure 11.6).

11.2.3. Adjustments Based on Health Conditions

Based on dietary recommendations for the elderly, adjustments based on an individual's health conditions are an important area of concern. As older individuals typically suffer from multiple chronic conditions, personalized diet treatment can be especially useful for their health. For instance, older adults with diabetes need to strictly control carbohydrate intake while ensuring that they incorporate healthy fats and proteins to keep blood sugar in check. In turn, patients with cardiovascular disease would find a diet high in saturated fat and low in omega-3 fatty acids beneficial to promote cardiovascular well-being. The use of tailored dietary changes attached to the specific challenges that aging and comorbid medical conditions present is the cornerstone of effective nutritional interventions among the elderly. The second key consideration is addressing sarcopenia syndrome, characterized by wasting and continuous decline of muscle function and mass common among older adults. Research indicates that fiber intake is significantlyly related to skeletal muscle mass, and therefore, its potential role in nutrition recommendations for this group. Among an older cohort, higher fiber intake was linked with higher skeletal muscle mass, particularly in women free from metabolic syndrome. This emphasizes the importance of incorporating sufficient fiber in the form of whole grains, fruits, and vegetables into the diet of elderly individuals because such an adjustment can be most important in hindering muscle loss and promoting functional independence. With these nutrient-dense foods, caregivers can make it relatively easy for the elderly to combat the physical decline of aging, thus enhancing their general quality of life. Finally, the dietary modifications for the elderly should also be informed by gastrointestinal health considerations. Aging is well established enough to produce an array of digestive issues, including constipation and poor nutrient absorption. Dietary modifications aimed at improving gut health in an effort to reverse these outcomes should thus be the primary consideration. This might include increased fiber intake, which can be shown to promote healthy bowel action and potentially cure constipation. Incorporating a combination of probiotics, which are found in fermented foods like yogurt and kefir, can also benefit digestive health. With these dietary alterations, caregivers will help older adults obtain adequate nutrition with less distress, promoting a more holistic style of dietary recommendations responsive to the complex interaction of health factors present in the elderly.

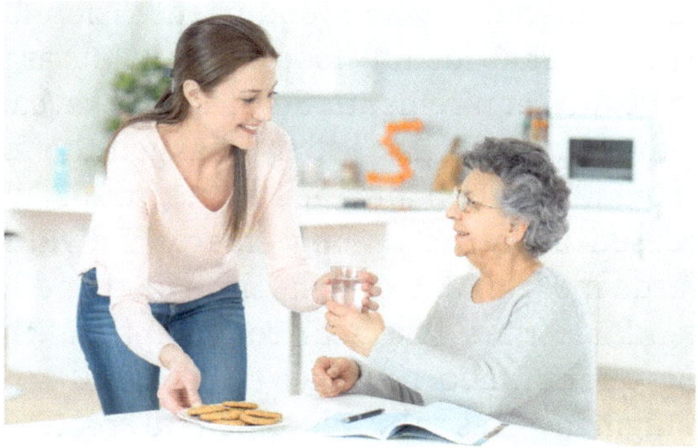

Figure 11.7. Hydration and injury prevention.

Source: https://www.coastalorthoteam.com/hs-fs/hubfs/Blog_photos/hydration-elderly-woman.jpg?width=960&name=hydration-elderly-woman.jpg.

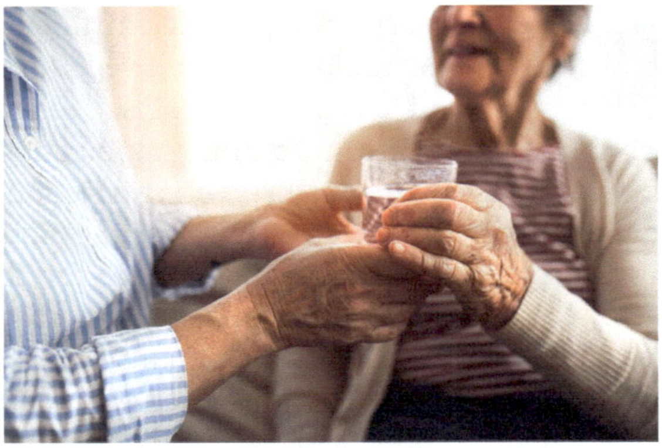

Figure 11.8. Study finds a lack of adequate hydration among the elderly.

Source: https://s3.amazonaws.com/cms.ipressroom.com/173/files/20192/5c7951112cfac2157702fe54_Elderly+woman-Halfpoint-iStock-915195294/Elderly+woman-Halfpoint-iStock-915195294_cf40b130-b581-4d23-8770-325ef7808dae-prv.jpg.

11.3. Dietary Patterns and Food Choices

Information regarding eating patterns and food habits is fundamental to the creation of effective dietary advice for the elderly. As the population is expanding, it often goes through fluctuations in metabolism, hunger, and food needs. Therefore, there is a need to identify food eating habits as per their health requirements. Studies have revealed that the pandemic has widely changed the food intake and eating habits of all age groups, with increased exposure among elderly individuals towards more intake of unhealthy food and less dependable time for meal consumption while being quarantined (Ammar et al., 2020). This paradigm involves the requirement to create new dietary guidelines in a way that supports well-balanced meals based on nutrient-dense food options that support general health, such as fruits and vegetables, whole grains, and lean meats. By means of an appreciation for psychological and social influences on food intake, it is now possible to design interventions to promote healthy eating and foster compliance with recommended dietary guidelines. Also, the understanding of food choices in preventing chronic diseases is included in shaping dietary advice for the elderly. The majority of elderly individuals are beset by diminished mobility, cognitive impairment, and social isolation that can influence their dietary habits. The need for precise nutritional interventions to stem the onset of diseases such as cardiovascular disease and diabetes is most important among this population. All these suggestions should include the addition of heart-healthy fats, a reduction in the sodium content, and the intake of low-glycemic index carbohydrates, among many others. It can clearly be seen that adherence to such dietetic principles can significantly enhance the nutritional health and well-being of the older population when they are educated on the long-term benefits of nutrition (Mach et al., 2019). Formulating good communication strategies around these dietary guidelines can also empower the elderly to make appropriate food decisions. Finally, integrating social and cultural factors into dietary practices is essential in promoting healthy dietary choices for the elderly. Mealtimes have the potential to enhance social interaction, imparting both nutritional and emotional value, essential in promoting mental well-being among the elderly. In addition, adopting culturally appropriate foods ensures that eating guidelines appeal to the diverse tastes of the older population to induce higher compliance and satisfaction. The impacts of isolation during the COVID-19 pandemic have demonstrated that alterations in communal eating habits result in unhealthy eating, making it imperative to guidelines addressing not only individual eating habits but also communal ones (Ammar et al., 2020). Through the sharing of food, social bonds can be promoted, and thus, dietary advice can foster physical and mental well-being, ultimately leading to an improved quality of life among elderly individuals (Figure 11.9).

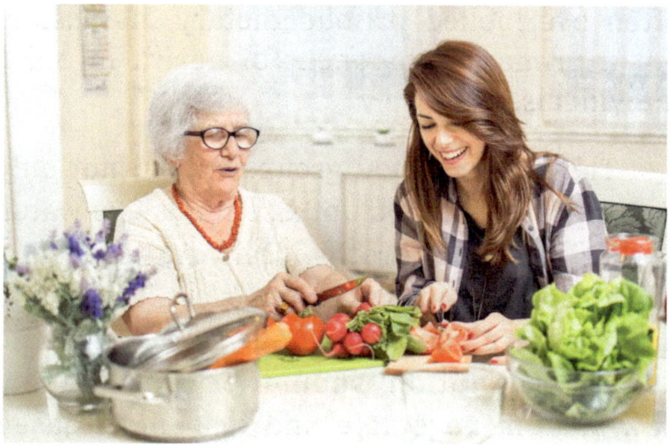

Figure 11.9. Dietary patterns and food choices for the elderly.

Source: https://www.elderly-homecare.com/wp-content/uploads/2020/02/Senior-Caregiver-Cutting-Vegetables.jpg.

11.3.1. Benefits of a Balanced Diet

A balanced diet is crucial for the elderly because it fosters overall health and prevents various age-associated diseases. With increasing age, physiological changes occur in important ways, including a declining metabolic rate and reduced effectiveness in nutrient utilization. All these changes necessitate that they consume diets high in nutrients required for bone density, muscle mass, and cardiovascular system function. It has been documented in literature that older people tend to experience a deficiency of important vitamins and minerals like vitamin D, which has been linked with bone density and reducing the risk of falls. The American Academy of Pediatrics recommends substantial consumption of vitamin D, highlighted by the necessity to address these diet-related deficiencies in older adults (Szu-Chang et al., 2019). Through emphasis on a healthy diet made of generous amounts of fruits, vegetables, lean protein, whole grains, and healthy fats, older adults can enhance their nutritional status and support better health outcomes. Consuming a combination of food groups in a total diet, in addition to providing essential nutrients, also helps promote mental health and cognition. Diets rich in antioxidants, healthy fats, and vitamins decrease oxidative stress and inflammation, which are factors that lead to cognitive decline. For instance, the Mediterranean diet, which emphasizes fruits, vegetables, whole grains, and omega-3 fatty acids, has been found to be at a lower risk of neurodegenerative disorders in the elderly. Moreover, adequate nutrient intake is associated with improved mood and reduced risk of depression, which is prevalent in the elderly (McGuigan et al., 2018). Ensuring that the old are on a balanced diet helps treat both physical and mental well-being, ultimately leading to their quality of life when older. The social aspect of meals also has a crucial role in the benefits of a balanced diet for the elderly. Eating together creates social relationships, which can help reduce any feelings of loneliness and isolation among older individuals. Involvement in shared meals, whether with family members or in senior living facilities, provides both dietary benefits and psychosocial benefits. Involving older adults in the process of preparing meals can promote independence and self-sufficiency and may allow for integration of personal food choices. Consequently, the healthy diet of the elderly is not only adequate nutrients but also the stimulation of social relationships and mental well-being, promoting overall health and well-being of this population (McGuigan et al., 2018) (Figure 11.10).

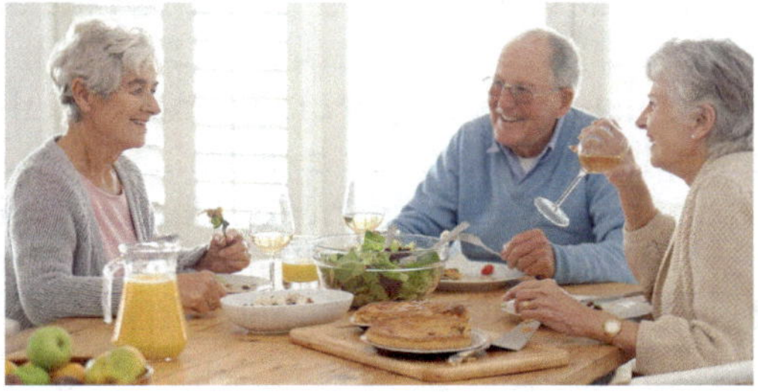

Figure 11.10. Nutrition guide for the aging and elderly.

Source: https://www.retailmenot.com/blog/wp-content/uploads/sites/2/2016/09/SeniorCitizenNutritionGuide-1473813427-1.jpg.

11.3.2. Recommended Food Groups

In developing guideline food groups for older people, they should consider the unique nutritional needs of the group that usually suffers from poor appetite, illnesses, and changes in metabolism. Elderly Food Based Dietary Guidelines (EFBDGs) are guidelines that emphasize balanced intake from all food groups, like fruits and vegetables, whole grains, lean meats, and low-fat milk. These groups not only supply basic nutrients but also help ensure the overall health of the elderly. Through enabling fruit and vegetable consumption, the guidelines ensure higher intake levels of vitamins, minerals, and fiber, which are important in ensuring digestion and preventing chronic diseases. In addition, whole grains offer complex carbohydrates that lead to long-term energy, which is of extreme importance to the dietary needs of elderly individuals as they engage in daily activities and maintain independence (Napier et al., 2018). Protein foods are heavily emphasized in diets, with adequate protein consumption being vital in the battle against age-related muscle loss, a condition known as sarcopenia. Recommended food groups include a range of lean protein sources such as poultry, fish, eggs, legumes, and low-fat dairy (EFBDGs). Research has indicated that increased consumption of fiber is linked with skeletal muscle mass, further highlighting the function played by these food groups in the diet of an older adult (Montiel-Rojas et al., 2020). The EFBDGs also encourage older individuals to include plant proteins as a sustainable means of boosting their dietary intake. The synergistic interaction of protein and fiber consumption of food can lead to improved muscle strength and physical functioning, thereby assisting older adults in maintaining their independence and quality of life. Lastly, the development of a richly varied and balanced diet through the aforementioned food groups is important for guaranteeing the nutritional needs of the elderly. Hydration is also a significant component often overlooked in food dietary discussion, but a primary component of health in older individuals.

The selected food groups should not only encompass solid food but also fluids like water, herbal tea, and broths. Dehydration leads to extreme health issues like confusion and urinary tract infections, and hence, adequate fluid consumption should be encouraged. Low-sodium vegetable and lean meat-based soups and stews may be used to feed while supplementing the daily intake with hydration. Also, the EFBDGs recommend limiting processed foods that are high in sugar and sodium since they have a negative effect on health conditions like hypertension and diabetes. By adhering to these guidelines, elderly individuals can ensure that they are consuming a well-balanced diet that will enhance their general health, keep them hydrated, and preserve their physical and mental functions as they age (Napier et al., 2018) (Figure 11.11).

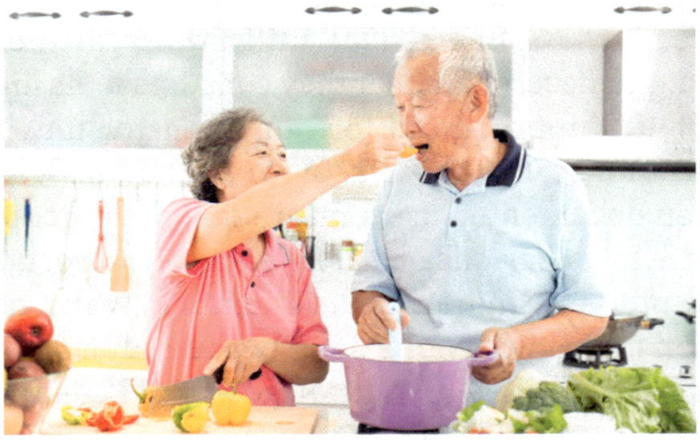

Figure 11.11. Elderly food based dietary guidelines (EFBDGs).

Source: https://images.squarespace-cdn.com/content/v1/56b5014d22482e764ea40f83/1563404270071-28CSIAEEW8ADBWV48SKD/Elderly+people+eating+healthy+oxford+healthcare+tulsa+healthy+food+prep.jpg.

11.3.3. Importance of Variety in Food Choices

The role of diversity of food selections becomes increasingly important as individuals become older, particularly for the elderly. Dietary variety is necessary for guaranteeing that older adults receive all the nutrients they require for health and the prevention of chronic disease. Vitamins, minerals, and antioxidants, which are most frequently found in fruits, vegetables, whole grain foods, and protein sources, are vital to health. Also, variety in the diet helps lower the risk of deficiency, particularly among groups such as dairy and fruits, which are commonly deficient in the diets of older adults. This is again supported by recent studies that determined that the majority of assisted living facilities fail to offer food variety as per the suggested nutritional requirements, thereby compromising the nutritional status of their populations (Schmir, 2018). Evidently, the cultivation of diversity in food choice is crucial to the improvement of health outcomes in the elderly. More than simply the presence of diverse food choices, the psychological and social aspects of a diverse diet need to be considered. Foods that provide a variety of flavors, textures, and colors are likely to stimulate appetite, enhance pleasure, and facilitate social interaction while eating. In the majority of cases, elderly individuals will have smaller appetites or will have difficulties eating; therefore, having stimulated and varied meal choices is paramount to ensure nutritional uptake. Eating meals together with others, particularly where meals consist of multiple dishes, not only raises nutritional levels but also reduces feelings of loneliness and depression typical at this stage of life. Therefore, integrating diversity in food intake not just implies good physical health but good emotional well-being and social contact as well, a general plan for healthy aging. In addition, present nutritional guidelines favor food intake variety based on a composite food pattern, focusing on the health potential of a balanced diet. The Dietary Guidelines for Americans suggest following a diverse diet and not only diversification of nutrients but also food selection from all food groups to improve the quality of the diet as a whole (Drewnowski et al., 2019). This combination of principles focuses on both individual nutrients and food groups in establishing dietary recommendations. By encouraging food variety, food policy will better assist public health objectives in the direction of quality in the older person's nutrition. Ultimately, variety adherence will not only ensure adequate nutrient requirements but also facilitate healthy eating habits that have been linked to longevity and quality of life in the elderly.

11.4. Special Dietary Considerations

Special dietary considerations among the elderly are highly critical to facilitate healthy growth and avoid chronic disease. As individuals grow older, their nutritional needs and metabolic levels shift, and therefore, malnutrition is increasingly likely to become an issue. This group of patients tends to require specific dietary strategies to control a variety of diseases such as diabetes, hypertension, and osteoporosis. For instance, older individuals may require a diet rich in vitamin D and calcium for bone strength, and diabetic patients require careful control of carbohydrate levels so that blood sugar levels can be maintained in check. Hence, it is essential that healthcare professionals know these specific dietary needs to create effective dietary plans so that older adults are able to gain maximum well-being and health. Besides, the function of food support programs cannot be undermined, particularly concerning the nutritional condition of the elderly group. These programs, like those offered by the USDA, aim to provide access to healthy food, which low-income elderly people might otherwise lack. Research has demonstrated that such program participants have enhanced food security, dietary adequacy, and nutritional status and, as a result, better quality of life. The findings highlight the importance of specialized diet interventions that consider budgetary limitations but ensure access to a required range of nutrients. They are not only important for the current diet but also for health status in later life in the older population, and their significance helps to reaffirm the importance of policy harmonization with dietary guidelines (Fox et al., 2004). Finally, special dietary needs are not just individual ones but also encompass community support systems that may impact old-age nutrition. Social isolation, a prevalent condition in the elderly, can negatively impact food choice and even well-being in general. Community-based interventions such as meal delivery and nutrition education can teach elderly people to improve their diet. Through enhancement of social relationships as well as provision of available resources, for example, food programs, CDC improves diet quality among the elderly and food security.

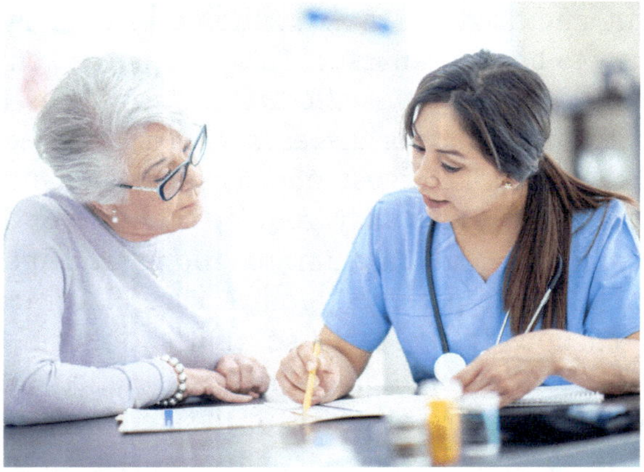

Figure 11.12. Special dietary considerations in geriatrics.

Source: https://westmontliving.com/wp-content/uploads/2024/11/Dietary-Considerations-for-Elderly-Vomiting.png.

The programs avoid deficiencies in diet, but through facilitating social contact, also ensure that elderly can live healthier lives. As research indicates that there is a correlation between social support and improved health outcomes, integrating social factors into older adult dietary recommendations for overall promotion of health is of utmost importance (Fox et al., 2004) (Figure 11.12).

11.4.1. Managing Chronic Diseases Through Diet

An effective diet plan for managing chronic diseases among the elderly is significant in terms of enhancing overall health and well-being. Among the chronic diseases that are prevalent among ageing individuals are diabetes, hypertension, and obesity. These diseases can have a critical impact on their nutritional status as well as metabolism. Use of diet guidelines among the elderly can enable weight management, normalize blood sugar levels, and maintain cardiovascular health. The inclusion of whole foods rich in nutrients and low in processed foods is greatly advised in order to provide the vitamins and minerals required for normal body functioning. Caloric consumption should also be modified while maintaining enough nutrient content; this balance helps minimize the chances of chronic diseases while enabling older adults to remain independent and have good health. Incorporating some food ingredients, such as synbiotics, may also enhance the management of chronic diseases among the elderly. Synbiotics, which consist of probiotics and prebiotics, promote gut health and may enhance immune function as well as metabolic status. Studies show that these foods control inflammation and promote a healthy microbiome, essential for elderly individuals with immune deficiency or gastrointestinal issues. A synbiotic-containing balanced diet not only helps in controlling diseases but is also a compatible approach to a total strategy to health because of its compatibility with digestive regularity. The health practitioners should hence make synbiotics a compatible choice when they are preparing the elderly person's diet, while ensuring that the diet under plan is safe and beneficial, according to guidelines and regulations as set by health organizations (Swanson et al., 2020). Secondly, incorporation of diet advice should be complementary to the integrated plans presented in reputable models of health, such as those suggested by the European Society of Cardiology (ESC) and the European Atherosclerosis Society (EAS). Such advice stresses the importance of individualized nutrition, with modifications based on individual health profiles and individual tastes. It is the duty of health professionals to translate and apply these recommendations responsibly, such that dietary changes made by them are flexible and sustainable. Periodic follow-ups and consultations can ensure adherence to these dietary changes while empowering geriatric patients by means of health education about their conditions and the role played by nutrition. Finally, by embracing a systematic approach to managing chronic conditions through diet, the overall efficiency of preventive and therapeutic care is amplified, which has a positive effect on the health trajectory of older individuals (Mach et al., 2019).

11.4.2. Dietary Restrictions and Allergies

As the population ages, dietary restrictions and food hypersensitivities come to play a growing role in the management of the elderly. Individuals may have a variety of dietary limitations due to long-term illnesses such as hypertension, diabetes, or cardiovascular diseases and must cut out specific foods that may exacerbate these issues. Apart from medical conditions, food allergies are also a significant concern. One prevalent food allergy to foods such as nuts, shellfish, or gluten may have an aggressive reaction and limit the food choices for the elderly individual. It is important that dietary recommendations account for these issues so that nutritional needs are addressed without adding foods that will provoke undesirable reactions. Generally speaking, a sensitive and tailored method of cooking can help older adults enjoy a healthy diet despite dietary limitations and food allergies. The health of the digestive system in older adults can be a determining factor in whether or not dietary limitations can be effectively managed. Aging also typically leads to alterations of the gastrointestinal tract, including decreased production of digestive enzymes, altered gut microbiota, and alteration of food transit times, resulting in impaired absorption of nutrients (Rémond et al., 2015). The aforementioned physiological alterations will augment the already present challenges for individuals with dietary restrictions or allergies because they will be disadvantaged in acquiring their nutritional requirements from limited food sources. Besides, malnutrition can also have the additional effect of aggravating existing health conditions, which expose older individuals to immune, musculoskeletal, and cardiovascular system maladies. To offset this, it is essential that dietary suggestions lean towards foods that, apart from being free of allergens, are rich in nutrients to address the unique digestive needs of the elderly in an effort to keep them well-stocked with nutrients and still enjoy a generally healthy quality of life. Food allergies and dietary restrictions management among elderly patients also entail careful attention to food additives. Sodium, potassium, and calcium salts of fatty acids are the most popular emulsifiers found in processed foods, posing issues to those with special dietary needs or food allergies (FSA ANS Panel et al., 2018). An understanding of the safety and tolerability of these additives is essential because older adults are more sensitive to changes in their diet. The European Food Safety Authority (EFSA) has reached the conclusion that these kinds of additives pose no significant safety concerns; however, they can still impact the nutritional value of foods for older adult populations (FSA ANS Panel et al., 2018). Hence, nutritional counselling should not just recommend avoiding allergens but also recommend eating less processed foods and limiting added constituents. In so doing, medical practitioners can help older individuals to stick to healthier foods while effectively managing their food allergies and restrictions (Figure 11.13).

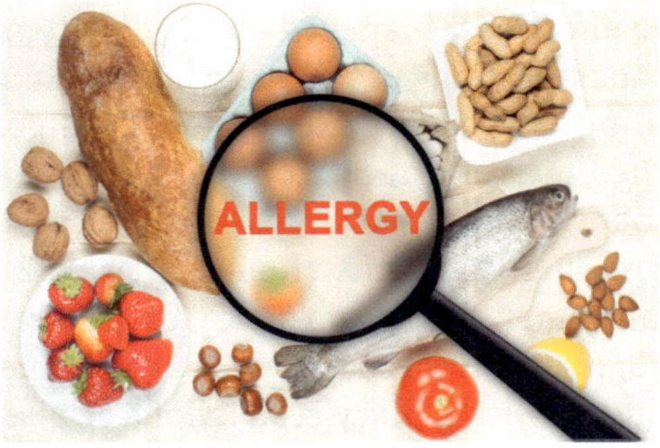

Figure 11.13. Dietary restrictions and allergies.

Source: https://www.icarehomehealth.ca/wp-content/uploads/2015/05/Food_Allergies.jpg.

11.4.3. Role of Supplements in Elderly Nutrition

As the population of older individuals grows, the role of dietary supplements in their diet has become increasingly important. Since the elderly naturally experience physiological changes that can impair nutrient absorption and metabolism, the supplements play an important role in enabling them to meet their nutritional needs. Illnesses such as loss of appetite, altered sense of taste, and chronic poor health can prevent the intake of essential vitamins and minerals, leading to potential deficiencies. Vitamin D and B12 in dietary supplements, along with minerals such as calcium, can compensate for these deficiencies and help to promote good health and well-being in older individuals. Besides, supplements such as omega-3 fatty acids are also gaining attention for their potential in mitigating inflammation and improving mental function, integral aspects of elderly care, complementing diet advice in building strength and vigor. Application of supplements as part of the elderly's diet needs to be undertaken with dignity and good counsel. Medical practitioners should consider individual needs and dietary habits and determine reasonable supplement intake. While some of the elderly may require additional nutrients due to some health conditions, others may receive sufficient from diet alone. Besides, the quality and efficacy of supplements could be extremely variable, necessitating the need to choose products that meet established safety and effectiveness standards. Past studies show that the synergistic action of the combination of probiotics and dietary fiber, known as synbiotics, can yield health-promoting effects specific to the elderly, enhancing gut well-being and immunity, an action most needed given the high prevalence of digestive diseases and compromised immunity in this group (Swanson et al., 2020). Besides, information on interactions between drugs and supplements is crucial in promoting the safe use of nutritional additives among older persons. Older persons tend to use more than one drug, and there are concerns about potential interactions between drugs and supplements that lead to unwanted effects. For instance, certain supplements have the potential either to interfere with drug absorption or to augment their effects and render therapeutic regimens difficult. Also, with caregivers coming up with supplements in a nutrition plan, the place of geriatric assessments is evident. Geriatric assessments can help guide the use of personalized dietary practice and supplement protocols so that older individuals receive integrated care to support their overall health. Keeping in mind cognitive problems, such as delirium risk, points to the importance of adopting a holistic approach to elderly nutrition (Livingston et al., 2020).

11.5. Practical Tips for Meal Planning

Effective meal planning is particularly important for the elderly because it has a direct impact on their health and well-being. To begin with, one should prioritize nutrient-dense foods that address the special dietary needs of older adults. A variety of fruit, vegetables, lean meats, and whole grains gives one a balanced diet with essential vitamins and minerals. For instance, foods rich in calcium and vitamin D, such as dairy products and leafy greens, ensure bone health that declines with age. Whole grains provide fiber essential for healthy digestion and prevent constipation, a highly prevalent issue among the elderly. Through creating a meal plan emphasizing these aspects, caregivers and older adults can facilitate maximum nutritional status, thereby enhancing their quality of life and reducing the risk of diet-related health issues. In a quest for easier meal planning, preplanning meals is also a valuable strategy. Older adults bear heavy burdens in terms of the daily effort of meal planning, leading to reliance on convenience foods that lack essential nutrients. By taking some time to prepare several meals simultaneously, older adults or their caregivers can have nutritious options ready for the week. Freezing single servings can even make it simpler to have meal options to open, with healthy meal choices available without the need for daily meal preparation. Additionally, utilizing options such as community programs with meal services can eliminate food insecurity and promote healthy consumption. This proactive approach not only minimizes stress at mealtimes but also promotes healthy eating habits that translate to general well-being. A second key component of successful meal planning for older adults is the integration of hydration planning. Dehydration is a danger that commonly goes unseen in older people, with changes in the body's sense of thirst, rendering it difficult to assess one's fluid needs. Encouraging fluid intake throughout the day, along with fluid-containing foods such as soup and fruit, can help to ensure adequate fluid levels. Encouraging a more visible water-drinking habit through the use of visually obvious aids, e.g., colored cups, or frequent reminders to drink can also be helpful. Additionally, offering a variety of drinks, including herbal teas or diluted juices, can increase pleasure and reduce the feeling of burdensome obligation. This priority on fluid intake facilitates meal planning exercises to ensure that elderly individuals not only eat a proper diet but also ensure proper hydration (Figure 11.14).

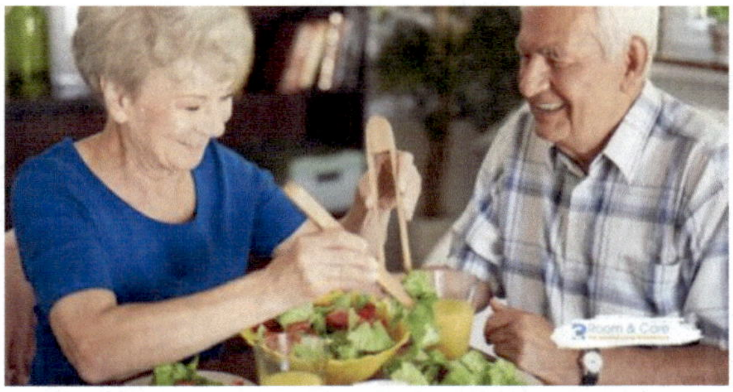

Figure 11.14. Healthy meals for the elderly.

Source: https://external-content.duckduckgo.com/iu/?u https%3A%2F%2Ftse4.mm.bi ng.net% 2Fth%2Fid%2FOIP.vSTirRsMX4igX2IXokOtEgHaD4%3Fpid%3DApi&f= 1&ipt=ee5b0f1bf194ad3c0c2e4f2 dcb9a3773cbbc89c07bab48485c49ccc2f6aa0e5e.

11.5.1. Strategies for Healthy Meal Preparation

As the promotion of optimal health of the elderly increases, healthy meal preparation methods are essential. The most critical of these is the inclusion in regular meals of a variety of foods so that the elderly will be able to access a good variety of essential nutrients. This aligns with the overall dietary recommendations that ensure food variety. By utilizing techniques such as batch cooking and meal preparation, caregivers will be able to incorporate healthier meals more conveniently, thereby being less reliant on processed foods. Similarly, individualizing meal plans to the cultural preferences of older people can promote increased acceptance and enjoyment of the food being consumed and, therefore, increased dietary adherence. As with other dietary recommendations, like Mach et al. (2019), incorporating a variety of food groups as well as individual choice helps with nutritional adequacy and cultural appropriateness and can be beneficial in maintaining the dignity and well-being of older individuals. Second, measures like the consumption of more fruits and vegetables as part of meals can significantly play a role in nutritional supply. The World Health Organization focuses on consuming a variety of foods, and this is particularly relevant in older cohorts who might have dietary restrictions or specific health concerns. For instance, including fruits and vegetables in new forms—like smoothies, soups, or stir-fries—can render them digestible and appealing. Cool planning can further support the retention of nutrients, particularly when employing cooking methods such as steaming and roasting instead of frying. All food preparation should also seek to reduce the use of sodium and unhealthy fats, as recommended by dietary guidelines. Preparation techniques such as spice and herb seasoning instead of salt can assist with heart health and general well-being, as advocated by Mach et al. (2019). Finally, portion control and eating mindfully are essential strategies in healthy meal preparation for elderly adults. As metabolism declines with age, appropriate portion sizes become critical to maintaining a healthy weight and preventing chronic diseases. Education on portion sizes and honoring hunger signals promotes autonomy in older adults, enabling them to assume responsibility for their food selection. Using smaller plates can also promote moderation at mealtimes without compromising on satisfaction. Apart from portion sizes, the habit of mindful eating—where one focuses on the meal process—can promote a more satisfying experience with food and better digestion. This concept agrees with advice provided throughout the majority of countries, as noted by Herforth et al. (2019), that focuses on mindful eating combined with nutrient-dense foods to ensure a systemic response to the elderly's healthy diet (Figure 11.15).

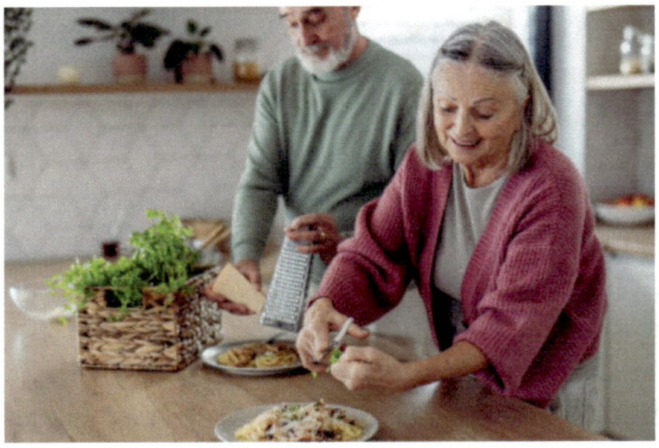

Figure 11.15. Strategies for healthy meal preparation.

Source: https://external-content.duckduckgo.com/iu/?u=https%3A%2F%2Fwww.elderlycaregivers.org%2Fwp-content%2Fuploads%2F2023%2F07%2Fbigstock-Senior-Couple-Cooking-Together-476666635-1536x1024.jpg&f=1&nofb=1&ipt=44e3db09042faa326f88046a963b6ce374efcb7e35f2d943f75606bda7db9864.

11.5.2. Importance of Portion Control

Portion control is particularly relevant among the elderly because it has immediate repercussions on health outcomes and the control of chronic diseases. As most older adults experience a decrease in metabolism as well as changes in appetite, understanding what portion sizes are acceptable can maintain a healthy weight and prevent overeating. This is vital as overconsumption of calories has the function of aggravates health disorders such as heart disease, diabetes, and hypertension, which are prevalent among aged citizens. Furthermore, portion control encourages even intake of nutrient-dense foods to prevent nutritional deficiencies due to imbalanced intake. Nutrient deficiency leads to compromised immune systems and muscle loss, thereby making disorders more complex. Therefore, the use of portion control not only inspires more mindful consumption patterns but also improves the general health of older adults by promoting healthier diets. Proper portion control can make a significant difference in modifying long-term dietary habits, supporting alterations towards healthier patterns of living among older adults. By educating older adults on proper servings, healthcare practitioners can allow them to prepare their own food in such a way that they minimize the chances of significant weight gain or undernutrition. This is particularly pertinent insofar as aging is generally accompanied by increased disease risk factors, including disease stages of cancer that involve diet, which the American Cancer Society's guidelines on colorectal cancer screening (Wolf et al., 2018) emphasize. Encouraging small, balanced meals with significant amounts of fruit, vegetables, lean proteins, and whole grains fosters a nutrition-driven approach in line with established dietary recommendations for the elderly. This prevention method can also decrease the risk of the development of chronic diseases, especially diet-related chronic diseases, and thus enhance the quality of life among this group. Portion control is also a successful method in addressing meal preparation and food consumption difficulties for an elderly population. Elderly people can have mobility or cognitive impairment issues hindering them from cooking nutritious meals. By following portion control, caregivers and medical professionals can supply edible portions of food that are easier to prepare and consume. This convenience can eliminate the intimidation typically felt when dealing with bulk food, thus improving a less stressful and more enjoyable dining experience. As evidenced by various research on the trend of health among the aging, including portion control in diets, can significantly reduce the workload of meal planning and preparation, but still be harmonious with a healthy diet (Zhou et al., 2019). Ultimately, a culture of mindful eating built by portion control can improve the dining experiences of older people to allow them to enjoy autonomy and health in their golden years.

11.5.3. Budget-Friendly Healthy Eating Options

Healthy eating under affordable circumstances is essential, particularly among the elderly who often have few resources. Economic downturn can restrict access to healthy foods, a key influence in helping older adults be healthy. The Dietary Guidelines for Older Adults emphasize how important balanced eating, such as fruits, vegetables, whole grains, lean protein, and good fats, is. Basic strategies, including the choice of meals based on seasonal produce and the use of sales or coupons at neighborhood supermarkets, can greatly support an elderly person's nutrition without excessively taxing their finances. In addition, the utilization of community assistance programs that work to reduce food insecurity can offer further funding, allowing dietary requirements to be met within budget. Coordination of food choice with resources at hand will ensure well-being as well as economic viability for older people, as indicated by the Food and Nutrition Guidelines Series. Also, being aware of the economic implications of an unhealthy diet can go a long way in highlighting the significance of affordable healthy consumption. Trends indicate that the economic downturn has hindered many individuals from accessing nutritious food, thereby affecting their health and increasing healthcare costs. To the elderly, who may already be struggling with fixed incomes, this is indeed a challenge. Prioritizing whole foods over processed is one strategy that results in better health outcomes but also yields dividends in terms of cost. Such foundational foods as beans, lentils, and grains can form a foundation for cheap meals. By prioritizing such foods, older adults are able to make healthy meals without resorting to more expensive convenience foods, hence adhering to nutritional guidelines without having to spend more. Finally, through the utilization of thrifty recipes, older individuals can be empowered to embrace healthy eating as a way of life. Passing on information about meals prepared from minimal ingredients, but rich in taste and nutrients, can motivate older individuals to be innovative in the kitchen. Neighborhood community centers and the internet also generally provide affordable cooking classes for this group of individuals that focus on simple yet healthy meal preparation. Group discussion or workshop participation in meal planning not only stimulates interpersonal interaction but also serves as an educational platform for sharing cost-saving advice. Because healthy nutrition is emphasized in the context of the Dietary Guidelines for the Elderly, these programs can potentially develop a positive environment where the elderly are enabled to choose healthier foods within their economic capacity.

SUMMARY

In a discussion of dietary guidelines for the elderly, there is a need to appreciate the interconnected aspects of nutrition, health, and well-being of the elderly. As the population ages, the importance of targeted diet recommendations is more evident than ever. Effective nutritional interventions can significantly enhance the overall health status and functional independence of older people. Metabolic changes, dietary restrictions, and increased prevalence of chronic diseases necessitate having a comprehensive overview of the nutritional needs of older individuals. Without proper guidance, this group is at risk of malnutrition and its consequences. Therefore, healthcare providers, caregivers, and policymakers must accord utmost importance to the implementation of evidence-based nutritional recommendations particular to this unique group. In addition, the implementation of principles such as synbiotics to nutritional protocols is the promise of new approaches in geriatric nutrition. According to recent expert consensus forums, the definition of synbiotics as a mixture that involves probiotics and prebiotics highlights the synergistic interaction between important nutrients. Rather than simply pondering these factors in isolation, recognizing their synergistic value identifies positive avenues for exploring the promotion of gut and general health in the elderly. This harmonizes with the new paradigm for the significance of microbial health and its impact on the aging population. Ensuring dietary guidelines encompass these advancements can decrease the effects of aging, enhance intestinal health, and enhance nutrient absorption, ultimately leading to improved health outcomes for the elderly. Finally, it is appropriate to touch on the broad implications of dietary guidelines that consider prevalent chronic conditions in older individuals, like dementia and delirium. As outlined in current literature, treatment of such illnesses through appropriate nutrition may improve cognitive function and health in sufferers. Through the practice of hydration-focused, nutrient-dense food and patient-specific meals, caregivers can create environments promoting wellness. Furthermore, the identification and understanding of disease complexity in conditions like dementia means that integrative dietary treatment must be considered more than mere physical sustenance. As society is facing an aging population, prioritizing nutrition for the elderly will not only enhance the health patterns of individuals but also eradicate social costs of aging and associated health conditions, as cited by Livingston et al. (2020).

The elderly have dietary guidelines that are a vital reference to facilitate health and wellness in the process of aging. These are all recommendations that point to the importance of an equilibrated diet rich in nutrients, one that responds to the individual physiological changes occurring during aging. The most significant among these recommendations is increasing the intake of fruits, vegetables, whole grains, and lean protein foods, collectively providing essential vitamins, minerals, and fiber needed to maintain health at its optimum. In addition, elderly people should control their caloric consumption, considering that metabolism slows as a result of aging. Complying with such recommendations not only aids people in achieving a healthy weight but also contributes to the body's ability to fight age-related disease and, therefore, enhances longevity and health among elderly people. Another equally important aspect of dietary recommendations among the elderly is highlighting fluid consumption. As one ages, he or she has the inability to sense thirst, which can lead to insufficient fluid consumption and subsequent dehydration. It is recommended by the guidelines that there be regular water and other fluid consumption throughout the day because optimal hydration is crucial to many of the body's functions, such as brain function, kidney function, and regulation of temperature. Food intake that is hydrating, such as fruits and vegetables, can also supplement fluid consumption. Moreover, observation of dietary modifications, such as reduction of sodium and added sugars, must be made in an attempt to reverse the risk from common chronic health conditions among elderly individuals, thus necessitating a tailored diet planning approach. Lastly, the guidelines stress the necessity of diet modifications reflective of the compromise of functional aging gastrointestinal tracts. Since older people may perceive changes in digestion, absorption, and bioavailability of nutrients, it is crucial that diets be designed to ensure optimal intake of nutrients. For instance, the addition of food with easy digestibility and supplementing dietary fiber can significantly improve digestion, which is generally compromised in the elderly. Using such factors in planning meals can prevent malnutrition—a relevant issue for this group since improper nutrition can lead to an enhanced risk of developing numerous diseases and impairments, including cardiovascular disease and cognitive impairment (Rémond et al., 2015; Lumbis, 2018). This thus forms a strong basis of knowledge of such guidelines, not just enhancing eating habits but also helping towards the general well-being and long life of older individuals.

A CLOSER LOOK

NUTRITION IN ELDERLY HEALTH

Nutrition is absolutely essential in the maintenance of health, functional independence, and quality of life among elderly individuals. With advancing age, there is a shift in nutritional requirements brought about by the physiological changes, such as reduced metabolic rate, altered gastrointestinal function, and changed taste and smell, that may affect appetite. Aging is also characteristically linked with chronic illnesses like diabetes, cardiovascular disease, osteoporosis, and cognitive impairment, which impact dietary limitations and requirements. Older people have the most common issues like dentition issues, restriction of movement, poverty, or social isolation, all negatively affecting food access and intake. Malnutrition in both undernutrition and overnutrition forms is common among the population and leads to muscle wasting, frailty, compromised immunity, and increased hospitalization risk. Adequate consumption of protein, calcium, vitamin D, B12, fiber, and fluids is especially important to sustain muscle mass, bone strength, and digestion. Nutrient-dense food is properly balanced with a variety of fruits, vegetables, whole grains, lean protein sources, and healthy fats that need to be eaten. Beyond this, nutritional interventions among older people need to be individualized, culturally appropriate, and responsive to individual preference and functional capacity. Close monitoring for unintended weight loss, dysphagia, and drug-nutrient interactions is essential. Overall, optimal nutrition is essential to promote healthy aging, halt disease worsening, and preserve physical and cognitive function in older adults.

REFERENCES

1. Brown, K. A., Timotijevic, L., Barnett, J., Shepherd, R., Lähteenmäki, L., & Raats, M. M. (2011). A review of consumer awareness, understanding and use of food-based dietary guidelines. *The British journal of nutrition, 106*(1), 15–26. https://doi.org/10.1017/S0007114511000250(accessed on 12th July 2025).
2. Madeira, T., Peixoto-Plácido, C., Goulão, B., Mendonça, N., Alarcão, V., Santos, N., de Oliveira, R. M., Yngve, A., Bye, A., Bergland, A., Lopes, C., Nicola, P., Santos, O., & Clara, J. G. (2016). National survey of the Portuguese elderly nutritional status: study protocol. *BMC geriatrics, 16,* 139. https://doi.org/10.1186/s12877-016-0299-x(accessed on 12th July 2025).
3. Ammar, A., Brach, M., Trabelsi, K., Chtourou, H., Boukhris, O., Masmoudi, L., Bouaziz, et al. (2020). Effects of COVID-19 home confinement on eating behavior and physical activity: Results of the ECLB-COVID19 international online survey. *Nutrients, 12,* 1583–1583. https://doi.org/10.3390/nu12061583 (accessed on 12th July 2025).
4. Mary Kay Fox, William Hamilton and Biing-Hwan Lin (2004). Effects of food assistance and nutrition programs on nutrition and health: Volume 3, literature review. https://www.ers.usda.gov/publications/pub-details?pubid=46574 https://core.ac.uk/download/pdf/6449553.pdf (accessed on 12th July 2025).
5. Ard, J., Atkinson, S., Bier, D., & Carriquiry, A. (2016). Options for basing dietary reference intakes (DRIs) on chronic disease endpoints: Report from a joint US-/Canadian-sponsored working group. https://core.ac.uk/download/323080977.pdf (accessed on 12th July 2025).
6. Montiel-Rojas, D., Nilsson, A., Santoro, A., Franceschi, C., Bazzocchi, A., Battista, G., de Groot, L. C. P. G. M., Feskens, E. J. M., Berendsen, A., Pietruszka, B., Januszko, O., Fairweather-Tait, S., Jennings, A., Nicoletti, C., & Kadi, F. (2020). Dietary Fibre May Mitigate Sarcopenia Risk: Findings from the NU-AGE Cohort of Older European Adults. *Nutrients, 12*(4), 1075. https://doi.org/10.3390/nu12041075(accessed on 12th July 2025).
7. Blanc Bisson, C., Bourdel Marchasson, I., Brigidi, P., et al. (2015). Impact of diet and nutraceutical supplementation on inflammation in elderly people: Results from the RISTOMED study, an open-label randomized control trial. https://core.ac.uk/download/54521140.pdf (accessed on 12th July 2025).
8. Rémond, D., Shahar, D. R., Gille, D., Pinto, P., Kachal, J., Peyron, M. A., Dos Santos, C. N., Walther, B., Bordoni, A., Dupont, D., Tomás-Cobos, L., & Vergères, G. (2015). Understanding the gastrointestinal tract of the elderly to develop dietary solutions that prevent malnutrition. *Oncotarget, 6*(16), 13858–13898. https://doi.org/10.18632/oncotarget.4030(accessed on 12th July 2025).
9. Bray, F., Laversanne, M., Sung, H., Ferlay, J., Siegel, R. L., Soerjomataram, I., & Jemal, A. (2024). Global cancer statistics 2022: GLOBOCAN estimates of incidence and mortality worldwide for 36 cancers in 185 countries. *CA: A Cancer Journal for Clinicians, 74,* 229–263. https://doi.org/10.3322/caac.21834 (accessed on 12th July 2025).
10. Carlson, B. B. (1991). History and analysis of food guides in the United States. https://core.ac.uk/download/270056278.pdf (accessed on 12th July 2025).
11. Chang, S. W., & Lee, H. C. (2019). Vitamin D and health–The missing vitamin in humans. *Pediatrics & Neonatology, 60,* 237–244. https://doi.org/10.1016/j.pedneo.2019.04.007 (accessed on 12th July 2025).

12. Drewnowski, A., Dwyer, J., King, J., et al. (2019). A proposed nutrient density score that includes food groups and nutrients to better align with dietary guidance. https://core.ac.uk/download/323080855.pdf (accessed on 12th July 2025).

13. Napier, C., Oldewage-Theron, W., & Grobbelaar, H. (2017). Testing of developed Food Based Dietary Guidelines for the elderly in South Africa. *South African Journal of Clinical Nutrition, 31*(3), 55–61. https://doi.org/10.1080/16070658.2017.1388560(accessed on 12th July 2025).

14. Herforth, A., Arimond, M., Álvarez-Sánchez, C., Coates, J., Christianson, K., & Muehlhoff, E. (2019). A global review of food-based dietary guidelines. *Advances in Nutrition, 10*, 590–605. https://doi.org/10.1093/advances/nmy130 (accessed on 12th July 2025).

15. LeBoff, M. S., Greenspan, S. L., Insogna, K., Lewiecki, E. M., Saag, K. G., Singer, A., & Siris, E. S. (2022). The clinician's guide to prevention and treatment of osteoporosis. *Osteoporosis International, 33*, 2049–2102. https://doi.org/10.1007/s00198-021-05900-y (accessed on 12th July 2025).

16. Livingston, G., Huntley, J., Sommerlad, A., Ames, D., Ballard, C., Banerjee, S., Brayne, C., et al. (2020). Dementia prevention, intervention, and care: 2020 report of the Lancet Commission. *The Lancet, 396*, 413–446. https://doi.org/10.1016/s0140-6736(20)30367-6 (accessed on 12th July 2025).

17. Lumbis, R. H. (2018). Nourishing dogs and cats through their twilight years. https://core.ac.uk/download/154422917.pdf (accessed on 12th July 2025).

18. Mach, F., Baigent, C., Catapano, A. L., Koskinas, K. C., Casula, M., Badimón, L., Chapman, M. J., et al. (2019). 2019 ESC/EAS guidelines for the management of dyslipidemias: Lipid modification to reduce cardiovascular risk. *European Heart Journal, 41*, 111–188. https://doi.org/10.1093/eurheartj/ehz455 (accessed on 12th July 2025).

19. McClinchy, J. (2018). Dietary management of older people with diabetes. https://core.ac.uk/download/287581385.pdf (accessed on 12th July 2025).

20. McGuigan, A., Kelly, P., Turkington, R., Jones, C., Coleman, H. G., & McCain, R. S. (2018). Pancreatic cancer: A review of clinical diagnosis, epidemiology, treatment and outcomes. *World Journal of Gastroenterology, 24*, 4846–4861. https://doi.org/10.3748/wjg.v24.i43.4846 (accessed on 12th July 2025).

21. Pelliccia, A., Sharma, S., Gati, S., Bäck, M., Börjesson, M., Caselli, S., Collet, J. P., et al. (2020). 2020 ESC guidelines on sports cardiology and exercise in patients with cardiovascular disease. *European Heart Journal, 42*, 17–96. https://doi.org/10.1093/eurheartj/ehaa605 (accessed on 12th July 2025).

22. Schmir, C. R. (2018). A nutritional analysis of food menus offered at local older adult assisted living facilities. https://core.ac.uk/download/215520909.pdf (accessed on 12th July 2025).

23. Swanson, K. S., Gibson, G. R., Hutkins, R., Reimer, R. A., Reid, G., Verbeke, K., Scott, K. P., et al. (2020). The International Scientific Association for Probiotics and Prebiotics (ISAPP) consensus statement on the definition and scope of symbiotic. *Nature Reviews Gastroenterology & Hepatology, 17*, 687–701. https://doi.org/10.1038/s41575-020-0344-2 (accessed on 12th July 2025).

24. Wolf, A. M. D., Fontham, E. T. H., Church, T. R., Flowers, C. R., Guerra, C. E., LaMonte, S. J., Etzioni, R., et al. (2018). Colorectal cancer screening for average-risk adults: 2018 guideline

update from the American Cancer Society. *CA: A Cancer Journal for Clinicians*, *68*, 250–281. https://doi.org/10.3322/caac.21457 (accessed on 12th July 2025).

25. Zhou, M., Wang, H., Zeng, X., Yin, P., Zhu, J., Chen, W., Li, X., et al. (2019). Mortality, morbidity, and risk factors in China and its provinces, 1990–2017: A systematic analysis for the Global Burden of Disease Study 2017. *The Lancet*, *394*, 1145–1158. https://doi.org/10.1016/s0140-6736(19)30427-1 (accessed on 12th July 2025).

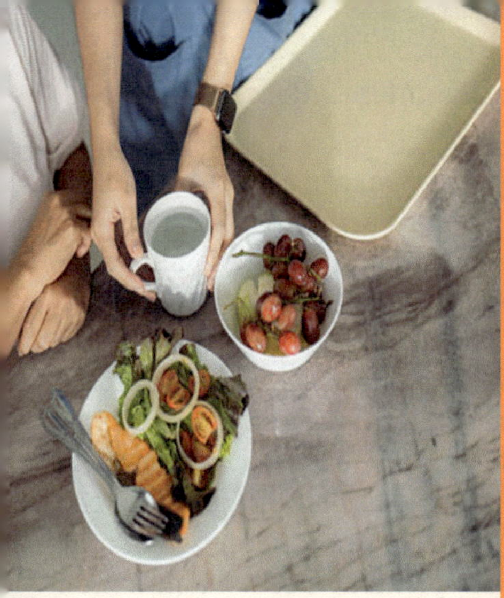

Chapter 12 SUPPLEMENT USE AND NUTRIENT INTERACTIONS IN GERIATRIC NUTRITION

Contents

Introduction

It is increasingly important to know the role of supplements in geriatric nutrition as the population ages and nutritional requirements increase. Older patients are likely to have a distinct constellation of nutrients that present nutritional challenges, including an increased risk for malnutrition and chronic disease. With aging comes loss of appetite, altered metabolism, and the potential for drug-nutrient interactions with polypharmacy. Older adults consequently tend to utilize dietary supplements as a means to supplement potential nutrient gaps. Supplement use may be both an attempt to correct deficiencies as well as an expectation that they will result in one being healthier and feeling better in general. As supplement use is on the rise, it is crucial to critically assess the interaction of the supplements and the essential nutrients among the elderly population. Nutrient and dietary supplement interactions are quite intricate and can contribute significantly to the well-being of the elderly. The majority of vitamins and minerals have essential functions in the prevention of diseases and sustaining body functions. For example, certain supplements can enhance or slow down the absorption of essential nutrients, and this can create potential imbalances that exacerbate current conditions. The concept of malnutrition among older adults is a more complex idea than calories being taken in; it is many deficiencies that are able to degrade immune systems, muscle endurance, and cognitive functions. Malnutrition has been identified by Reber et al. (2019) as a standalone risk factor that adversely impacts the clinical outcomes of patients, and individualized nutritional management is needed to overcome it. Understanding such nutrient interactions is essential for healthcare providers to develop inclusive nutritional management techniques that ensure better health in older adults. Second, the implementation of systematic nutritional risk screening can enhance the assessment of geriatric patients' dietary needs for timely interventions. In accordance with Reber et al. (2019), early detection of malnutrition during the course of illness through simple screening can lead to more comprehensive assessments of dietary intake and nutrient status to deliver individualized nutrition interventions.

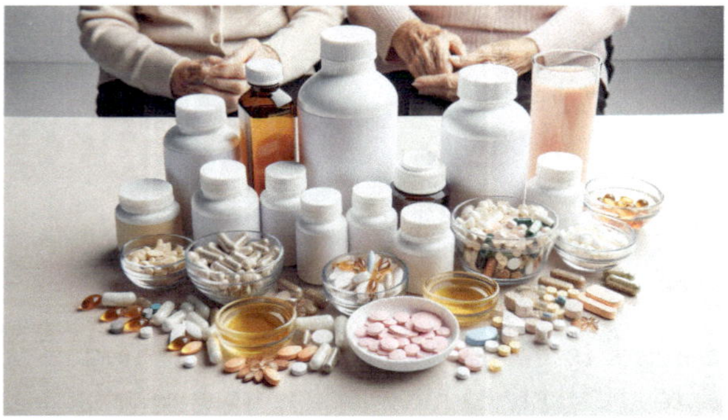

Figure 12.1. Potential benefits of nutrition supplements for elderly.

Source: https://cdn.growtha.dev/6516de5dbcce181d2bd88c56/65d71cfae37d465273ee24f7_1695575082593x234550197059517630-1708596065318x823133269475698800-dalle-WYPY5.png.

Interplay of various supplements necessitates an interdisciplinary strategy for the optimal optimization of geriatric nutrition, as healthcare providers from various specialties can assist in adequate choice of diet and supplementation methods. Such integration is necessary in the correction of nutritional status, increased quality of life, and reduced costs of healthcare for complications of aging. As the geriatric nutrition scenario keeps changing, awareness of supplement use and nutrition interaction will become part of helping the health of the elderly population (Figure 12.1).

Role of Supplements in the Elderly

With aging, the nutritional needs of an individual change because of various physiological and lifestyle aspects, and therefore, a shortage of required nutrients is possible. The majority of elderly people suffer from diminished nutrient uptake, changes in appetite and sense of taste, and the development of chronic disease that makes eating difficult. The result is heightened vulnerability to many conditions of illness, such as osteoporosis and cognitive impairment, which are abated by adequate supplementation. For instance, vitamins D and B12 are particularly important in older adults since vitamin D supports bone and immune function, while B12 is needed for mental health and the formation of red blood cells. With a growing awareness of the significance of supplements, it has become increasingly clear that supplements will play the most significant role in addressing these nutritional gaps and enhancing overall health, solidifying the need for diet interventions among older adults. The prevalence of chronic diseases in elderly individuals further underscores the role of individualized supplement use. Chronic diseases such as osteoporosis increase the risk of fractures, which can have severely disabling long-term consequences for the well-being of an elderly individual. Osteoporotic fractures, for example, could lead to a vicious cycle of repeated injuries and poor health outcomes. Given the fact that clinical or subclinical vertebral fractures may significantly increase the risk of subsequent fracture, the integration of calcium and vitamin D supplementation into the health regimen of older adults is crucial in measures to prevent fractures. Individualized diet therapy with supplementation lowers fractures and improves the general well-being of older adults, making the regular maintenance of bone health through nutrient intervention a significant guideline by leading health organizations (LeBoff et al., 2022). Geriatric nutrition also takes into perspective the mental aspect, highlighting the role of supplements in potentially delaying or preventing disorders such as Alzheimer's. As statistics foretell a drastic rise in Alzheimer's patients, the health implications stretch far beyond individual patients to catastrophic family and social burdens with each passing year. Recent research is now pointing towards the function of specific nutrients like omega-3 fatty acids and antioxidants in sustaining healthy neurons and combating the onset of mental deterioration. Supplements may be a strategic component of the dietary regimen of at-risk older adults, thereby improving quality of life and maintaining function. With the aging population increasing, the role of supplements in clinical practice is important for maximizing the health status of older adults and managing the complex issues of aging-related nutrition.

Overview of Nutrient Interactions

The interaction among various nutrients is important to maintain physiological activities, particularly within geriatric populations, where nutrient absorption and metabolism may be compromised. Nutrient interaction can significantly influence bioavailability and health effects. Calcium and vitamin D, for instance, interact synergistically; adequate vitamin D ensures greater absorption of calcium from food and supplements, thereby for bone health. A lack of vitamin D can lead to reduced calcium absorption, which can further exacerbate illnesses such as osteoporosis. As older adults are particularly susceptible to both osteoporosis and lack of vitamin D, it is worth studying these interactions to inform best practice supplementation strategies with which to maximize nutrient use and reduce fracture risk, particularly in the face of multiplicities of health issues in elderly, as illustrated in the latest studies with regard to the importance of optimal nutrient pairs in favoring better outcomes (LeBoff et al., 2022). The second major interaction is that of antioxidants with an ability to modulate oxidative stress and inflammation, the two driving forces of aging. Nutrition essentials such as vitamins E and C, along with selenium, possess potent antioxidant effects, and they can inhibit aging-related cell damage. Given in combination, micronutrients possess the capability of enhancing one another's action and hence maximize protective effects against common chronic diseases that occur in the aged. This harmony-synergy nexus is underscored by the significance of a balanced diet with a range of antioxidants and no supplements in isolation, as food sources may provide ancillary benefits that single supplementation cannot provide. Additionally, studies show that diets rich in fruits and vegetables are associated with reduced frailty, which emphasizes the role of eating habits in preventing deleterious health outcomes of nutrient interaction (Lochlainn et al., 2021). Lastly, macronutrient balance—carbohydrates, proteins, and fats—comes into play in nutrient interactions that impact total health among older adults. For instance, protein intake is crucial for protein synthesis, which is crucial to sustain mobility and prevent the risk of frailty. Meanwhile, adequate fat intake is crucial for nutrient absorption, namely fat-soluble vitamins A, D, E, and K. These interactions highlight the importance of providing aged people with a balanced diet that not only provides the required caloric supply but also the correct proportion of macronutrients to meet their body's requirements. Besides, upcoming evidence favors the adoption of an interdisciplinary approach, involving diet intervention together with exercise and supplements, to manage the complexities of nutrient interactions in an optimal way, thereby ensuring optimal health among aging adults (LeBoff et al., 2022; Lochlainn et al., 2021) (Figure 12.2).

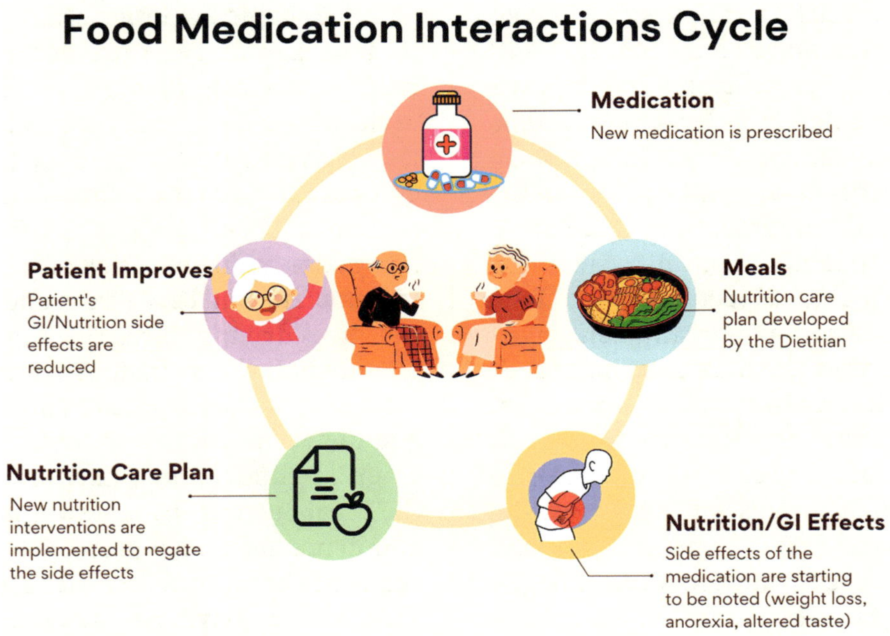

Figure 12.2. Food and medications interactions.

Source: https://longtermcarerd.com/wp-content/uploads/2022/07/Medication-1.png.

12.1. Common Supplements Used by Older Adults

The aging population increasingly relies on dietary supplements to deal with specific ailments and to supplement nutritional levels. Supplements that are most prevalent in the elderly are vitamin D, calcium, and omega-3 fatty acids. Vitamin D is particularly crucial because it allows for the absorption of calcium, thereby performing a central role in bone maintenance, which is critical due to the greater susceptibility of postmenopausal women and elderly men to osteoporosis. Calcium supplements stave off age-related fracture risks owing to loss of bone density. Furthermore, omega-3 fatty acids, which are usually found in fish oil, have been a target of interest due to their properties to reduce inflammation as well as promote cardiovascular health. Given that the incidence of chronic disease is higher with advancing age, these supplements will also play a critical role in improving the health and well-being of older adults, and it is essential to know about them in geriatric nutrition. In addition to vitamins and minerals, other supplements for mental health, like ginkgo biloba and omega-3 fatty acids, are widely used among elderly people. Loss of cognitive function, as exemplified by conditions like Alzheimer's disease, is an important health issue, as evidenced by the growing incidence of dementia among the elderly. Ginkgo biloba, an herbal supplement, has been widely speculated to possess a cognitive benefit, with research yielding inconclusive findings. Similarly, omega-3 fatty acids are believed to support brain function and may play a role in reducing the risk of cognitive impairment. Increased focus on maintaining cognitive capacity in older age demands balanced evaluation of such supplements, as they possess the possibility to interfere with standard drugs, influencing efficacy and safety. Correct understanding of the nutritional interactions involved with supplement use is hence vital to sustain safe and valuable nutritional practices. While the benefits of supplementation may be significant, they are also encumbered by some risk that must be acknowledged, most notably with respect to interactions with prescribed medications. For example, older adults take medications for chronic conditions like hypertension, diabetes, and cardiovascular disease, and some supplements will increase or decrease these risks of drug action. These risks are also to falls and fall-related injuries, which are an issue for this population due to the fact that supplementation has implications for balance and proprioception. Montero-Odasso et al. (2022) state that the consequences of falls are significant, leading to increased morbidity and mortality, which also complicates geriatric care. Caregivers need to be current on supplement intake to ensure older adults both gain the intended benefits and minimize adverse effects. Creating a sophisticated understanding of the interaction between supplements and medications is essential in maximizing health in older adults (Figure 12.3).

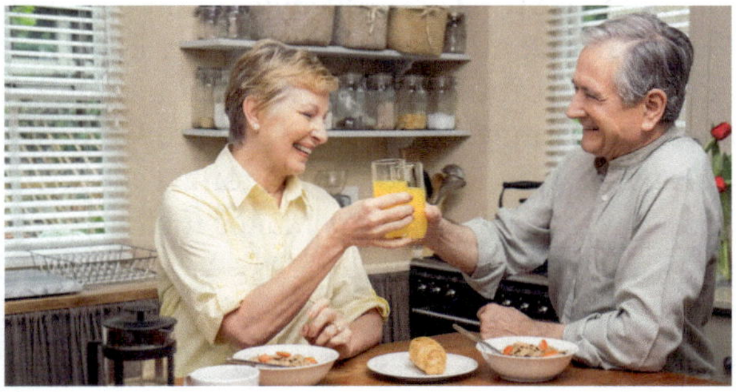

Figure 12.3. Nutritional drinks for the elderly.

Source: https://www.mealvillage.com/blog/nutritional-drinks-for-elderly.jsp.

12.1.1. Vitamins and Minerals

The role of vitamins and minerals in the nutrition of older people cannot be overlooked because they not only play a part in the well-being of a person but also act against age-related diseases. Aging is accompanied by a decrease in the body's physiological function, which can lead to a heightened risk of chronic diseases such as cardiovascular and neurodegenerative diseases. Adequate consumption of major minerals and vitamins such as calcium and Vitamin D has been observed to improve bone density and immune function. Some nutrients among older adults can act as protective factors against the development of age-related disorders. While continued research is revealing the complex interplay between individual nutrients and outcomes, it is becoming more apparent that supplementation is required in the case of individuals whose dietary intake is not quite sufficient to meet accepted standards, especially among the population often found in geriatric communities and characterized by a declining absorption capacity (Guo et al., 2022). Among the spectrum of nutritional treatments, the concomitant application of minerals and vitamins has both positive and negative aspects. Some pairs of vitamins and minerals enhance one another's activity because vitamin D, for example, promotes the absorption of calcium from the intestine, which is critical in osteoporosis prevention. There is also a risk of hypervitaminosis and cross-reactions. For instance, excessive intake of certain fat-soluble vitamins has the potential to lead to toxicity and worsen underlying conditions. Elderly patients must, therefore, exercise utmost caution in supplementation with proper monitoring and consultation with healthcare professionals. This underscores the importance of embracing personalized supplementation strategies considering diverse health conditions, dietary habits, and prevailing medical conditions. By addressing such nuances, health care providers can enhance the long-term well-being of elderly individuals in a manner that equips them with the nutritional needs to perform at their best without inadvertently causing harm (LeBoff et al., 2022). In further offering nutrition support for elderly individuals, it is critical to consider the impact of overall dietary planning as opposed to supplementation. A diet of whole foods is able to provide naturally the essential vitamins and minerals required, and in most instances, these function better in their food form than that of isolated supplements. Leafy greens, nuts, seeds, and fortified foods are capable of not only providing the necessary nutrients but also beneficial phytochemicals that work synergistically for improved health outcomes. In addition to this, social interactions, cooking abilities, and financial situation can also contribute to an older individual's diet, which is best met with a holistic approach to nutrition. Attending nutrition classes tailored for the elderly can help them adopt healthy diets, thereby reducing reliance on supplements and establishing a wellness culture based on whole-food consumption as the cornerstone of geriatric management (Guo et al., 2022) (Figure 12.4).

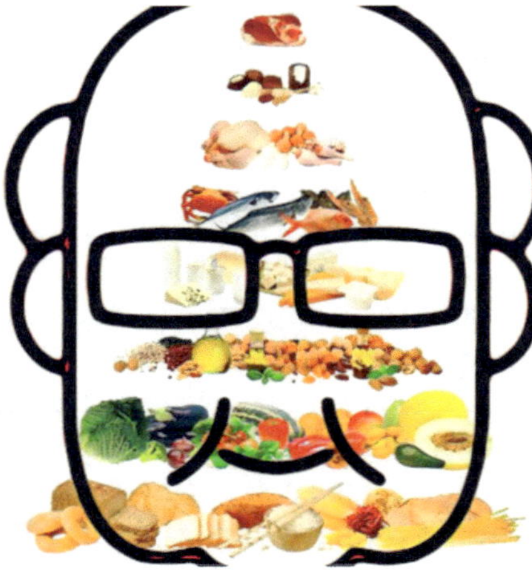

Figure 12.4. Vitamins and minerals in geriatric nutrition.

Source: https://www.foodtimes.eu/wp-content/uploads/2022/04/nutrizione-anziano.jpg.

12.1.2. Herbal Supplements

The consumption of herbal supplements in the diets of elderly adults presents both opportunities and challenges in geriatric nutrition. Elderly adults suffer from a variety of age-related diseases, leading them to seek alternative medications to improve their condition. Herbal supplements, derived from plants, have been linked with great benefits for health, including anti-inflammatory properties and cognitive function, for centuries. Yet the effectiveness and safety of these supplements are bound to be inconsistent on account of variability in metabolism among individuals and the possibility of interactions with medication. With more than 60% of elderly individuals said to use supplements, it becomes essential to gauge the consequences of adding herbal products to their diet, especially since their immune systems and overall health could already be weakened by chronic ailments. A holistic evaluation is thus needed to determine the impact of these supplements on geriatric health. In particular, the interaction of the herbal supplements with conventional drugs is a matter of concern in the context of geriatric nutrition. Elderly individuals are also likely to be on multiple drugs for various ailments and hence at risk for drug interactions. For instance, certain herbal supplements such as ginkgo biloba and garlic have the potential to interfere with blood clotting or anticoagulant metabolism. This interaction is likely to result in increased bleeding susceptibility, particularly among the elderly who may already have susceptibilities. Moreover, the lack of stringent regulation among herbal supplements makes it challenging to ensure safety and quality. While herbal supplements may be regarded by some older adults as natural replacements, their absence of comprehensive research and standardized dosing necessitates the interference of healthcare professionals to facilitate safe supplementation regimens. In addition, potential benefits of herbal supplements must be weighed in relation to the context of holistic geriatric practice. Although these products may be of therapeutic value, e.g., improved cognitive function or reduction in the symptoms of anxiety and depression, they should not substitute regular nutrients and balanced diets that elderly individuals require. Because nutritional deficiencies in elderly individuals are common, relying on herbal supplements alone can overlook significant dietary needs. Therefore, healthcare providers are required to have comprehensive consultations with the patient regarding their supplement use, considering the holistic interaction between their entire diet, lifestyle, and health conditions. Emphasizing teamwork in nutritional planning can lead to informed choices that optimize health outcomes, allowing older adults to manage the complexities of supplement use in their overall health (Guo et al., 2022) (Figure 12.5).

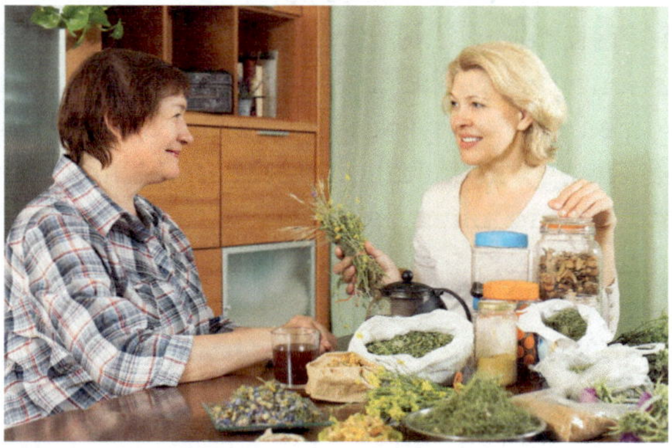

Figure 12.5. Geriatric nutrition in ayurveda.

Source: https://i0.wp.com/theancientayurveda.com/wp-content/uploads/2023/10/old-ayurveda.png?fit=1238%2C826&ssl=1.

12.1.3. Protein Powders and Amino Acids

The use of protein powders in geriatric nutrition has been increasing due to the fact that older individuals have unique dietary requirements that influence their health experience. Protein consumption is imperative in maintaining well-strengthened and well-maintained muscles, particularly among aging people who are prone to the sarcopenia condition, characterized by the loss of muscle mass. Protein powders may provide a ready solution for increasing dietary protein intake as a highly concentrated source of essential amino acids that the body needs to repair and build muscle. Of these amino acids, leucine stands out because of its ability to stimulate muscle protein synthesis, which becomes increasingly important in overcoming the age-related loss of muscle strength and function. Therefore, the incorporation of protein powders into the diet of elderly individuals can be an effective step to neutralize the risks of malnutrition as well as promote overall health (Solval & Estuardo, 2015). Amino acids, which are building blocks of protein, play a very important part in numerous physiological processes like metabolic regulation and tissue preservation. With age, the body loses its ability to synthesize certain amino acids, and hence it is more and more important to consume protein foods and supplements. The literature reveals that not all protein foods are equal in eliciting anabolic responses and therefore, a necessity for high-quality protein, such as whey or egg-based powders. For instance, egg-derived protein powders not only contain all the amino acids necessary but are also rich in bioactive compounds that can improve immunity and gut health by exerting beneficial interactions with healthy gut microbiota (Solval & Estuardo, 2015). With the high vulnerability of undernutrition in the aged population, consuming high-quality protein powders via supplementation can ensure the effective provision of necessary nutrients and support enhanced health benefits. Also not to be overlooked is the interaction of the protein with other nutrients, which can potentially influence protein supplementation efficiency. For instance, protein and carbohydrate co-ingestion has been claimed to enhance amino acid uptake and produce a more desirable metabolic pattern. This is particularly relevant in geriatric nutrition, where ensuring proper nutrient balance is significant in maintaining muscle function and overall well-being. Additionally, the presence of chronic diseases can influence nutrient metabolism and utilization, consequently influencing the method of supplementation employed in this group. As much as healthcare professionals attempt to optimize nutritional status in the elderly patient, the entire nutritional environment which protein powders are taken must be considered. By encouraging an equal nutrition plan that favors appropriate protein supplementation along with other essential nutrients, practitioners can more efficiently assist the health and well-being of the elderly (Cederholm et al., 2017).

12.2. Nutritional Needs of the Elderly

The nutritional needs change significantly with age, and hence, there is a rise in deficiencies aggravating age-related illnesses. Elderly individuals require a balanced diet supplemented with essential nutrients such as protein, vitamins, and minerals to support their physiological as well as cognitive functions. Increased hunger, dysgeusia and anosmia, and impairment of mastication can restrict the consumption of essential nutrients. Nutritionists, therefore, emphasize that foods that are calorie-dense and nutrient-dense and designed specifically for the elderly are the priority. Dietary interventions to enhance phytochemical consumption and enhance variety can provide a guarantee of enhanced health benefits and counteract risks of aging, including chronic disease. Recommended dietary allowances also endorse supplement use when food alone does not provide sufficient resources, especially in situations where nutrition is compromised or malnutrition prevails. The connection between medical conditions present and nutritional supplementation cannot be overlooked, particularly with the elderly population, who possess more than one chronic illness. A great example of this is osteoporosis, a huge issue with the elderly population, which requires appropriate calcium and vitamin D consumption in order to maintain bone density as well as prevent fractures (LeBoff et al., 2022). Absence of these nutrients can lead to brittle bones, undermining the higher fracture risk in older people following a minor fall. Also, in the treatment of osteoporosis, supplementation must be done with careful consideration of the potential interaction with other medications and diseases.

Medical practitioners must ensure that nutritional supplementation is done within the context of an overall treatment plan to enhance the strength of bones without adding the risk of adverse effects. Protocol-based plans can ultimately result in enhanced clinical outcomes, with an emphasis on prevention for reducing the incidence of osteoporotic fractures. Understanding the dynamic interactions of nutrients is crucial in maximizing the dietary regimen of elderly people. During aging, there is a change in metabolic processes and some vitamins and minerals, such as B12, magnesium, and zinc, become even more crucial in maintaining an individual in good overall health (Guo et al., 2022). These personal deficits have the potential to lead to cognitive impairment, fatigue, and immune compromise and therefore worsen other medical complications. Gastrointestinal changes also affect the absorption of these nutrients, and therefore supplementation and dietary manipulation become a priority. A baseline of nutritional status needs to be established through aggressive screening and monitoring so that healthcare providers can create individualized nutritional care plans. Appreciation of the intricate interplay between supplements and medications can further enhance integration approaches so that older patients can enjoy optimal health and vitality through adequately controlled nutrition (Figure 12.6).

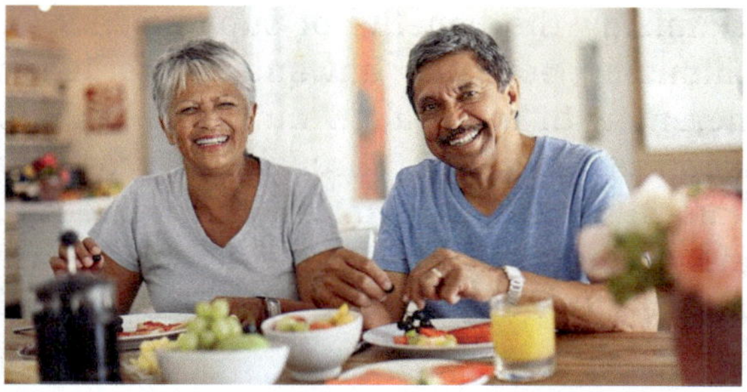

Figure 12.6. Primary nutrition needs for elderly people.

Source: https://www.tribecacare.com/wp-content/uploads/2022/07/blogs-1-2.png.

12.2.1. Changes in Metabolism with Age

With advancement in age, there are remarkable changes that take place in metabolic functions affecting nutrient needs and utilization. One of the noticeable changes is the reduction in energy expenditure that has a direct effect on dietary requirements. Aging is related to the reduction of lean muscle mass and consequent lowering of resting metabolic rates. This metabolic loss necessitates adjustments to consumption and consequently calls for greater attention to high-quality nutrient consumption to meet evolving caloric needs. Supplements would therefore be part of standard geriatric diets and assist in filling new nutritional gaps. Detection of such metabolic changes is crucial in the formulation of effective dietary interventions to achieve well-being among the elderly and avoid malnutrition. In addition to energy metabolism changes, the aging process has effects on the physiological responses of the body to nutrients. Specifically, elderly individuals have problems with the absorption and metabolism of a number of vitamins and minerals. For instance, reduced production of gastric acid might inhibit vitamin B12 absorption, whereas alterations in the gastrointestinal tract can impede the absorption of calcium and magnesium. Such changes can necessitate supplementation so that nutrient status is ensured. Also, nutrient interactions become increasingly important with age, as some vitamins may enhance or inhibit the action of others. It is important for optimizing supplement consumption in geriatric nutrition to know these interactions to ensure better outcomes and a greater quality of life among the elderly. Age-related illnesses also impose metabolic changes on top, making it all the more complex for nutritional needs. Long-term diseases such as diabetes, cardiovascular disease, and osteoporosis have the ability to reshape how the body utilizes and processes nutrients. For instance, inflammation resulting from such diseases has been proven to impact energy metabolism and the efficiency of nutrient. Research has established this through its studies on how immune function influences metabolism, with the aim of targeted nutritional therapy among the elderly with these conditions. Thus, supplementing with some nutrients may not only complete the deficits but also assist in metabolic processes that decline with age, hence emphasizing the importance of personalized meal planning. Understanding how metabolism and interactions between nutrients occur, health care providers are in a better position to counter the unique needs of the elderly to benefit them with optimal health through ideal nutrition.

12.2.2. Common Deficiencies in Older Adults

The prevalence of nutrient deficiencies among older people continues to be a significant public health problem, mainly due to the physiological changes that come with aging. With advancing age, the body demonstrates decreased absorption of key vitamins and minerals, combined with alterations in food habits that are perhaps not capable of providing sufficient nutrients. These deficiencies usually include critical vitamins such as B12, D, and calcium, all of which are necessary for overall health and well-being. The effects of these deficiencies can be particularly debilitating since they cause the onset of diseases such as osteoporosis and cognitive decline that are directly responsible for reducing quality of life. To this end, understanding the nutritional requirements of the elderly is essential for health care workers to be able to effectively introduce interventions that address these widespread deficiencies and optimize the health of the elderly. The connection between nutritional deficiencies and chronic illnesses in the elderly cannot be overstressed. For instance, vitamin D deficiency has been implicated as causing osteoporosis, which increases the risk of fracture, posing an enormous threat to the independence of older adults. Osteoporosis, often spoken of as a silent disease until a fracture occurs, can result in disabling complications and is prevalent among this age group, particularly women. Furthermore, the cognitive manifestations of vitamin B12 deficiency may involve memory loss and confusion, which adds to the challenges faced by elderly people with neurodegenerative conditions like Alzheimer's disease. The conditions demand an interdisciplinary intervention, including dietary modification as well as the possible use of supplements. Encouraging regular screening for nutritional deficiency among this age category could permit early interventions that reduce the perils that entail aging and health decline. Incorporating supplements into the dietary regimen of the elderly might be important in preventing the effects of nutritional deficiencies. Based on the evidence, regular supplementation with vitamins and minerals that are typically under-consumed can significantly enhance overall health and immune function. For instance, calcium and vitamin D supplements can be employed to reverse the risks of osteoporosis and optimize bone health, as advised in various guidelines on health. However, it is critical to include such interventions within the context of a more inclusive understanding of nutrient interactions; for instance, calcium absorption is contingent on vitamin D availability. Therefore, promoting individualized treatment based on the individual needs of every older person is important for maximizing the benefits of supplements and minimizing potential unwanted interactions inherent with multivalent nutritional therapy (LeBoff et al., 2022). Through the promotion of an environment of informed intervention, clinicians can improve the nutritional status and quality of life of older adults significantly (Figure 12.7).

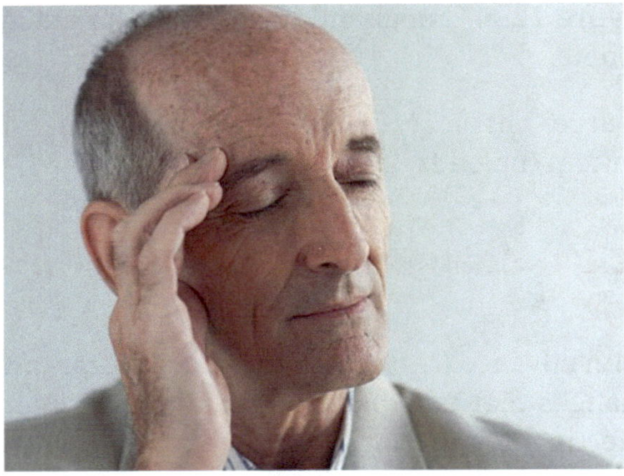

Figure 12.7. Nutrient deficiency in older adults.

Source: https://getopt.com/wp-content/uploads/2024/06/A-bald-old-man-stress.jpg.

12.2.3. Role of Dietary Guidelines

Dietary guidelines play a critical role in health promotion and disease prevention due to diet, particularly in the elderly. Guidelines serve as a foundation for recommended nutrient intakes established in terms of what will be needed to meet the unique metabolic needs of the geriatric population. With aging, there are certain physiological changes that might alter the absorption, metabolism, and utilization of nutrients, and hence standard dietary recommendations will need to be modified. Hence, guidelines do not merely aim to provide an overall overview of required nutrients but also point to the importance of eating patterns in favoring general well-being, so they agree with evidence showing that certain diet patterns have the potential to delay functional decline in older people, like the Mediterranean diet. As more data is put forward, the guidelines must continue to change to address the specific nutritional needs of this age group so that the elderly can receive the recommendations they require for improved health. In geriatric dietetics, the use of dietary guidelines extends beyond recommendations; they also have a role in guiding the correct use of dietary supplements. Given that elderly individuals may not have all of the essential vitamins and minerals due to impaired food intake or inadequate absorption, dietary advice advises careful supplementation where appropriate. However, the interaction of diet and supplements must also consider potential interactions of nutrients that could adversely affect the health of elderly individuals. It has been observed that while some supplements complement nutritional status, others may lead to imbalances or interfere with the effectiveness of prescribed medication (Inzitari et al., 2011). Therefore, the careful addition of supplements must be grounded on dietary counseling with consideration of such interactions, seeing in the process the necessity for comprehensive nutritional assessment in geriatric practice. The implementation of diet recommendations necessitates collaboration between health professionals, dietitians, and policymakers to ensure that older adults are able to access and maintain proper nutritional advice. Education and continued training are essential for both practitioners and patients, particularly in the integration of whole foods to supplementation. While dietary guidelines create a solid foundation for healthy diets, personal taste, cultural values, and economic constraints could influence the selection of foods. Correspondingly, individually tailored interventions considering these special characteristics must be done to enforce dietary advice compliance among older adults. Through encouraging an environment that promotes informed food choice and valuing the intricate roles of supplements in the diet, the quality of life and functional ability among the elderly can be attained.

12.3. Benefits of Supplement Use

The inclusion of dietary supplements in the diet of the aged can have many positive effects on health, particularly in offsetting the exact nutritional deficiencies most common in the aged. As people get older, the body may become less efficient at absorbing nutrients. The consequences of this can result in deficiencies of important vitamins and minerals, which are needed for long-term health and the avoidance of chronic disease. Supplements are therefore a convenient and effective method of replenishing these nutrients, hence supplementing dietary intake. With targeted supplementation, older people can potentially enhance their immune functions, thinking ability, and overall well-being, particularly when diets tend to become suboptimal because of loss of appetite or a shift in food choices. These are not the only roles of supplementation, as the purpose of supplementation extends beyond the restoration of only deficiencies in nutrients. Certain supplements have been known to have specific physiological effects most suited to the elderly. Omega-3 fatty acids, for instance, may improve cardiovascular function and reduce inflammatory reactions, while vitamin D is important in ensuring bone health and preventing osteoporosis. As the geriatric population is apt to develop more comorbidities, incorporating these supplements may avoid or treat some illnesses associated with age. It is important, however, to introduce supplementation with an individual approach considering the specific health profiles and needs, so the advantages of use are maximized and future interactions with existing medicines or illness are prevented, particularly in elderly individuals. In addition, the ongoing research on the impact of nutritional supplementation sustains a comprehensive approach in the case of elderly nutrition. The COVID-19 pandemic has revealed susceptibilities within this group, proving the effect of compromised health on multiple systems, as evidenced by studies linking poor nutrition to higher morbidity and mortality rates within the elderly (Woods et al., 2020). These findings provide a strong case for proactive dietary supplement use as a means of not only enhancing nutritional status but also enhancing overall resilience to health. In a world dominated by the increasing incidence of chronic disorders and demographic shifts toward aging populations, the benefits of employing supplements are a priority for health care professionals to be considered when establishing individual treatment strategies, especially in the management of the complexities surrounding Alzheimer's and other dementias (Figure 12.8).

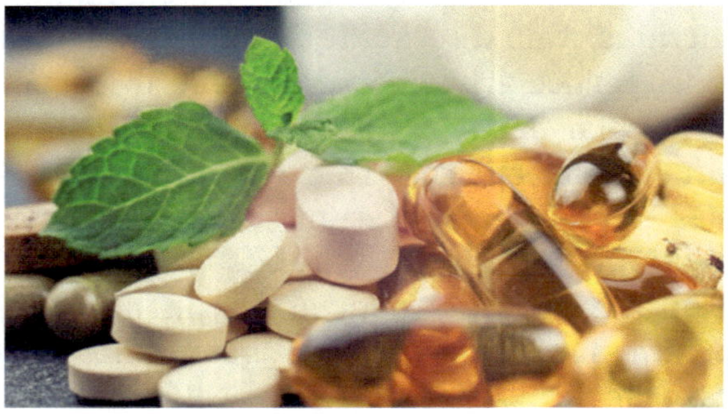

Figure 12.8. Dietary supplements elderly.

Source: https://www.nia.nih.gov/sites/default/files/inline-images/dietary-supplements-elderly-inline.jpg.

12.3.1. Improved Bone Health

The importance of improved bone health in the elderly cannot be overstated, particularly as aging can be characterized by declining skeletal integrity. Osteoporosis is the most prevalent metabolic bone disease, and preventive strategies towards bone density improvement and maintenance are therefore necessary among the elderly. This concern for bone health is synergistic with efforts to prevent the risks of fractures, which can lead to a cascade of adverse health outcomes. Scientific evidence demonstrates that intervention with nutritional supplementation and dietary modification has promise for making important improvements in bone health. Nutrients like vitamin D and calcium play a decisive role in maintaining bone strength and preventing osteoporosis, thereby promoting the importance of holistic dietetic practices in treating the population of older adults with inadequate nutrition status due to age-related complications (Guo et al., 2022). In addition to the promotion of the proper consumption of necessary nutrients, value for supplement utilization is paramount in geriatric diets. Various studies have demonstrated that some supplements can complement dietary consumption in order to enhance the body's ability to absorb necessary minerals that contribute to bone health. For instance, supplementation of calcium and vitamin D has been effective in upgrading bone mineral content in older individuals, thereby decreasing their vulnerability to fractures. However, such supplement application must be considered with regard to the distinct individual profiles of health, including existing illness and other drugs impacting the intake of nutrients. To prevent drug-nutrient interactions that might exacerbate deficiencies or compromise bone integrity, healthcare providers must monitor elderly patients receiving such therapy closely (Guo et al., 2022). Lifestyle also dictates the degree to which nutritional supplements can enhance bone health. Weight-bearing and resistance-training exercises are important aspects of a comprehensive approach to bone density preservation, particularly when combined with adequate nutrient feeding. Physical exercise stimulates bone remodeling and improves muscle strength, contributing to the prevention of fractures. Educational interventions directed towards the elderly must highlight interdependencies between nutrition, the use of supplements, and exercise. By raising awareness about such interdependencies, health care professionals can help enable older persons to apply self-managed strategies to enhance their bone health, thereby better preserving their quality of life in response to aging processes. A multifaceted approach that includes diet change, supplementation, and physical activity can go a long way in overcoming the risks of osteoporosis for healthy aging (LeBoff et al., 2022).

12.3.2. Enhanced Cognitive Function

Enhanced cognition is a significant area of study in geriatric nutrition, with the high prevalence of degenerative conditions such as Alzheimer's. There is increasing evidence to indicate that certain nutrients and supplements may have significant impacts on older adults' cognitive health. Omega-3 fatty acids, for instance, which are commonly found in fish oil, have been shown to positively impact brain function and recall. Because cognitive decline is a progressive disease, the alleviation of nutritional deficiencies through supplements may be a way of minimizing potential impairments. This proactive emphasis is particularly so in light of the predicted increase in Alzheimer's cases, projected to affect 13.8 million people by 2060 if no preventative measures are achieved, which highlights the priority of food-based interventions to optimize intellectual resilience in older populations (Damluji et al., 2023). In addition, antioxidants such as vitamins C and E play a role in protecting neural tissues from oxidative stress, a major cause of cognitive loss. Supplementation with these nutrients has been linked with deferred progression of cognitive impairment, particularly in individuals at risk for neurodegenerative disorders. Aging is often accompanied by reduced absorption of vital nutrients, which contributes to the risk of cognitive loss. Therefore, awareness of how various nutrients interact with one another is required during the formulation of effective nutritional plans for aged individuals. These interactions can impact the availability and functioning of supplements, thus making the correct formulation and delivery of nutrient supplements crucial to maximizing cognitive wellness. With the complex interplay between nutrition and cognitive capacity, targeted supplementation can be a cornerstone for the prevention of cognitive impairment in aging populations (Damluji et al., 2023). In addition to vitamins and omega-3s, B vitamins, particularly B12, B6, and folate, have been on the table for their role in cognitive capacity. These vitamins play a significant role in homocysteine metabolism, and elevated levels of homocysteine have been associated with increased risk of cognitive impairment as well as Alzheimer's disease. Because vitamin B can reduce the concentration of homocysteine, supplementation may be protective. The efficacy of such interventions, however, largely depends upon the individual's existing concentrations of these nutrients, which vary in the elderly. As has been well documented that deficiencies of nutrients have the tendency to exacerbate the susceptibility to cognitive impairments, it is essential to incorporate complete diet assessments with the supplementation regimen. Such a comprehensive approach not only seeks to delay cognitive impairment but also allows for a holistic understanding of geriatric nutrition, where enhanced cognitive function is a core goal.

12.3.3. Support for Immune System

The immune system plays a crucial role in health preservation, particularly in the geriatric group, who are more susceptible to declines in immune function due to old age. Immunosenescence refers to the loss of immune function, which results in increasing vulnerability to infections and chronic diseases, and therefore, there is a requirement for specific nutritional interventions. Vitamins C and D, zinc, and omega-3 fatty acids are nutrients that have been shown to enhance immune function and decrease the effect of aging on immunity. Older adults can build immune resilience through supplementation and dietary interventions, leading to improved health outcomes and quality of life. Just as in research on the emerging issues of aging, optimizing nutritional use is central to turning around the biological changes that result in immune function loss in the elderly. Furthermore, the role of dietary supplements in immunity gain becomes increasingly relevant with increasing chronic disease and loss of mental acuity in the elderly. The action of varying nutrients on each other can enhance their individual effect, creating a synergistic environment for better results. For instance, the interaction between vitamin D and calcium strengthens not only bone health but may also positively affect immune function, thereby performing a dual function to optimize geriatric nutrition. Evidence has documented that overall nutritional regimens involving a set of micronutrients can increase immune defense, particularly in susceptible populations at risk of deficiency from suboptimal dietary intake or defective absorption. This is particularly pertinent in light of the disturbing statistics indicating escalating rates of death attributed to long-term conditions in older populations. Besides, specific strategies in geriatrics emphasize the importance of personalized dietary regimens incorporating evidence-based supplementation. As the number of elderly people continues to swell with more instances of such conditions as Alzheimer's disease, adaptable intervention is necessary to augment immune status. An understanding of immune function and interaction among single nutrients can empower health professionals to enhance support for the elderly population with improved dietary practices. For example, dietary addition of antioxidants reduces oxidative stress, a widely reported causative factor for impairments in cognition as well as immune dysregulation. In general, the establishment of an overall strategy towards supplementation and interaction of nutrients is important to improve longevity and health in geriatric populations, particularly given that they are more susceptible to most chronic conditions (Guo et al., 2022) (Figure 12.9).

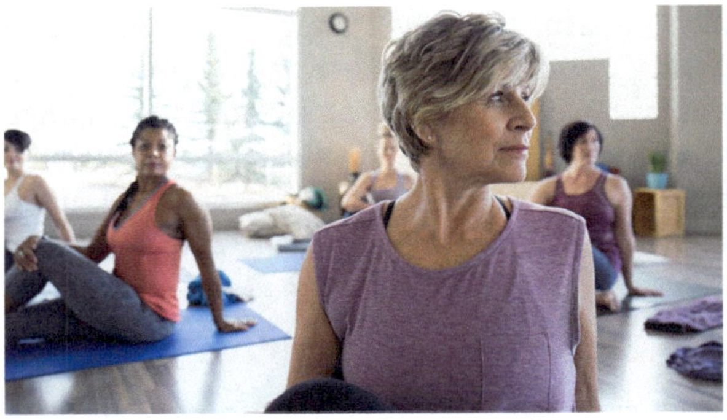

Figure 12.9. Immune system boosting tips for older adults.

Source: https://i0.wp.com/images-prod.healthline.com/hlcmsresource/images/topic_centers/sponsored-programs/age-well/female_senior_doing_yoga_stretch-1296x728-header.jpg?w=1155&h=1528.

12.4. Risks and Side Effects of Supplements

Increased consumption of dietary supplements by older individuals is a cause for concern regarding the risk and side effects that can be produced as a result of the consumption of supplements. Older individuals, consuming multiple drugs for chronic illnesses, are more likely to have unfavorable interactions with supplements that complicate their illness course. These interactions can range from the reduced efficacy of prescribed medication to enhanced side effects that can require hospitalization. For instance, certain vitamins and herbs, such as St. John's Wort, were shown to interact negatively with some medications administered for the treatment of dementia and other neurodegenerative diseases, which attests to the pressing need of medical professionals to assess the consumption of supplements among the population. The complexities of supplement-drug interactions call for integrative management strategies that focus on optimal use of these products in the process of geriatric nutritional treatment. Also, side effects accompanying supplements affect the overall health of older adults. Side effects like gastrointestinal discomfort, nausea, or allergic reactions discourage adherence to healthy nutritional interventions. Moreover, the psychological impact that accompanies experiencing unwanted effects causes elderly patients to lose their trust in supplements as well as normal treatments. More and more evidence suggests that elderly individuals lack the correct information on the perceived and actual dangers of nutritional supplementation. This unawareness can result in a lack of adherence to dietary recommendations and worsening of already existing conditions. Hence, it is important to impart education to aged people about how crucial it is to choose quality supplements and identify possible side effects of their intake, particularly since they are trying to navigate the complexities of managing their changing health. Further, the prevalence of unregulated markets for supplements also tends to elevate the dangers that geriatric patients are exposed to. Many supplements have exaggerated claims and contain unlabeled or harmful substances that present a significant risk to seniors. Such an unregulated environment discourages healthcare professionals from ensuring supplements taken are not only safe but also effective for patients' unique health statuses. Poorly produced bottled supplements may lead to contamination or incorrect dosage, further risking seniors with undeserved adverse effects on their health. Therefore, caregivers and older adults should approach decisions about supplements by consulting trustworthy sources and obtaining consultation from healthcare practitioners to guide their application in the broader context of geriatric care and nutritional management. Chronic disease, as it becomes increasingly prevalent in the aging population, is something that one must stay current with in terms of threat to safe nutrition (Figure 12.10).

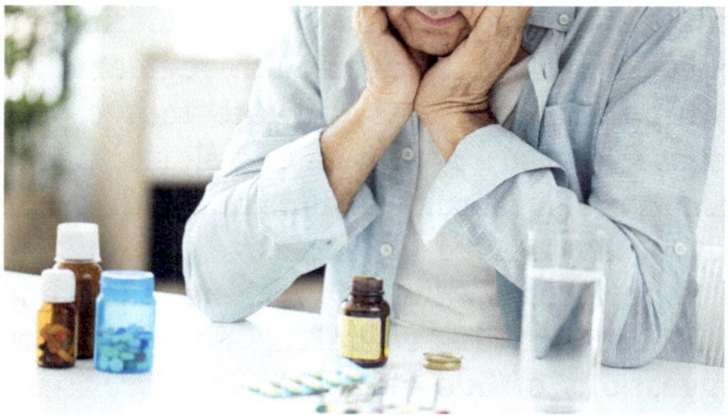

Figure 12.10. Risks and side effects of supplements in older adults.

Source: https://images.ctfassets.net/4f3rgqwzdznj/4Anf2TKZz24ovWwCRzd21x/0e46613cfbf3009a7bd89df159cd1ee2/senior_man_looking_down_at_pills_thinking_842975468.jpg.

12.4.1. Potential for Toxicity

While the elderly population increasingly relies on dietary supplements to fill nutritional gaps, it becomes essential to know their toxicity potential. Not all elderly people might be aware that even though supplements are known to be safe since they are natural, they can be incredibly detrimental to health if taken in excess or with other medicines. The complexity of nutrient interactions can lead to unwanted results, such as imbalance of nutrients or adverse interaction with prescribed drugs. For instance, excessive consumption of fat-soluble vitamins A, D, E, and K can result in body tissue accumulation and toxicity, especially among patients with liver disease or taking anticoagulants. Therefore, prudent recommendations by health care professionals regarding supplement intake remain essential in minimizing health risk to this vulnerable population. The toxic risk issue is further magnified by the physiological aging process itself, whereby the body can alter its ability to metabolize and excrete some of the supplements. With progressive age, there is also impairment of liver and kidney function, with attendant reduced elimination of drugs from the body. Such a condition could enhance the likelihood of accumulation and consequent toxicity even with regular doses of supplements. Facts indicate that chronic diseases that are typical among elderly people, such as cardiovascular and metabolic disorders, may be aggravated by excessive consumption of supplements, thereby making underlying conditions more complex. Following the suggestions of Guo et al (2022), there is also considerable emphasis placed on the description of aging-associated physiological changes that can inform maximal dietary guidance, with a need for careful and personalized approaches in supplement use to counteract the threat of toxicity. Also, nutrient interactions themselves create situations that favor increased risks of toxicity in older adults. For example, overuse of zinc will hamper copper absorption, leading to deficiency and, in turn, neurological and hematological symptoms. Similarly, high intakes of dietary supplements may be desirable but can also disturb the fine balance between interactions among nutrients, which might have undesirable effects on health. At a time when the aging population is increasing, it is not an intellectual exercise to appreciate these interactions; it's crucial in ensuring the total well-being of elderly people. By prioritizing education and ongoing research regarding the consumption of supplements, healthcare providers can assure geriatric nutrition safety while minimizing the possibility of toxicity as patients navigate through the maze of dietary supplements.

12.4.2. Drug-Supplement Interactions

The interaction between prescription medications and supplements is a significant consideration in geriatric nutrition, particularly against the background of the typical elderly patient's complex health profile. The older a person gets, the more multimorbidity they experience and therefore need to use different drugs to meet their health requirements. This polypharmacy is prone to escalating the risk of adverse drug interactions, as read from research that showed 81.2% of the elderly patients presented with potential drug interactions with an average of 4.24 interactions for every patient (Błeszyńska-Marunowska et al., 2022). The compounding effect of taking both over-the-counter supplements, vitamins, and prescription medication at the same time results in increased susceptibility to harmful side effects, a good reason for close scrutiny of all substances these older patients consume. Because increasing reliance on supplements by this group necessitates it to be aware of the necessity to monitor such interactions. Furthermore, the growing popularity of complementary and integrative medicine (CIM) in older adults complicates the model of drug-supplement interaction further. Older adults tend to view such alternative therapies, including dietary supplements, as more culturally acceptable or safer compared to conventional drugs. Although some supplements might be therapeutically helpful, evidence remains conflicting, particularly regarding their efficacy and safety in conjunction with conventional pharmaceutical drugs (Nguyen & Lavretsky, 2020). Problems of herb-drug interactions are particularly pertinent since they can significantly alter the pharmacokinetics and pharmacodynamics of prescribed medication. Health care practitioners, therefore, must balance the potential benefit of supplement use with the risk of possible interactions, in which proper explanations and assessment need to be made with patients. With such considerations in mind, it is critical that healthcare systems adopt more systematic and automated approaches towards the handling of drug-supplement interactions in geriatric medicine. The use of technology, for instance, automated analysis platforms that evaluate pharmacological interactions, can be utilized to identify potential risks that can be linked with the use of supplements in conjunction with prescribed medication (Błeszyńska-Marunowska et al., 2022). These systems not only support clinical decision-making but also increase patient safety in a more complicated therapeutic context. Furthermore, informing the healthcare providers regarding the implications of CIM and the specifics of dietary supplements improves their capacity to provide quality care. Lastly, an active role in realizing and coordinating drug-supplement interactions is necessary to maximize the outcome of nutrition in older adults and enhance their well-being (Figure 12.11).

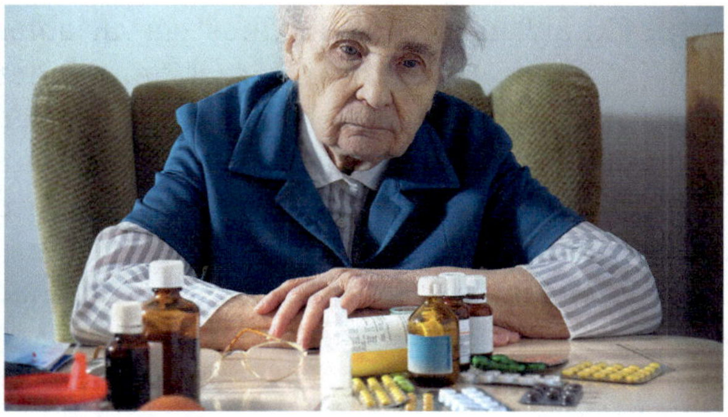

Figure 12.11. Pharmaceutical drugs and dietary supplements pose a significant concern in geriatric nutrition.

Source: https://www.seniorcarelifestyles.com/wp-content/uploads/2017/09/senior-multiple-medicines-1200x675.jpg.

12.4.3. Misleading Marketing Claims

In the context of geriatric nutrition, the overuse of supplements has brought about significant concern regarding misleading marketing claims. Such claims have the potential to overstate the benefit of certain nutraceuticals to treat complex health conditions like frailty and cognitive impairment. For older people, who might already have several health issues to contend with, the dependence on such products can divert attention away from overall dietary and lifestyle measures. The temptation of quick fixes can override the value of evidence-based measures, including having a balanced diet and engaging in periodic physical exercise. Deceptive promotion may exploit vague terminology—e.g., "maintains brain health" or "enhances immunity"—without adequate scientific backing, leaving clients more exposed to useless or even harmful alternatives. It serves to emphasize the necessity of well-informed decision-making on the basis of sound facts instead of sensationalized sales stories. Furthermore, nutraceutical advertising specifically targets a group eminently susceptible to misleading information: the elderly. These individuals can be exposed to additional health problems and might have a strong desire to enhance their general level of well-being through comparatively accessible avenues. Consequently, they might overlook serious evaluations of product performance and safety. For example, claims that a supplement decreases the incidence of chronic disease inherent in elderly populations can neglect to offer rigorous clinical data to support them, building unrealistic expectations. As described in recent literature, the addition of nutraceuticals to therapeutic regimens does have some positive effects, particularly with their antioxidants, that may benefit disorders like Parkinson's disease and elderly frailty (Montanari et al., 2024). When irresponsibly promoted, however, the focus is taken away from other key health interventions, decreasing the overall holistic regimen to effective geriatric care. Regulatory authorities are constantly grappling with the problem of deceptive marketing claims in the supplement industry. The current laws governing dietary supplements in the United States give manufacturers a lot of leeway in making health claims, and it often results in imprecise terminology that may be misleading to consumers. Not having stringent pre-market testing for effectiveness means that many products remain in circulation on the shelves even though the claims are dubious. This requires an integrated strategy for safeguarding elderly individuals against misinformation. Agenda 2030 emphasizes health and well-being throughout all stages, demanding universal health protection that encompasses accurate information about interventions in health, such as supplements. By embracing stricter regulation and improving transparency in marketing, stakeholders can help ensure geriatric groups are provided with accurate and useful information pertaining to the intake of supplements to enhance their health outcomes and quality of life.

12.5. Nutrient Interactions

In gerontology nutrition, understanding nutrient interactions is crucial to optimizing older adults' health outcomes. Age advancement tends to lead to physiological changes that may affect the absorptive process and metabolism of nutrients. For instance, the interaction between minerals and vitamins is an important aspect since certain nutrients can enhance or inhibit each other's bioavailability. General assessment of such interactions indicates that supplementary use of nutrients must be properly calculated. For example, calcium can inhibit the absorption of magnesium and iron, which are both important for supporting muscle structure and cognitive functions in older adults. Therefore, doctors should be careful to recommend dietary supplements so that they do not unknowingly interfere with the absorption of other nutrients important for our body, lowering the risk of deficiency and ensuring overall wellness (Mohankumar et al., 2021). The delicate control of interactions of nutrients is also used in the impact that dietary supplements exert on elderly diseases. Chronic illnesses such as osteoporosis, cardiovascular disease, and diabetes typically require subtle nutritional care. In particular, the interaction between minerals such as calcium, phosphorus, and vitamin D is of utmost significance with regard to bone health. If older people are placed on vitamin D supplements to ensure proper absorption of calcium, it is essential to evaluate the overall diet intake so that imbalances do not take place due to excessive supplementation. The complementarity among nutrients not only optimizes their effectiveness but also helps in mitigating adverse effects commonly linked to taking them into isolation. This underscores the critical need for an individualized approach in geriatrics nutrition, whereby the synergy of nutritional intake and supplements is given comprehensively in personal health plans (Mohankumar et al., 2021). Moreover, supplement consumption in geriatric nutrition must be considered in the context of a larger body of knowledge regarding lifestyle variables that influence nutrient interactions. Older adults are often challenged with impaired diet, functional disability, and impaired appetite and digestion, all of which contribute to altering nutrient utilization. Certain dietary practices, such as whole foods versus isolated supplements, can maximize nutrient synergy, ultimately resulting in improved overall health. In addition, drug interactions with prescribed drugs are likely to make the nutritional situation more complicated. For example, certain diuretics are likely to enhance potassium loss and, hence, dietary modification involving the inclusion of potassium-rich foods or supplementation might be indicated. These kinds of intricate interactions demand an integrated nutrition approach that considers not only the probable benefit of supplements but also their effect on nutrient interactions, medication adherence, and individualized dietary needs of the elderly (Mohankumar et al., 2021).

12.5.1. Synergistic Effects of Nutrients

Synergistic effects of nutrients should be understood in the context of geriatric nutrition because aging, as with any other process, is accompanied by certain challenges and degeneration of various body functions. Interactions among nutrients are an important factor in determining supplement efficacy and thereby promoting health benefits among elderly individuals. For example, the combination of vitamins B12, B6, and folic acid has been proven to lower homocysteine, a variable that is associated with increased risks of cognitive decline and cardiovascular diseases among the older population. The relationship not only suggests the importance of individual nutrients but also how they can interact to strengthen nutritional interventions to prevent age-related deterioration. Further, targeting these synergy effects supports more advanced supplementation regimens tailored to older adults, ultimately aiming to improve overall health and longevity (Guo et al., 2022). Beyond synergy with vitamins, ketogenic interventions offer convincing insight into nutrient interactions that support improving cognitive function in older adults. Increased brain energy from ketone bodies may be able to reverse decreasing glucose metabolism—a prevalent condition among geriatric populations with cognitive impairment.

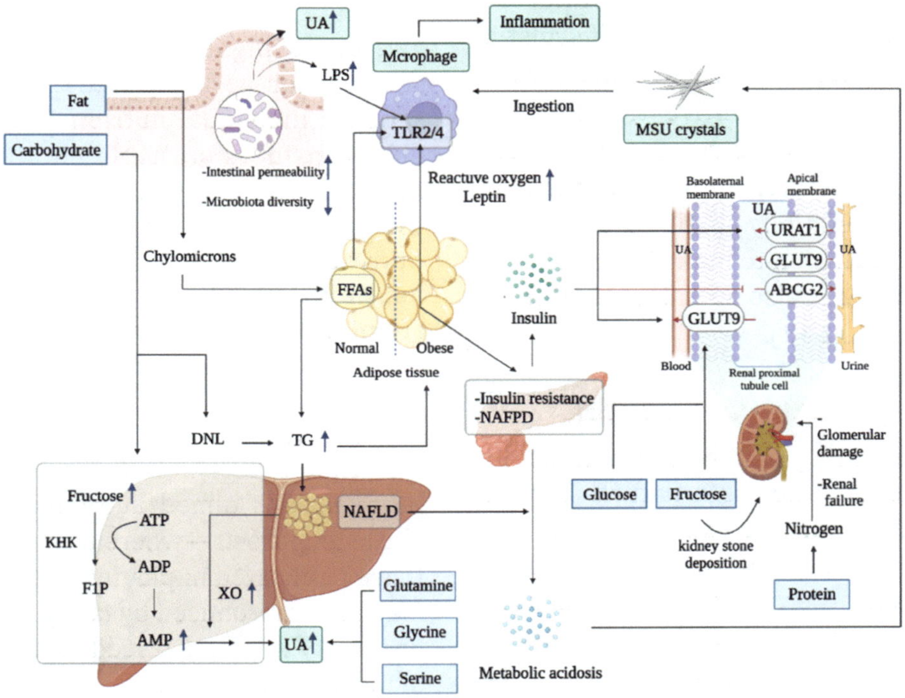

Figure 12.12. Nutrient interactions.

Source: Zhang, Y., Chen, S., Yuan, M., Xu, Y., & Xu, H. (2022). Gout and Diet: A Comprehensive Review of Mechanisms and Management. Nutrients, 14(17), 3525. https://doi.org/10.3390/nu14173525

Research shows that the union of ketogenic medium-chain triglycerides (kMCT) and aerobic exercise results in enhanced cognitive functioning through the support of brain ketone uptake and the availability of a backup source of energy when glucose metabolism is not optimal. Such findings highlight that the cumulative effects of lifestyle treatment and dietary supplements can strategically alleviate cognitive impairments associated with disorders like mild cognitive impairment or Alzheimer's disease. Such identification of synergistic interactions not only guides nutritional recommendations but also reveals avenues for more effective interventions in elderly nutrition (Cunnane et al., 2022). Furthermore, the interaction between lifestyle conditions and nutritional supplements reveals the necessity of the multidisciplinary management of geriatric health. The combination of nutritional therapy, such as kMCT and B vitamins, with aerobic exercise may be more effective, but it is still important to understand the mechanisms of these interactions in order to maximize treatment protocols. The Finnish Geriatric Intervention Study to Prevent Cognitive Impairment and Disability (FINGER) is the most striking demonstration of how multifaceted approaches included can produce tangible benefits in the cognitive abilities of the elderly population. The trial reinforces that holistic strategies adopting synergistic interactions of different nutrients along with physical activity and cognitive training are crucial in managing age-related diseases. Eventually, more research into these nutrient interactions will definitely shape paradigms of future geriatric nutrition to make interventions not only effective but also sustainable (Guo et al., 2022) (Figure 12.12).

12.5.2. Antagonistic Interactions

The variety of antagonistic interactions in nutrient supplementation is a natural part of geriatric nutrition, and it can be potentially complex in older populations. As the aging process progresses, there are molecular changes that affect the metabolism and absorption of nutrients, making them more susceptible to interactions that can reduce the effectiveness of dietary supplements. When taken together, some vitamins and minerals may hinder the absorption of one another, causing imbalances that may exacerbate existing conditions or develop new issues. For instance, eating too much calcium may hinder the body's ability to absorb magnesium and zinc, which play a pivotal role in many facets of bodily processes, such as immune function and repair of tissues. It is vital that these interactions are realized by healthcare providers, particularly in the choice of supplement regimens for optimizing health and preventing deficiencies in older adults. Furthermore, some of these antagonist interactions take place in the context of pharmacological therapies that are routinely prescribed for the elderly, and thus nutrition management becomes much more challenging. Medications for the treatment of chronic illness may interact negatively with nutrient supplements, further undermining their benefits. For example, some diuretics can lead to the depletion of potassium, requiring supplementation but possibly being antagonistic if too much sodium is ingested at the same time. This relationship between food, supplements, and drugs highlights the value of a holistic strategy for geriatric nutrition that not only satisfies individual nutrient requirements but also considers possible interactions. Thus, medical personnel must undergo thorough assessments to ascertain the patient's overall nutrition status with their keen attention to possible antagonistic effects between their supplements and drugs. The implications of antagonistic interactions extend beyond individual nutrient supplementation to public health advice and nutritional recommendations for the elderly. For example, nutrition interventions aimed at remedying conditions like osteoporosis—wherein calcium and vitamin D are implicated in playing such pivotal roles—may be compromised by faulty supplementation or dietary habits that lead to imbalanced levels of nutrients. As indicated in recent studies, aging individuals are found to be characterized by increased vulnerability for fractures and bone loss insofar as there is an intricate interplay of numerous nutrients, absorption, and biological activity on bone condition (LeBoff et al., 2022). Having proper measures of prevention for such interactions is of significance so that an even more specific and positive approach can be made towards geriatric nutrition. Educating for such interactions can provide patients and professionals with informed decisions, promoting healthier aging and preventing complications related to chronic disease (Figure 12.13).

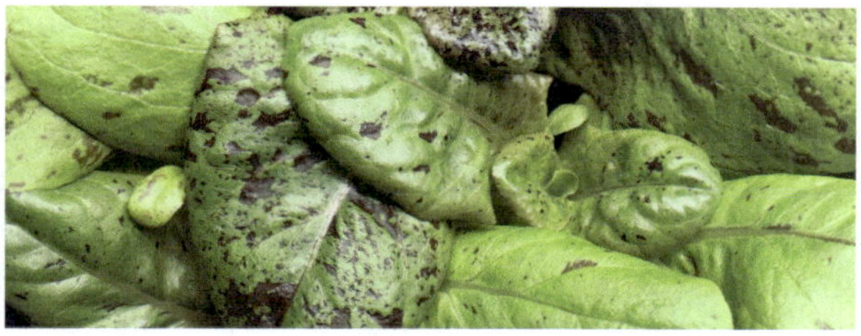

Figure 12.13. Nutrient interactions & antagonism.

Source: https://aptus-holland.com/wp-content/uploads/2020/02/nutrient-interactions-blog.jpeg.

12.5.3. Impact on Absorption and Bioavailability

The role of absorption and bioavailability in geriatric nutrition supplementation is an important factor that must be considered very seriously. Age alters the physiological functions, and these altered physiological functions influence the gastrointestinal system and the metabolic functions. With increasing age, the surface area of the intestine can decrease, and thus the efficiency of absorption of various nutrients decreases. Therefore, in addition to the normal decrease in organ function, supplement use becomes more complicated with more complexity, requiring an appreciation of how these alterations influence the bioavailability of dietary nutrients and supplements. This decreased capacity to consume nutrients can also potentially have a very significant effect on the general health and well-being of older people, especially within the context of persistent disease in this group and therefore highlights the significance of optimizing supplemental intake methods in geriatrics (Guo et al., 2022). In addition to the physiological alterations that accompany aging, the pharmacokinetics of supplements are largely influenced by food-drug interaction, which is also very critical when the nutritional needs of the elderly are being considered. The bioavailability of some foods tends to enhance or suppress the absorption of certain nutrients, providing additional layers of complexity to supplementation effects. For example, fat-soluble vitamins require dietary fat for their optimal absorption, and certain minerals may be impaired by the consumption of fiber or phytates in certain foods, causing potential nutrient deficiencies. In addition, one must also know how drugs typically given to elderly individuals may impact nutrient absorption to provide effective supplementation. This showcases the importance of constructing personalized nutritional regimens that consider not just the typical diet patterns but also the medication regimen of geriatric patients (Vinarov et al., 2021). Finally, constructing effective guidelines for supplement use in geriatric patients depends on a complex grasp of absorption and bioavailability processes. By incorporating knowledge of age-related physiological changes, gastrointestinal function, and potential interactions among nutrients, healthcare providers are able to maximize the therapeutic effectiveness of supplement interventions. It is not just a case of writing prescriptions for more nutrients but establishing the circumstances for older adults to be at optimal nutrient status and health outcome. This plan calls for ongoing study of the elderly's unique absorption mechanisms and the investigation of the complicated interrelationships among food components and drug treatment, thus setting the stage for future study in geriatric nutrition (Guo et al., 2022).

12.6. Recommendations for Supplement Use

In the context of geriatric nutrition, supplement use has been the focus of much discussion due to ongoing interests in the area of micronutrient deficiencies in older adults. With physiological changes, such as lowered nutrient utilization and altered metabolism, such patients are, in all likelihood, deprived of basic vitamins and minerals. Prescriptions for the use of supplements must thus be founded on intimate knowledge of each patient's individual diet and overall health status. For instance, the elderly may require higher levels of calcium and vitamin D to offset the threat from osteoporosis, an extremely prevalent condition among this population, where bones are compromised and more susceptible to fractures. These interventions can preserve the integrity of the skeleton and general well-being, supporting the necessity for individualized nutrition strategies that weigh both intake through food and physiological requirements. Aside from bone health, supplementation is also essential to cognitive function among the elderly. There is evidence to suggest an uptrend in the prevalence of neurodegenerative diseases, such as Alzheimer's disease, that affect millions of elderly people and have serious personal and social costs. Cognitive support through dietary supplements like omega-3 fatty acids and antioxidants could potentially ensure a healthier brain and reduce the risk of cognitive decline. These supplements are frequently recommended in conjunction with a well-balanced diet to maximize their impact on mental function. Notably, clinicians and dietitians have the responsibility to ensure that the selection of supplements matches overall health objectives and individual requirements, underscoring the value of an integrated model of geriatric nutrition focusing on both physical and mental health. In addition, in formulating suggestions for supplements, the interplay among different nutrients cannot be ignored. For example, calcium and vitamin D have synergistic interactions, whereby vitamin D enhances the absorption of calcium to exert beneficial effects on bone condition (LeBoff et al., 2022). Interactions between supplements, on the other hand, may have adverse effects or decreased effectiveness if properly controlled. Physicians should, therefore, conduct thorough assessments of patients' existing drug regimen and potential nutrient interactions before prescribing supplements. Identification of such interactions is particularly vital in the older adult, who might have numerous medications for chronic diseases, further complicating their nutritional status. Individualized counseling, which considers both nutrient-nutrient interactions and individual health profiles, is imperative to ensure proper application of supplements in geriatric nutrition, ultimately enhancing quality of life in older adults (Figure 12.14).

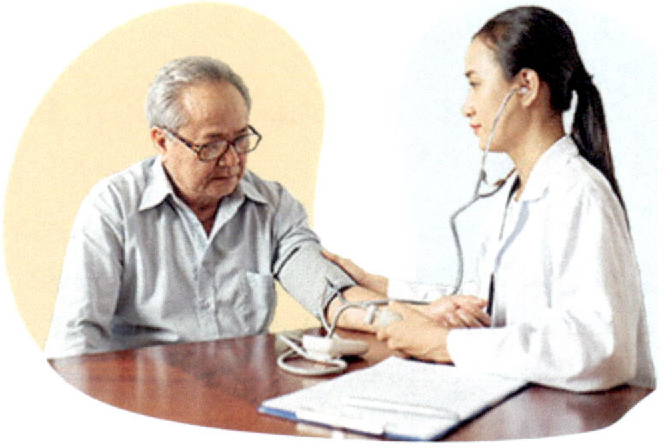

Figure 12.14. Nutrient deficiencies related to healthy aging.

Source: https://7dvariety.com/wp-content/uploads/2023/08/L00078_American-nutrient-deficiencies-related-to-healthy-aging-850x560.jpg.

12.6.1. Consultation with Healthcare Providers

The role of healthcare workers in the consultation process for supplement use in the nutrition of the elderly cannot be overstated. Given that older individuals experience various physiological changes related to nutritional status, health care professionals are important assets for determining individual needs and potential interactions of nutrients. For instance, by virtue of age, the absorption of certain vitamins and minerals is reduced, making individualized supplementation more important. Besides, the interaction between supplements and prescription medications can also be complex, necessitating intensive counseling. Medical professionals can assist geriatrics to demystify such complexities to ensure that the intake of supplements is best timed relative to the ongoing treatments. As a result, not only is nutrient absorption maximized, but also the risk of deleterious interaction is avoided, thereby maximizing the welfare of the elderly patients. Effective communication between older adults and their health care professionals is required for making informed choices about dietary supplements. A few older adults may base their choices on hearsay advice or advertising rather than scientific evidence when selecting supplements. This dearth of information may lead to improper choices that complicate an already unstable nutritional balance. Through open discussion, healthcare providers can make patients aware of the pros and cons of specific supplements, considering dietary restrictions, lifestyle, and comorbidities. For example, considering that older patients are at higher risk of developing diseases like osteoporosis, health workers have a key role in prescribing sufficient calcium and vitamin D supplements. Consultation not only enables older adults to become active participants in their own health care but also ensures that their use of supplements is based on sound clinical evidence. Effective communication with health care providers improves the likelihood of older adults completing their prescribed nutritional regimens, including the use of supplements. If patients are comfortable discussing their health concerns and desires, they will be more willing to engage in collaborative decision-making, and this will enhance the effectiveness of tailored nutrition advice. Also, health practitioners can employ frequent checks to monitor how well supplements work, enabling early recommendations to be altered if needed. As there is a rising prevalence of diseases like Alzheimer's and osteoporosis among the elderly, it becomes increasingly vital to have proactive consultation with healthcare professionals. Not only does regular consultation contribute in the long term to optimizing the utilization of supplements, but it also facilitates achieving an environment to serve the overall health issues of the elderly and thereby providing effective geriatric care and nutrition (LeBoff et al., 2022).

12.6.2. Importance of Personalized Nutrition Plans

In geriatric nutrition, there cannot be enough stress placed on individualized nutrition plans. As elderly people typically have multiple nutritional issues and dietary restrictions, nutrition plans must be especially tailored to an individual's needs. Personalized nutrition does not merely consider the nutritional requirements identified by alterations in metabolism due to age, but also considers specific health conditions that may affect diet choices. This customized approach facilitates more accurate monitoring of nutrient intake, which is likely to minimize malnutrition-associated risks and optimize overall health outcomes in elderly populations. One illustration is the development and implementation of personalized nutritional care interventions during hospital admissions, which can lead to a major decline in complications caused by malnutrition among polymorbid patients, thereby improving the recovery process and overall patient well-being (Wunderle et al., 2023). In addition, inclusion of customized nutrition plans is essential when tackling the complex interactions of supplement use with nutrient absorption in geriatric patients. Some elderly people consume supplements to complete gaps in their diet, but without a customized plan, the potential for adverse interactions is greater. For example, certain supplements may compete with the bioavailability of prescription medications, which is prevalent among the elderly who typically have polypharmacy problems. Effective nutrition plans, therefore, must incorporate a complete assessment of a patient's existing medication and overall health to determine that supplementation is safe and beneficial. Such tailoring ensures the optimal use of nutrients alongside decreased adverse interactions, thereby attaining enhanced health outcomes and quality of life in the elderly (Wunderle et al., 2023).

Moreover, the ongoing evolution of dietary guidelines also points towards the importance of personalized nutrition in disease prevention as well as cognitive well-being among older adults. With diseases like Alzheimer's reaching epidemic proportions, it is more important to understand the dietary components that can influence initiation and progression alike. Personalized nutrition plans can be developed to put into prominence nutrient-dense foods that support cognitive function, thus managing or even delaying such disorders. By establishing diet recommendations in terms of individual health profiles, geriatric nutrition can evolve from a one-size-fits-all policy to a diversified and strategic approach. This shift not only acknowledges the unique dietary needs of the aged but also empowers them as active participants in their own health care through intelligent nutritional decision-making tailored to their individual circumstances (Figure 12.15).

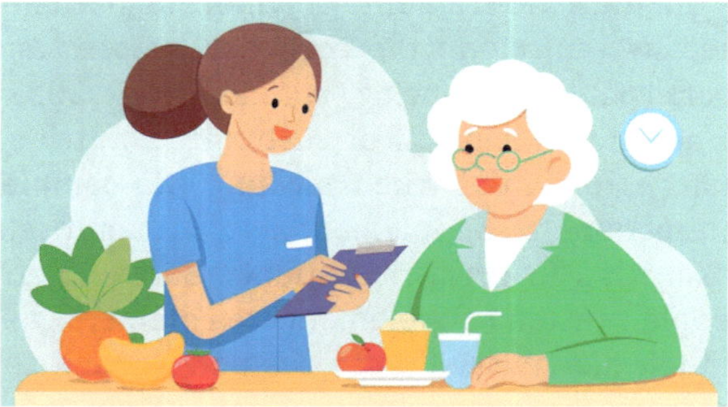

Figure 12.15. A nurse helping an elderly woman with her meal planning.

Source: https://img.freepik.com/premium-vector/nurse-helping-elderly-woman-with-her-meal-planning-teaching-her-about-proper-nutrition_216520-109018.jpg.

12.6.3. Monitoring and Adjusting Supplement Intake

Regulation and modification of supplement use are crucial in maximizing the nutritional status of aging individuals, particularly because they experience numerous physiological changes and ailments affecting nutrient metabolism and uptake. As people age, their dietary requirements are altered, typically requiring greater intakes of specific vitamins and minerals to maintain bone density, muscle power, and health. For instance, calcium and vitamin D are key in preventing osteoporosis, a condition of high prevalence among aged populations. Regular monitoring of the performance of supplements and nutrient levels can aid in the detection of deficiencies or toxicities that may occur due to abuse of supplements, so that the elderly will be given maximum benefits without toxicity. The use of organized monitoring is evident in the context of the prevalence of osteoporosis and fractures among the elderly, necessitating specific interventions supporting bone strength and overall nutritional balance (LeBoff et al., 2022). The inter-relationship between nutrients further emphasizes the need for careful monitoring and control over supplement use. Some vitamins and minerals interact to facilitate or inhibit uptake. For example, overconsumption of calcium can inhibit the absorption of magnesium, leading to deficiency and aggravating pre-existing muscle weakness or neuromuscular impairment that already occurs in older patients. Similarly, the action of certain medications that are commonly prescribed to older adults may affect the metabolism of nutrients or amplify nutritional requirements. Such synergistic action among supplements, nutrients, and medications highlights the importance for health professionals to review an individual's supplement regimen on a regular basis and adjust depending on their personal health profile and treatment plan. The tailoring of these adjustments is important in addressing the compounded needs of older adults to their nutritional care (Lai et al., 2021). In addition, encouragement of patient education and adherence to supplement regimens are key elements of successful nutritional management. Older adults experience difficulties learning and following complicated dietary recommendations, so it is extremely important to make recommendations simple and easily understandable and to ensure monitoring processes are conveyed in equally simple language. Healthcare providers are extremely important to the process by sitting down with patients and discussing their supplement use, the possible side effects, and the need for persistent adherence to recommended regimens. Tailored interventions with regular follow-up consultations and easy-to-understand education tools can immensely optimize the efficacy of supplement consumption among geriatric patients. It finally results in improved health outcomes, reducing the likelihood of nutrient-related complications, and enhancing the quality of life of the geriatric population (LeBoff et al., 2022).

SUMMARY

Research on supplement use and nutrient interaction within elderly nutrition unwraps a complex situation that warrants careful consideration. Since older adults usually undergo changes in metabolism, gastrointestinal health, and use of drugs, their nutritional needs vary drastically compared to those in younger age groups. Additionally, the development of chronic illnesses in the elderly population makes dietary planning more complex since some nutrients might either contribute to or mitigate health disorders. As has been documented, close to 6.7 million Americans over the age of 65 have Alzheimer's dementia, highlighting the fundamental importance of individualized nutritional strategies that address both cognitive and overall health. In light of these factors, however, the role of nutritional supplements must be examined with particular care in the context of personal risk and health profiles. Apart from that, nutritional status assessment is also crucial in developing effective dietary management in the elderly. Repeated screening for nutrition should become routine practice in order to reveal susceptible subjects and to determine the appropriate requirement of supplementation. Prompt detection of malnutrition, a risk factor per se with a negative impact on outcomes and quality of life, can maximize the effectiveness of care delivered to geriatric patients (Reber et al., 2019). A systematized approach to nutritional assessment not only facilitates tailored care plans but also encourages interdisciplinary collaboration to ensure that the heterogeneous needs of older adults are tackled holistically within the healthcare system. In conclusion, the interplay of supplement consumption, nutrient interactions, and geriatric diet presents challenges and opportunities to effectively handle this age group's health. Strategic incorporation of adequate dietary supplementation can serve as an aid to healthier measures, reduced healthcare spending, and better quality of life among the elderly. But healthcare professionals must exercise utmost care through rigorous assessment and consideration of the unique nutrient interactions that define the geriatric population. The increasing rate of diseases like Alzheimer's disease underscores the necessity of incorporating systematic nutritional care focusing on the prevention and treatment of malnutrition to ensure that older individuals receive the best possible care and maintain independence in their aged years (Reber et al., 2019).

In gerontological nutrition, the importance of supplement intake cannot be overstated since it addresses the unique nutritional requirements of older individuals who are afflicted with various health conditions. Evidence repeatedly indicates that deficiencies in principal micronutrients can have unfavorable impacts on health outcomes, particularly for those with chronic conditions such as heart failure. As illustrated in recent studies, for example, very high rates of deficiency exist for vitamins A and D, calcium, and magnesium in older adults, stressing the importance of specific supplementation to reverse these effects. Additionally, deficiency conditions become compounded by pre-existing medical conditions, increasing rates of hospitalization and making diseases like heart failure harder to treat (Alves et al., 2020). Therefore, supplements used to meet the needs for deficiency conditions illustrate a critical element of geriatric nutrition strategies, which works in support of a wide goal of improving health and quality of life for the elderly population. In addition, knowing the interactions of nutrients is essential in geriatric nutrition, especially regarding the interaction of supplements with the medications already taken by them. Older people are often prescribed a variety of drugs, and therefore, they can become victims of nutrient insufficiency or worsen their deficiencies. This is especially relevant for people suffering from heart failure, where diuretics, traditionally used to control fluid status, can cause massive depletion of water-soluble vitamins like thiamine (Alves et al., 2020). Therefore, the addition of these vitamins might not only rectify the imbalance but also enhance the efficacy of heart failure management programs by alleviating these drug-nutrient interactions. Moreover, more recent studies indicate that certain supplements, like glycine, enhance metabolic function and insulin sensitivity in the older population, revealing a complex relationship between nutrient supplementation and overall health care (Alves et al., 2020). Evaluation of these interactions provides a foundation for the development of multifaceted diet interventions in older adults. Finally, the development of diet interventions must be evidence-based, considering individual variation in nutrient requirements and health status among older adults. For example, a multicenter study highlighted the prevalence of micronutrient deficiencies in patients with heart failure and their correlation with poor health outcomes and demanded specific dietary strategies (Alves et al., 2020). Furthermore, trials like GOURMET-HF demonstrate the worth of complete nutritional support in the management of heart failure, emphasizing the promise of tailored meal plans to reduce rates of hospitalization and improve quality of life (Alves et al., 2020). Therefore, the incorporation of these findings emphasizes the significance of an unobtrusive strategy of supplementation and food quality in geriatric nutrition. As science evolves, the determination of these factors will guide healthcare practitioners about how to optimally maximize nutrition care for elderly patients in order to ultimately enhance their health and well-being through informed dietary habits.

A CLOSER LOOK

VITAMIN B12

Vitamin B12, or cobalamin, is a water-soluble vitamin involved in a vitally important role in neurological function, red blood cell formation, and DNA synthesis. It plays a critical function to maintain the nervous system in a healthy state by helping to produce myelin, the sheath that wraps over nerve fibers. Vitamin B12 also plays a crucial role in homocysteine metabolism; elevated levels of homocysteine are often seen in states of B12 deficiency and are associated with cardiovascular risk. Natural source foods that have vitamin B12 include meat, eggs, milk, and fish. Accordingly, individuals on strict vegan or vegetarian diets are more apt to be deficient (Figure 12.16).

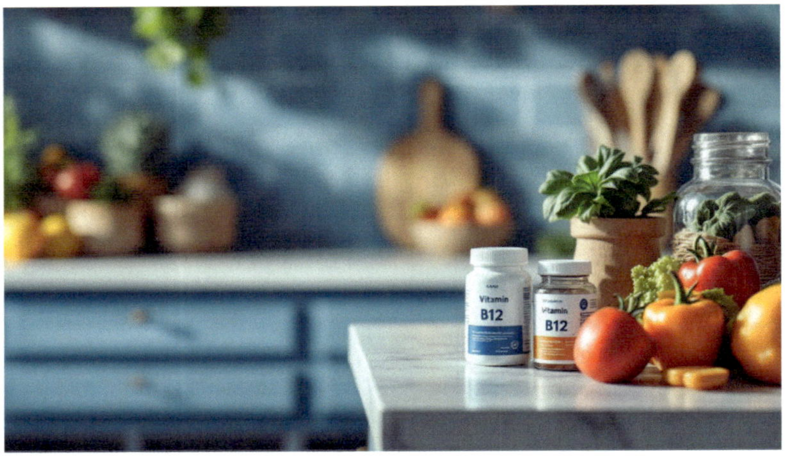

Figure 12.16. Vitamin B12 for the elderly diet.

Source: https://cdn.growtha.dev/65aa488862a2dc298476c66a/677eb7efdcdb88ba4774ce5e_tmpzz5e7rmn.jpeg.

Vitamin B12 deficiency among elderly individuals is relatively common due to age-related conditions such as atrophic gastritis, reduced gastric acid secretion, and the use of medication, including proton pump inhibitors or metformin, that blocks B12 absorption. Symptoms of deficiency can include weakness, forgetfulness, numbness and tingling of the hands and feet, mood changes, and even permanent neurological damage with advanced deficiencies. Early detection by laboratory studies during deficiency and immediate oral or injectable supplementation are vital to prevent long-term consequences. Maintaining proper vitamin B12 levels is especially important in the elderly to enhance mental function, energy metabolism, and health.

REFERENCES

1. Alves, A., Bulteau, A., Pirola, L., Rieusset, J., & Morio, B. (2020). Glycine contributes to the control of hepatic response to insulin by promoting mitochondrial-endoplasmic reticulum interactions. *Proceedings of the Nutrition Society, 79.* https://www.semanticscholar.org/paper/f3aab7366136d2fce22f941fa04f17a7582d013f (accessed on 12th July 2025).
2. Cederholm, T., Barazzoni, R., Austin, P., Ballmer, P., Biolo, G., Bischoff, S. C., Compher, C., Correia, I., Higashiguchi, T., Holst, M., Jensen, G. L., Malone, A., Muscaritoli, M., Nyulasi, I., Pirlich, M., Rothenberg, E., Schindler, K., Schneider, S. M., de van der Schueren, M. A., Sieber, C., ... Singer, P. (2017). ESPEN guidelines on definitions and terminology of clinical nutrition. *Clinical nutrition (Edinburgh, Scotland), 36*(1), 49–64. https://doi.org/10.1016/j.clnu.2016.09.004(accessed on 12th July 2025).
3. Błeszyńska-Marunowska, E., Wierucki, Ł., Jagiełło, K., Rewiuk, K., Mitręga, K., & Kalarus, Z. (2022). Prevalence and factors predisposing to potential drug-drug interactions in a Polish community-dwelling geriatric population: An observational, cross-sectional study. *Advances in Clinical and Experimental Medicine, Official Organ Wroclaw Medical University*. https://www.semanticscholar.org/paper/68eba14507be0a366256936702e8c2d37410a349 (accessed on 12th July 2025).
4. Cascino, T., & Hummel, S. (2018). Nutrient deficiencies in heart failure: A micro problem with macro effects? *Journal of the American Heart Association: Cardiovascular and Cerebrovascular Disease, 7.* https://www.semanticscholar.org/paper/54369632d26dec8c0756674fd91eedcd2d1abbca (accessed on 12th July 2025).
5. Cunnane, S. C., Swerdlow, R. H., Inzitari, M., Olaso-Gonzalez, G., & Viña, J. (2022). Multimodal strategy to rescue the brain in mild cognitive impairment: Ketogenic oral nutrition supplementation with B vitamins and aerobic exercise. *European Journal of Clinical Investigation, 52.* https://doi.org/10.1111/eci.13806 (accessed on 12th July 2025).
6. Damluji, A. A., Alfaraidhy, M., Alhajri, N., Rohant, N., Kumar, M., Al Malouf, C., Bahrainy, S., et al. (2023). Sarcopenia and cardiovascular diseases. *Circulation, 147,* 1534–1553. https://doi.org/10.1161/circulationaha.123.064071 (accessed on 12th July 2025).
7. Forteguerri, E. B. R. (2016). Síntesis endógena de ácidos grasos en la glándula mamaria y síndrome de baja grasa en la leche en ovejas. https://www.semanticscholar.org/paper/794a6ea49ecac53ff09b0791288a8e1bcbf861e0 (accessed on 12th July 2025).
8. Guo, J., Huang, X., Dou, L., Yan, M., Shen, T., Tang, W., & Li, J. (2022). Aging and aging-related diseases: From molecular mechanisms to interventions and treatments. *Signal Transduction and Targeted Therapy, 7.* https://doi.org/10.1038/s41392-022-01251-0 (accessed on 12th July 2025).
9. Inzitari, M., Doets, E., Bartali, B., Benetou, V., Bari, M., Visser, M., Volpato, S., et al. (2011). Nutrition in the age-related disablement process. *The Journal of Nutrition, Health & Aging, 15,* 599–604. https://www.semanticscholar.org/paper/c605cb85042d015de702bb1f0cc73301164b5368 (accessed on 12th July 2025).
10. Lai, J. C., Tandon, P., Bernal, W., Tapper, E. B., Ekong, U. D., Dasarathy, S., & Carey, E. J. (2021). Malnutrition, frailty, and sarcopenia in patients with cirrhosis: 2021 practice guidance by the American Association for the Study of Liver Diseases. *Hepatology, 74,* 1611–1644. https://doi.org/10.1002/hep.32049 (accessed on 12th July 2025).

11. LeBoff, M. S., Greenspan, S. L., Insogna, K., Lewiecki, E. M., Saag, K. G., Singer, A., & Siris, E. S. (2022). The clinician's guide to prevention and treatment of osteoporosis. *Osteoporosis International, 33*, 2049–2102. https://doi.org/10.1007/s00198-021-05900-y (accessed on 12th July 2025).

12. Meer, Y. (2017). Nutrition of pigs kept under low and high sanitary conditions: Effects on amino acid and energy metabolism and damaging behavior. https://www.semanticscholar.org/paper/aa8d59142af8277c5a6e5c37e7c673ee27a3b0c5 (accessed on 12th July 2025).

13. Mohankumar, T., Park, J., Mun, S., & Kim, I. (2021). Influence of the supplementation of *Achyranthes japonica* extracts on the growth performance, nutrient digestibility, gas emission, fecal microbial, and meat quality traits of finishing pigs with different nutrition concentrations in the diet. *Korean Journal of Agricultural Science.* https://www.semanticscholar.org/paper/e9582b89edd748fb2b869a7cdd7024348388d186 (accessed on 12th July 2025).

14. Montanari, M., Mercuri, N. B., & Martella, G. (2024). Exceeding the limits with nutraceuticals: Looking towards Parkinson's disease and frailty. *International Journal of Molecular Sciences, 26*, 122–122. https://doi.org/10.3390/ijms26010122 (accessed on 12th July 2025).

15. Montero-Odasso, M., van der Velde, N., Martin, F. C., Petrović, M., Tan, M. P., Ryg, J., Aguilar-Navarro, S. G., et al. (2022). World guidelines for falls prevention and management for older adults: A global initiative. *Age and Ageing, 51*. https://doi.org/10.1093/ageing/afac205 (accessed on 12th July 2025).

16. Nguyen, S. A., & Lavretsky, H. (2020). Emerging complementary and integrative therapies for geriatric mental health. *Current Treatment Options in Psychiatry, 7*, 447–470. https://www.semanticscholar.org/paper/83721c1c3fdff36f41293cb9b9e605864e71f90e (accessed on 12th July 2025).

17. Ní Lochlainn, M., Cox, N., Wilson, T., Hayhoe, R., Ramsay, S. E., Granic, A., Isanejad, M., et al. (2021). Nutrition and frailty: Opportunities for prevention and treatment. *Nutrients, 13*, 2349–2349. https://doi.org/10.3390/nu13072349 (accessed on 12th July 2025).

18. Reber, E., Gomes, F., Vasiloglou, M. F., Schüetz, P., & Stanga, Z. (2019). Nutritional risk screening and assessment. *Journal of Clinical Medicine, 8*, 1065–1065. https://doi.org/10.3390/jcm8071065 (accessed on 12th July 2025).

19. Mis Solval, Kevin Estuardo, "Developing Co-current and Counter-current Spray Drying Computational Fluid Dynamics (CFD) Simulation Studies to Predict the Quality of Microencapsulated Fish Oil with Egg White Hydrolysates Powders" (2015). LSU Doctoral Dissertations. 295. https://repository.lsu.edu/gradschool_dissertations/295(accessed on 12th July 2025).

20. Vinarov, Z., Abrahamsson, B., Artursson, P., Batchelor, H., Berben, P., Bernkop-Schnürch, A., Butler, J., et al. (2021). Current challenges and future perspectives in oral absorption research: An opinion of the UNGAP network. *Advanced Drug Delivery Reviews, 171*, 289–331. https://doi.org/10.1016/j.addr.2021.02.001 (accessed on 12th July 2025).

21. Woods, J. A., Hutchinson, N. T., Powers, S. K., Roberts, W. O., Gómez-Cabrera, M. C., Radák, Z., Berkés, I., et al. (2020). The COVID-19 pandemic and physical activity. *Sports Medicine and Health Science, 2*, 55–64. https://doi.org/10.1016/j.smhs.2020.05.006 (accessed on 12th July 2025).

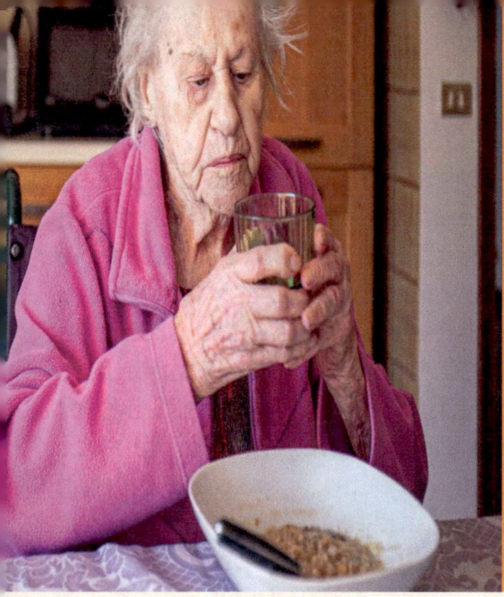

Chapter 13

SCREENING FOR GERIATRIC NUTRITIONAL RISK

Contents

Introduction

As the population of the world is getting older and older, addressing nutritional risk in older individuals has gained significant momentum both clinically and in the field of public health. Geriatric nutritional risk screening is an attempt to identify elderly individuals at risk of developing complications from inadequate dietary intake or malnutrition. This is particularly significant as a blend of factors, from physical and social to mental disorders, impacts nutritional status in this population. With more individuals becoming increasingly sensitized to the effects of malnutrition on health outcomes, researchers and clinicians have increasingly advocated for systematic screening protocols that can facilitate early discovery and intervention. By way of efficient screening methods, it is possible to not just enhance the quality of life of elderly people but also reduce healthcare costs associated with nutrition-related diseases and complications. Another aspect that makes the nutritional scenario more complicated in older people is the presence of co-morbid medical conditions, chronic illnesses, and depressive disorders. For example, research has established that depression that is undiagnosed depression among the elderly is prevalent, tending to affect their capacity for memory retention of important healthcare information, such as eating instructions (Wynn-Grundy, 2016). These co-morbidities often accentuate malnutrition risks since cognitive impairment or physical deficits can deter people from learning proper nutrient consumption. Moreover, the severity of these problems often gets underestimated, preventing timely interventions. Accordingly, it becomes imperative to develop comprehensive assessments incorporating nutrition needs as well as mental health concerns to develop integrated care plans for elderly patients. Subsequently, inclusion of systematic screening tools in clinic practice remains challenging, being sidelined by time constraints faced by health professionals (Lampugnane, 2017). Despite the need for an understanding of geriatric assessment in the identification of vulnerable populations, there are knowledge-practice gaps. Proper education programs that educate healthcare professionals, such as Physician Assistants and Medical Students, in the skill of understanding the multidimensional aspect of nutritional risk are important. This training will allow future clinicians to perform quality assessments and hence improve surgical outcomes as well as general health in the elderly. As geriatric nutrition continues to grow, directed and actionable screening instruments become more important and, therefore, an important target of interest in geriatric practice (Figure 13.1).

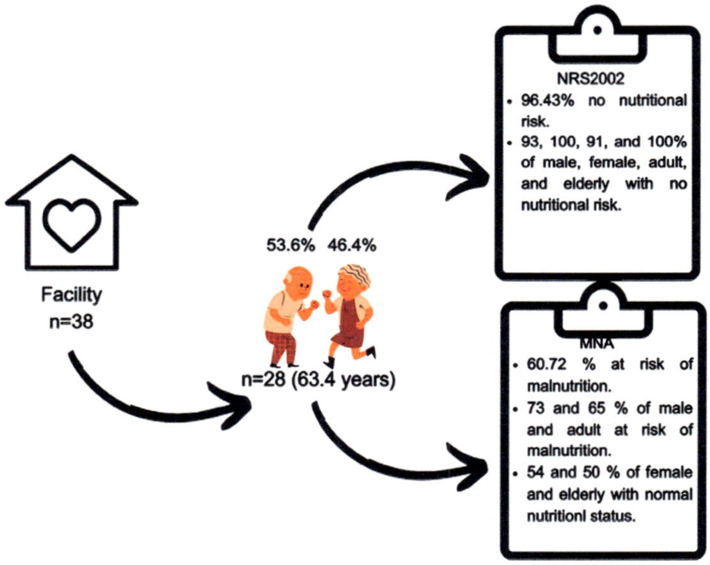

Figure 13.1. Nutritional screening tools for institutionalized people.

Source: https://html.scirp.org/file/2703904-rId15.jpeg?20240717030946.

Definition of Geriatric Nutritional Risk

Geriatric nutritional risk is essential knowledge in order to address the specialized nutrition needs of elderly people, particularly because malnutrition can impact their overall health and convalescence. Geriatric nutritional risk is the potential to experience adverse health effects due to inadequate nutrient intake by older persons and may be caused by many determinants, such as chronic illness, drug side effects, or social isolation. These risks can potentially lead to frailty, immune system dysfunction, and risk of infection or perioperative complications. The importance of detecting and acknowledging these risks implies the need for extensive nutritional evaluation, possibly allowing interventions that are done on a timely basis to maximize health outcomes among older adults, particularly those undergoing surgery or rehabilitation. To be able to properly assess and reduce geriatric nutritional risk, screening tools such as the Mini-Nutritional Assessment (MNA) play an important role. The MNA helps clinicians determine the nutritional status of older adults based on considerations such as dietary intake, weight loss, and body mass index. The case for earlier diagnosis is particularly important, as evidenced by work that demonstrated that the incidence of malnutrition can be unrealistically high at 18.7% in hip fracture patients who are elderly. More sophisticated criteria reveal even greater figures, underlining the fact that nutritional deficiency is likely to be underdiagnosed. Evaluation of such factors is crucial in the development of effective nutrition interventions that can optimize recovery and reduce hospital complications and thus the risks incurred due to malnutrition in the elderly population (Malafarina et al., 2017).

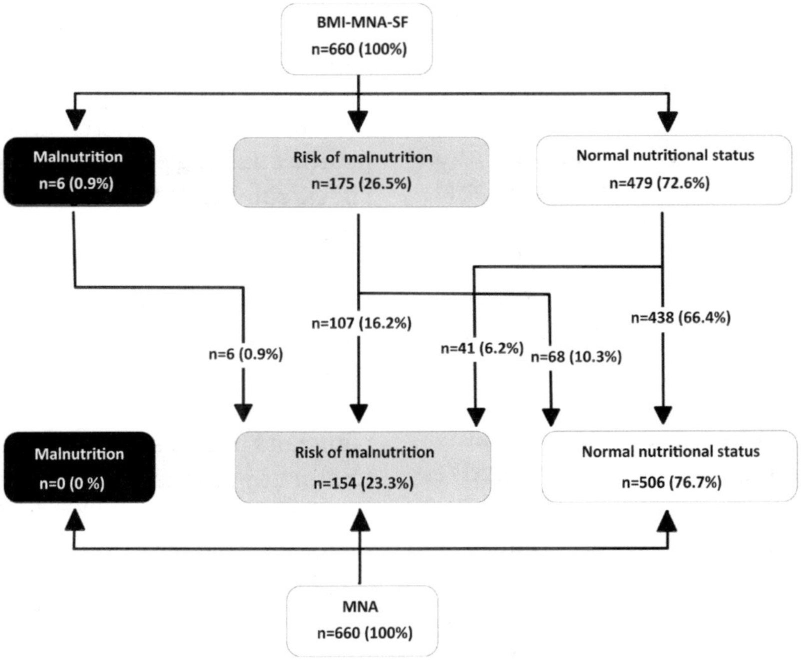

Figure 13.2. Mini-nutritional assessment (MNA).

Source: https://peerj.com/articles/3345/.

The consequences of geriatric nutritional risk extend beyond the acute health complications to affect long-term recovery and mortality. Poorly nourished elderly individuals are often linked with increased complications during the process of hospitalization, along with delayed functional recovery. For instance, studies have shown that malnutrition correlates with a high rate of mortality, suggesting an urgent need for intervention. Such issues must be addressed in an integrated approach to involve the care proficiency of medical practitioners in geriatric evaluation and nutritional treatment. As argued in the literature, implementation of systematic pre-surgical assessment of the geriatric patient based on their nutritional needs has the ability to improve the surgical outcome as well as the quality of life (Lampugnale, 2017). Hence, detection and intervention in geriatric nutritional risk through systematic screening and early intervention are essential in improving the health standards of this growing population segment (Figure 13.2).

Importance of Nutrition in Older Adults

The importance of ideal nutrition in older adults cannot be overestimated, especially in connection with their unique physiological and psychological needs. As age advances, the body is exposed to underlying changes that compromise nutrient absorption and metabolism. These changes in most instances result in a deficit of essential vitamins and minerals, which may lead to numerous health complications, including osteoporosis, cognitive dysfunction, and cardiovascular diseases. Therefore, nutritional screening is significant in identifying older adults at risk of malnutrition. Research has shown that nutritional interventions for increasing intake can be beneficial to overall health consequences and quality of life in this population. For instance, proactive management of diets will promote immune function and decrease frailty risk, consequently leading to a more active and independent life. Implementing efficient screening strategies is required to ensure that older individuals receive the nutritional support they require to thrive. Furthermore, social determinants are a significant part of older adults' nutrition since social determinants establish older adults' ability to receive proper types of nutrition. Various elderly individuals have impediments such as poor mobility, mental impairments, or social isolation that prevent them from eating a healthy diet. Such identification through extensive assessments can direct healthcare providers to the support systems required to meet the nutritional needs of the elderly patients. Such interventions may include personalized meal delivery, community programs to enable social meals, or workshop-based training emphasizing nutrition. By integrating these strategies, health workers are not only able to enhance the nutritional health of older adults but also their social health, which translates into improved mental health and reduced loneliness. Defeating these multifaceted issues directly correlates to better health outcomes, showing the power of nutrition on total geriatric practice. Lastly, the interplay of nutrition and chronic disease in older patients necessitates astute screening and intervention methods. Increasing literature outlines how a nutritionally inadequate diet can exacerbate underlying disorders of health, thereby furthering morbidity and mortality within this group. Nutritional screening, such as the Mini-Nutritional Assessment, has been proven to be a useful tool for the identification of at-risk malnourished patients and resultant loss of health, enabling early intervention. Furthermore, specifically tailored diets to the unique health patterns of the elderly can greatly improve the overall course of their health. For example, diet modification to include anti-inflammatory foods decreases symptoms for those with arthritis or cardiovascular disease. Hence, systematic screening for nutritional risk can ensure that clinicians possess the data that will enable them to aim at personalized interventions, ultimately resulting in enhanced health outcomes in aging populations (Madeira et al., 2016; Lampugnale, 2017).

Overview of Screening Methods

Geriatric nutritional risk screening techniques are important to identify older adults that could be subjected to heightened vulnerability due to inadequate nutritional supply. Multidimensional screening tools, such as the Mini-Nutritional Assessment (MNA), are a mainstay in this area. The MNA facilitates clinicians to evaluate several aspects of nutritional status ranging from intake to weight loss and body mass index. Universal application has been justified by several studies, which have established that older persons are likely to manifest inadequate nutrient intake, further exacerbating their risk for malnutrition. Consequently, through the application of screening instruments like MNA, practitioners can identify individuals who require intervention in terms of nutrition, specifically, thus addressing this multifaceted issue proactively. Beyond the MNA, there are additional screening instruments that provide complementary data regarding what constitutes a patient's nutritional environment. These include instruments like the Frailty Index and the Social Support Survey that quantify additional sociopsychological factors that may contribute to nutritional status. As such, social isolation can affect an older adult's ability to access or prepare healthy food, such that these elements need to be addressed in a holistic approach. Although the application of multiple screening tools helps enhance the general assessment, however, it is still that numerous healthcare practitioners still find it difficult to incorporate these tools into their everyday work due to time and resource constraints. Overcoming these challenges is crucial for the enforcement of comprehensive assessments on a regular basis. Despite the obstacles that exist in implementing strict screening processes, strong evidence shows that early detection of risk of nutritional issues can yield substantial health gains. Research has shown that intervening to correct malnutrition can reduce hospital admissions and enhance recovery, especially among older adults recovering from surgery like hip fractures. Research indicates that malnourished inpatients are at higher risk of death, and it is necessary to implement efficacious screening measures. As the significance of nutritional assessment comes to the attention of more healthcare professionals, efficacious, streamlined geriatric assessment strategies are required. Practical teaching programs for healthcare workers can encourage familiarity with these screening tools, therefore better enabling them to assist older individuals in maintaining their nutritional status.

13.1. The Aging Population

As the aging population increases, so do their special health care needs. Nutritional risk is a significant problem for older adults, and this can compound the severity of existing medical conditions and accelerate further complications. The complexities of aging, such as decreased appetite, dental conditions, and metabolic alterations, contribute to higher rates of malnourishment. This is particularly worrisome since malnutrition can lower the well-being of older adults and increase their susceptibility to many other complicating health conditions. Improved knowledge and foresight are imperative in developing screening tools that can accurately identify nutritional risk in older persons, hence allowing intervention in a timely fashion and consequently improving health outcomes. Screening for geriatric nutritional risk is an essential method of averting malnutrition among older people. Various areas of geriatric assessment, such as the Mini-Nutritional Assessment and the Frailty Index, have proven to be sensitive predictors of morbidity and mortality among this population. However, despite their significance, the implementation rate is low, primarily due to the time constraints faced by healthcare workers. As a result, many patients do not receive the comprehensive evaluation necessary to guide effective nutritional interventions. Encouraging greater awareness of nutritional risk factors among health professionals can mean greater utilization of these vital screening techniques, ultimately enhancing the overall treatment provided for elderly patients. The consequences of overlooked nutritional risk in the elderly are broad and multifaceted. Malnutrition has been demonstrated by studies to be associated with important adverse outcomes, including increased hospitalization rates, susceptibility to infection, and lower functional capacity. These problems are particularly pertinent in residential aged care facilities, where malnutrition rates can be as much as 50%. By applying systematic screening for nutrition and effective management plans that cater to the needs of this group, stakeholders can enhance quality of life and health equity. A multi-disciplinary approach involving educational campaigns, inter-professional collaboration, and aggressive monitoring can significantly reduce the severity of malnutrition in older people, thus driving healthier aging in our population (Agarwal et al., 2016; Lampugnale, 2017) (Figure 13.3).

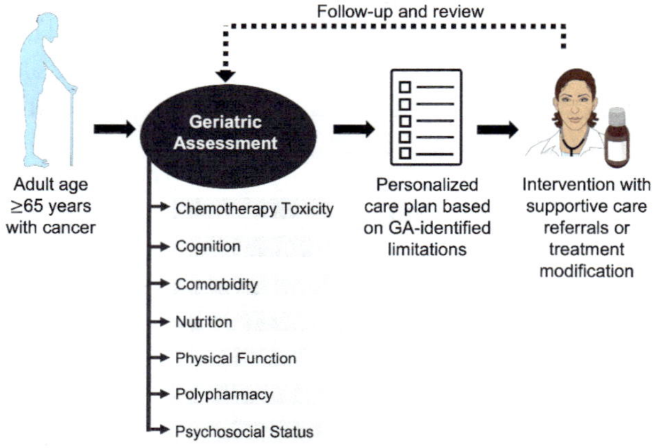

Figure 13.3. Geriatric assessment in older adults.

Source: https://www.frontiersin.org/files/Articles/1124309/fonc-13-1124309-HTML/image_m/fonc-13-1124309-g001.jpg.

13.1.1. Demographic Trends in Aging

Aging demographic trends present special challenges and opportunities in public health, notably in the area of geriatric risk of malnutrition. The world is experiencing unprecedented expansion of the elderly population as a result of improved healthcare and scientific advancements in disease management. As life expectancy is on the rise, the proportion of individuals aged 65 and older is projected to increase exponentially. This demographic transition also comes with many physiological changes that have the potential to adversely affect nutritional intake and status. Older individuals are prone to difficulty in digestion and absorption of necessary nutrients due to age-related declines in gastrointestinal function. It is essential to address such special dietary requirements since it can mitigate the negative risk of malnutrition, which deeply impacts the overall well-being and functional condition of the elderly, making the strength of screening programs within geriatric medicine (Rémond et al., 2015). The relationship between age and other lifestyle factors has a significant impact on nutritional status. Physical activity patterns among older adults have been identified to have immediate influences on such medical conditions as muscle strength and bone mass that are critical in promoting independence and mobility. Sedentary behavior in this age group has been found to enhance the rise in chronic diseases and potentially worsen nutritional deficiencies. For example, research shows that older adults who are less physically active demonstrate a shocking reduction in bone density, which can further deteriorate their nutritional status and well-being (Rodríguez-Gómez et al., 2018). Recognition of these associations emphasizes the imperative for effective screening and intervention measures specifically tailored to this population's unique lifestyle and health profile, with a focus on encouraging physical activity as a means of reducing nutritional risk. The implications of demographic aging extend from individual health to social and economic domains. Countries all over the world are facing the challenge of adapting healthcare systems and social infrastructure to meet the needs of an aging population. Effective nutritional screening programs will be a significant driving force in reducing the prevalence of malnutrition in older adults, and through this, may contribute to saving healthcare costs for other age-related conditions. Furthermore, a concerted effort towards the development of focused nutritional interventions that are grounded in an aging individual's changing physiology and lifestyle can be highly beneficial. Such strategies need to incorporate nutrition education as well as physical activity, thereby advocating for a holistic approach to health among older people. Through understanding demographic trends in aging, we can more effectively guide policy and practice that support the well-being of older people, leading to healthier, higher-quality lives (Rémond et al., 2015).

13.1.2. Nutritional Challenges Faced by Older Adults

As age increases, there are multiple physiological changes that have a significant impact on the nutritional status of individuals, leading to great challenges for the elderly. Likely the most applicable symptom is loss of appetite and changed taste, both of which may be influenced by hormonal alterations and drug side effects. Such anorexia of aging results in insufficient caloric and nutrient intake, further complicating malnutrition. Thus, elderly people are more likely to develop nutrition-related health problems such as osteoporosis and sarcopenia, which will have an additional effect on their quality of life. Nutritional risk screening is necessary in order to identify individuals who may require intervention in order to be given well-balanced and adequate diets that meet their specific health needs. Addressing these short-term nutritional requirements is a key step towards optimizing the health of this vulnerable population. Cognitive impairment, such as Alzheimer's disease, places additional nutritional requirements on older individuals. With an estimated 6.7 million people aged 65 years and over living with Alzheimer's dementia, the effect on nutritional status is considerable. Cognitive impairment can cause issues in food preparation, meal forgetfulness, and decreased ability to establish a healthy food environment, propagating a cycle of nutritional deficiency that further exacerbates health consequences. Moreover, family caregivers also assume responsibility for adequate nutrition, contributing to their own stress and health-related issues as they navigate the complexities of care. Awareness of cognitive well-being in terms of nutrition emphasizes the value of multi-domain screening tools that measurably assess one's eating habits and nutritional needs when experiencing cognitive impairment at an older age. Physical disabilities that typically occur during old age also challenge nutritional status among the elderly. Discomforts such as loss of mobility, ongoing pain, and sensory loss make grocery shopping and cooking a challenging endeavor.

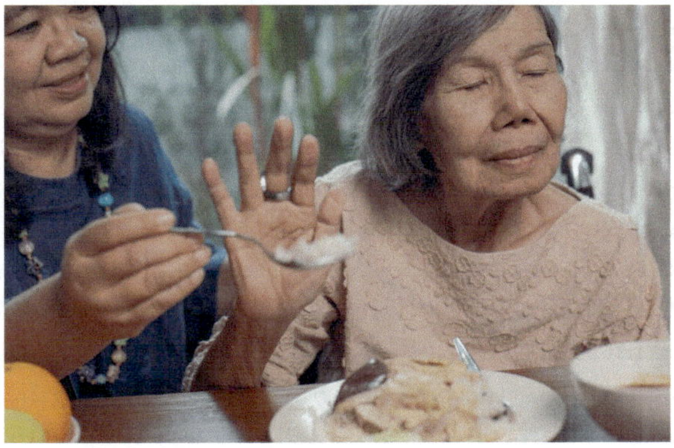

Figure 13.4. Nutritional challenges faced by older adults.

Source: https://meetcaregivers.com/wp-content/uploads/2023/02/Senior-nutrition-Caregiver-holding-spoon-of-rice-to-elderly-woman-waving-it-away-with-her-hand-MeetCaregivers.png.

Additionally, the prevalence of comorbidities, including diabetes and cardiovascular complications, calls for the expertise in specialized diet management that can be difficult to achieve without professional consultation. According to assertions, mortality and morbidity in older populations are significantly associated with nutritional deprivation via diet, resulting in adverse health consequences. Thus, successful geriatric nutrition risk screening has to involve physical capability and access to food resources assessment. Through the identification of these impediments, health professionals can apply evidence-based interventions that promote nutritional adequacy and overall well-being among older adults, addressing the multifaceted challenges they face in maintaining healthy eating (Montero-Odasso et al., 2022) (Figure 13.4).

13.1.3. Assessing Nutritional Needs

Systematic assessment of nutritional needs of the elderly is important in maintaining maximum health and preventing malnutrition. The elderly have unique diet-related needs resulting from physiological alterations, chronic illnesses, and alterations in appetite and metabolism. To aid in addressing such issues, routine nutritional screening and assessment examining dietary intake, nutritional status, and general health status are important. Effective nutritional screening identifies patients at risk of malnutrition, giving them an early chance for intervention that improves their well-being. Nutrition guidelines incorporating regular assessments by multidisciplinary teams are essential in the detection of potential carb, fat, and fluid deficits, ultimately leading to the development of individualized diet interventions in older individuals in various settings of care, including residential aged care facilities (Agarwal et al., 2016). Adding technology to nutritional screening can further improve our understanding of older adults' specific dietary needs. Advanced systems, such as the expert systems designed for nutrition care, have been developed to facilitate individualized care planning. Based on an examination of older adults' self-feeding behaviors, such systems are capable of identifying unhealthy eating behaviors that can lead to malnutrition. This evidence-based approach enables healthcare professionals to create dynamic nutrition care plans specific to each individual's health condition and eating behavior. For instance, an ontology-based system can logically describe dietary knowledge and tailor nutritional treatments, i.e., education and diet orders, therefore enhancing dietary compliance and general well-being among the elderly (Cioara et al., 2017). The effects of accurate nutritional assessment extend far beyond immediate health gains. The satisfaction of the nutritional needs of older people is directly related to long-term health outcomes, such as less hospitalization, improved quality of life, and decreased health costs. Malnutrition is a key risk factor for adverse health events, like infection and falls, and may lead to the development of additional complications and institutionalization. The regular assessments are therefore of the most importance not only in individual care of the elderly but also in public health care for the elderly. Since the weight of malnutrition and its complications presses heavily on the need for nutritional interventions, integration of holistic screening and personalized eating plans will be vital to the welfare and health of the elderly (Agarwal et al., 2016) (Figure 3.14).

13.1.4. Methods for Evaluating Dietary Intake

Assessment of dietary consumption among older people is a critical component in the calculation of their nutritional needs. There are various means by which this can be accomplished, each with varying advantages and limitations. The 24-hour dietary recall is a common approach that measures food types and amounts consumed over the course of the day before to allow examination of macronutrient intake. This method can potentially provide patterns of eating behavior but relies strongly on the participants' memory and integrity. Food frequency questionnaires (FFQs) also provide a general estimation of the usual long-term diet. While FFQs are good at showing trends, they are not precise when assessing true daily intakes. Consequently, scientists and clinicians prefer a package of approaches together to best understand the eating habits of older people so that any nutrition assessment is in consonance with their unique nutritional demands. Malnutrition detection is the other significant characteristic of dietary intake assessment among the elderly, as it is unfortunately common among them. Measurement of food consumption can be such a robust determinant for designing interventions to manage malnutrition. With systematic analysis of these elements, health practitioners can recognize inappropriate dietary habits and implement personal intervention programs based on the individual needs and preferences of the elderly with the end goal of enhancing their nutritional status and well-being. Technological advances have also broadened the choices for determining dietary intake among older people.

13.2. Nutritional Assessment Tools

In applying good nutritional assessment instruments among the geriatric population, one should consider the multifaceted nature of nutritional risk. The Mini-Nutritional Assessment (MNA) has been noted to provide valuable information, especially among the elderly. The instrument examines various aspects such as dietary habits, weight loss, and anthropometric values to determine nutritional status in its entirety.

Research indicates that MNA is a valid way of detecting malnutrition among geriatric patients, particularly considering the high rate of nutritional inadequacies within this group. Employing such a tool allows clinicians to risk-stratify patients and implement proper interventions in a timely fashion. In a bid to continue enhancing patient outcomes, increased awareness and systematic application of these assessment instruments in clinical practice are necessary, particularly with patient population and a shift in their nutritional needs. Secondly, the incorporation of comprehensive nutrition assessment instruments in clinical practice is often undermined by time constraints among health professionals. While the validity of screening instruments like the Frailty Index and the Geriatric Depression Screening has been determined, many clinicians are unable to finish thorough evaluations because of the weight of their workload. Of concern is that most oncogeriatric patients do not receive full pre-surgical geriatric assessments, even though they have been shown to be associated with favorable postoperative outcomes.

The lack of widespread application of these essential tools is alarming, especially knowing that a proper evaluation can greatly improve the quality of care provided to geriatric patients. Education that equips future medical caregivers with the skills needed to effectively perform these evaluations is the basis for bridging this gap, ultimately enhancing geriatric nutritional care. In addition, malnutrition in older patients has serious consequences that are backed by studies in geriatric groups undergoing surgery, such as hip fractures. Malnutrition prevalence in these groups has been shown to be highly correlated with higher morbidity and mortality. Especially, in a systematic review, it was quoted that the older subjects with hip fractures had 18.7% malnutrition prevalence according to MNA criteria, 45.7% when different diagnostic criteria were applied. The harsh statistics only highlight the increasing significance of the implementation of credible nutritional assessments for early detection of people at risk. Nutritional interventions, among other early treatments, have been shown to increase the recovery rate and lower hospitalization complications risk. Therefore, enabling the use of nutritional assessment tools to a larger extent is not so much an issue of clinical best practice but one of imperative towards maximizing the overall health outcome for the older adults (Figure 13.5).

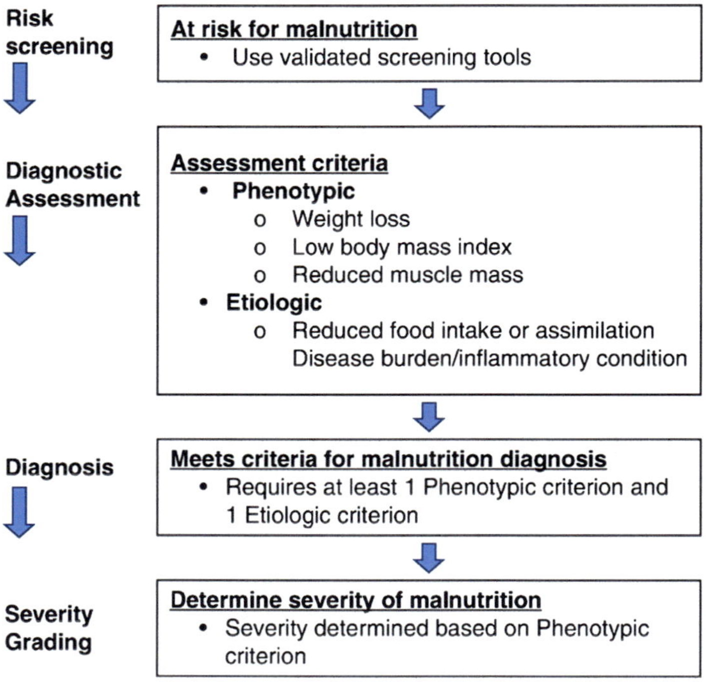

Figure 13.5. Nutritional assessment, diagnosis, and treatment in geriatrics.

Source: https://media.springernature.com/lw685/springer-static/image/chp%3A10.1007%2F978-3-030-63892-4_3/MediaObjects/497744_1_En_3_Fig4_HTML.png.

13.2.1. Common Screening Tools Used in Geriatrics

Screening tools in geriatrics are necessary for the identification of nutrition risk factors that can have a detrimental effect on the well-being and health of older individuals. The most critical of these tools is MNA. Designed specifically for use with the elderly, the MNA is a comprehensive examination that considers the anthropometric information, the eating pattern, and the overall health status. The multi-dimensional method enables healthcare professionals to detect malnutrition and risk of malnutrition in the best possible way. The MNA has also demonstrated excellent validity and reliability in both clinical and community settings and is therefore a cornerstone tool in the arsenal of nutritional screening of the older person. Its continued use in such a wide range of fields serves to highlight its relevance in early intervention and preventative care efforts, eventually with the aim of enhancing the quality of life for elderly individuals. Another widely used screening tool is the Nutritional Risk Screening 2002 (NRS 2002), which utilizes both clinical and nutritional factors to assess the risk of malnutrition among geriatric patients. This tool is very effective in hospital settings and assists healthcare workers in identifying the patients who would gain the most from nutritional therapy. The NRS 2002 considers several factors, such as body mass index, loss of weight, and severity of disease, and therefore gives a full description of the nutritional status of the patient. Of importance is that the tool is versatile enough to be employed in different care settings, including acute hospitals and long-term care facilities. By enabling targeted nutritional intervention, the NRS 2002 works significantly towards the alleviation of the ill effects of malnutrition, advancing better health among elderly groups and improving their overall quality of care. Besides the above-mentioned tools, the Geriatric Nutritional Risk Index (GNRI) is an effective tool for the identification of the risk of malnutrition in the elderly. The GNRI has a simple formula that considers serum albumin level and body weight relative to height, enabling clinicians to quantify nutritional deficits that otherwise would not be evident. It is of greatest value in the inpatient setting and has been demonstrated to be linked to hospital stay length and risk of complications. GNRI is important because it emphasizes the importance of early nutritional screening and intervention among older individuals since malnutrition can lead to serious decline in health. The integration of such tools as the GNRI into geriatric care pathways will allow healthcare providers to enhance active interventions on nutrition risk, thereby enhancing the overall health of older people and potentially decreasing healthcare costs associated with malnutrition complications.

13.2.2. Validity and Reliability of Assessment Methods

The evaluation of the nutritional risk in older adults calls for the use of valid and reliable assessment tools. Validity is the quantification of the accuracy with which a measure estimates what it is meant to assess, while reliability is the quantification of the consistency of the outcome of the tools over time and across different populations. Referring to the screening of nutrition in geriatrics, several instruments have been developed, varying in their levels of validity and reliability. Among these instruments, Nutritional Risk Screening (NRS) and the Mini-Nutritional Assessment (MNA) have proven more sensitive and specific in identifying malnutrition among the elderly, compared to others. For instance, studies indicated that the NRS had 93.88% sensitivity and 96.77% specificity, proving its potential superiority to the Malnutrition Universal Screening Tool (MUST), which showed much lower values (Nasreen et al., 2020). Other than validity, the reliability of the screeners is an essential requirement for effective clinical application in geriatric nutrition. The reliability of these instruments is confirmed by their ability to provide consistent results if applied in the same conditions. When contrasting various instruments, the MNA was more reliable than the NRS, which indicates that even though the NRS might be more valid in certain respects, the MNA can provide more reliable identification of malnutrition risk when applying them at varying times.

This nuance indicates that sole reliance on a single tool will not do, but rather the implementation of several tests or the usage of the most suitable tool for the population one is looking at is the optimal solution (Nasreen et al., 2020). Therefore, awareness of the nuances of validity and reliability highlights the need for a tailored response to nutritional screening in the elderly age group of the elderly. In addition, the comparison of various screening tools underscores the need for the proper choice of assessment methods that are not just effective but also clinically feasible. Research findings indicate that older adults with cancer, for instance, suffer from malnutrition with a profound impact on their therapy and recovery. The MNA has been noted for its excellent validity and reliability, that render it a suitable instrument for this group. Its holistic approach allows for more comprehensive evaluation of a patient's nutritional status, which results in improved clinical decision-making. In general, continuous scrutiny of the validity and reliability of nutritional screening tools is essential to ensure effective and correct nutritional risk assessment in older individuals. This enhances the capacity of healthcare professionals to make early interventions, consequently improving the well-being and health of this vulnerable population (Figure 13.6).

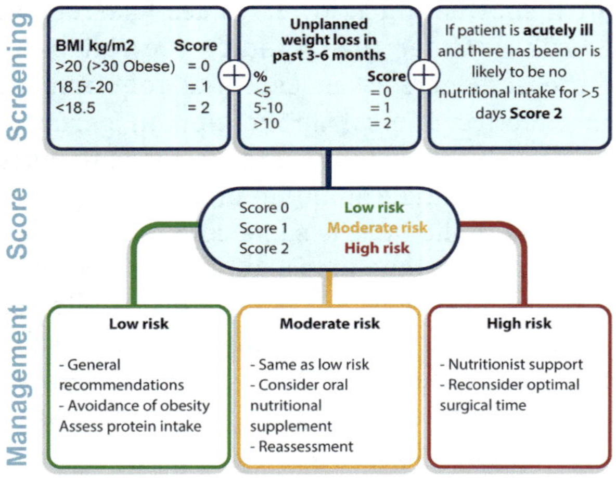

Figure 13.6. Malnutrition universal screening tool (MUST).

Source: https://www.researchgate.net/publication/374393453/figure/fig3/AS:11431281199316566@1697564321129/Malnutrition-universal-screening-tool-MUST-77-78.tif.

13.2.3. Role of Healthcare Professionals in Assessments

The role of healthcare professionals in assessments is central, particularly in terms of the nutritional risk among the elderly population. Because elderly individuals may possess various health problems, including cognitive impairment and diseases, a comprehensive assessment is required to ascertain their specific nutritional needs. Healthcare professionals may develop customized meals to offer sufficient carbohydrates, fats, and fluid consumption in addition to changes in texture depending on chewing difficulty or special food inclination. This team approach not only enhances the accuracy of nutritional assessments but also offers a healthy environment where older individuals actively participate in their food choices. By considering the diversified capacities and needs of older people, healthcare professionals can improve health results and promote quality of life by well-organized nutrition care plans. The multi-factorial assessment allows more customized interventions, which are essential to avoid malnutrition and its consequences. Moreover, involvement of caregivers and family members can complement these assessments with a balanced view of patients' interests and needs. Synchronization of the same with evidence-based guidelines, as stressed in healthcare literature, will not only enhance nutritional status but also overall health in this group of patients (The Stern Center for Evidence-Based Policy, 2015). Along with standard nutritional assessments, clinicians must also include cognitive status in the assessment. Cognitive impairment can have a direct effect on an individual's geriatric ability to adequately provide for their nutrition. The National Academy of Neuropsychology convened a summit to debate whether cognitive status in elderly individuals needs to be assessed and, if so, who should be screened and how the screenings can be integrated into routine medical practice. Participants at the summit emphasized that possessing a baseline of cognitive function and detecting changes over time are critical in the management of nutritional risk (Perry et al., 2018). Not only does this collaboration among various healthcare stakeholders result in improved screening processes, but it also informs treatment in addition to enhancing the general quality of care given to older individuals suffering from nutritional challenges. Furthermore, technology has also altered the means by which nutritional risk is determined among the geriatric population. Electronic health records (EHRs) could facilitate it to be easier to track patients' mental and nutritional status so that healthcare staff are able to conduct more effective follow-ups and screenings. Since different populations have their own assessment measures refined and validated, cultural, educational, and linguistic differences must be considered. Through the utilization of EHRs with standardized screening tools, healthcare providers are in a position to mitigate some of the associated risks of nutritional deficiency. In doing so, they not only improve individual health status but also support public health endeavors at large for improved overall well-being among older adults (The Stern Center for Evidence-Based Policy, 2015). Understanding the intersectionality of the factors influencing geriatric health is essential to effective assessment and accompanying interventions, resulting in healthier aging populations.

13.3. Factors Contributing to Nutritional Risk

The complexity of the nutrition in geriatric patients is influenced by a range of factors that contribute to nutritional risk in the aging population. As humans age, they are likely to experience a number of physiological changes that influence their appetite, digestion, and metabolic processes. These age-related changes can increase the risk of malnutrition, especially in residential aged care facilities where the incidence is significantly elevated. A study showed that about half of all residents in these facilities are malnourished owing to obstacles such as reduced appetite, restricted dietary consumption, and compromised nutrient absorption (Agarwal et al., 2016). The implications of these nutritional deficiencies extend beyond mere weight loss; they are linked with high infection, fall, and hospitalization risks, all of which add to the overall health challenge of aging populations. In addition, the presence of multi-morbidities makes it even harder to manage nutritional status in elderly individuals. Most chronic diseases, such as diabetes or cardiovascular disease, tend to demand dietary restrictions or alterations that add to the limitation of nutrient supply. Such nutritional alterations can inadvertently lead to deficiencies in essential nutrients, further adding to the medical history of older individuals. In addition, cognitive impairment that accompanies age may invalidate one's ability to prepare or to eat enough food, further aggravating nutritional risk. The impact of socioeconomic status on nutrition is beyond individual-level issues and incorporates more systemic problems. For instance, communities with limited access to supermarkets usually lead to the expansion of food deserts, where individuals have little opportunity to access healthy nutrition. This gap is particularly prominent among older people, who are already prone to mobility and transport limitations and thus more limited in accessing healthy food. According to research, the high prevalence of protein-energy malnutrition among the elderly is also exacerbated by these socioeconomic underlying determinants and hence, point interventions for screening and assessment are required (Agarwal et al., 2016). Nutrition interventions to address such inequalities, hence, need to be multifaceted, targeting both food access and education, and involving health care providers, community organizations, and public policy actively A multidisciplinary approach is therefore paramount in addressing such challenges, through routine nutrition screening and assessment for the identification of at-risk individuals at an early stage (Agarwal et al., 2016). By way of understanding and intervening in the intricate issues of nutritional problems, interventions can be tailored specifically to enhance the health status of residents. The provision of proper nutritional intervention is imperative to minimizing risks associated with malnutrition in the elderly. Effective food and nutrition interventions are not merely about adding more nutrients to meals; they require an interprofessional collaboration among healthcare professionals, dietitians, and caregivers. The installation of a comprehensive nutritional protocol within residential aged care facilities can make long-term improvement in dietary and nutritional levels possible. The protocol has to include frequent screening, prompt assessments, and targeted interventions based on the individual needs of each resident. Since the older population is generally known to have some dietary requirements and needs, these measures have to be appropriately designed (Agarwal et al., 2016). Ultimately, by facilitating a culture of nutritional well-being, health care providers are able to significantly enhance the quality of life and the health of older individuals (Figure 13.7).

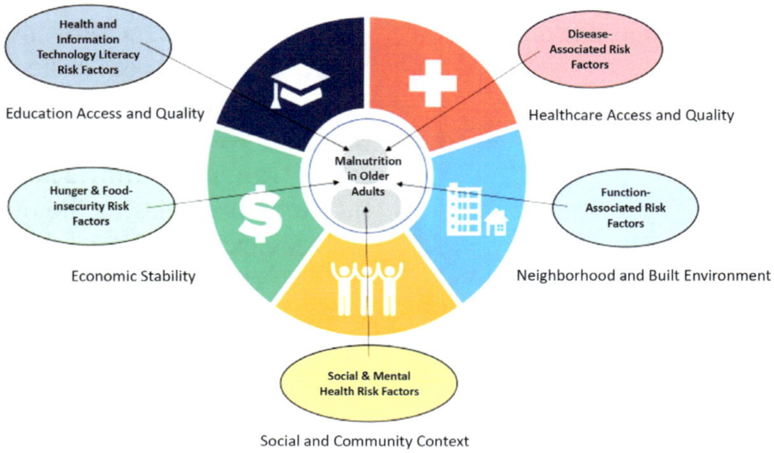

Figure 13.7. Factors contributing to nutritional risk by older adults.

Source: https://www.researchgate.net/publication/359087227/figure/fig1/AS:11431281141692427@1681077577168/Overlay-of-older-adult-malnutrition-risk-factors-and-social-determinants-of-health.tif.

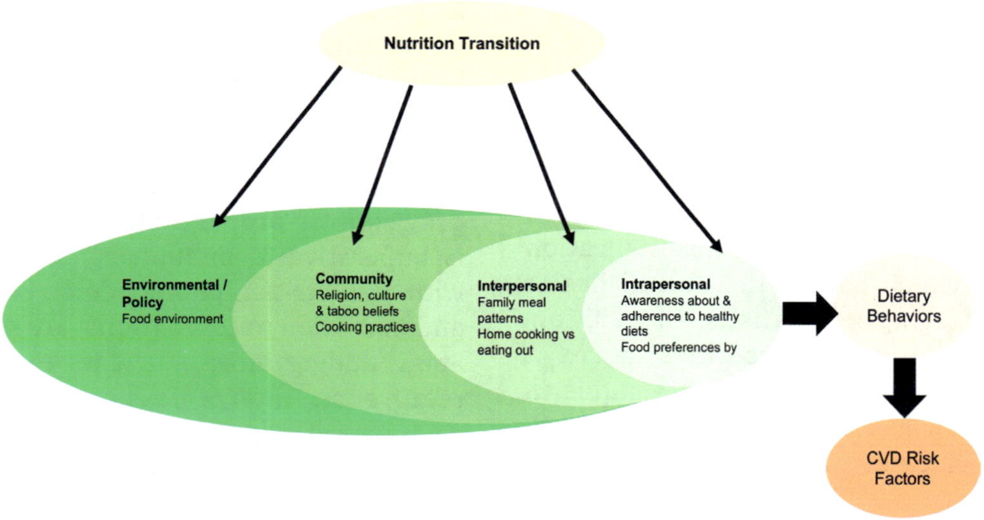

Figure 13.8. Socio-ecological model of the impacts of nutrition.

Source: https://www.researchgate.net/publication/366513733/figure/fig1/AS:11431281212417311@1702618556868/Socio-ecological-model-of-the-impacts-of-nutrition-transition-on-dietary-behaviors-and.tif.

13.4. Consequences of Poor Nutrition

In the older population, the consequences of poor nutrition may be most significant, not just impacting physical health but also general quality of life. Malnutrition, which is prevalent in older individuals, leads to a failure to resist infection, a rise in risk of falls, and the development of pressure ulcers. Such outcomes lead to a vicious circle of ill health, as increased morbidity equals more hospital admissions and increased healthcare costs. Most of the older residents in aged care homes are afflicted with these issues due to conditions of appetite, food consumption, and utilization of nutrients. During the time of literature review, it seems nearly half of the population residing in aged care homes are malnourished, which indicates the gravity of having optimal screening and management measures in place to counteract the consequences of poor nutrition among such a group of susceptible persons (Agarwal et al., 2016). The aging gastrointestinal tract experiences a number of alterations that further complicate nutrient consumption and assimilation, which can exacerbate the effects of poor nutrition. Physiological and anatomic changes, such as reduced gastrointestinal motility and modified digestive processes, reduce the supply of nutrients in older individuals. The alterations can lead to deficiencies in essential vitamins and minerals and thus give rise to consequent health disorders involving more than one organ system. The implications of such shortcomings are impaired immune systems, impaired musculoskeletal systems, and mental deterioration, making it a highly difficult problem for geriatrics. Hence, understanding these changes is crucial to establishing specialized dietary interventions that address both the physiological constraints of aging and the nutritional needs of the aged to prevent the accompanying risk of malnutrition (Rémond et al., 2015). To best respond to the impact of malnutrition in the elderly, it is necessary to have thorough screening protocols in geriatric facilities. Regular nutritional evaluation can help detect those at risk of malnutrition at an early stage and result in timely interventions. The protocols should incorporate interdisciplinary methods using physicians who specialize in nutrition and geriatrics. By focusing on individualized nutritional care according to the unique dietary needs and desires of older people, facilities can optimize nutritional intake and improve overall health outcomes. Multidisciplinary practice among healthcare professionals is critical because it enables the planning and monitoring of individualized nutritional regimens that address not just diet but also the underlying physiological changes that accompany aging. This proactive approach of screening and intervention is critical in the protection of the health and wellbeing of at-risk older individuals from malnutrition (Agarwal et al., 2016) (Figure 13.9).

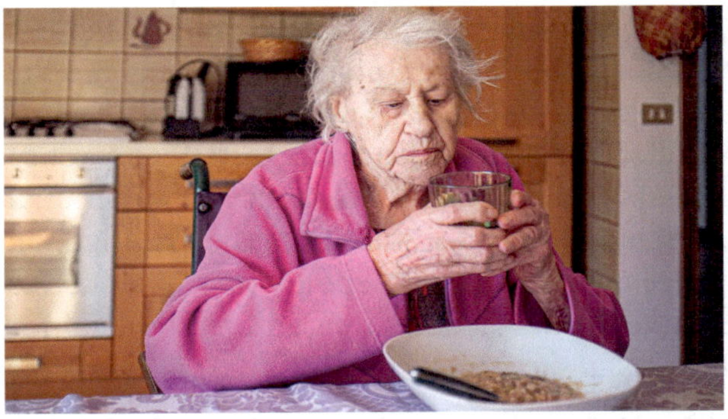

Figure 13.9. Consequences of poor nutrition.

Source: https://www.mealvillage.com/mvimages/blog/senior-woman-struggling-with-malnutrition-at-home.jpg.

13.4.1. Health Complications Related to Malnutrition

Malnutrition in the elderly can cascade into a chain of health complications that significantly jeopardize the quality of life and outcomes in this age group. Inadequate nutrient intake typically manifests as loss of weight, muscle wasting, and frailty, all of which combined contribute to increased morbidity. Malnutrition and functional decline go together very strongly; older individuals may experience longer recovery times from hospitalizations and surgeries for acute medical illnesses. For instance, in hip fracture-admitted geriatric patients, literature reports malnutrition not only to impede healing but also to pose a higher risk of hospitalization complication, which highlights the immediate need for effective nutritional screening practices to address this issue (Malafarina et al., 2017). Recognition of malnutrition risk patients can guide early interventions that might forestall fatal health emergencies. Moreover, the effects of malnutrition extend beyond physical illnesses; the psychological and social aspects are affected, too. As nutritional status declines, the elderly can become socially isolated due to weakness or depression, worsening their situation further. Nutritional risk screening can thus serve as a core first step towards a comprehensive geriatric assessment, assisting practitioners to establish holistic care plans that determine the individualized needs of older patients. A study of oncogeriatric patients suggests that intense pre-surgical assessments, such as nutritional screenings, may optimize the risk stratification process to actually respond in a productive manner towards health parameters crucial for successful surgery (Lampugnale, 2017). It calls for the inclusion of nutritional screening in geriatric care models. Management of malnutrition is achievable with a properly organized framework that includes screening in early stages and appropriate interventions, which can positively impact the health outcomes of older people. Nutritional interventions, grounded in evidence-based practices, have been shown to be effective in providing enhanced functional recovery after surgeries and lower mortality among individuals who are malnourished. Because the prevalence of malnutrition in the elderly is generally underreported, implementation of standardized tools such as the Mini-Nutritional Assessment will enable proper identification of high-risk patients. Raising awareness and routine nutritional screening may enable healthcare professionals to prevent adverse effects of malnutrition and promote better recovery and overall survival in the elderly (Malafarina et al., 2017). This proactive approach is important to achieve optimal care for an age group at growing risk of both malnutrition and associated health issues.

13.4.2. Impact on Quality of Life

The quality of life of elderly patients is intrinsically linked with their nutrition, and this highlights the important part that screening for nutritional risk has to play in this age category. Aging leads to physiological changes that can cause malnutrition, which exacerbates comorbid illness and deteriorates well-being. Malnutrition is actually underdiagnosed in most cases, which can lead to widespread declines in physical function, worsening of comorbidities, and increased caregiver dependence. The intersection of nutrition and health outcomes calls for an integrated assessment to address the unique challenges that aging poses. Correct screening can identify at-risk patients, enabling timely intervention not only to enhance health but also to promote quality of life and autonomy. Perhaps most importantly, the interrelationship between nutritional status and recovery from illnesses such as hip fractures cannot be overestimated. Evidence suggests that nutrient uptake deficiencies will lead to higher rates of hospitalization complications, increased recovery time, and higher death rates—elements sharply diminish the well-being of the elderly. For instance, older adults with hip fractures are highly malnourished, and this impacts their functional outcomes and overall prognosis negatively. With the inclusion of nutritional assessment in standard care protocols, medical professionals can better develop personalized interventions based on individual needs and hence ensure optimal recovery as well as lower the chances of post-operative complications. This critical approach can potentially pave the way to improved health histories among geriatric patients. In addition, early nutrition interventions not only ensure healthier recovery outcomes but also translate into significant cost-effectiveness in terms of healthcare spending.

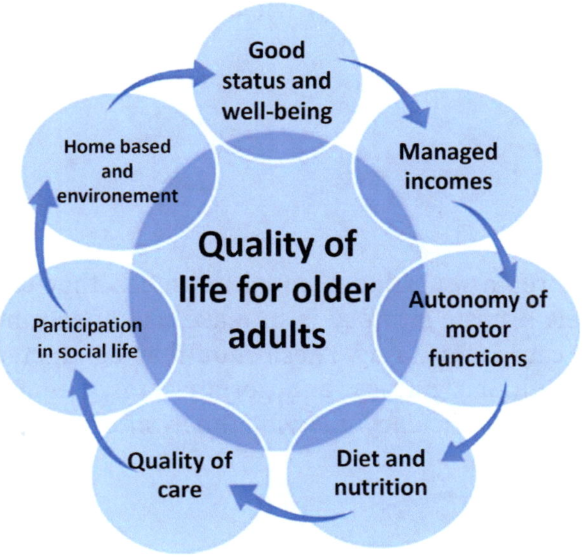

Figure 13.10. Quality of life for geriatric patients.

Source: https://www.researchgate.net/publication/362163476/figure/fig1/AS:1182715751735336@1658992817899/Multimodal-approach-of-Quality-of-Life-in-older-adults.png.

As malnutrition has also been shown to result in a lot of mortality and morbidity, which can be resolved by preventive measures, considerable improvements in the quality of life are attained. Studies show that patients receiving appropriate nutritional interventions show better functional recovery, resulting in a generally better quality of life satisfaction. Thus, geriatric nutritional risk screening becomes part of the overall comprehensive geriatric care, in alignment with the perception that good nutrition is at the heart of positively affecting health and well-being in older adults. These preventive interventions may enable individuals to remain independent and have a more dignified quality of life, which is an applicable aim in the geriatric patient (Figure 13.10).

13.4.3. Economic Burden of Nutritional Deficiencies

The cost to the economy of nutritional deficiencies among the elderly is significant, impacting both healthcare systems and society as a whole. With aging comes multiple long-term diseases, and inadequate nutrition is a risk factor that adds to the increased costs of care associated with hospitalization, long-term care, and outpatient visits. For instance, malnutrition can cause frailty, decreased mobility, and compromised cognition, which ultimately necessitate more invasive medical interventions and extended care. It is crucial for healthcare workers, especially in geriatric care, where the risk of nutritional deficiency is higher, to understand the fiscal implications of these deficiencies. By implementing screening initiatives for nutritional risk, healthcare professionals can identify at-risk patients early, ultimately reducing the financial strain on both individuals and the national healthcare system. Furthermore, the implications of nutritional deficiencies extend beyond immediate healthcare costs, influencing broader societal concerns, including productivity and mental health. When elderly people suffer from malnutrition, their ability to carry out day-to-day tasks declines, leading to a decrease in overall living standards. This decline not only affects the person but also adds to the burden of carers and relatives who may be compelled to provide more support. Further, food insecurity, one of the most potent causes of nutritional deficiencies, has a broader economic effect. According to recent research, food insecurity has downstream costs that entail the allocation of charitable aid, mental health treatment, and long-term consequences of impaired educational attainment and workforce productivity (Shepard et al., 2007). Intervention on these variables through targeted nutritional intervention is a necessity in mitigating their economic burden. Finally, the integration of holistic nutritional assessment into the geriatric model can significantly alleviate the economic burden of nutritional deficiency. Effective screening tools, such as the Mini-Nutritional Assessment, can assess the nutritional status of elderly adults and initiate early dietary interventions. Although these screens are helpful, their use in practice has been inconsistent due to time demands on practitioners (Lampugnale, 2017). But if the healthcare systems place priority on educating medical professionals to perform such evaluations in an economical way, then they can significantly contribute towards enhancing the quality of care provided to the elderly. Not only will this cut down healthcare costs for the complications of malnutrition, but also enable healthier ageing, which will result in an improved life for the elderly and a lighter economic burden on society.

13.5. Strategies for Effective Screening

Effective screening for geriatric nutritional risk requires a multidimensional approach that can navigate the complications of aging and comorbidities. A basic strategy is to make use of routine nutrition screening on admission and throughout the care facility stay. These should be conducted by a multidisciplinary team with the expertise of dietitians, nurses, and geriatricians. Regular screening will identify early evidence of potential nutritional deficiency, allowing timely intervention.

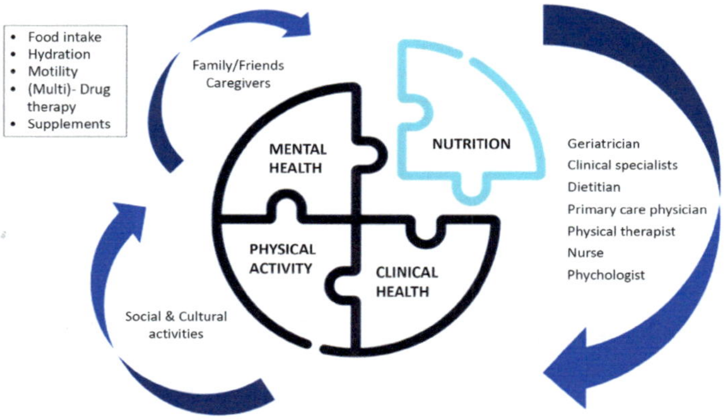

Figure 13.11. Nutritional strategies for ageing populations.

Source: https://care24.co.in/wp-content/uploads/2020/10/Elderlycare1200x600-Transparent.png.

By the use of quantifiable tools such as the Mini-Nutritional Assessment, facilities can properly estimate the nutritional status of residents, minimizing the occurrence of malnutrition that otherwise goes undetected and untreated in older adults with severe illnesses (Agarwal et al., 2016). The implementation of full nutritional protocols is another essential practice in geriatric facilities. Such procedures must incorporate not only systematic screening but also targeted interventions tailored to the residents' individual needs. An example would be upgrading the food service systems to offer appealing meals and adding supplements that could have a significant impact on the nutritional well-being of the residents. Moreover, personnel should be trained to recognize indicators and consequences of poor nutrition. Through the establishment of a well-being culture based on nutritional well-being, care institutions are able to avoid the adverse effects associated with malnutrition, such as increased hospitalizations and reduced quality of life for older people (Lampugnani, 2017). Finally, technology and educational interventions in screening make it more efficient. The application of telehealth and mobile platforms enables constant monitoring and follow-up of geriatric patients, therefore, within the constraints of traditional health models. Training programs aimed at educating caregivers and clinicians about the most predictive aspects of geriatric assessment can also promote enhanced screening practice. Focusing on developing a strong curriculum based on these approaches can play an integral role in better training future clinicians to respond effectively to geriatric nutritional risk. Last but not least, a comprehensive proactive approach with these interventions can lead to improved health status and quality of life for this vulnerable population (Agarwal et al., 2016; Lampugnale, 2017) (Figure 13.11).

13.5.1. Best Practices for Conducting Nutritional Screenings

The process of conducting nutritional screenings in elderly patients involves a multi-aspect approach with attention to detail and sensitivity. Among the best practices is the application of validated screening tools, such as the Mini-Nutritional Assessment (MNA), which has been found to be useful in identifying at-risk status for malnutrition among the elderly. These devices, apart from aiding in the early detection of nutritional deficiency, also facilitate enhanced communication among healthcare workers for an integrated care approach. Most importantly, through the application of such assessments, healthcare workers can tailor interventions better to address the individual nutritional needs of elderly individuals, thus enhancing overall health outcomes. The incorporation of these evidence-based tools into daily practice is essential, as it forms a preventive regimen in geriatric care that can effectively reduce the incidence of complications arising from malnutrition, thereby improving the quality of life in this setting. Another essential component of effective nutritional screening is the incorporation of a comprehensive geriatric assessment (CGA) that extends beyond routine diet evaluation. A CGA takes variables like physical function, psychological status, and social support into account, as it acknowledges that nutrition is closely entwined with the health of older adults as a whole. By looking at the multi-dimensional nature of a person's health, healthcare providers can more accurately gauge factors that might affect nutritional health, like social isolation or depression, which tend to be overlooked in routine screenings. Furthermore, the combined effort of dietitians and geriatricians in conducting such assessments makes it possible for an individualized approach, hence individualized care planning. As pointed out in existing literature, such complexity demands a scrupulous attention to methodology, which can potentially revolutionize the effectiveness of nutritional intervention among geriatric patients (Lampugnale, 2017). Healthcare professionals' education and training are key to the attainment of best practice for the delivery of nutritional screening in geriatrics. By virtue of proper skills and knowledge empowerment, professionals are able to identify risk factors of malnutrition and implement effective interventions. Education interventions need to address teaching professionals on how to educate on predictive areas like frailty and social support that influence dietary needs. Continuing professional development in this regard can guarantee that health professionals are current with the most recent evidence-based practice, ultimately reflecting better screening procedures. Encouraging an interdisciplinary model can also fill patient care gaps and enhance the delivery of nutritional services. Consequently, with the increasing aging population, appropriate training and best practice in nutritional screening become the priority in alleviating nutritional deficiency-related health hazards among older populations (The Stern Center for Evidence-Based Policy, 2015).

13.5.2. Importance of Interdisciplinary Collaboration

Interdisciplinary teamwork continues to be a central component in addressing the challenges affecting geriatric nutritional risk. As nutrition in the elderly is a multifaceted issue, diverse expertise is essential in developing a general framework that adequately responds to this issue. Experts such as dietitians, geriatricians, social workers, and nurses must work together to find and establish nutritional risks. With their shared specialist knowledge, such experts can develop individualized interventions that consider the numerous aspects of a person's health, way of life, and nutritional needs in old age. This kind of collaborative strategy not only enhances the quality of nutritional assessment but also creates interventions as responsive as possible to the unique needs of older adults, ultimately leading to improved health outcomes. Moreover, good interdisciplinary collaboration also facilitates enhanced communication among health practitioners, which is crucial in the case of geriatric care. The several comorbidities of the nutrition issues of the elderly typically involve input from multiple disciplines, and effective collaboration is thus paramount. Regular interdisciplinary meetings can facilitate learning between parties and ensure an integrated approach to nutrition assessment and intervention. By effective collaboration, potential barriers to effective nutritional care are addressed and integrated care plans are encouraged. Furthermore, as recognized through evidence, favorable policies towards interprofessional practice can lead to revolutionary improvement in patient outcomes, revealing the necessity for concerted collaboration in closing the gap between various disciplines in the care of the elderly (The Stern Center for Evidence-Based Policy, 2015). Finally, interprofessional collaboration is crucial in policy design and implementation on the topic of geriatric nutritional risk. Through the collective might of various experts, research findings can be effectively converted into evidence-based policies that ensure enhanced nutritional care for the elderly. Not only do these policies emphasize prevention, but they also encourage integrated care plans that tackle the multidimensional needs of the elderly. Stern Centers' work emphasizes that the research must be linked with possible policies, promoting programs that support family caregivers and long-term financing (Khezrian et al., 2017). With the emphasis placed on interdisciplinary practice within clinical care as well as in policy formulation, the health system can improve its responsiveness to the nutrition requirements of the elderly to maximum benefit, thereby improving their quality of life (Figure 13.12).

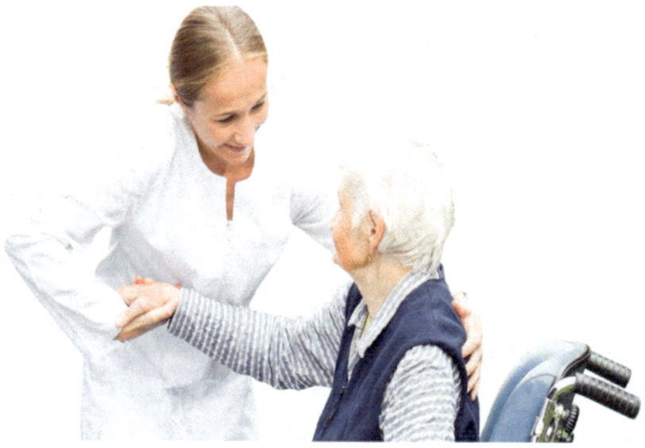

Figure 13.12. Elderly people are healthy in geriatric populations.

Source: https://care24.co.in/wp-content/uploads/2020/10/Elderlycare1200x600-Transparent.png.

13.5.3. Tailoring Screening Approaches to Individual Needs

Geriatric nutritional risk screening entails a tailored approach that considers every patient's specific needs. The growing size of the aging population makes the complexity of trying to solve nutritional problems for older individuals more apparent. A one-size-fits-all strategy is insufficient; rather, screening processes must be adaptable in a way that allows for consideration of variability in health status, comorbidities, and personal preferences. Comprehensive assessments, like pre-surgical geriatric assessment, provide a foundation to establish specific nutritional needs and risks of aging patients undergoing surgery. Unfortunately, the lack of utilization of these assessments can compromise optimal intervention plans despite acknowledgment of applicability. As stated, few patients receive thorough assessments, recognizing the necessity of including sensitive and responsive screening protocols that address the unique requirements of the geriatric population (Lampugnane, 2017). Proper screening also requires understanding the complexity of older adults' nutritional requirements. Mental health, social support, and physical frailty intersect to influence nutritional status and overall well-being among this group. The most informative areas of geriatric evaluation, like the Mini-Nutritional Assessment and Geriatric Depression Screening, play a critical role in formulating individualized approaches to nutritional intervention. By individualizing screening techniques to encompass these important considerations, healthcare providers can maximally enhance the detection rates of vulnerable individuals. Implementation of strategies that respect the physical and mental components of aging will not only increase the relevance of nutritional assessments but also improve compliance with dietary intervention required to attain better health for elderly people (Lampugnane, 2017). The addition of tailored screening strategies translates to a commitment to ongoing education and training of healthcare practitioners. As highlighted in geriatric training guidelines, educational interventions that address the exact areas predictive of nutritional risk can enhance clinicians' skills in conducting the evaluations. Competency- and simulation-based education focus on providing an impetus to foster confidence among future healthcare professionals to conduct these crucial evaluations. The knowledge gained through interprofessional learning, especially involving geriatricians and other medical experts, can provide improved insight into nutritional needs. Lastly, creating a culture of individualized screening, led by practice and education, enables clinicians to cope with the complexities of geriatric nutritional risks in an efficient manner, such that individualized care protocols directly respond to the unique needs of the elderly age group.

13.6. Interventions to Mitigate Nutritional Risk

The nutritional risk among the geriatric population is one that is increasingly at the forefront, especially with the older population typically being plagued by an array of comorbidities that influence their food requirements. Interventions to mitigate nutritional risk must be holistic in approach and include nutritional assessment as part of routine healthcare practices. Assessment must not just be derived from dietary intake but also consider such problems as polypharmacy, which greatly affects nutritional status. Effective screening will help in the identification of those at higher risk and permit interventions aimed at their unique health profiles. Various methods exist for the evaluation of nutritional risk, but the protocols need to be standardized in order to allow for consistency and replicability of results. All of these variables are essential in the formulation of interventions that hold promise for improving health outcomes and quality of life in older adults. One of these methods with potential for mitigating nutritional risk is the delivery of community-based nutrition education programs.

These programs aim to provide older adults with the education and knowledge to make improved nutritional choices. Through a focus on self-management and experiential cooking demonstrations, one can acquire the skill set necessary to prepare nutritious meals based on their specific nutritional requirements. Not only does this serve to address the nutritional gaps prevalent in the geriatric population, but it also provides socialization and mental stimulation. Nutrition education can also be most effective when supplemented by policies that encourage regular health checks and care coordination, establishing a comprehensive support system for older adults. Policies backing such training programs can establish an environment where nutritional well-being is prioritized, ultimately reducing the incidence of malnutrition and its associated healthcare complications among this vulnerable group (The Stern Center for Evidence-Based Policy, 2015). Also, efforts to optimize medication usage, that is, deprescribing harmful-to-beneficial medicines, can have a big impact on nutritional status. As polypharmacy is such a pressing geriatric issue, systematic elimination and scrutiny of potentially more-harm-than-benefit medications are necessary. These efforts need to be coupled with multidisciplinary collaborative efforts among healthcare professionals, like physicians, pharmacists, and dietitians. These health providers can work together to assess patients' medication, with a special focus on the overall impact on nutritional health and general well-being. It cannot be overstated that there is a need for standardized practice in polypharmacy assessment because such guidelines would ensure that all aspects of an older individual's nutritional and healthcare needs are regularly addressed systematically. By integrating these methods, healthcare systems can efficiently reduce nutritional risk and enhance overall health outcomes for the elderly (Sharma et al., 2016).

13.6.1. Nutritional Education and Counseling

Nutrition education and counseling are key parts of the management of geriatric nutritional risk, particularly because older individuals tend to have personalized physiological changes that make their nutritional needs more complex. Such changes usually result in alternative metabolism, loss of appetite, and risk for long-term diseases, and hence, proper nutrition education becomes essential. Good nutritional guidance should be on a one-to-one basis with regard to an individual's medical history, lifestyle, and preferences. By providing them with individualized advice, health care providers can bring about older individuals' understanding of nutrients and help them make improved food choices. These interventions have been shown to improve the overall health outcome, reduce the risk of malnutrition, and even enhance the quality of life among the elderly. Furthermore, ongoing education helps in the development of sustainable dietary practices that can prevent certain age-related diseases, such as osteoporosis and cardiovascular disease, prevalent among them. Cognitive and motivational factors play an important role in determining the success of nutritional education and counseling among the elderly. Many older people will have trouble with information processing because of cognitive impairment or sensory loss, such as decreased taste and smell. Therefore, healthcare professionals must utilize effective teaching strategies such as the use of simple language, visual presentation, and demonstration of food preparation techniques to facilitate clear communication of key nutritional information. Moreover, adding motivational interviewing can empower older adults by alleviating their anxiety and involving them in goal setting about what they eat. Not only is this client-driven approach a way of feeling ownership over dietary choices, but it is also a means of adhering to nutritional principles. By nurturing both the educational and emotional aspects of counseling, practitioners can play a significant role in encouraging older adults to adopt healthier dietary practices and thus mitigate their nutritional risks more effectively. The integration of nutrition education and counseling into routine screening protocols for geriatric nutritional risk is an aggressive approach to healthcare. For instance, according to recent guidelines, effective identification of nutritional issues must be woven into overall health assessments so that at-risk patients can garner the benefits of early intervention. With the use of standardized tools in routine assessments, clinicians can identify those who need additional support from the beginning. Again, collaboration among interprofessional personnel—dietitians, physicians, and mental health professionals—offers an overall plan for nutrition management. This dual method not only underlines the relevance of nutritional counseling but also addresses factors that lead to malnutrition, such as socioeconomic status or psychiatric illness. Lastly, the inclusion of educational programs into screening protocols is central to improving geriatric nutritional well-being and fostering a culture for prevention among the elderly (Figure 13.13).

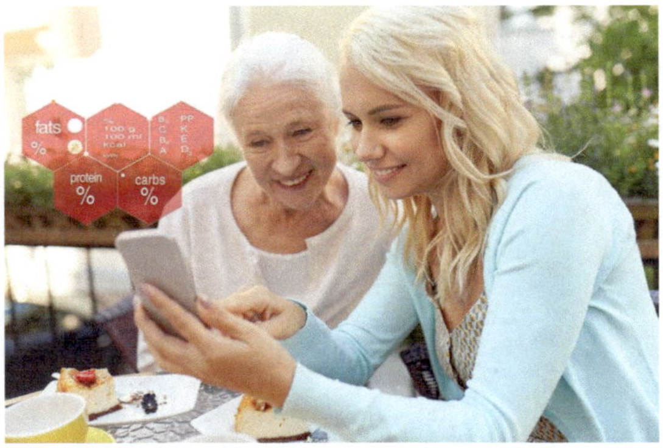

Figure 13.13. Nutritional education and counseling for geriatrics.

Source: https://bucknerretirement.org/wp-content/uploads/2022/05/What-are-the-Benefits-of-Nutrition-Counseling-for-Seniors-1024x683.jpg.

13.6.2. Community Resources and Support Systems

Community resources and support systems are critical in addressing the nutritional susceptibilities of older individuals. As the number of elderly people increases, there must be sufficient support mechanisms that facilitate easy access to diet resources. Many communities have developed meal programs, advisory nutrition services, and grocery assistance programs for seniors, which provide nutrition aid. These resources can play a role in mitigating food insecurity, a condition prevalent among older individuals, and thus improving their general health status. Moreover, community facilities are likely to serve as information centers, connecting older individuals to various services for healthier living and thus finally confirming the value of social support in mitigating nutritional risk due to aging. Integration of community resources into health care systems is required for effective geriatric nutritional risk screening. Healthcare facilities can refer patients to neighboring resources that offer nutritional education and counseling and thereby develop a more comprehensive strategy of old age care. Such collaboration lightens the burden of work on healthcare centers and enhances the delivery of specialized services targeting the individualized needs of the elderly. For instance, evidence-based policy enabling prevention as well as care coordination can impact the nutritional health of older adults significantly. Interests that enhance awareness of dietary requirements and cooking abilities can make the elderly choose healthier diets, which translates to better management of age-related diseases and improving their quality of life (The Stern Center for Evidence-Based Policy, 2015). Moreover, interventions at the community level help improve the quality of life among older people with nutritional problems. Family caregivers, who are often the primary caregivers of elderly relatives, can benefit from community-based resources that encourage education and respite care. Increased support for family caregivers not only increases their capacity to provide care in terms of nutritional needs but also improves the health of the elderly person who is being cared for by them. Enlargement programs in terms of self-management and palliative care, and reinforcing the social connections' role, can lead to more effective screening processes for nutritional risk among aged populations. These integrative approaches mean that older patients are not only being treated by healthcare professionals but also by their community to enable them to survive (Lampugnane, 2017).

13.6.3. Role of Technology in Monitoring Nutrition

Technology incorporation in the tracking of nutrition is the solution to the nutritional problems among the elderly, particularly in residential aged care (RAC) facilities. High-tech technologies, such as mobile phone-based programs and wearable devices, enable real-time tracking of food intake and nutritional status. They enable carers to track eating patterns and identify areas of potential for deficiencies in the consumption of nutrients, which is significant as it has been documented that almost half of all RAC residents are malnourished due to various factors affecting appetite and the absorption of nutrients (Agarwal et al., 2016). Along with this, these technologies encourage active participation of residents in their nutrition management and empower them to choose healthier alternatives while creating a feeling of autonomy in their nutritional lives. Incorporation of digital platforms encouraging regular screening and assessment of nutrition can give nutritional care in aged care a huge boost. For instance, electronic health records (EHRs) with nutrition-assessment tools allow the healthcare provider to monitor weight changes, dietary habits, and overall health measurements over time. Such systemic practice not only makes it possible for early detection of malnutrition but also allows timely intervention, which is imperative in preventing residents' nutritional declines (Agarwal et al., 2016). Furthermore, the use of data analytics can identify food use and preference trends and patterns, making it possible to design targeted dietary interventions and more effective food service systems. By implementing these technologies, facilities can respond to both individualized care and systemic nutritional issues. Furthermore, the technological role supports a multi-disciplinary care model through the involvement of numerous stakeholders, like dietitians, nurses, and relatives, in nutritional care among older adults. Systematic research-based policy guidelines highlight the need to prioritize care coordination and patient self-management tool integration. Technology that facilitates communication amongst members of the multidisciplinary team can lead to holistic care plans that consider the individual nutritional needs of older residents. With electronic communication tools, caregivers can quickly share information regarding an individual's nutritional status and adjust interventions accordingly, enhancing overall quality of care. Lastly, embracing trends in nutritional monitoring with technology is not only a matter of responding to immediate needs but also a matter of guaranteeing long-term health and well-being among the elderly population (Figure 13.14).

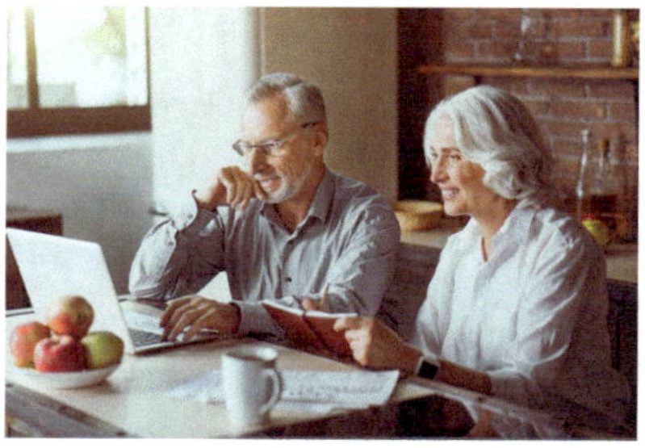

Figure 13.14. The role of technology in monitoring geriatric nutrition.

Source: https://bucknercalderwoods.org/wp-content/uploads/2023/01/The-Importance-of-Nutritional-Education-for-Seniors.jpg.

SUMMARY

Geriatric nutritional risk screening becomes a key element in the promotion of health and well-being among older adults. The importance of nutrition cannot be overstressed, given the devastating consequences of poor nutrition on health, including malnutrition, immunocompromised status, and reduced quality of life. The fact that these conditions are known but screening practices differ highlights an acute need for sound nutritional risk management. A concerted effort towards the application of validated assessment tools, such as the Mini Nutritional Assessment (MNA), must be made in order to screen for risk among the geriatric population. The need for evidence-based protocols that cut across community settings is further enhanced by research demonstrating the predictive validity of the instruments in measuring health outcomes. Therefore, assigning utmost importance to comprehensive nutritional screening must be a part of a core protocol for ensuring healthy aging of the aged population (Marshall et al., 2017). Further studies on this matter also seem evident, particularly with the countermeasures against built-in limitations with existing instruments of nutritional assessment. The general absence of heterogeneous studies establishing the validity of varied screening tools poses a hindrance to developing the best practices in geriatric nutrition. Specifically, while MNA has moderate predictive validity for certain outcomes of health, existing evidence supporting its use falls short for more widespread usage in various community settings. Follow-up studies should then focus on the concurrent and predictive validity of diverse evaluation tools so as to provide practitioners a reliable source of data to guide their interventions. Through improving the knowledge of these tools and their effectiveness, the healthcare field can solidify its practice in managing nutritional risk in the elderly (Marshall et al., 2017). Finally, the impact of enhanced nutritional screening extends beyond patient health; it extends to healthcare systems and social aging population costs. By identifying nutritional deficiencies early, medical practitioners can implement timely interventions that can reduce the occurrence of conditions such as frailty, hospitalization, and long-term care admission. Not only does this retrospective action guarantee better health outcomes, but it also envisions significant economic benefits by reducing the total burden on healthcare resources. As the population continues to age, efficient screening processes will be instrumental in maintaining health and independence in older age. Cooperation among clinicians, researchers, and policymakers will be necessary to bring these efforts forward to ultimately enhance the quality of life for an aging population. Geriatric nutrition screening is a critical component of a comprehensive health assessment of the elderly. Because this group is particularly susceptible to nutritional deficiencies, identification of at-risk individuals by systematic screening can permit early intervention. Identification in the early stages addresses not only immediate nutritional needs but also prevents associated comorbid conditions of health, such as frailty and decline in functional capacity. Standardized screening tools can enhance the reliability and validity of the results. These instruments should record a number of parameters, including medical history, dietetics, and social determinants of health, in order to make an integrated assessment of nutritional risk among elderly patients and ensure a culture of proactivity in health care. Additionally, the guidelines issued by trustworthy institutions emphasize the importance of individualized assessment methods with regard to the specific situation of older people. Geriatric populations similarly present with varying levels of cognitive function, mobility, and comorbid health statuses and so necessitate individualized screening protocols. Recommendations stress the need for healthcare providers to integrate these assessments as part of routine practice, utilizing evidence-based instruments and protocols. Training practitioners in the utilization of instruments and the interpretation of results is necessary since misinterpretation can yield suboptimal care planning. Jean-Ricco et al. (2017) advocate for the responsibility of health professionals to integrate these guidelines with patient contexts in a bid to achieve maximum health outcomes as well as to ensure informed decision-making regarding nutritional care. Moreover, the ongoing incorporation of interdisciplinary teams is also vital in ensuring the efficient use of nutritional risk screening. Interdisciplinary collaboration between dietitians, doctors, nurses, and social workers is required in order to effectively address the multifaceted needs of older people. Interdisciplinary care facilitates comprehensive care: not only do team members share professional views on nutrition, but they all work together to plan individual interventions suitable to the specific needs of each patient. Knowledge of the effect of exposure to nutritional risk in this population directs expected lifestyle modifications and therapeutic interventions. By using an interprofessional approach, health professionals can further the conversation in geriatric nutrition and ensure that patient-driven care remains at the forefront of intervention strategies. Eldridge et al. (2016) address the need for confirmation of pilot study efficacy in this field in an effort to pave the way for upcoming large-scale research studies.

A CLOSER LOOK

PROGNOSTIC ROLE OF GERIATRIC NUTRITIONAL RISK INDEX (GNRI)

GNRI has been shown to be a helpful prognostic factor in the assessment of nutritional status and in the prediction of outcome in the elderly. On the basis of serum albumin levels and actual/ideal body weight ratio, GNRI provides a rapid, objective, and reproducible index to categorize elderly patients into different categories of nutritional risk. Its utility extends beyond its role in conventional nutritional assessment because studies have increasingly shown it to be a strong prognostic factor in a wide range of clinical states, such as chronic diseases like heart failure, chronic kidney disease, malignancy, and postoperative convalescence. Low GNRI scores have independently been associated with increased morbidity, increased hospital length of stay, greater susceptibility to infection, and greater mortality. Such a relation underlines the very important role of nutrition in predicting the potential for recovery and resilience among the elderly. GNRI functions as an early warning sign, allowing clinicians to initiate early nutritional interventions and individualize care plans. In geriatric oncology, for instance, low GNRI has been shown to predict poor tolerance of chemotherapy and reduced survival. Similarly, in patients with cardiovascular disease, GNRI helps in risk stratification and sets the intensity of treatment (Figure 13.15).

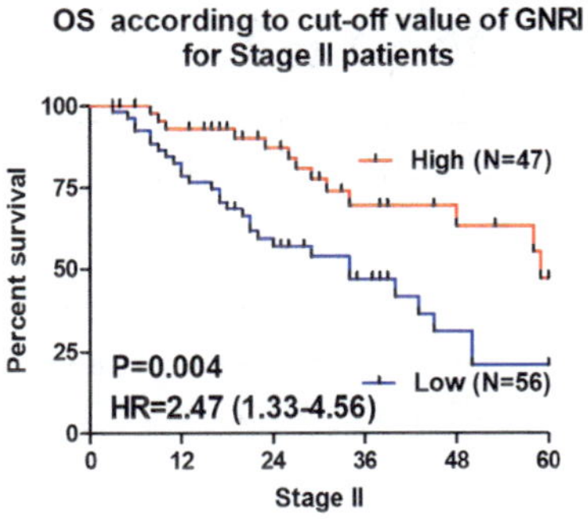

Figure 13.15. Geriatric nutritional risk index as a potential prognostic marker for patients.

Source: https://media.springernature.com/lw685/springer-static/image/art%3A10.1038%2Fs41598-022-18077-z/MediaObjects/41598_2022_18077_Fig3_HTML.png.

The index is of particular use in conditions where comprehensive nutritional assessments are not feasible due to time or resource constraints. In its simplicity, GNRI captures important aspects of both energy and protein malnutrition and thus appears to be an effective marker of diminished health status. With the aging of the world's population, the addition of standard geriatric assessment can enhance clinical decision-making and outcome by the early detection of at-risk individuals. Future studies can continue to refine GNRI thresholds or combine them with other markers to further enhance prediction in different elderly populations. Ultimately, GNRI's prognostic role reinforces the importance of routine nutritional monitoring in elderly care as a cornerstone for maintaining function, independence, and quality of life.

REFERENCES

1. Perry, W., Lacritz, L., Roebuck-Spencer, T., Silver, C., Denney, R. L., Meyers, J., McConnel, C. E., Pliskin, N., Adler, D., Alban, C., Bondi, M., Braun, M., Cagigas, X., Daven, M., Drozdick, L., Foster, N. L., Hwang, U., Ivey, L., Iverson, G., Kramer, J., ... Golden, T. (2018). Population Health Solutions for Assessing Cognitive Impairment in Geriatric Patients. *The Clinical neuropsychologist*, *32*(7), 1193–1225. https://doi.org/10.1080/13854046.2018.1517503(accessed on 12th July 2025).
2. Agarwal, E., Isenring, E., Marshall, S., et al. (2016). Optimizing nutrition in residential aged care: A narrative review. https://core.ac.uk/download/196601588.pdf (accessed on 12th July 2025).
3. Madeira, T., Peixoto-Plácido, C., Goulão, B., Mendonça, N., Alarcão, V., Santos, N., de Oliveira, R. M., Yngve, A., Bye, A., Bergland, A., Lopes, C., Nicola, P., Santos, O., & Clara, J. G. (2016). National survey of the Portuguese elderly nutritional status: study protocol. *BMC geriatrics*, *16*, 139. https://doi.org/10.1186/s12877-016-0299-x(accessed on 12th July 2025).
4. Rodríguez-Gómez, I., Mañas, A., Losa-Reyna, J., Rodríguez-Mañas, L., Chastin, S. F. M., Alegre, L. M., García-García, F. J., & Ara, I. (2018). Associations between sedentary time, physical activity and bone health among older people using compositional data analysis. *PloS one*, *13*(10), e0206013. https://doi.org/10.1371/journal.pone.0206013(accessed on 12th July 2025).
5. Ambrosetti, M., Abreu, A., Corrà, U., Davos, C. H., Hansen, D., Frederix, I., Iliou, M. C., et al. (2020). Secondary prevention through comprehensive cardiovascular rehabilitation: From knowledge to implementation. 2020 update. A position paper from the Secondary Prevention and Rehabilitation Section of the European Association of Preventive Cardiology. *European Journal of Preventive Cardiology*, *28*, 460–495. https://doi.org/10.1177/2047487320913379 (accessed on 12th July 2025).
6. Sharma, M., Loh, K. P., Nightingale, G., Mohile, S. G., & Holmes, H. M. (2016). Polypharmacy and potentially inappropriate medication use in geriatric oncology. *Journal of geriatric oncology*, *7*(5), 346–353. https://doi.org/10.1016/j.jgo.2016.07.010f (accessed on 12th July 2025).
7. Bagg, J., Bowie, L., Langhorne, P., et al. (2007). Risk factors for chest infection in acute stroke: A prospective cohort study. https://core.ac.uk/download/110683.pdf (accessed on 12th July 2025).
8. Bisnar, R. R. (2024). Nursing management in the prevention of malnutrition in elderly homes. https://core.ac.uk/download/638724337.pdf (accessed on 12th July 2025).
9. Rémond, D., Shahar, D. R., Gille, D., Pinto, P., Kachal, J., Peyron, M. A., Dos Santos, C. N., Walther, B., Bordoni, A., Dupont, D., Tomás-Cobos, L., & Vergères, G. (2015). Understanding the gastrointestinal tract of the elderly to develop dietary solutions that prevent malnutrition. *Oncotarget*, *6*(16), 13858–13898. https://doi.org/10.18632/oncotarget.4030(accessed on 12th July 2025).
10. Marshall, S., Craven, D., Kelly, J., & Isenring, E. (2018). A systematic review and meta-analysis of the criterion validity of nutrition assessment tools for diagnosing protein-energy malnutrition in the older community setting (the MACRo study). *Clinical nutrition (Edinburgh, Scotland)*, *37*(6 Pt A), 1902–1912. https://doi.org/10.1016/j.clnu.2017.09.022(accessed on 12th July 2025).

11. Eldridge, S., Chan, C., Campbell, M. J., Bond, C., Hopewell, S., Thabane, L., & Lancaster, G. (2016). CONSORT 2010 statement: Extension to randomized pilot and feasibility trials. *BMJ*. https://doi.org/10.1136/bmj.i5239 (accessed on 12th July 2025).

12. Khezrian, M., McNeil, C. J., Murray, A. D., et al. (2017). A review of frailty syndrome and its physical, cognitive and emotional domains in the elderly. https://core.ac.uk/download/131025041.pdf (accessed on 12th July 2025).

13. LeBoff, M. S., Greenspan, S. L., Insogna, K., Lewiecki, E. M., Saag, K. G., Singer, A., & Siris, E. S. (2022). The clinician's guide to prevention and treatment of osteoporosis. *Osteoporosis International*, *33*, 2049–2102. https://doi.org/10.1007/s00198-021-05900-y (accessed on 12th July 2025).

14. Malafarina, V., Reginster, J. Y., Cabrerizo, S., et al. (2017). Nutritional status and nutritional treatment are related to outcomes and mortality in older adults with hip fractures. https://core.ac.uk/download/pdf/212756692.pdf (accessed on 12th July 2025).

15. Montero-Odasso, M., van der Velde, N., Martin, F. C., Petrović, M., Tan, M. P., Ryg, J., Aguilar-Navarro, S. G., et al. (2022). World guidelines for falls prevention and management for older adults: A global initiative. *Age and Ageing*, *51*. https://doi.org/10.1093/ageing/afac205 (accessed on 12th July 2025).

16. The Stern Center for Evidence-Based Policy (2015). The Stern Center for Evidence-Based Policy, 2015. The Stern Center for Evidence-Based Policy ("Stern Center"), University of Pittsburgh's Health Policy Institute. The Stern Center for Evidence-Based Policy, 2015. https://core.ac.uk/download/75783019.pdf (accessed on 12th July 2025).

17. Nasreen, S., Saraf, M., & Nabeela, S. (2020). Evaluation of efficacy of nutritional screening tools to assess malnutrition among elderly patients in a tertiary hospital in Telangana, India. *International Journal of Food and Nutritional Sciences*, *9*, 54–57. https://www.semanticscholar.org/paper/d1cb9ef0bf86b47f0168098a47b5e3d410e67bff (accessed on 12th July 2025).

18. Ricco, J. B., Bartelink, M. L., Björck, M., Brodmann, M., Cohnert, T., Czerny, M., De Carlo, M., et al. (2017). 2017 ESC guidelines on the diagnosis and treatment of peripheral arterial diseases, in collaboration with the European Society for Vascular Surgery (ESVS). *European Heart Journal*, *39*, 763–816. https://doi.org/10.1093/eurheartj/ehx095 (accessed on 12th July 2025).

19. Shepard, D., Brown, J. L., Orwat, J., & Martin, T. (2007). The economic cost of domestic hunger: Estimated annual burden to the United States. https://core.ac.uk/download/71358043.pdf (accessed on 12th July 2025).

20. Wynn-Grundy, N. J. (2016). Undiagnosed depression in the elderly and healthcare education. https://core.ac.uk/download/70426926.pdf (accessed on 12th July 2025).

21. Zhang, X., Pang, L., Sharma, S. V., Li, R., Nyitray, A., & Edwards, B. (2019). The validity of three malnutrition screening markers among older patients with cancer. *BMJ Supportive & Palliative Care*, *10*, 363–368. https://www.semanticscholar.org/paper/0831ca3c2e81498469a027d17a8bba71fd55bb39 (accessed on 12th July 2025).

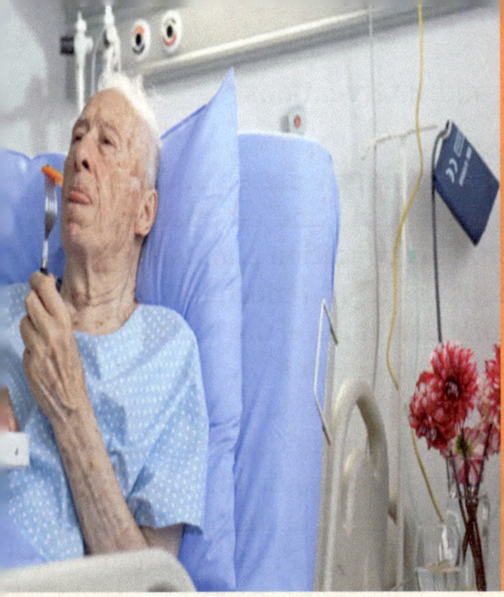

Chapter 14

GERIATRIC SARCOPENIA AND NUTRITION IN THE CASE OF CACHEXIA BEFORE EXITUS

Contents

Introduction

The increasing prevalence of sarcopenia in the geriatric population, particularly in cases of cachexia, underscores the critical interplay between muscle mass, mobility, and nutritional status. Sarcopenia, defined as the age-related loss of muscle mass and strength, can significantly impact an individual's quality of life and functional independence. This deterioration often occurs alongside chronic diseases, such as cancer and heart failure, which can exacerbate nutritional deficiencies and further contribute to muscle wasting. The connection between poor physical performance and adverse health outcomes has been highlighted in studies of patients with colorectal neoplasia, demonstrating a higher incidence of postoperative complications in those with lower physical performance measures like the Short Physical Performance Battery (SPPB) (Carrasco-Campos et al., 2022). Understanding these relationships is vital as they provide insight into designing effective interventions that could mitigate the effects of geriatric sarcopenia and improve overall patient outcomes. In the realm of cachexia, the multifaceted nature of this syndrome poses additional challenges for nutritional management in elderly patients. Cachexia not only entails significant weight loss but also manifests as a loss of muscle and adipose tissue, compounded by systemic inflammation and metabolic dysregulation. This condition stands in stark contrast to simple malnutrition, as cachexia involves complex pathophysiological mechanisms that require a targeted approach to treatment. As indicated by research on heart failure, the relationship between nutritional status and patient prognosis serves as a critical reminder of the importance of comprehensive assessments (Laiglesia R et al., 2019). Addressing cachexia in geriatric patients necessitates a nuanced understanding of how nutritional interventions, specifically tailored to individual needs, can effectively counteract the progression of sarcopenia and related health risks, ultimately optimizing care for this vulnerable population. To combat geriatric sarcopenia and the associated complications of cachexia, a multidisciplinary approach is essential. Combining nutritional support with physical therapy and medical treatment can facilitate a comprehensive strategy that addresses both muscle wasting and nutritional deficiencies. The role of standardized assessment tools for evaluating physical performance and nutritional status cannot be overstated, as these tools allow for timely intervention and tailored management plans (Carrasco-Campos et al., 2022). Furthermore, studies indicate that early identification of malnutrition and physical decline is vital in reducing morbidity and improving functional outcomes in elderly patients facing surgery or chronic illness (Laiglesia R et al., 2019). As the healthcare landscape evolves, a deeper understanding of the intricate connections between sarcopenia, nutrition, and cachexia will be imperative for enhancing the quality of life in geriatric patients and optimizing healthcare resources.

Definition of Geriatric Sarcopenia

The concept of geriatric sarcopenia has emerged as a critical area of study within geriatrics, particularly due to its implications for health outcomes in older adults. Sarcopenia is defined as the progressive and generalized loss of skeletal muscle mass and strength, culminating in reduced physical performance. This condition not only affects mobility but also increases the risk of falls, fractures, and morbidity among elderly populations. It becomes particularly concerning in patients experiencing comorbidities such as cancer, where the interplay with cachexia—a syndrome characterized by involuntary weight loss and muscle wasting—can exacerbate the clinical picture, leading to a more complicated therapeutic landscape. Understanding these relationships is vital, especially in geriatric patients, as they face unique physical and nutritional challenges that can significantly influence their quality of life and overall health outcomes. Research highlights that the intersection of geriatric sarcopenia with cachexia necessitates a nuanced approach to diagnosis and management. As noted, individuals with sarcopenia often display overlaps with malnutrition, which may complicate their clinical assessments and treatment plans. Misapplication of diagnostic criteria can hinder timely intervention, resulting in adverse health effects and decreased efficacy of rehabilitation strategies. The Global Leadership Initiative on Malnutrition (GLIM) framework has been proposed as a standard for assessing malnutrition in older adults, aiming to clarify the diagnostic criteria and treatment priorities. Within this context, addressing geriatric sarcopenia entails not only nutritional interventions but also comprehensive assessments to tailor management strategies that facilitate better clinical outcomes for patients grappling with both sarcopenia and cachexia. This multifaceted approach is essential for improving life quality in this vulnerable population. Furthermore, the understanding of geriatric sarcopenia must include considerations of underlying mechanisms and patient-centered interventions that target both nutrition and physical activity. Nutritional therapies tailored to combat sarcopenia show promise; however, their effectiveness can be hindered by the presence of acute inflammation or end-stage diseases associated with cachexia. Interventions such as targeted exercise programs combined with nutritional support may foster improvements in muscle mass and functionality in older adults, as long as they are adapted to the individual's overall health status. Moreover, integrating non-nutritional strategies, such as pharmacologic agents or comprehensive care plans, can further enhance patient outcomes. As the literature reveals, successful management of geriatric sarcopenia, particularly in cases complicated by cachexia, demands a holistic approach that encompasses multiple therapeutic modalities (Mortellaro S et al., 2024) (G Jensen et al., 2024).

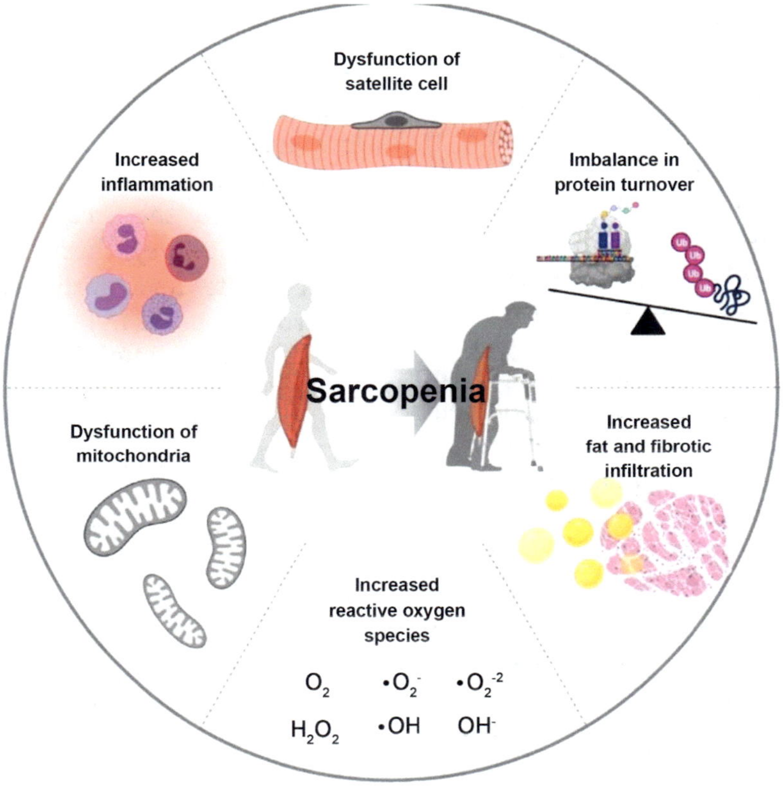

Figure 14.1. Geriatric Sarcopenia.

Source: https://media.springernature.com/lw685/springer-static/image/art%3A10.1007%2Fs10354-022-00927-0/MediaObjects/10354_2022_927_Fig1_HTML.png

Overview of Cachexia

Cachexia is a complex metabolic syndrome characterized by severe muscle wasting, often seen in individuals suffering from chronic illnesses such as cancer, heart failure, and chronic obstructive pulmonary disease (COPD). This multifactorial condition transcends simple malnutrition, involving an imbalance between muscle protein synthesis and degradation driven by inflammatory processes. In geriatric populations, cachexia not only contributes to physical frailty but also diminishes quality of life, leading to increased disability and dependency. Recent insights into the underlying mechanisms have highlighted the role of pro-inflammatory cytokines, which stimulate catabolic pathways while inhibiting anabolic pathways essential for muscle maintenance. Understanding these interactions is crucial for developing therapeutic strategies to combat cachexia in older adults and can inform the design of intervention programs aimed at the prevention and management of this debilitating condition. Given the significant relationship between nutrition and cachexia, dietary interventions play a vital role in the management of this syndrome. Malnutrition, which often accompanies cachexia, exacerbates its effects and leads to further muscle loss. Aging itself influences nutrient metabolism, as the gastrointestinal tract undergoes changes that impair nutrient intake, digestion, and absorption. The decline in GIT functionality can hinder the elderlys ability to gain sufficient nourishment, contributing to the vicious cycle of cachexia and malnutrition. To address these challenges, it is essential to design dietary guidelines tailored to the unique needs of the aging population. This includes not only enhancing caloric intake but also focusing on protein quality and nutrient bioavailability, which are crucial in promoting muscle preservation and overall health in older adults affected by cachexia (Bordoni et al., 2015). Moreover, the potential for exercise as an adjunctive therapy presents an emerging avenue for mitigating the effects of cachexia in the geriatric population. Physical activity has been shown to counteract muscle wasting by stimulating muscle protein synthesis and improving overall physical function. Exercise interventions can mitigate the adverse effects of cachexia and improve prognostic outcomes. Studies suggest that combining exercise with nutritional supplementation, such as creatine, may amplify benefits by promoting lean body mass and strength gains. This synergistic approach is particularly important for older adults, who are at higher risk for muscle loss due to aging-related sarcopenia and cachexia. Understanding these interactions lays the groundwork for optimizing treatment protocols that not only target nutrition but also incorporate physical activity, ultimately enhancing the quality of life in patients facing the challenges of cachexia before exitus (Fairman et al., 2018).

Importance of Nutrition in Elderly Patients

Nutrition plays a pivotal role in the health and well-being of elderly patients, particularly in mitigating the effects of sarcopenia and cachexia. As individuals age, physiological changes can compromise their nutritional status, leading to muscle loss, reduced strength, and increased frailty. The European Working Group on Sarcopenia in Older People (EWGSOP) emphasizes the need for a nuanced understanding of sarcopenia, which is defined by low muscle mass in conjunction with diminished muscle function. Adequate nutrition is essential in preventing these conditions, as it supports muscle protein synthesis and overall health in older adults. Specifically, ensuring a diet rich in protein, essential vitamins, and minerals can assist in maintaining muscle mass, thereby enhancing physical performance and quality of life during the aging process (Baeyens et al., 2017). Furthermore, malnutrition is alarmingly prevalent among the geriatric population, exacerbating the risks associated with chronic conditions, and contributing to poor recovery from illness or injury. A significant study highlights the connection between malnutrition and adverse outcomes in elderly individuals with hip fractures, revealing that nearly 19% of these patients are classified as malnourished using standard assessments. More concerning is that this prevalence can rise to 45% under stricter diagnostic criteria. Malnutrition not only hinders the recovery efforts of these patients but also correlates with heightened mortality rates, underscoring the critical importance of early nutritional intervention strategies (Malafarina et al., 2017). Therefore, healthcare providers must prioritize nutritional assessments in this demographic to enhance treatment outcomes and improve overall survival rates. The implications of inadequate nutrition extend beyond immediate physical health; they also impact mental and emotional well-being. Malnourished elderly patients often experience increased feelings of isolation, depression, and anxiety, which can further deteriorate their health status. This psychological dimension is particularly salient in those suffering from sarcopenia and cachexia, as the loss of independence and physical ability can corrode their sense of self-worth and quality of life. Health practitioners must adopt a comprehensive approach that includes nutrition as a cornerstone of geriatric care, tailoring dietary interventions to individual preferences and needs. By fostering a supportive environment where elderly patients are encouraged to maintain proper nutrition, healthcare providers can promote resilience against illness and enhance both physical and mental well-being, thereby diminishing the overall burden of age-related conditions (Baeyens et al., 2017).

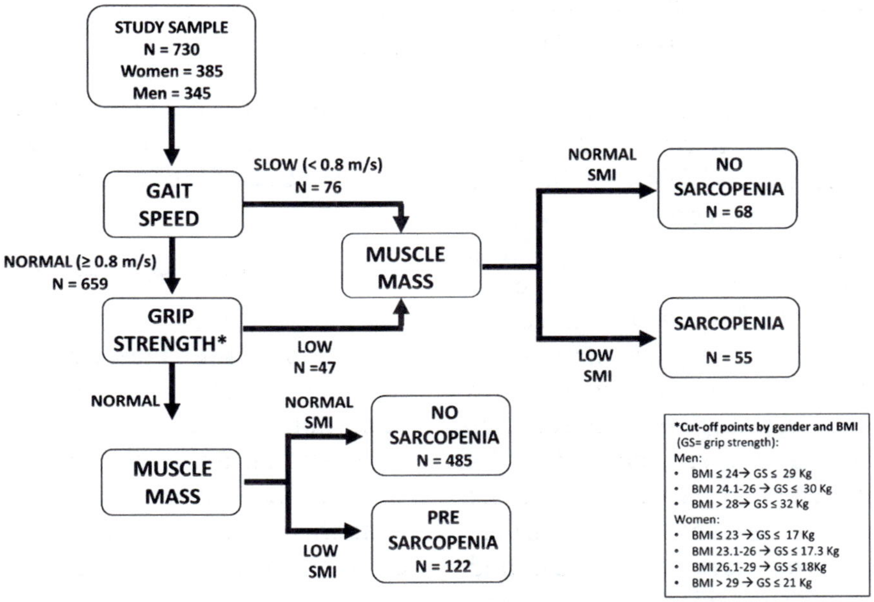

Figure 14.2. Application of the European Working Group on Sarcopenia in Older People.

Source: https://www.researchgate.net/profile/Marcello-Maggio/publication/257301474/figure/fig1/AS:297330910744576@1447900621250/Application-of-the-European-Working-Group-on-Sarcopenia-in-Older-People-algorithm-for-the.png

14.1 Understanding Geriatric Sarcopenia

Geriatric sarcopenia, characterized by progressive loss of muscle mass and strength, poses a significant health challenge for the elderly population. This condition is often exacerbated by factors such as malnutrition, chronic diseases, and reduced physical activity, making it a multidimensional issue that requires comprehensive understanding and intervention. Older adults suffering from sarcopenia frequently experience complications such as impaired mobility, increased risk of falls, and a higher likelihood of hospitalization. Moreover, the negative outcomes associated with sarcopenia extend beyond physical health, impacting psychological well-being and overall quality of life. Timely identification and intervention strategies are crucial in mitigating the adverse effects of geriatric sarcopenia and promoting healthier aging. Nutrition plays a pivotal role in managing geriatric sarcopenia, particularly given the interplay between inadequate dietary intake and muscle degradation. A diet rich in proteins, vitamins, and essential nutrients is vital for maintaining muscle health and combating sarcopenia. Research indicates that the elderly may require higher protein intake than younger adults to effectively promote muscle synthesis and maintenance. In some cases, nutritional supplementation can aid in addressing deficiencies that contribute to the onset of sarcopenia. Furthermore, the relationship between nutrition and muscle health is reinforced by findings that indicate malnutrition can exacerbate sarcopenic symptoms, highlighting the necessity for a tailored nutritional approach in elder care. Thus, a comprehensive dietary plan becomes essential in the management of sarcopenia, providing a foundation for improved health outcomes. Understanding the integrative aspects of sarcopenia involves recognizing its association with cachexia, particularly in the context of terminal illness. Cachexia, a syndrome characterized by involuntary muscle loss and weight reduction, can significantly accelerate the progression of sarcopenia, ultimately leading to adverse health outcomes such as increased mortality. Studies have demonstrated that patients with advanced conditions experience heightened muscle wasting due to metabolic changes, which are further complicated by poor nutritional status. In this light, it becomes evident that managing nutritional deficiencies is crucial in elderly patients presenting with both sarcopenia and cachexia. Implementing effective nutritional interventions not only slows the progression of these conditions but also enhances the overall quality of life for affected individuals prior to exitus. Addressing the dual challenges of sarcopenia and cachexia through an integrated nutritional framework can offer a promising pathway to improve health management in geriatric populations.

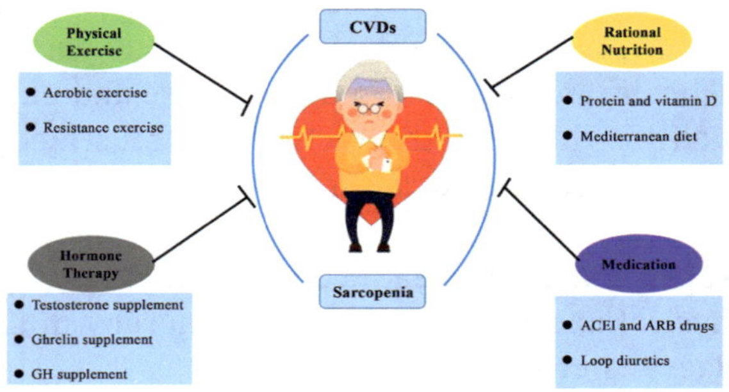

Figure 14.3. Sarcopenia (Muscle Loss): Symptoms.

Source: https://www.yorkrehabclinic.ca/media/mediahub/generic-media/1692876567882.png

14.1.1 Causes of Sarcopenia in the Elderly

Sarcopenia, the age-related loss of muscle mass and strength, is a multifactorial condition primarily attributed to physiological changes that occur with aging. One significant contributing factor is the gradual decline in anabolic hormones, such as testosterone and estrogen, which play crucial roles in muscle protein synthesis. This hormonal imbalance leads to decreased muscle regeneration and repair following physical exertion. Additionally, aging is accompanied by a reduction in satellite cell activity, which negatively impacts the body's ability to maintain and build muscle tissue. Research has shown that this decrease in cellular regeneration capacity can significantly compromise muscle quality and size, ultimately resulting in sarcopenia. Also, physical inactivity, exacerbated by an aging lifestyle, contributes to muscle wasting, highlighting the importance of maintaining an active regimen to counteract these physiological declines. Another major cause of sarcopenia in the elderly is nutritional deficiency, specifically inadequate protein intake. As individuals age, a combination of reduced appetite and altered taste perception can lead to insufficient nutrient consumption, particularly protein, which is vital for muscle maintenance and growth. Studies indicate that older adults often consume protein levels below the recommended dietary allowance, impairing their ability to preserve muscle mass. Furthermore, malnutrition increases the risk of developing cachexia, a severe condition characterized by muscle wasting and weight loss, which is frequently encountered in patients with chronic diseases. Improved nutritional strategies, including the emphasis on higher protein intake and the consumption of rich nutrient sources, are essential for ameliorating the effects of sarcopenia and preserving muscle health in the elderly population (Tacar SY et al., 2022). Additionally, comorbidities such as chronic inflammation and metabolic disorders play a substantial role in the development of sarcopenia among the elderly. Conditions like diabetes and renal failure can exacerbate muscle wasting by disrupting metabolic processes and fostering chronic inflammatory states, which have been associated with muscle degradation. The presence of systemic inflammation not only hinders muscle protein synthesis but also promotes the breakdown of muscle tissue, creating a vicious cycle that leads to further decline. Consequently, understanding the interplay between chronic diseases and sarcopenia is vital in developing targeted interventions that address both nutritional and medical needs. For example, effective management of underlying health conditions can diminish their impact on muscle health and contribute to a better overall prognosis for elderly individuals (Jos Fé Sánchez-Torralvo et al., 2024).

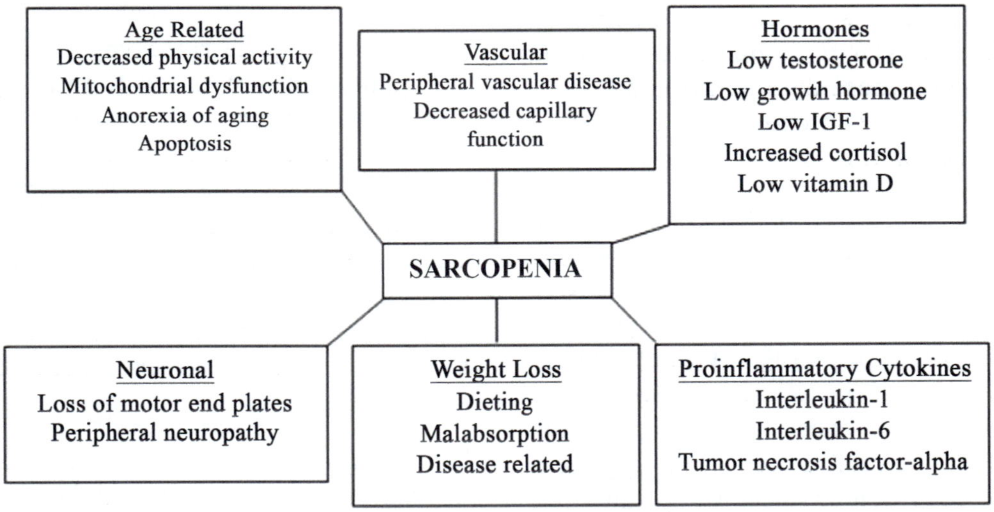

Figure 14.4. The Cause of Sarcopenia.

Source: https://www.researchgate.net/profile/Igp-Aryana-2/publication/323414461/figure/fig2/AS:609137943662592@1522241211603/The-Cause-of-Sarcopenia-1.png

14.1.2 Symptoms and Diagnosis

The manifestations of geriatric sarcopenia, particularly when it intersects with cachexia, encompass a range of symptoms that complicate diagnosis. Typically characterized by a progressive loss of muscle mass and strength, sarcopenia significantly affects older adults functional status, leading to increased frailty and vulnerability. The initial indications often include fatigue, reduced physical performance, and unintentional weight loss. As these symptoms advance, they may escalate into more severe stages of malnutrition, perpetuating a cycle that exacerbates overall health decline and significantly reduces quality of life. Importantly, identifying sarcopenia requires a thorough assessment that considers not just muscle mass but also strength and functional performance, which are critical in evaluating the prognosis of affected individuals. Addressing these symptoms through early and comprehensive evaluation is crucial to developing effective management strategies tailored to the individual's unique health status and needs, aligning with the multifaceted nature of this syndrome (Chao C-T et al., 2025). Diagnosis of sarcopenia presents its own set of challenges, primarily due to the overlap of symptoms with other geriatric syndromes such as frailty and malnutrition. Clinicians must employ a combination of clinical assessments and diagnostic criteria, including measurements of muscle mass via imaging techniques and strength assessments through standardized tests like the handgrip dynamometer. However, reliance solely on these data points can lead to misdiagnosis if not contextualized within the broader clinical picture.

The complexity is further heightened in older individuals who often present multiple comorbidities that can obscure definitive diagnosis. As such, a comprehensive geriatric assessment, incorporating evaluations of nutritional status, physical function, and comorbid conditions, is essential. Only through this thorough and multidimensional approach can healthcare providers accurately diagnose sarcopenia and its contributing factors, thereby facilitating timely intervention strategies that can greatly enhance patient outcomes (N/A, 2025). Interventions focused on managing symptoms of sarcopenia and cachexia necessitate an equally nuanced diagnostic framework to address underlying nutritional deficiencies and physical activity limitations. The interrelationship of these conditions with chronic illnesses underscores the importance of identifying early signs of deterioration in muscle health. To promote a personalized management plan, clinicians must delve into the patients nutritional intake, physical activity levels, and functional capacity. Evidence suggests that integrating nutritional support—especially high-quality protein intake—alongside tailored exercise regimens can combat the loss of muscle strength and mass. Notably, the significance of individual lifestyle factors cannot be overstated; psychosocial aspects impacting an individual's motivation to engage in physical activities can also play a critical role in recovery. Thus, comprehensive management of sarcopenia demands both a thorough understanding of its symptoms and proactive engagement in multidisciplinary approaches that include nutritional and rehabilitative strategies (Chao C-T et al., 2025).

14.1.3 Impact on Quality of Life

The impact of geriatric sarcopenia and cachexia on quality of life is profound, significantly influencing functional capacity and overall well-being. Sarcopenia, characterized by the loss of muscle mass and strength, adversely affects elderly individuals' abilities to carry out daily activities, ultimately leading to increased dependence on caregivers. This reliance can result in feelings of helplessness and diminished self-worth, which can exacerbate depression and anxiety.

The combination of physical decline and psychological distress not only hinders one's ability to maintain independence but can also create a cycle of further physical deterioration, as individuals may withdraw from social interactions and physical activities due to their condition. Moreover, nutritional deficiencies commonly associated with cachexia further compound these challenges, making it vital to address both physical and psychological aspects to enhance quality of life in this vulnerable population (Rodr Íguez-Sánchez et al., 2022). Nutritional interventions play a critical role in mitigating the adverse effects of sarcopenia and cachexia on quality of life.

Adequate nutrient intake, particularly protein and essential vitamins, is crucial for muscle preservation and functional status. Malnutrition can accelerate muscle loss and exacerbate the symptoms of sarcopenia, leading to a rapid decline in physical capabilities and social engagement. In this context, the implementation of personalized nutrition programs becomes essential, as they not only aim to combat malnutrition but also to improve energy levels, mood, and cognitive function. Studies reveal that targeted nutritional strategies, when combined with structured physical activity regimens, can foster improvements in both muscle strength and psychological well-being. By adopting a multifaceted approach to tackle sarcopenia and cachexia, healthcare providers can significantly enhance older adults' quality of life and functional outcomes as they navigate the complexities of aging (Míkel Izquierdo et al., 2021). Furthermore, social and environmental factors significantly influence the quality of life for older adults experiencing sarcopenia and cachexia. Social isolation, a common challenge faced by this demographic, may result in reduced social participation, leading to emotional distress and exacerbating feelings of loneliness. This isolation often impedes access to nutritional resources and physical activity, creating a vicious cycle that perpetuates functional decline. Community-based programs designed to encourage social interaction, physical participation, and nutritional education can be transformative by fostering a supportive network for older adults. Such initiatives can counteract the detrimental impacts of sarcopenia and cachexia, promoting a sense of belonging and enhancing overall well-being. Ultimately, by addressing these interrelated aspects, including physical health, nutrition, and social engagement, it is possible to reclaim and improve quality of life for older individuals facing these challenges in aging (Rodr Iíguez-Sánchez et al., 2022).

14.2 The Role of Cachexia in Elderly Patients

In the context of geriatric care, cachexia emerges as a complex syndrome characterized by involuntary weight loss, muscle wasting, and a decline in physical function, all of which are particularly detrimental for elderly patients. This condition complicates pre-existing health issues and is often seen in conjunction with chronic diseases such as cancer or heart failure, making its management increasingly vital for this demographic. Cachexia not only contributes to a decreased quality of life but also poses significant challenges to treatment outcomes, as it can worsen the patients overall prognosis. Research indicates that a low phase angle, obtained through bioelectrical impedance analysis, serves as a prognostic indicator for mortality in elderly patients, specifically those suffering from fragility hip fractures, highlighting the urgent need to address the underlying mechanisms of cachexia and its impact on survival rates in older adults (Jos Fé Sánchez-Torralvo et al., 2024). The physiological consequences of cachexia are profound, as it involves an imbalance between energy intake and expenditure, leading to the breakdown of muscle tissue. This process is further exacerbated by the interplay of inflammatory cytokines and metabolic changes characteristic of chronic illnesses. As cachexia progresses, elderly patients may experience a rapid decline in their abilities to perform daily activities, leading to increased dependency on caregivers and healthcare systems. Evidence suggests that those who present with low muscle mass, indicative of sarcopenia, demonstrate shorter overall survival rates, as observed in studies on patients with metastatic renal cell carcinoma receiving nivolumab. Such findings reinforce the critical link between muscle mass and patient outcomes, urging the need for targeted nutritional interventions to halt or reverse the downward trajectory associated with cachexia (Tacar SY et al., 2022). Addressing cachexia in elderly patients thus necessitates a multifaceted approach that combines nutritional support with strategies aimed at improving muscle strength and function. Nutritional interventions tailored to individual dietary needs can help mitigate weight loss and promote muscle preservation, which is essential for maintaining independence and improving overall survivability. Furthermore, integrating physical rehabilitation and resistance training alongside nutritional strategies has shown promise in enhancing muscle mass and functional performance. As healthcare providers become more aware of cachexias role in the health of elderly patients, interdisciplinary teamwork will be crucial in managing this pervasive issue. Therefore, both awareness and practical interventions in the realms of nutrition and physical activity can pave the way for better health outcomes and improved quality of life for older adults facing the challenges of cachexia.

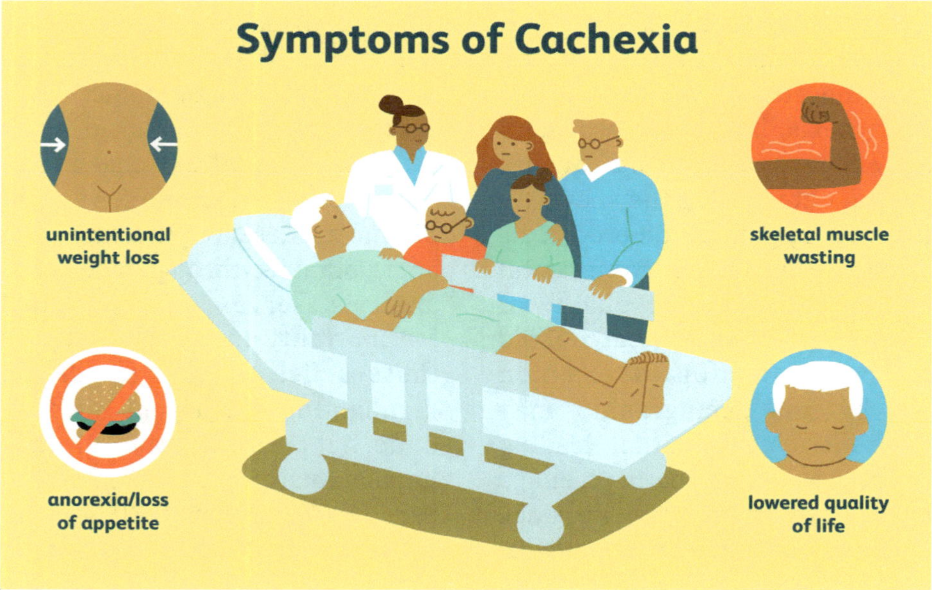

Figure 14.5. Cachexia: Causes, Symptoms, Diagnosis, and Treatments.

Source: https://www.verywellhealth.com/thmb/7o1uJkIghv-UIcjhqeCXn0xFV4M=/1500x0/filters:no_upscale():max_bytes(150000):strip_icc()/understanding-cachexia-symptoms-causes-and-treatments-2249008-01-f720df8f199c40f69770d108ac8a9b95.png

14.2.1 Definition and Characteristics of Cachexia

Cachexia is a complex metabolic syndrome characterized primarily by severe weight loss and muscle wasting, often occurring in conjunction with chronic illnesses, particularly in geriatric populations. Unlike simple malnutrition, cachexia involves systemic inflammation and a notable alteration in body composition that extends beyond mere caloric deficiency. The condition is intricately linked to factors such as poor appetite, elevated energy expenditure, and the release of pro-inflammatory cytokines, all of which contribute to the disintegration of lean body mass and muscle function. As the European Working Group on Sarcopenia in Older People (EWGSOP) delineates, the presence of both low muscle mass and diminished muscle strength or performance is critical for diagnosing sarcopenia and cachexia, underscoring the relationship between these two conditions and reinforcing the importance of accurate identification in clinical practice (Baeyens et al., 2017). A critical aspect of cachexia is its differentiation from other conditions such as sarcopenia and anorexia of aging. While sarcopenia refers specifically to the age-related loss of muscle mass and strength independent of underlying disease, cachexia arises from disease-related metabolic dysfunction that prominently affects energy balance and muscle protein metabolism. The interplay between cachexia and anorexia of aging, characterized by decreased appetite and altered taste, further complicates nutritional interventions in elderly patients. Studies indicate that addressing these factors through targeted nutritional strategies can significantly improve outcomes, affecting not only body weight but also overall quality of life. By understanding the unique features of cachexia, healthcare providers can develop more effective treatment protocols aimed at mitigating its severity and enhancing nutritional status in vulnerable older adults (LM D et al., 2018). In terms of clinical implications, early detection and diagnosis of cachexia are imperative for implementing timely interventions that can slow its progression. The characteristics of cachexia must be integrated into geriatric assessments to formulate comprehensive care plans that address both nutritional needs and concurrent medical conditions. This involves utilizing diagnostic tools to evaluate muscle mass, strength, and performance, as recommended by EWGSOP, which lays the groundwork for further research aimed at establishing effective therapeutic options. The recognition of cachexia not only facilitates better management of caloric intake and nutritional support but also encourages a multidisciplinary approach in treating elder patients, thus promoting healthier aging and improved survival outcomes prior to exitus (Baeyens et al., 2017).

14.2.2 Differences between Cachexia and Sarcopenia

The distinction between cachexia and sarcopenia is crucial in the understanding of muscle wasting conditions, particularly in geriatric patients. Cachexia is characterized by systemic inflammation and metabolic dysregulation, resulting in significant weight loss, muscle atrophy, and fat loss, often linked to underlying chronic conditions such as cancer or heart failure. In contrast, sarcopenia primarily refers to the age-related loss of muscle mass and strength, occurring without the inflammatory component seen in cachexia.

This delineation is significant for healthcare providers aiming to tailor nutritional and therapeutic strategies for elderly patients. It is essential to recognize that while both conditions involve muscle degradation, their underlying mechanisms and implications for treatment differ markedly, thereby requiring specialized intervention approaches (Fernandes et al., 2017). Another key difference lies in the physiological underpinnings and clinical manifestations of cachexia and sarcopenia. Cachexia stems from a complex interplay of neurohormonal changes, cytokine production, and increased catabolism, leading to profound systemic effects that extend beyond mere muscle loss. In contrast, sarcopenia is often attributed to aging-related factors, including decreased physical activity, hormonal changes, and nutritional deficiencies.

Although sarcopenia may manifest primarily as diminished muscle mass and strength, it does not typically present the profound systemic implications seen with cachexia. This variation in clinical presentation calls for a nuanced understanding and a comprehensive assessment of nutritional status to effectively combat the detrimental impacts of either condition (Bover J et al., 2017). In light of these differences, nutrition plays a pivotal role in addressing both cachexia and sarcopenia among geriatric populations. Tailored nutritional interventions must be considered, focusing on not only caloric intake but also the quality of nutrients consumed. For sarcopenia, strategies such as increased protein intake combined with resistance training can help to mitigate muscle loss and restore functional capacity. Conversely, in the context of cachexia, addressing underlying inflammatory processes through anti-inflammatory dietary strategies may prove beneficial. Furthermore, supplementing with vitamin D may play a significant role in promoting overall musculoskeletal health, taking into account its influence on muscle function and metabolism (Bover J et al., 2017). As the geriatric population continues to grow, understanding the distinctions between these two conditions will enhance nutritional approaches and improve patient outcomes in older adults at risk.

14.2.3 Prevalence of Cachexia in Geriatric Populations

The phenomenon of cachexia, characterized by significant weight loss and muscle wasting, is a critical concern within geriatric populations, particularly as it often complicates the management of chronic illnesses. As older adults frequently experience multimorbidity, conditions such as cancer, chronic obstructive pulmonary disease (COPD), and heart failure may elevate the risk of cachexia. The multifactorial nature of this syndrome underscores the importance of understanding its prevalence among the elderly. Research indicates that approximately 5-15% of older patients in community settings experience cachexia, with this figure rising significantly in those residing in long-term care facilities or hospitalized patients, where prevalence rates can exceed 30%. This growing incidence emphasizes the need for early identification and intervention. Moreover, inadequate nutritional intake exacerbates the development of cachexia, creating a vicious cycle that further impacts overall health outcomes in this vulnerable population. Sarcopenia, the age-related loss of muscle mass and strength, is often closely linked with cachexia in geriatric patients. The European Working Group on Sarcopenia in Older People has established that low muscle mass, coupled with impairments in muscle function, is indicative of sarcopenia, and the interaction between these conditions is increasingly recognized. This overlap exacerbates the risk for complications and contributes to higher morbidity and mortality rates among older adults. For instance, the presence of sarcopenia in patients suffering from cachexia can lead to decreased functional mobility, increased frailty, and a decline in quality of life. Furthermore, targeted interventions focusing on both nutritional support and physical activity can be crucial. By integrating strategies to manage sarcopenia and cachexia, healthcare providers can significantly improve the clinical outcomes for older adults facing these debilitating conditions (Baeyens et al., 2017). Malnutrition remains a significant factor influencing the prevalence and management of cachexia among geriatric populations. Studies have demonstrated that malnutrition can contribute to the deterioration of nutritional status, exacerbating the challenges associated with cachexia, particularly in patients with complex medical histories, such as those recovering from hip fractures. The prevalence of malnutrition can be alarming, with figures reaching over 18% to 45%, depending on the criteria applied. This high prevalence correlates with poor functional recovery and elevated mortality rates, highlighting the critical need for nutritional assessments as part of comprehensive geriatric evaluations. Furthermore, evidence suggests that implementing early nutritional interventions can lead to improved outcomes, including reduced complications and enhanced recovery trajectories. Therefore, integrating nutritional strategies into the overall treatment framework for older adults with cachexia is essential to mitigate the impacts of malnutrition and improve quality of life before exitus (Malafarina et al., 2017).

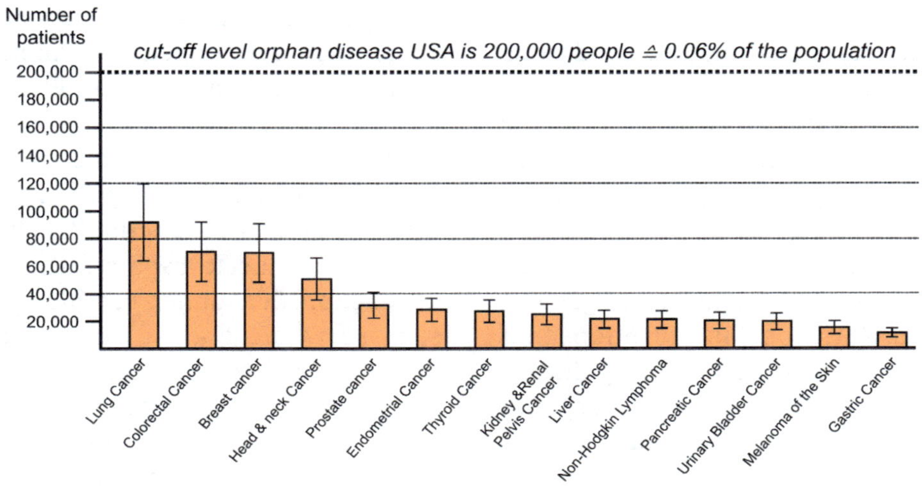

Figure 14.6. Prevalence of cancer cachexia.

Source: https://www.researchgate.net/publication/332064049/figure/fig2/AS:11431281180804016@1691711161678/Prevalence-of-cancer-cachexia-in-the-USA-2014-with-30-error-bars-to-indicate-the.png

14.3 Nutritional Requirements for the Elderly

The nutritional requirements for the elderly are crucial as they face unique challenges that affect their overall health and well-being. As individuals age, physiological changes, such as reduced metabolic rates and decreased appetite, can lead to insufficient nutrient intake. Many older adults exhibit inadequate consumption of essential nutrients, which exacerbates health conditions and may contribute to the deterioration of muscle mass. A study focusing on geriatric patients with hip fractures found that nearly 19% met the criteria for malnutrition, a significant factor that negatively impacted recovery outcomes and increased mortality risk. Interventions that prioritize nutritional adequacy are essential not only for recovery in acute situations but also for improving quality of life in the aging population. Addressing these nutritional deficits through tailored dietary plans involves a comprehensive understanding of individual dietary needs and lifestyles. The role of nutrition in preventing and managing sarcopenia among the elderly cannot be overlooked, as it directly influences muscle health and functional capacity. Sarcopenia, the age-related loss of muscle mass and strength, is profoundly affected by nutritional status and physical activity. Factors contributing to sarcopenia include inadequate protein intake, less physical activity, and underlying health issues, all of which can be mitigated by proper nutritional strategies. For instance, nutrition rich in protein, particularly from sources that are easily digestible, plays a vital role in muscle synthesis. Researchers have indicated that a balanced diet combined with resistance training is key to enhancing muscle strength and mitigating sarcopenia effects. Addressing nutritional deficiencies through dietary modifications can not only improve muscle mass but may also enhance functional independence among the elderly population. Furthermore, understanding the intricate relationship between nutrition and conditions such as cachexia is imperative in elderly care. Cachexia, often observed in patients with chronic diseases, leads to pronounced weight loss and muscle wasting that significantly impairs health outcomes. The complex interplay between inflammation, reduced appetite, and metabolic changes complicates nutritional management for such patients. Nutritional interventions that counteract malnutrition have shown significant benefits in improving functional recovery and minimizing complications. Individuals with a cachectic state often exhibit altered nutrient absorption and increased energy expenditure, necessitating a recalibration of their dietary intake. Consequently, early nutritional interventions and continuous monitoring are critical to manage not only sarcopenia but also the multifaceted challenges posed by cachexia in geriatric care settings, ultimately enhancing patient outcomes and quality of life.

14.3.1 Macronutrient Needs

The aging process often precipitates a decline in muscle mass and function, conditions collectively referred to as sarcopenia. This deterioration is frequently exacerbated by cachexia, a multifactorial syndrome characterized by severe weight loss and muscle wasting. In managing these conditions, understanding macronutrient needs becomes essential, as proper nutrition plays a pivotal role in mitigating muscle loss.

A focus on a balanced distribution of carbohydrates, proteins, and fats can optimize energy intake while providing the necessary building blocks for muscle repair and synthesis. Proteins, in particular, are crucial as they supply amino acids that stimulate muscle protein synthesis, which is often impaired in elderly populations suffering from cachexia . Thus, ensuring adequate protein intake—often recommended at levels higher than those for younger adults—is vital in effectively addressing sarcopenia and cachexia . Carbohydrates, while sometimes overlooked, are another essential component in formulating a nutritional strategy for elderly individuals facing sarcopenia and cachexia. They serve not only as a primary energy source but also play a crucial role in preserving muscle function by sparing protein for use in muscle repair rather than energy production. Consuming complex carbohydrates, such as whole grains, fruits, and vegetables, contributes to sustained energy levels throughout the day, thereby enabling older adults to engage in physical activities that are integral for maintaining muscle mass .

Furthermore, the glycemic index of carbohydrates can influence satiety and overall dietary habits, impacting caloric intake. Therefore, a deliberate focus on carbohydrate quality and quantity is necessary to support the nutritional requirements of aging individuals (Institute of Medicine et al., 2010-11-29). Fats, often maligned in dietary discussions, also hold importance in fulfilling the macronutrient needs of older adults facing sarcopenia and cachexia. Healthy fats, particularly mono- and polyunsaturated fats found in foods such as avocados, nuts, and olive oil, can provide dense caloric content and essential fatty acids that are crucial for overall health. These fats not only assist in nutrient absorption but also serve as a necessary energy source, especially when caloric intake needs to be increased without overwhelming the digestive system (Institute of Medicine et al., 2010-11-29). Additionally, the anti-inflammatory properties of omega-3 fatty acids, commonly found in fatty fish, have been shown to play a role in combating muscle loss and promoting muscle anabolism. As such, an intentional inclusion of healthy fats into the diet is significant in the overall nutritional strategy for elderly individuals experiencing sarcopenia and cachexia (Institute of Medicine et al., 2010-11-29).

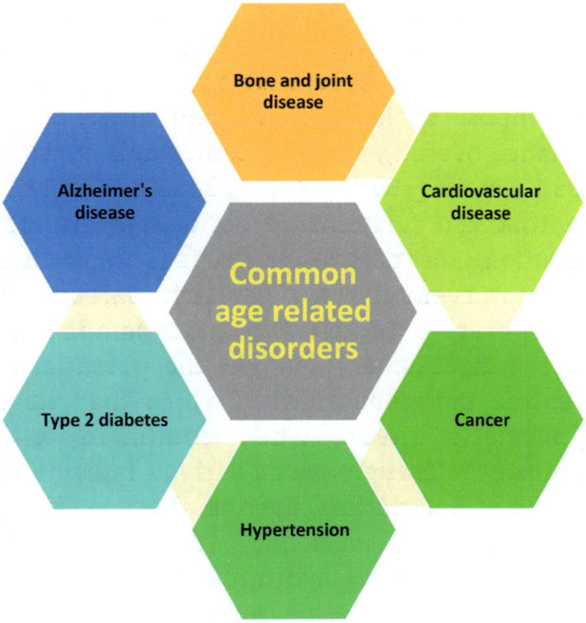

Figure 14.7. Macronutrients and Their Roles in Aging.

Source: https://media.springernature.com/lw685/springer-static/image/chp%3A10.1007%2F978-981-99-0534-8_8/MediaObjects/521606_1_En_8_Fig1_HTML.png

14.3.2 Micronutrient Considerations

The intricate relationship between micronutrients and their impact on muscle health is particularly significant in the context of geriatric populations suffering from sarcopenia and cachexia. Micronutrients, including vitamins and minerals, play essential roles in various physiological processes such as energy metabolism, muscle contraction, and repair. For instance, vitamin D is integral to muscle function and strength, with deficiencies linked to increased falls and mobility issues in older adults. Similarly, certain B vitamins, like B12 and folate, are crucial for metabolic processes and the maintenance of nerve function, which are essential to physical performance and overall quality of life in aging individuals. Understanding the specific micronutrient needs of this demographic is key for developing effective nutritional interventions that may alleviate the adverse effects of sarcopenia and cachexia, ultimately prolonging functional independence and improving the overall health outcomes for older adults facing these challenges . The complexities of micronutrient absorption and utilization in older adults further compound the risks associated with sarcopenia and cachexia. Aging often leads to physiological changes that can hinder the absorption of various nutrients; for example, decreased gastric acid production can significantly affect the bioavailability of essential vitamins such as B12, a nutrient vital for red blood cell formation and neurological function. Additionally, chronic diseases prevalent in older populations may exacerbate these absorption issues, leading to a cycle of deficiency that complicates muscle maintenance.

Moreover, those experiencing cachexia may have altered metabolic rates and increased metabolic demands, which can exacerbate existing deficiencies. Therefore, a comprehensive understanding of these interactions is essential for healthcare providers to devise tailored nutritional strategies that address both micronutrient deficiencies and the underlying conditions contributing to sarcopenia and cachexia (Institute of Medicine et al., 2010-11-29). Incorporating a diverse range of whole foods rich in micronutrients into the diets of older adults becomes paramount in combating sarcopenia and cachexia. Evidence points to the importance of dietary patterns that prioritize fruits, vegetables, lean proteins, and whole grains, as these food groups are comprehensive sources of essential vitamins and minerals. For instance, antioxidants found in fruits and vegetables may play a role in reducing inflammation, which is often heightened in chronic illness, potentially benefiting muscle preservation and function. Additionally, the inclusion of zinc and magnesium-rich foods supports muscle recovery and protein synthesis, both critical components for maintaining muscle mass. By promoting dietary diversity, practitioners can not only address immediate nutritional deficiencies but also contribute to enhanced well-being and longevity among older adults experiencing these debilitating conditions (Institute of Medicine et al., 2010-11-29)(Institute of Medicine et al., 2010-11-29).

14.3.3 Hydration and Its Importance

Hydration plays a critical yet often overlooked role in maintaining overall health, particularly among the elderly population. As individuals age, their bodys physiological mechanisms for sensing and regulating hydration become less efficient, leading to a higher risk of dehydration. This risk is exacerbated in cases of cachexia, where nutritional intake is compromised and muscle mass is significantly reduced. Proper hydration is essential for optimal muscle function and performance; it assists in the synthesis of proteins and supports the transport of nutrients throughout the body. Moreover, adequate fluid intake can mitigate some associated symptoms of sarcopenia, providing a foundation for interventions aimed at muscle maintenance and restoration. By prioritizing hydration, healthcare professionals can address a critical component in the comprehensive management of geriatric sarcopenia, ensuring patients are equipped to engage with therapeutic practices effectively. In the context of geriatric patients experiencing cachexia, hydration takes on even greater significance due to its array of physiological benefits. Dehydration can lead to a cascade of complications, including decreased physical performance, cognitive impairment, and increased morbidity and mortality. Studies have indicated that maintaining optimal hydration levels can improve muscle strength and endurance, which are particularly crucial for seniors facing muscle degeneration associated with aging and chronic illness. Furthermore, proper hydration supports gastrointestinal health, which is vital for nutrient absorption, particularly when considering the dietary restrictions and challenges that often accompany aging. The alteration of gastrointestinal function in the aging population complicates nutrient intake, necessitating strategies that encompass both hydration and nutrition to enhance overall health outcomes and improve quality of life ((Bordoni et al., 2015)). Given the multifaceted relationship between hydration, nutrition, and muscle health, it is imperative that interventions for geriatric sarcopenia incorporate a robust hydration component. Recent discussions highlight the potential of creatine supplementation, which may have synergistic effects when combined with sufficient hydration, particularly in individuals at risk of muscle loss, such as those suffering from cancer or cachexia ((Fairman et al., 2018)). Integrating hydration strategies with nutritional rehabilitation can lead to substantial improvements in functional status and longevity for older adults. Efittingly addressing hydration, alongside other components of diet and exercise, may safeguard against the debilitating consequences of sarcopenia. Ultimately, recognizing the importance of hydration not only enhances the therapeutic potential for geriatrics but also empowers both patients and caregivers to achieve better health outcomes in the face of age-related challenges.

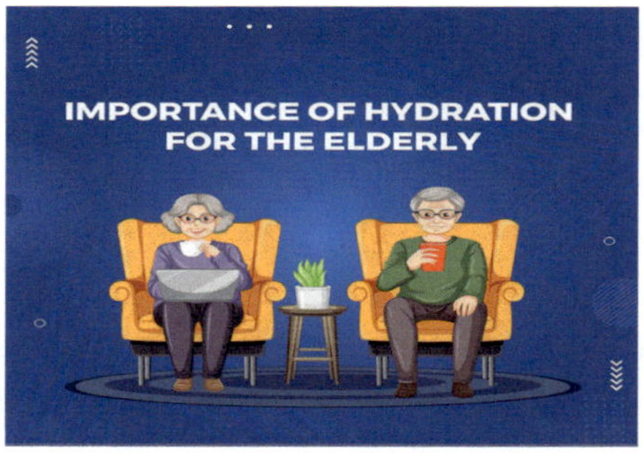

Figure 14.8. Importance Of Hydration For The Elderly.

Source: https://static.wixstatic.com/media/4e00cf_0bc333c7f71f41a6b4afc2c93e584061~mv2.jpeg/v1/fill/w_1000,h_1000,al_c,q_85,usm_0.66_1.00_0.01/4e00cf_0bc333c7f71f41a6b4afc2c93e584061~mv2.jpeg

14.4 Nutritional Interventions for Sarcopenia

Nutritional interventions play a crucial role in addressing sarcopenia, particularly in the geriatric population suffering from cachexia. As muscle mass declines with age, tailored dietary strategies become essential to counteract the effects of this condition. A high-protein diet is often recommended, as it promotes muscle protein synthesis and helps mitigate functional decline. Additionally, the inclusion of essential amino acids, particularly leucine, has been shown to enhance muscle recovery and growth. A systematic approach to meal planning that incorporates these dietary elements can significantly improve outcomes in older adults. By focusing on nutrient-dense foods and appropriate caloric intake, healthcare providers can create individualized nutrition plans that address the unique needs of patients grappling with sarcopenia and cachexia, ultimately improving their quality of life before the terminal phase of their illness. To assess the effectiveness of nutritional interventions in managing sarcopenia, it is essential to understand the interaction between dietary intake and muscle health. Recent studies have demonstrated that deficiencies in protein can exacerbate muscle loss, especially in older adults already affected by frailty and cachexia. Moreover, specific micronutrients, such as vitamin D and omega-3 fatty acids, have been identified as pivotal in muscle preservation and regeneration. These nutrients contribute not only to muscle strength but also to overall metabolic health, influencing various physiological pathways that support muscle function. Therefore, it is critical for clinicians to evaluate the nutritional status of their patients and address any deficiencies through dietary modifications or supplementation as part of a comprehensive treatment strategy for sarcopenia. In addition to dietary modifications, resistance training has been shown to synergistically enhance the benefits of nutritional interventions in combating sarcopenia. Engaging in regular physical activity, particularly strength training, can lead to significant improvements in muscle mass and strength. Studies suggest that when combined with an adequate protein intake, such exercises can help reverse the effects of sarcopenia, significantly enhancing the abilities of older adults to perform daily activities. Consequently, a multidisciplinary approach that incorporates both nutritional strategies and exercise regimens is vital for managing sarcopenia in geriatric patients facing cachexia. This dual strategy not only addresses the muscle wasting associated with sarcopenia but also improves overall functional status, ultimately contributing to a better quality of life during the later stages of life as indicated in findings linking low muscle mass with poorer survival outcomes (Jos Fé Sánchez-Torralvo et al., 2024) (Tacar SY et al., 2022).

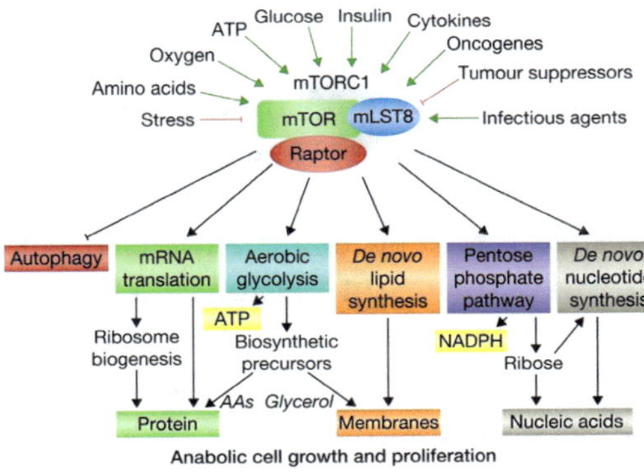

Figure 14.9. Nutrition interventions for frailty and sarcopenia.

Source: https://image.slidesharecdn.com/02nutritioninterventionsfrailtyandsarcopenia30sept15mhickson-151013054214-lva1-app6892/95/nutrition-interventions-for-frailty-and-sarcopenia-3-638.jpg?cb=1444740780

14.4.1 Protein Supplementation

Protein supplementation plays a critical role in mitigating the effects of geriatric sarcopenia and cachexia, particularly in vulnerable elderly populations. As individuals age, the natural decline in muscle mass and strength can lead to significant functional impairments and increased risk of morbidity. Protein, serving as a fundamental building block for muscle tissue, can counteract these effects by promoting muscle protein synthesis. Research suggests that adequate protein intake, particularly through supplementation, can help restore muscle mass and improve physical function in older adults experiencing sarcopenia or cachexia. The timing, quantity, and type of protein consumed are essential factors to consider, as they can influence muscle recovery and overall health outcomes. Thus, implementing a tailored protein supplementation strategy is vital to enhancing nutritional intake and mobilizing the body's adaptive responses against the muscle-wasting processes common in the aging population. The significance of protein supplementation is emphasized in contexts where patients face increased catabolic stress, such as during illness or after hospitalization. Elderly individuals recovering from acute conditions, like those resulting from SARS-CoV-2 infection, may experience exacerbated sarcopenia and malnutrition, complicating their recovery trajectories. Studies indicate that nutritional interventions, including protein supplementation, can enhance recovery rates and reduce mortality risks among hospitalized older adults. For instance, monitoring simple anthropometric measures like calf circumference can provide insights into nutritional status and correlate with outcomes such as mortality (N/A). In these scenarios, a strategic approach to protein supplementation can yield significant benefits, helping to stabilize nutritional intake and support muscle mass preservation during critical illness phases, thereby promoting better overall prognosis. Nevertheless, the implementation of protein supplementation must account for individual variations in nutritional status, comorbidities, and the patients specific rehabilitation needs. The intersection of pain management and nutritional status necessitates a holistic approach to care. Factors influencing the effectiveness of rehabilitation programs, such as pain intensity and psychosocial factors, also play a crucial role in outcomes (Abaunza U et al., 2022). Thus, healthcare providers should assess these variables meticulously to formulate individualized nutrition plans that incorporate adequate protein supplies to enhance patient resilience. By integrating protein supplementation within broader nutritional strategies tailored to enhance the elderly patient's overall health, it becomes possible to address the deleterious effects of sarcopenia and cachexia effectively, ultimately improving quality of life and longevity for this vulnerable population.

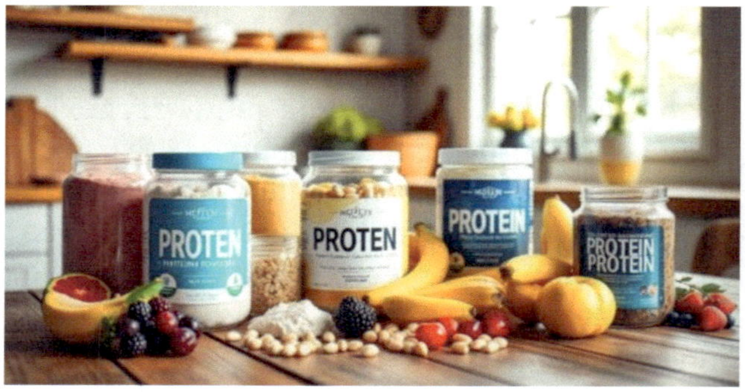

Figure 14.10. Protein supplements.

Source: https://comfortalife.com/wp-content/uploads/2025/02/protein_supplements_for_seniors-560x300.jpg

14.4.2 Role of Omega-3 Fatty Acids

The role of omega-3 fatty acids in nutrition is increasingly recognized, particularly concerning geriatric sarcopenia and cachexia. Omega-3 fatty acids are essential fats that possess anti-inflammatory properties, which can significantly benefit elderly individuals suffering from muscle wasting conditions. In the context of cachexia, characterized by considerable weight loss, muscle atrophy, and decreased appetite, these fatty acids may offer therapeutic advantages by modulating inflammatory cytokines and promoting muscle protein synthesis. Clinical studies have shown that omega-3 supplementation can enhance overall energy intake and improve muscle mass, thereby potentially mitigating some adverse outcomes associated with sarcopenia, such as increased mortality and decreased quality of life (N/A). Thus, incorporating omega-3 fatty acids into the diet of elderly individuals presents a promising strategy to combat the dual burden of sarcopenia and malnutrition. Moreover, the efficacy of omega-3 fatty acids extends to their synergistic effects with other nutritional interventions. For instance, combining omega-3 supplementation with adequate protein intake can lead to more significant improvements in muscle strength and mass. Recent research indicates that elderly patients who participate in structured nutritional programs, including omega-3 fatty acids and sufficient protein, demonstrate increased handgrip strength and improved physical performance (Cervera Díaz et al., 2023). These findings suggest that omega-3s play a crucial role not only in enhancing nutritional status but also in fostering physical resilience among the elderly, which is vital for maintaining mobility and independence. Addressing the nutritional needs of this population, particularly in the context of cachexia, underscores the importance of incorporating omega-3 fatty acids as a potential key component in comprehensive care strategies for geriatric patients. In addition to their nutritional value, omega-3 fatty acids have implications for improving the overall health trajectory of aging individuals. The accumulation of evidence suggests that these fatty acids may help reduce the risk of chronic diseases commonly seen in older adults, such as cardiovascular disease and arthritis, which can compound the effects of sarcopenia. By minimizing inflammation and promoting cardiovascular health, omega-3s may help to sustain an active lifestyle longer, thus allowing seniors to maintain muscle function and prevent further declines associated with sarcopenia. Therefore, the integration of omega-3 fatty acids into dietary approaches for older adults dealing with sarcopenia and cachexia is not merely about addressing immediate nutritional deficiencies. It is about enhancing long-term wellness and functional capacity as these individuals navigate the complexities of aging (N/A).

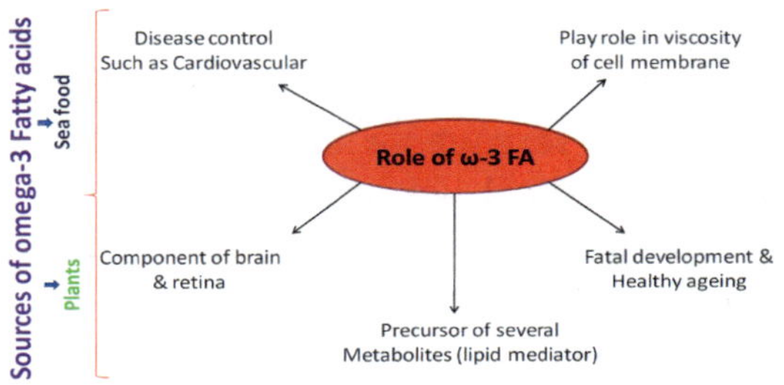

Figure 14.11. Role of omega-3 fatty acids.

Source: https://www.researchgate.net/profile/Avinash-Marwal/publication/330586281/figure/fig1/AS:722114072031232@1549176819586/Role-of-omega-3-fatty-acids.png

14.4.3 Importance of Vitamin D

In the context of geriatric care, the significance of Vitamin D transcends mere nutritional value, positioning itself as a paramount factor influencing muscle health and functional ability among older adults. This fat-soluble vitamin plays a critical role in calcium absorption, which is essential for maintaining muscle function and bone health.

A deficiency in Vitamin D is linked to various adverse outcomes in the elderly, including increased risk of falls, fractures, and sarcopenia. Studies have indicated that adequate levels of Vitamin D may enhance muscle strength and prevent deteriorative conditions often associated with aging, reinforcing the idea that nutritional interventions that include Vitamin D supplementation could serve as a preventive strategy against sarcopenia in older populations, particularly among those experiencing cachexia before exitus (N/A). Research has established a connection between Vitamin D levels and sarcopenia, highlighting the importance of this nutrient in managing and potentially reversing muscle loss in the elderly. The prevalence of sarcopenia and malnutrition in older adults necessitates a comprehensive approach that integrates dietary assessment and specialized interventions. Vitamin D, through its regulatory effects on muscle protein synthesis and function, plays a crucial role in the prevention of sarcopenia and the enhancement of overall physical performance. For instance, the Comprehensive Geriatric Assessment (CGA) has shown that older patients exhibiting low levels of Vitamin D are more susceptible to frailty and muscle weakness, suggesting a direct correlation between Vitamin D deficiency and the progression of sarcopenia (Cervera Díaz et al., 2023).

Furthermore, the implementation of nutritional strategies that include Vitamin D supplementation could significantly improve outcomes for elderly individuals facing cachexia. Evidence suggests that addressing malnutrition and deficiencies is imperative for optimizing muscle health and reducing mortality risk associated with geriatric syndromes. Specifically, older patients suffering from fragile fractures and experiencing sarcopenia are often found to have inadequate Vitamin D levels, thus reinforcing the necessity for routine screening and supplementation protocols. By prioritizing Vitamin D intake within nutritional plans, healthcare providers can better support muscle preservation and mobility in the geriatric population, consequently mitigating the impacts of cachexia and ensuring improved health trajectories as they approach end-of-life care (N/A).

14.5 The Relationship Between Cachexia and Sarcopenia

The intricate relationship between cachexia and sarcopenia is crucial in understanding the nutritional and physiological challenges faced by the geriatric population. Cachexia, characterized by severe weight loss, muscle wasting, and metabolic dysfunction, often coexists with chronic illnesses, significantly impacting the quality of life in older adults. Conversely, sarcopenia is defined as the age-related decline in skeletal muscle mass and strength, which can exacerbate the effects of cachexia. The shared mechanisms underlying both conditions include inflammation, hormonal changes, and alterations in protein metabolism, leading to a compounded risk of disability and mortality in elderly patients. As geriatric individuals may already be predisposed to sarcopenia due to age-associated physiological changes, the presence of cachexia can quickly accelerate muscle loss, necessitating novel therapeutic approaches aimed at preserving muscle mass and enhancing nutritional intake in this vulnerable demographic . Nutritional interventions play a pivotal role in addressing the dual challenges presented by cachexia and sarcopenia. Adequate dietary intake, particularly proteins, is essential for muscle preservation and recovery. Yet, the metabolic imbalances inherent in cachexia often lead to decreased appetite and nutrient absorption, complicating dietary management strategies. Supplements such as branched-chain amino acids (BCAAs) and omega-3 fatty acids have demonstrated potential benefits in stimulating muscle protein synthesis and reducing inflammation, thus serving as adjuncts to conventional dietary approaches. Furthermore, personalized nutrition plans that consider individual preferences, nutritional status, and disease progression can significantly improve adherence and outcomes. Importantly, a multidisciplinary approach, encompassing dietitians, physicians, and exercise specialists, can yield comprehensive management strategies targeting muscle depletion while addressing the underlying causes of cachexia (Crucitti A, 2018-05-08). Understanding the interplay between cachexia and sarcopenia emphasizes the necessity for early diagnosis and intervention in geriatric care. With the aging population increasingly affected by chronic illnesses alongside these muscle-wasting syndromes, healthcare professionals must prioritize screening and risk assessment in older adults. Enhanced awareness and education surrounding the signs and symptoms of both conditions are vital for timely intervention.

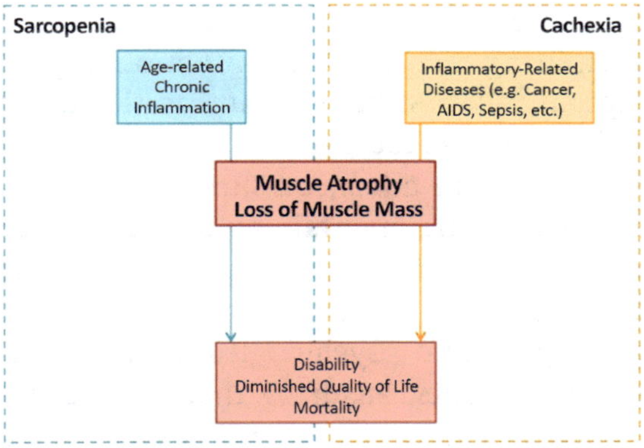

Figure 14.12. Relationship between Cachexia and Sarcopenia.

Source: https://external-content.duckduckgo.com/iu/?u=https%3A%2F%2Fwww.researchgate.net%2Fprofile%2FSergio_Marco%2Fpublication%2F51562514%2Ffigure%2Ffig1%2FAS%3A216422744629248%401428610611317%2FSarcopenia-and-cachexia-represent-two-distinct-diseased-states-though-both-can-result.png&f=1&nofb=1&ipt=56399fde40471792a958294bfff80916712062f5062d9293606c4c6605b1b7e6

Moreover, public health initiatives that advocate for nutritional education and accessible resources can further empower seniors and caregivers to combat these challenges. Ultimately, addressing the relationship between cachexia and sarcopenia within a geriatric population signifies a critical advancement in improving health outcomes and prolonging quality of life, particularly as individuals approach end-of-life care (Crucitti A, 2018-05-08)(Crucitti A, 2018-05-08).

14.5.1 Pathophysiological Links

The emergence of sarcopenia in geriatric populations is closely linked to the pathophysiological processes underlying cachexia, particularly as both conditions manifest through progressive muscle loss. Sarcopenia refers specifically to the age-related decline in skeletal muscle mass and function, while cachexia is characterized by unintentional weight loss and systemic inflammation, often exacerbated by other diseases. This nuanced distinction is vital for understanding treatment implications; sarcopenia can exist independently, but when combined with cachexia, it leads to significantly worsened functional outcomes and diminished quality of life. As skeletal muscle is critical for mobility and overall health, interventions aimed at preserving or enhancing muscle mass in older adults can directly impact their resilience against cachexia-related complications, ultimately leading to improved clinical outcomes. Furthermore, the intersection of nutrition and pathophysiological alterations plays a crucial role in managing sarcopenia and cachexia in elderly patients. Inadequate nutritional intake can trigger a cascade of metabolic changes that exacerbate muscle loss. Investigating parameters such as body composition via bioelectrical impedance analysis has unveiled significant relationships between fat mass and muscle deterioration. For instance, individuals diagnosed with sarcopenic obesity demonstrate how increased adiposity correlates with muscle mass decline, illustrating the complexities inherent in managing these syndromes. This correlation underscores the necessity for thorough nutritional evaluations to inform dietary strategies tailored for individuals at risk of both conditions, thereby promoting muscle protein synthesis, which is essential in counteracting the deleterious effects of aging and disease progression on physical function (T Moga et al., 2022). In addition to nutritional interventions, understanding the frailty syndrome is essential, especially when considering surgical and critically ill geriatric patients. Frailty, often characterized by a reduction in physiological reserve and increased vulnerability to stressors, is intrinsically linked to both sarcopenia and cachexia. The frailty index serves as a dynamic tool to assess the multifaceted risks associated with surgical procedures, allowing for tailored preoperative nutritional management aimed at stimulating muscle protein synthesis. Such interventions can mitigate postoperative complications, thereby enhancing recovery and survival rates among elderly surgical patients. Ultimately, a multifactorial approach that addresses the pathophysiological links governing sarcopenia and cachexia, alongside effective nutritional strategies, is vital for optimizing health outcomes within this vulnerable population (Y Sakurai, 2020).

14.5.2 Clinical Implications

The clinical implications of geriatric sarcopenia and cachexia are critical in shaping patient management strategies for older adults approaching the end of life. Sarcopenia, characterized by a decrease in skeletal muscle mass and strength, can significantly exacerbate the functional decline seen in aging individuals. The condition often coexists with cachexia, a syndrome defined by muscle wasting related to underlying illnesses, such as cancer and chronic obstructive pulmonary disease (COPD). Identifying sarcopenia in patients with cachexia can be challenging due to the limitations inherent in traditional diagnostic tools. Therefore, employing more accessible and practical assessments, such as the SARC-F questionnaire and bioelectrical impedance analysis, is essential in this clinical context. These methods allow for a more comprehensive evaluation of patients nutritional status and physical function, ultimately influencing therapeutic decisions and quality of life as patients navigate palliative care (S Go et al., 2025). Nutritional intervention plays a pivotal role in managing both sarcopenia and cachexia, aiming to mitigate muscle loss and enhance patients overall well-being. Tailoring nutritional support to the individual patients prognosis and needs is essential, especially as aggressive interventions are typically avoided during end-of-life care. Intervening with adequate caloric intake, protein supplementation, and micronutrient enrichment can help counteract the progression of sarcopenia and cachexia, contributing to improved functionality and symptom relief. Although the traditional focus has been on muscle mass restoration, the primary goal in advanced illness is symptom management and maintaining quality of life (D Floriano et al., 2017). This approach emphasizes the importance of understanding both the physiological and psychological dimensions of geriatric patients, ensuring that interventions are not only clinically effective but also aligned with their personal preferences and values. Lastly, a multidisciplinary approach is critical in addressing the clinical implications of sarcopenia and cachexia among older adults. Collaborative efforts among healthcare providers, including nutritionists, physical therapists, and palliative care specialists, facilitate comprehensive management plans that target the multifaceted nature of these conditions. Continuous evaluation and monitoring of body composition, functional performance, and nutritional status are necessary to make timely adjustments to care plans. Research highlights the heightened risk of disability and comorbidities in aging populations, which underscores the urgency to refine diagnostic and therapeutic strategies. As the prevalence of sarcopenia and cachexia continues to rise, particularly among patients with terminal illnesses, a concerted effort in clinical practice will be vital in enhancing patient outcomes and ensuring dignity in care before exitus (S Go et al., 2025).

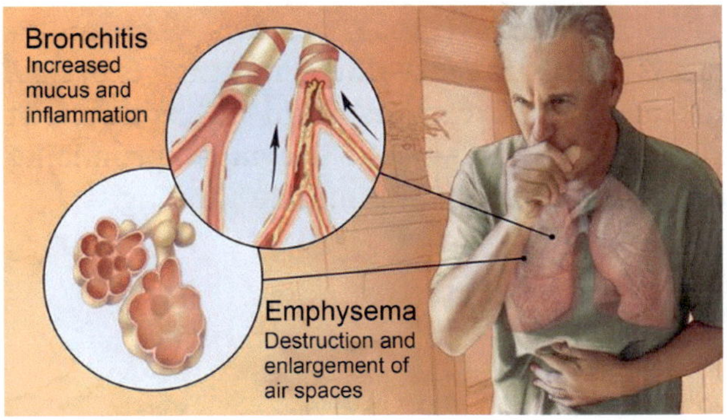

Figure 14.13. Chronic Obstructive Pulmonary Disease (COPD).

Source: https://www.airphysio.com/wp-content/uploads/2015/12/COPD.jpg

14.5.3 Management Strategies

Effective management strategies for geriatric sarcopenia, particularly in the context of cachexia, require a multifaceted approach incorporating nutrition, physical intervention, and monitoring of patient health. Nutrition plays a pivotal role in addressing the anabolic resistance characteristic of muscle wasting conditions in elderly patients. Evidence shows that older adults often exhibit inadequate nutrient intake, exacerbating their compromised nutritional state, especially following events such as hip fractures (Malafarina et al., 2017). The implementation of tailored nutritional interventions can lead to significant improvements in muscle mass and functional recovery. This strategy emphasizes not only increasing caloric intake but also enhancing the quality of nutrients, such as protein, to facilitate muscle synthesis. Identifying individuals at risk for malnutrition through assessments can further guide intervention strategies, ensuring that nutritional support aligns with patient needs during recovery phases and beyond. In addition to nutritional management, incorporating strength and resistance training is crucial in addressing sarcopenia in elderly patients. Physical interventions help rebuild muscle strength and functional independence, which are often diminished due to aging and prolonged inactivity. The synergy between nutrition and regular physical activity amplifies the benefits of both interventions, leading to enhanced muscle mass and better health outcomes. Studies suggest that engaging in targeted resistance training can stimulate muscle hypertrophy and improve metabolic health, contributing to an overall reduction in complications associated with sarcopenia and cachexia (Bover J et al., 2017). Moreover, a structured exercise regimen paired with proper nutritional counsel creates a holistic management plan that promotes optimal mobility and quality of life in geriatric patients, which is particularly critical in the context of chronic illnesses that may accelerate muscle degradation.

Monitoring the effectiveness of these management strategies through regular assessments is essential to ensure that interventions are meeting their intended goals. Clinicians should utilize comprehensive assessments, focusing on dietary intake and physical performance metrics to adjust nutritional and exercise regimens as needed. Additionally, monitoring bone health through vitamin D levels can furnish valuable insight, as deficiencies in this nutrient directly correlate with muscle and bone integrity (Bover J et al., 2017). By establishing a continuous feedback loop, healthcare professionals can identify potential setbacks and tailor interventions accordingly. Such proactive management not only addresses immediate concerns of sarcopenia and cachexia but also fosters a long-term strategy aimed at enhancing the resilience and overall health of geriatric patients facing the challenges associated with frailty and muscle wasting conditions.

14.6 Case Studies and Clinical Evidence

In exploring the interface between geriatric sarcopenia and nutritional interventions, case studies provide crucial clinical evidence highlighting the multidimensional aspects of muscle loss in older adults. For instance, longitudinal studies have reported significant correlations between declining muscle mass and factors such as inadequate protein intake and vitamin deficiencies, particularly in the context of cachexia—a metabolic syndrome often observed in chronic diseases. Such findings underscore the rationale proposed by the European Working Group on Sarcopenia in Older People (EWGSOP), which emphasizes an operational definition of sarcopenia involving low muscle mass coupled with diminished muscle function. This stratification implies that clinical assessments must consider not only muscle size but also the physiological capacity of elderly patients, thereby informing tailored nutritional strategies to mitigate sarcopenias progression (Baeyens et al., 2017). Moreover, clinical evidence illustrates the importance of targeted nutritional interventions for older adults experiencing cachexia. In various case studies, the administration of vitamin D, alongside other essential nutrients, has demonstrated potential benefits in improving muscle health and overall physical performance. Vitamin Ds role extends beyond calcium regulation—it appears to influence muscle metabolism directly by engaging the vitamin D receptor in skeletal muscle tissue. Observations in older adults indicate that increased levels of circulating 25-hydroxyvitamin D are associated with enhanced muscle morphology and functionality (Bover J et al., 2017). These findings suggest a critical need for healthcare providers to evaluate and potentially supplement vitamin D and other nutrients as part of a comprehensive approach to manage geriatric sarcopenia and its related conditions effectively. As the body of case studies continues to grow, it becomes increasingly evident that interventions aimed at addressing sarcopenia and cachexia must consider the complex interplay of nutritional factors and physiological responses. Analysis of these case studies reveals a pattern where multifaceted approaches—incorporating exercise, dietary modifications, and micronutrient supplementation—yield the most promising outcomes in mitigating muscle wasting.

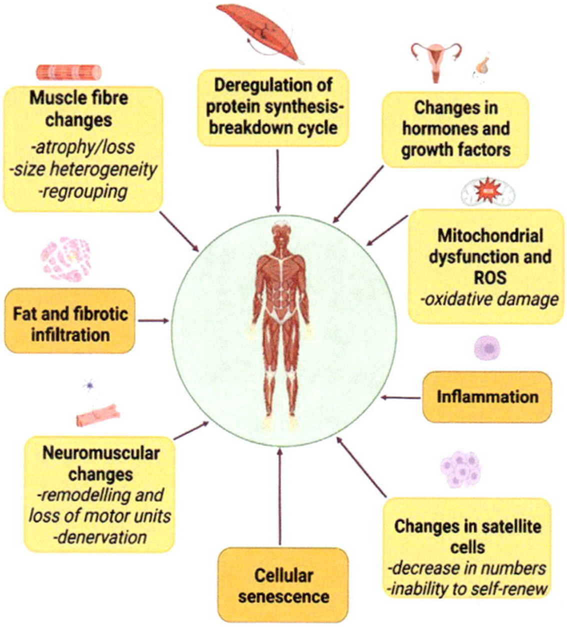

Figure 14.14. The role of nutrition in the prevention of sarcopenia.

Source: https://ajcn.nutrition.org/cms/10.1016/j.ajcnut.2023.08.015/asset/e1d6a280-aec8-43c4-889d-86e624d08195/main.assets/gr1_lrg.jpg

The integration of objective measurement tools outlined by the EWGSOP, which includes assessments of gait speed and grip strength, facilitates a systematic approach to identifying at-risk populations. Ultimately, refining our understanding of the interrelationship between nutrition and skeletal muscle health in geriatric patients will enhance clinical practices, leading to better outcomes for individuals facing the dual challenges of sarcopenia and cachexia before exitus (Baeyens et al., 2017).

14.6.1 Review of Relevant Research

The intersection of geriatric sarcopenia and nutritional deficiencies highlights a pressing issue in the health management of older adults. The European Working Group on Sarcopenia in Older People (EWGSOP) has established comprehensive criteria for diagnosing sarcopenia, emphasizing the coexistence of low muscle mass and low muscle function as critical indicators. This consensus approach aids clinicians in identifying at-risk populations, particularly those experiencing cachexia, a syndrome characterized by significant weight loss and muscle wasting. The identification of sarcopenia stages—presarcopenia, sarcopenia, and severe sarcopenia—enables targeted interventions tailored to the degree of muscular decline, which is essential for improving health outcomes. Incorporating these definitions into geriatric assessments provides a structured avenue for addressing both sarcopenia and the therapeutic implications of nutritional support, setting the stage for more effective management in older individuals facing multiple health challenges (Baeyens et al., 2017). Research underscores the prevalence and impact of malnutrition among geriatric patients, particularly those with conditions such as hip fractures, which can exacerbate the decline into sarcopenia and cachexia. A review that analyzed 44 studies indicated an alarming malnutrition rate of 18.7% among older individuals, with figures rising to 45.7% when additional criteria were considered. Such malnutrition frequently leads to poorer health outcomes, including increased hospital complications and reduced functional recovery, ultimately either preventing recovery or compromising survival rates. Not surprisingly, the findings revealed high one-year mortality rates, emphasizing the urgency of integrating nutritional interventions in clinical practice. The evidence suggests that timely nutritional assessments and tailored interventions can significantly enhance recovery processes, illustrating the need for a holistic treatment approach that encompasses both nutritional status and muscle health in geriatric populations (Malafarina et al., 2017). The implication of these findings is multifaceted, demonstrating that addressing nutritional deficiencies can be a cornerstone in combating geriatric sarcopenia and cachexia. As the aging population continues to grow, the operationalization of the diagnostic criteria for sarcopenia, as proposed by EWGSOP, should be prioritized within geriatric care frameworks. This strategy should be complemented by evidence-based nutritional interventions aimed at improving dietary intake and muscle health. Incorporating strategies such as protein supplementation and tailored nutrition plans based on individual needs can facilitate better muscular health and mitigate the risks associated with sarcopenia. Ultimately, a concerted focus on managing malnutrition and sarcopenia as intertwined facets of geriatric care will not only improve quality of life but also enhance survival rates among the aging population, aligning closely with contemporary healthcare objectives (Baeyens et al., 2017) (Malafarina et al., 2017).

14.6.2 Analysis of Treatment Outcomes

The analysis of treatment outcomes for geriatric sarcopenia, particularly in the context of cachexia, necessitates a multifaceted approach that includes both nutritional intervention and physical activity. As individuals age, the loss of muscle mass and strength, known as sarcopenia, often intersects with conditions such as cachexia, characterized by severe weight loss and muscle wasting. The European Working Group on Sarcopenia in Older People (EWGSOP) provides a foundation for understanding this intersection, indicating that effective treatments must address both low muscle mass and diminished muscle function to achieve meaningful outcomes in older patients. Evaluating the results of various therapeutic interventions, including resistance training and protein supplementation, is critical for establishing a comprehensive treatment protocol that targets the unique needs of the geriatric population suffering from these conditions. Interactions between cachexia and anorexia of aging further complicate treatment outcomes, as they contribute to reduced appetite and energy intake in elderly patients. Recent systematic reviews, including meta-analyses of interventions for anorexia of aging, suggest that targeted nutritional strategies can significantly improve outcomes like body weight and energy intake in affected individuals. The studies reviewed showed an average increase of 1.59 kg in body weight and a notable uplift in caloric intake, underscoring the importance of adapting treatment approaches to the specific manifestations of anorexia of aging. Such findings highlight the necessity of not only addressing nutritional deficiencies but also promoting an overall increase in dietary engagement to counteract the deleterious impacts of cachexia and sarcopenia, facilitating a holistic recovery strategy for older adults. In assessing treatment outcomes, it is also crucial to analyze the broader implications of sarcopenia and cachexia on quality of life and overall health in elderly patients. Evidence indicates that decreases in muscle mass significantly correlate with increased frailty, functional decline, and heightened mortality risk. By utilizing the diagnostic criteria set forth by EWGSOP, healthcare providers can better identify patients at risk and implement prevention strategies that focus on nutritional intake and physical activity. Effective management of sarcopenia and its associated conditions can lead to improved functional capacities and enhanced quality of life. Furthermore, understanding the unique pathways linking these conditions not only aids in crafting more effective interventions but also aligns therapeutic goals with the general aim of maintaining independence and dignity in aging populations impacted by these debilitating health issues.

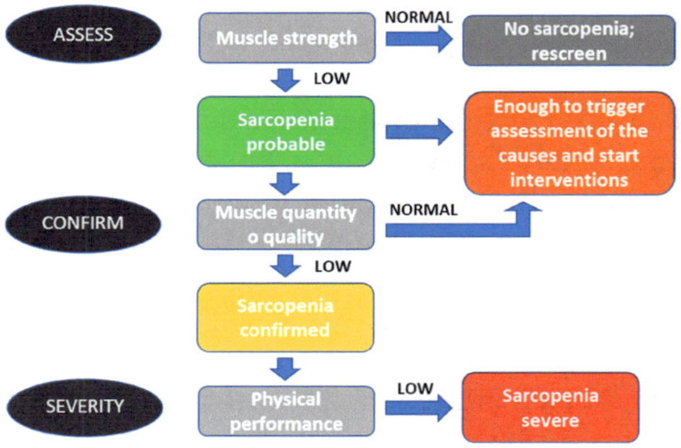

Figure 14.15. Sarcopenia Diagnosis and Management in Hematological Malignancies and Differences with Cachexia and Frailty.

Source: https://pub.mdpi-res.com/cancers/cancers-15-04600/article_deploy/html/images/cancers-15-04600-g001.png?1694868717

14.6.3 Lessons Learned from Clinical Practice

Clinical practice provides essential insights into the multifaceted nature of geriatric sarcopenia, particularly in the context of cachexia. One notable lesson stems from the nutritional challenges faced by older adults with chronic conditions such as chronic kidney disease (CKD). The intersection of geriatric nutrition guidelines and nephrology recommendations highlights the need for tailored dietary approaches that both combat malnutrition and slow CKD progression. Increased life expectancy and the prevalence of sarcopenia necessitate innovative strategies in nutritional assessments and interventions. (Avesani C M et al., 2023) underscores the complexity of protein intake recommendations in this demographic, illustrating the delicate balance between enhancing nutritional status and managing renal health. Consequently, employing interdisciplinary strategies that incorporate dietary preferences and individual risk assessments is paramount in developing effective nutritional interventions for older patients experiencing cachexia. The recruitment and management of participants with sarcopenia in clinical trials further reflect the lessons learned from practice. Notably, the shift from hospital-based to primary care recruitment has shown promising results in enhancing participatory rates for those with sarcopenia. This transition allowed for better identification and management of patients who might otherwise go untreated, facilitating more comprehensive care pathways. Evidence from studies indicates that localized telephone pre-screening, as opposed to centralized methods, improves conversion rates to trial participation. This practical insight emphasizes the necessity of adapting recruitment strategies to the clinical setting, ensuring that interventions are effectively deployed and that participants needs are foregrounded in the clinical trial process. The findings from (Achison et al., 2021) demonstrate that optimizing engagement with the population can foster better research outcomes, informing rehabilitation frameworks for sarcopenia. Understanding the nuances of muscle mass estimation is another critical lesson learned from clinical practice. The use of bioimpedance analysis, while prevalent in estimating muscle mass, can yield systematically biased results, necessitating recalibration for accuracy. This key insight sheds light on the importance of employing precise measurement techniques when screening for sarcopenia, especially in geriatric patients exhibiting signs of cachexia. The emergence of refined equations for estimating lean mass, coupled with comprehensive assessments of physical function, ensures a more stable and reliable approach to identifying at-risk individuals. (Achison et al., 2021) accentuates how improving bioimpedance techniques correlates with more effective screening processes, ultimately guiding clinical decisions in nutritional therapy and rehabilitation. Thus, by integrating precise measurement methodologies into clinical practice, healthcare providers can deliver better-targeted interventions and improve outcomes for elderly patients facing the challenges of sarcopenia and cachexia.

SUMMARY

Addressing geriatric sarcopenia and nutrition is imperative in managing older adults experiencing cachexia. The considerable alterations in body composition and functionality highlighted in recent studies emphasize the connection between malnutrition and sarcopenia, particularly in this vulnerable population. Findings indicate that many elderly individuals experience a decline in skeletal muscle mass, which exacerbates their physical disability risks, particularly as demonstrated in the gender-specific disparities observed over a three-year span. Consequently, early and targeted interventions are crucial to counteract these effects and enhance the quality of life for older adults afflicted with cachexia. This approach must encompass both physical rehabilitation and nutritional strategies to foster muscle retention and overall health among this demographic. The challenges posed by aging, particularly in the context of gastrointestinal changes, further complicate the path to optimal nutrition for older adults. As the aging gastrointestinal tract (GIT) undergoes mechanical and functional changes, the absorption and digestion of essential nutrients become increasingly impaired. This ultimately contributes to malnutrition, which further aggravates the issues associated with geriatric sarcopenia. A comprehensive understanding of these physiological changes is essential for developing effective dietary guidelines and nutritional interventions that cater specifically to the elderly population's needs. By recognizing the interplay between aging, malnutrition, and sarcopenia, health practitioners can formulate more effective strategies aimed at enhancing nutritional intake and mitigating the decline in muscle mass and, consequently, functional capability in older adults affected by cachexia. Moreover, it is vital to continue research in this area to establish standardized interventions that prioritize the nutritional needs of the elderly. Future studies should focus on identifying biomarkers that can signal nutrient deficiencies and the onset of sarcopenia, allowing for timely interventions. Additionally, exploring tailored dietary solutions that improve nutrient bioavailability while accommodating the reduced functionality of the aging GIT will be paramount. As the prevalence of geriatric sarcopenia and malnutrition continues to rise globally, collaborative efforts involving nutritionists, geriatricians, and caregivers are essential to implement holistic care strategies. Ultimately, improving the nutritional status of older adults will not only combat sarcopenia but also significantly diminish the risk of comorbidities, enhancing the overall health and well-being of this population before exitus occurs.

In the study of geriatric sarcopenia, particularly in the context of cachexia before exitus, key points emerge regarding the relationship between muscle mass and overall health outcomes in elderly patients. Sarcopenia, characterized by the loss of skeletal muscle mass and function, poses significant risks for older adults, especially those facing critical conditions such as hip fractures. Evidence illustrates that a low phase angle, as assessed through bioelectrical impedance analysis, significantly correlates with mortality rates in this demographic. Specifically, patients with a low phase angle exhibit markedly higher mortality rates at intervals of one to twelve months post-surgery, underscoring the need for early identification and intervention in those with diminished muscle integrity (Jos Fé Sánchez-Torralvo et al., 2024). Such findings emphasize the importance of nutritional support and rehabilitation strategies to mitigate the adverse effects associated with sarcopenia, especially in frail elderly patients. Furthermore, understanding the implications of low muscle mass extends beyond immediate post-operative concerns, particularly in the context of cancer-related cachexia. Recent studies focusing on metastatic renal cell carcinoma indicate that low muscle mass is associated with poorer clinical outcomes, including reduced overall survival and progression-free survival among patients undergoing treatment with nivolumab. This suggests that the maintenance of muscle mass could be vital not only for recovery from acute events like fractures but also in chronic conditions involving advanced malignancies (Tacar SY et al., 2022). The insights garnered from these findings highlight the need for tailored nutritional approaches designed to preserve lean body mass and enhance physical resilience in older patients, ensuring their quality of life remains a primary goal in geriatric healthcare. Lastly, the interplay between nutrition, muscle mass, and health outcomes in older adults serves to delineate the critical role of multidisciplinary intervention strategies in addressing sarcopenia. A comprehensive approach that incorporates nutritional assessment and intervention is essential for mitigating the risks associated with inadequate muscle mass, particularly in frail elderly populations confronting serious health challenges. By integrating dietary modifications, physical activity, and possibly therapeutic supplementation, healthcare providers can potentially improve muscle function and overall prognosis in at-risk populations (Jos Fé Sánchez-Torralvo et al., 2024)(Tacar SY et al., 2022). Consequently, acknowledging and addressing the nutritional needs of geriatric patients is not merely an ancillary consideration; it is a foundational component of effective patient management strategies aimed at countering the detrimental effects of sarcopenia and cachexia leading to exitus.

CLOSER LOOK

ROLE OF NUTRITION IN THE PREVENTION OF GERIATRIC SARCOPENIA

Nutrition plays a critical role in the prevention and management of geriatric sarcopenia, a condition characterized by progressive loss of skeletal muscle mass, strength, and function that commonly occurs with aging. Adequate nutritional intake supports muscle metabolism and preserves muscle tissue, thus mitigating the onset or severity of sarcopenia. Protein intake is particularly important, as dietary protein provides essential amino acids necessary for muscle protein synthesis. Older adults often require higher protein intake than younger individuals, with current recommendations suggesting at least 1.0–1.2 grams of protein per kilogram of body weight per day, distributed evenly across meals. Additionally, nutrients such as vitamin D, omega-3 fatty acids, and antioxidants like vitamin C and E contribute to muscle health by modulating inflammation, enhancing calcium absorption, and supporting mitochondrial function. Vitamin D deficiency, common in the elderly, is associated with impaired muscle strength and increased risk of falls, making supplementation essential in deficient individuals.

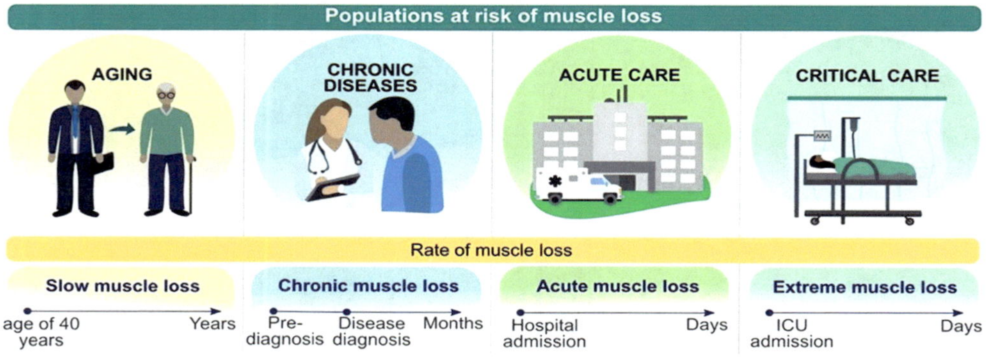

Figure 14.16. The role of nutrition in prevention and management of frailty.

Source: https://pavilionhealthtoday.com/wp-content/uploads/2023/11/Frality-2.jpg

Moreover, the timing and quality of nutrients—such as leucine-rich proteins from dairy or legumes—play a role in stimulating muscle synthesis more effectively. Malnutrition or inadequate caloric intake accelerates muscle loss, especially during illness or periods of physical inactivity. Hence, preventing undernutrition through balanced, nutrient-rich diets is crucial. Combining nutrition with resistance training further amplifies its benefits by stimulating muscle anabolism and improving functional outcomes. Screening tools like the Mini Nutritional Assessment (MNA) help identify those at nutritional risk early, allowing for prompt intervention. In summary, nutrition serves as both a preventive and therapeutic strategy in combating sarcopenia in the elderly. By ensuring adequate intake of protein, essential micronutrients, and total calories, and integrating dietary strategies with physical activity, older adults can maintain muscle health, physical independence, and overall quality of life.

REFERENCES

1. Achison, Marcus, Aspray, Terry J., Avenell, Alison, Band, et al. (2021) Recruitment strategies for sarcopenia trials – lessons from the LACE randomised controlled trial. doi: https://core.ac.uk/download/437567413.pdf
2. Antonio Crucitti (2018-05-08) Surgical Management of Elderly Patients. Springer. doi: https://play.google.com/store/books/details?id=qk5aDwAAQBAJ&source=gbs_api
3. Avesani C. M., Bakker S. J. L., Barazzoni R., Bellizzi V., Carrero J. J., Cederholm T., Cuerda C., et al. (2023) Nutritional status and the risk of malnutrition in older adults with chronic kidney disease – implications for low protein intake and nutritional care: A critical review endorsed by ERN-ERA and ESPEN. doi: https://core.ac.uk/download/614215078.pdf
4. Baeyens, Jean Pierre, Bauer, Jürgen M., Boirie, Yves, Cederholm, et al. (2017) Sarcopenia: European consensus on definition and diagnosis: Report of the European Working Group on Sarcopenia in Older People. doi: https://core.ac.uk/download/85210827.pdf
5. Bordoni, Alessandra, Dupont, Didier, Gille, Doreen, Kachal, et al. (2015) Understanding the gastrointestinal tract of the elderly to develop dietary solutions that prevent malnutrition. doi: https://core.ac.uk/download/286575279.pdf
6. Burton, Louise A., Sumukadas, Deepa (2010) Optimal management of sarcopenia. doi: https://core.ac.uk/download/20453974.pdf
7. Carrasco-Campos, Joaquín, García-Olivares, María, Gonzalo-Marín, Montserrat, González-Poveda, et al. (2022) Poor Physical Performance Is Associated with Postoperative Complications and Mortality in Preoperative Patients with Colorectal Cancer. doi: https://core.ac.uk/download/533907002.pdf
8. Cervera Díaz, Maria Carmen (2023) Estudio de sarcopenia en pacientes mayores de 74 años con fractura de la extremidad proximal del fémur.. doi: https://core.ac.uk/download/570983825.pdf
9. Chia-Ter Chao, Csaba P. Kovesdy, R. A. Merchant (2025) Sarcopenia, sarcopenic obesity, and frailty in individuals with chronic kidney disease: a comprehensive review.. Kidney research and clinical practice. doi: https://www.semanticscholar.org/paper/2cced26845d113ebc47b1770ce9802f9027345b2
10. D. Floriano, B. Cruz, Laís, Rosa Viana, C. Salgado, R.D Santos, L. Ramos, et al. (2017) Abstracts of the 10th International Conference on Cachexia, Sarcopenia and Muscle Wasting, Rome, Italy, 8–10 December 2017 (Part 1). Volume(8), 999 - 1080. Journal of Cachexia, Sarcopenia and Muscle. doi: https://www.semanticscholar.org/paper/4a164a1b27dea3098fe5db8531433a0421df88f7
11. Donini LM, Lenzi A, Perna S, Poggiogalle E., Rondanelli M, Spadaccini D (2018) Are the therapeutic strategies in anorexia of ageing effective on nutritional status? A systematic review with meta-analysis. doi: https://core.ac.uk/download/188830393.pdf
12. Fairman, C M, Galvao, D A, Hart, Nicolas H, Kendall, et al. (2018) The potential therapeutic effects of creatine supplementation on body composition and muscle function in cancer. doi: https://core.ac.uk/download/213607833.pdf
13. Fernandes, Beatriz, Galán-Mercant, Alejandro, Tomás, Maria Teresa (2017) Body composition changes over three years in older adults: a descriptive longitudinal analysis. doi: https://core.ac.uk/download/143415359.pdf

14. Francisco José Sánchez-Torralvo, Verónica Pérez-del-Río, Luis Ignacio Navas Vela, María García-Olivares, Nuria Porras, Jose Abuín Fernández, Manuel Francisco Bravo Bardají, et al. (2024) Phase Angle as a Predictor of Mortality in Older Patients with Hip Fracture. Volume(Vol 16), 2221. Nutrients. doi: https://doi.org/10.3390/nu16142221

15. G. Jensen, T. Cederholm (2024) Exploring the intersections of frailty, sarcopenia, and cachexia with malnutrition.. Nutrition in clinical practice : official publication of the American Society for Parenteral and Enteral Nutrition. doi: https://www.semanticscholar.org/paper/d4f2963f2044eb723c9b8bcaece9895ab526b7e7

16. Institute of Medicine, Food and Nutrition Board, Food Forum (2010-11-29) Providing Healthy and Safe Foods As We Age. National Academies Press. doi: http://books.google.com/books?id=HopeAgAAQBAJ&dq=Geriatric+sarcopenia+nutrition+macronutrient+needs+cachexia+exitus&hl=&source=gbs_api

17. Isabel Rodríguez-Sánchez, Leocadio Rodríguez-Mañas, Olga Laosa (2022) Long COVID-19. Volume(38), 533-544. Clinics in Geriatric Medicine. doi: https://doi.org/10.1016/j.cger.2022.03.005

18. Jordi Bover, Juan J. Carrero, null null, Pablo Molina, Pablo Ureña Torres, Philippe Chauveau, Sandro Mazzaferro (2017) Vitamin D, a modulator of musculoskeletal health in chronic kidney disease. doi: https://core.ac.uk/download/153367338.pdf

19. Malafarina, Vincenzo, Reginster, J. Y., Cabrerizo, Sonia, Bruyère, et al. (2017) Nutritional status and nutritional treatment are related to outcomes and mortality in older adults with hip fracture. doi: https://core.ac.uk/download/pdf/212756692.pdf

20. Míkel Izquierdo, Reshma Aziz Merchant, John E. Morley, Stefan D. Anker, Iván Aprahamian, Hidenori Arai, Mylène Aubertin-Leheudre, et al. (2021) International Exercise Recommendations in Older Adults (ICFSR): Expert Consensus Guidelines. Volume(25), 824-853. The journal of nutrition health & aging. doi: https://doi.org/10.1007/s12603-021-1665-8

21. Ruiz Laiglesia, Fernando José, Tarí Ferrer, Lucía (2019) Malnutrición y pronóstico en pacientes con insuficiencia cardiaca. doi: https://core.ac.uk/download/521879695.pdf

22. S. Go, M. Kang, Hoon-Gu Kim (2025) Sarcopenia in Terminally Ill Patients with Cancer: Clinical Implications, Diagnostic Challenges, and Management Strategies. Volume(28), 10 - 17. Journal of Hospice and Palliative Care. doi: https://www.semanticscholar.org/paper/27c3fbba75cf96df80af1e68823d0a7bea42f93e

23. Seher Yildiz Tacar, Mesut Yilmaz, Deniz Tural, Ilkay Gulturk, Mustafa Orhan Nalbant, Ercan Inci, Gulistan Bahat (2022) Association of Low Muscle Mass as a Marker of Sarcopenia with Survival in Metastatic Renal Cell Carcinoma Patients Receiving Nivolumab. Volume(6(3)), 374–382. EJMI. doi: https://www.ejmi.org/pdf/Association%20of%20Low%20Muscle%20Mass%20as%20a%20Marker%20of%20Sarcopenia%20with%20Survival%20in%20Metastatic%20Renal%20Cell%20Carcinoma%20Patients%20Receiving%20Nivolumab-66227.pdf

24. Sveva Mortellaro, Sonia Triggiani, Federica Mascaretti, Micol Galloni, O. Garrone, G. Carrafiello, M. Ghidini (2024) Quantitative and Qualitative Radiological Assessment of Sarcopenia and Cachexia in Cancer Patients: A Systematic Review. Volume(14). Journal of Personalized Medicine. doi: https://www.semanticscholar.org/paper/4a01ba6d8fdebd86d81e36fc5ec75731270fa64c

25. T. Moga, Ioana Moga, M. Sabau, A. Venter, D. Romanescu, Erika Bimbo-Szuhai, L. Costas, et al. (2022) Evaluation of Geriatric Sarcopenia and Nutrition in the Case of Cachexia before Exitus: An Observational Study for Health Professionals. Volume(7). Geriatrics. doi: https://www.semanticscholar.org/paper/a770b35516667e213eb3e778ae207559c87f41d5

26. Urquiza Abaunza, Miriam (2022) Errekuperazio funtzionaleko unitate bateko adinduetan minaren, nutrizio egoeraren eta ebaluazio geriatriko integraleko parametroen arteko erlazioa: errehabilitazioaren eraginaren eta gertakarien arrisku faktoreen analisia. doi: https://core.ac.uk/download/547401998.pdf

27. Y. Sakurai (2020) Tissue loss syndrome as an important predictor of survival and clinical outcome in surgical patients. The Japanese Journal of SURGICAL METABOLISM and NUTRITION. doi: https://www.semanticscholar.org/paper/703e56c7236ffbac444e306a4bf451b64f0fec0c

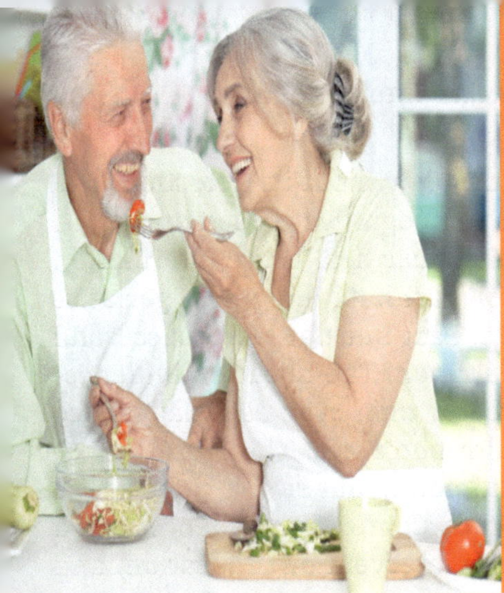

Chapter 15

GERIATRIC NUTRITION IN THE PREVENTION AND TREATMENT OF DISEASE

Contents

Introduction

As the aging population increases, nutrition plays a significant role in the overall health and well-being of older people. With age, nutritional needs are modified, and proper food consumption is essential in preventing and treating many conditions related to age. Geriatric nutrition is the field of study and practice focusing on dietary habits specifically for the older population with the purpose of improving quality of life, promoting independence, and reducing the threat of chronic diseases. Considering that demographic projections show that by 2029, 20% of the United States will be made up of people aged 65 and above (The Stern Center for Evidence-Based Policy, 2015), it is important to know the nutritional needs of this group. Furthermore, coordination of geriatric nutrition and mental health cannot be overlooked, as such factors as depression could readily undercut one's access to nutritional knowledge and practices. Studies have confirmed that depression, particularly when left undiagnosed, is prevalent among the elderly population, with estimates that up to 40% of older adults who are diagnosed with chronic illness carry this condition without its detection. The ramifications of this are far-reaching, with depression tending to impair cognitive processes such as concentration, such that elderly people may not be able to hold onto basic healthcare information as diet advice. Treating these mental health problems will ultimately facilitate integrated geriatric nutrition policy and practice for disease prevention and treatment. Last but not least, successful policy and community action are key to disseminating geriatric nutrition. The need for evidence-based policy to support nutritional programs for the elderly is greater than ever, especially since research continues to identify promising avenues to enhance health outcomes. The Stern Center report identifies the need for prevention and care coordination and points out severe policy gaps in areas like patient self-management and palliative care (The Stern Center for Evidence-Based Policy, 2015). Hence, encouraging a healthy eating culture through intervention, education, and community services will help bridge these gaps. Implementing the schemes properly not only addresses the nutritional needs of the elderly but also contributes to overall healthcare strategies that will improve their health and quality of life (Figure 15.1).

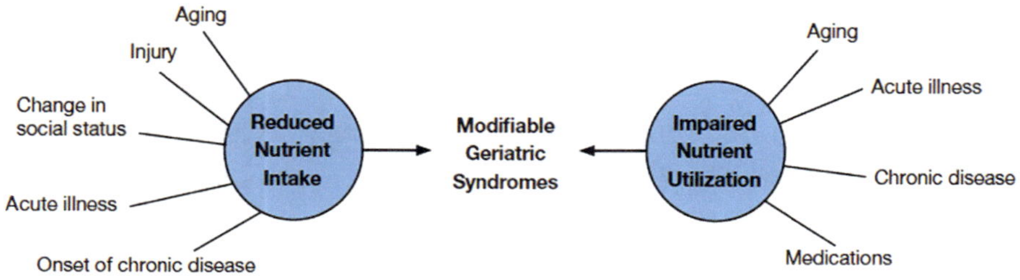

Figure 15.1. The role of nutrition in modifiable geriatric syndromes.

Source: https://s3.amazonaws.com/HMP/hmp_ln/imported/inline-images/Screen%20Shot%20 2019-05-31%20at%2012.39.02%20PM.png.

Importance of Nutrition in Older Adults

Nutrition is an important element of the health and well-being of the elderly, as it is an enabling factor for functional independence and quality of life. With increasing age, there are physiological changes that undermine their ability to absorb nutrients effectively, leading to increased vulnerability to malnutrition. Increased vulnerability can exacerbate chronic diseases and contribute to a worsening of health status. Of particular note is the fact that proper nutritional intake not only sustains basic requirements of health but also sustains dynamic processes such as immune processes and wound healing. Proactive control of such nutritional needs by health practitioners can be a way to avert age-related diseases, hence emphasizing the importance of nutrition in attaining longevity and better health status among elderly individuals. The effects of malnutrition among the elderly are especially significant for older individuals with certain medical conditions. For example, it has been reported through research that malnutrition has a significant effect on the outcome of recovery in patients who have hip fractures, which is a common injury within this age group. Evidence reports that nearly 18.7% of older hip fracture patients suffer from malnutrition, and morbidity during hospital stays is significantly greater among those with low nutrition. The high prevalence of malnutrition warrants targeted nutritional intervention in this population. Active detection and treatment of malnutrition by health professionals can improve functional recovery and decrease the incidence of post-operative complications and ultimately enhance the quality of care and independence of older adults. Other than short-term health complications, long-term consequences of a poor diet among the elderly can lead to increased mortality and reduced quality of life. Malnutrition has been shown to directly cause increased mortality, with statistics indicating 30% mortality within one year of hip fracture among malnourished patients (The Stern Center for Evidence-Based Policy, 2015). This sobering fact highlights the need for integrated care strategies that place nutrition high on the list of priority concerns in the broader context of comprehensive geriatric care. By introducing evidence-based policy that promotes nutrition intervention among older populations, such as that promoted by the Stern Center, we can promote improved health status and quality of life for older adults (The Stern Center for Evidence-Based Policy, 2015). Generally, the important relationship between nutrition and health outcomes highlights the necessity for ongoing research and policy development devoted to addressing the nutritional needs of older individuals.

Overview of the Relationship Between Nutrition and Disease Prevention

The multifaceted relationship between nutrition and disease prevention gains a unique value in the context of older adults' health. With age, as chronic diseases such as heart disease, diabetes, obesity, and hypertension become common, one has to adopt a cautious approach towards food consumption. Nutritional interventions play an important role in the health status of the elderly, not only in controlling prevailing conditions but also in preventing new conditions from arising. For instance, a healthy diet that includes a variety of fruits, vegetables, whole grains, and lean proteins can help build a strong immune system and promote improved health. Thus, having knowledge of how nutrition is linked to disease management is crucial when creating effective health interventions for the elderly population. Field-level implementation of nutritional interventions is also crucial in geriatrics. Several studies have confirmed that adherence to nutritional recommendations can reduce disease risk factors in the elderly. For example, consumption of omega-3 fatty acids has been associated with decreased occurrence of cardiovascular diseases, which points to the role of dietary factors in disease prevention. However, poorly synchronized nutrition policies often compromise the effective passing of such information to the elderly. As suggested by current research, interventions designed to improve the nutritional status of older people, such as tailored dietary recommendations and improved delivery of nutritional education, are needed at once to achieve maximum health benefit within this population (The Stern Center for Evidence-Based Policy, 2015). Through this approach, not only are healthier diets encouraged, but also self-care of chronic disease by increasing dietary awareness. Finally, mental health, by depression, emphasizes the importance of incorporating nutrition in disease prevention among the elderly even further. Evidence is such that undiagnosed depression is highly prevalent in older adults living with chronic diseases and typically translates into lower motivation for eating well (Wynn-Grundy, 2016). The ramifications of such interaction are significant, with depression capable of impairing cognitive function negatively, for example, memory for health care education, which is necessary for ensuring one's nutritional requirements. Therefore, an interdisciplinary approach combining nutritional education with identification of mental illness is able to empower older individuals to take charge of their well-being. By recognizing and responding to these interdependencies, healthcare professionals and caregivers can establish an environment in which geriatric nutrition is an essential component of disease prevention and treatment (Figure 15.2).

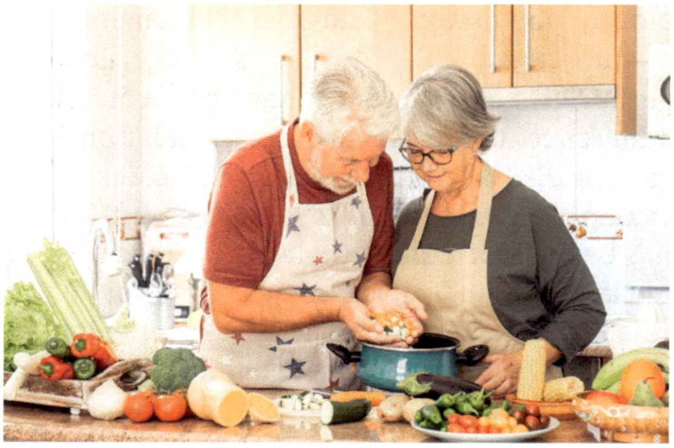

Figure 15.2. Role of nutrition in disease-prevention.

Source: https://disabilitydenials.com/wp-content/uploads/2024/07/the-role-of-nutrition-in-disease-prevention.jpg.

15.1. Nutritional Needs of the Elderly

The nutritional needs of the elderly are complex and multifarious, resulting from physiological alterations that occur with aging. As people age, their metabolism and nutrient absorption may decrease, calling for changes in dietary consumption. Protein consumption becomes especially important, as older adults tend to lose muscle mass, a process referred to as sarcopenia. Proper protein intake can help to counteract loss and preserve global strength and function. Furthermore, vitamins and minerals such as vitamin D, calcium, and vitamin B12 are crucial for bone health and cognitive function, respectively.

Studies have established that the lack of these nutrients causes increased morbidity and mortality among the elderly, and, therefore, the need for targeted nutritional interventions to control corresponding health risks accompanying aging. Additionally, mental well-being is a significant factor in the eating habits of older adults, particularly in conditions such as depression, which usually remains undiagnosed among the elderly. Wynn-Grundy (2016) identifies the impact of depression on the elderly's ability to take in healthcare information, including nutrition. Mental well-being is intrinsically linked with food choices; consequently, depressed people who do not receive their depression treated have no interest in preparing nutritious meals, and so they resort to convenience foods that, in most instances, have few or no necessary nutrients. Social loneliness that can result from aging can also lead to unhealthy diets because the dining experience would change from being social to an isolating one.

Therefore, both nutritional education and mental health should be addressed so that effective intervention programs can be in place to improve the diet of the elderly. Comprehensive geriatric assessment plays an extremely vital role, particularly in surgical management as well as in the treatment of cancer among the elderly.

Lampugnale (2017) reaffirms that, although pre-surgical assessment has the capability to influence patient outcomes, it remains underutilized due to limited time in clinical practice. It can be possible for these assessments to provide important information about the complicated nutritional requirements of elderly patients, frailty, and post-operative recovery failure probability. Highlighting the Mini-Nutritional Assessment and adjoining areas can provide healthcare professionals with information on how to develop personalized nutrition therapy that addresses the individual physiological and psychological needs of older patients immediately. By the integration of comprehensive geriatric assessment in healthcare practice, better nutritional health can be fostered by clinicians, thus enhancing recovery rates and overall quality of life in elderly individuals (Figure 15.3).

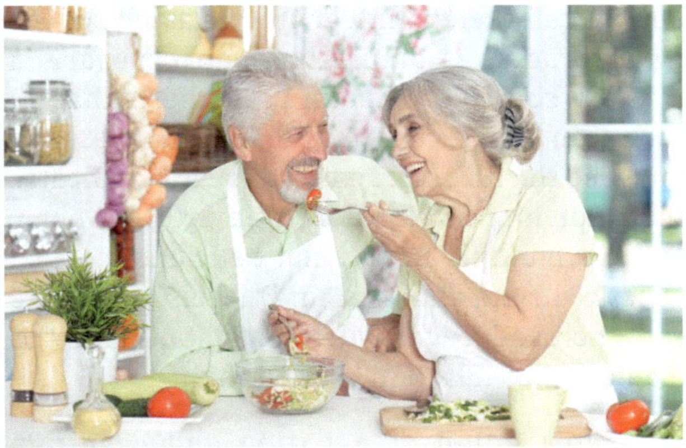

Figure 15.3. Nutritional needs for elderly health.

Source: https://greentreewestwood.com/wp-content/uploads/2024/10/Portrait-of-a-senior-couple-co.jpg.

15.1.1. Essential Nutrients for Older Adults

As people age, their nutritional demands become significantly different due to physiological changes that influence the digestion and absorption of nutrients. The ageing gastrointestinal system undergoes changes that affect the mechanical breakdown of food and efficiency in digestion, ultimately leading to compromised capacity to absorb nutrients. Malnutrition from gastrointestinal dysfunction has the potential to increase the risk of a variety of health issues, including compromised immune function and muscle wasting and loss of strength. Consequently, older adults require more emphasis on nutrient-dense food that can provide the requisite vitamins and minerals for the maintenance of health and well-being. Establishment of certain guidelines for aging is very crucial in the prevention of problems that result from these digestive changes, ultimately guiding diet to the very unique nutritional needs of the elderly (Rémond et al., 2015). Among the major nutrients that are essential in advanced age, protein stands out due to its function in avoiding wasting and frailty of muscle. It has been discovered to trigger muscle repair and enhancement, which reverses the effects of sarcopenia—loss of muscle mass and physical functionality with increasing age. Apart from protein, vitamins D and B12 are significant with regard to maintaining healthy bones and the brain. Vitamin D assists in the absorption of calcium, which is essential in preventing osteoporosis among older people, and vitamin B12 assists in the manufacturing of red blood cells and the brain.

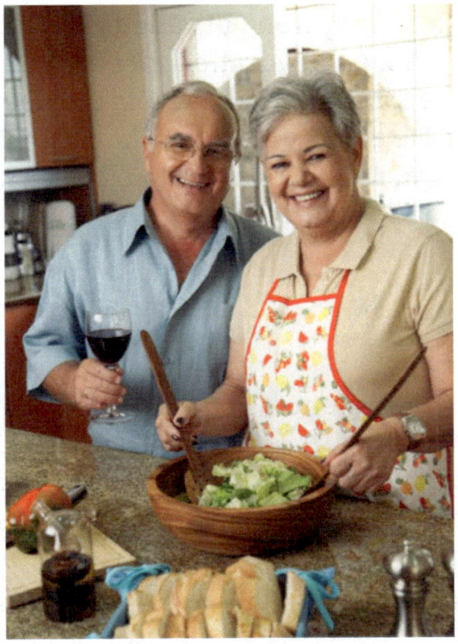

Figure 15.4. Healthy aging in the Hispanic population caring for Abuelita.

Source: https://grainfoodsfoundation.org/wp-content/uploads/2022/01/image-1.jpeg.

Since older adults are likely to experience difficulty in obtaining sufficient sources of these nutrients from diet, more stress on supplementation or fortified foods with high protein levels can prove to be a feasible solution in bridging gaps in nutritional deficiencies and maintaining overall health gains (The Stern Center for Evidence-Based Policy, 2015). Furthermore, hydration turns out to be an essential but relatively overlooked aspect of geriatric nutrition. Dehydration can lead to serious health issues, such as urinary tract infection, kidney stones, and decreased mental function. Older people are typically at higher risk due to changes in the physiology of thirst perception and renal function. Therefore, prevention of dehydration is not just about suggesting continuous fluid intake but adding water-containing foods to their diet, such as fruits and vegetables. Emphasizing the call to maintain fluid balance, namely through the consumption of nutrient-rich, hydrating foods, helps counteract threats posed by dehydration. Thus, the adoption of adequate nutrient consumption and hydration measures amounts to a whole system for addressing the nutritional needs of the elderly, ultimately to facilitate their well-being and quality of life to old age (Rémond et al., 2015) (Figure 15.4).

15.1.2. Common Dietary Deficiencies in the Elderly

Dietary deficiencies become a common occurrence with aging, underpinned by alterations in the physiology of the gastrointestinal tract. The aging process naturally alters nutrient absorption efficiency because mechanical and chemical food breakdown is reduced. Thus, elderly individuals are bound to experience deficiencies of key nutrients such as vitamins B12, D, and calcium, which are required for the maintenance of physical health and mental abilities. Malnutrition, moreover, in the elderly is not just a result of less food intake but also due to a lesser digestive capacity, which prevents the delivery of nutrients at the cellular level. Meeting the nutritional needs of older people is a selective procedure that acknowledges such age-related alterations and proposes dietary guidelines aimed at maximizing nutrient consumption and minimizing the hazards of unfavorable health outcomes due to malnutrition while enhancing quality of life (Rémond et al., 2015). Among the common dietary deficiencies present in the elderly, vitamin D and calcium are particularly noteworthy due to their effects on bone density and overall skeletal integrity. One aspect of the aging process is diminished sun exposure, a primary source of vitamin D synthesis that, in turn, can result in osteoporotic changes and increase the risk of fracture. Research indicates that individuals with dementia are less likely to have multiple nutritional deficiencies, such as low calcium and vitamin D levels, and these can increase cognitive impairment and the likelihood of falls and related injury.

The intersection of nutrition and cognition indicates a necessity for the incorporation of comprehensive dietary protocols into the elderly practice. Through promoting the elderly's intake of such vitamins and minerals through food modification and potential supplementation, health professionals can play a significant role in preventing such conditions as osteoporosis and supporting brain function simultaneously (Downey et al., 2017). The relationship between nutritional deficiency and overall medical outcomes in the elderly is also complicated by the multi-factorial nature of malnutrition. The majority of older individuals suffer from disability, exclusion, and economic constraints, making it hard for them to enjoy a balanced diet. More often than not, these conditions lead to a lack of an adequate intake of essential nutrients, and this will cumulatively affect the health condition of the person in question. To address this problem, one needs an integrative approach comprising nutritional education together with economic and social support systems. Most importantly, the linkage of vitamin D and K deficiencies with increased risks of diseases such as dementia and osteoporosis underscores the imperative necessity for integrative geriatric nutrition practices. Through the identification and treatment of deficiencies, caregivers and medical professionals can contribute significantly to enhancing the well-being of elderly groups, resulting in disease prevention and enhanced quality of life (Rémond et al., 2015).

15.2. Impact of Nutrition on Chronic Diseases

The relationship between diet and chronic disease is most acute in geriatric patients, where the diet severely impacts health. Adequate nutrition is at the hub of the treatment and prevention of chronic diseases such as diabetes, cardiovascular disease, and obesity that define elderly subjects. Because the conditions all co-exist, the need for a well-balanced diet is twice over. Evidence indicates that the adoption of some food trends—high in lean meats, fruits, vegetables, and whole grains reverses or prevents factors for these chronic diseases. Furthermore, such dietary approaches are in tandem with policy recommendations to increase older adult health through prevention and care planning, namely integral components for keeping this population healthy (The Stern Center for Evidence-Based Policy, 2015). Lastly, the emphasis on nutritional education can enable older adults to make the necessary food choices that are very important to enhance their quality of life. Nutrition, however, extends beyond physical health as it is intricately related to mental health as well. Undiagnosed health conditions, such as depression, can disrupt the eating patterns of older people and further complicate health conditions. Literature indicates that undiagnosed depression is prevalent among elderly patients with chronic conditions, with as many as 40% of them having gone undetected (Wynn-Grundy, 2016). Such psychosocial impairment has the capability to impair concentration and memory of important health information, such as nutritional guidance. Thus, promotion of mental health through regular screening for depression is essential in providing effective nutritional education. By psychologically supporting geriatric patients, their memory and compliance with nutritional recommendations are enhanced, which facilitates the circular relationship between mental and physical health results. Additionally, policy recommendations for improving geriatric nutrition must incorporate integrative strategies in meeting physical and mental health concerns. Evidence-based policies can markedly improve the overall well-being of the elderly through evidence-targeted interventions. For instance, patient self-management and family caregiver educational programs can enhance dietary environments for health among older people. Education programs coupled with sufficient healthcare resources can enhance retention of nutritional information and support better compliance with the recommended diets. More importantly, these combined programs can lower the burden of chronic disease in older adults and eventually enhance health outcomes. With the build-up of evidence, what is evidently observed is the need for nutrition-focused strategies to be integrated into healthcare policies as a whole in an attempt to improve the well-being and health of our aging population (The Stern Center for Evidence-Based Policy, 2015) (Figure 15.5).

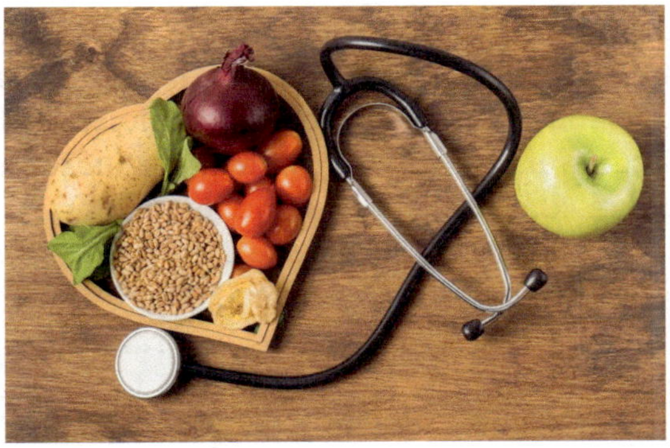

Figure 15.5. Nutrition and chronic diseases.

Source: https://www.euroschoolindia.com/blogs/wp-content/uploads/2024/04/nutrition-chronic-diseases.webp.

15.2.1. Role of Nutrition in Cardiovascular Health

Nutrition is critical to maintain cardiovascular well-being, particularly in the aged, where the incidence of heart disease is significantly on the increase. Dietary patterns directly influence risk factors such as hypertension, hyperlipidemia, and obesity, all of which are key drivers of cardiovascular disease. The aged become subject to alterations in metabolism and usage of nutrients and hence require an eating strategy dedicated to nutrient-dense foods with regulated calorie consumption. Overall, nutrition plans emphasizing fruits, vegetables, whole grains, and lean protein sources can decrease chronic disease risks. Furthermore, dietary intervention can not only be used to prevent cardiovascular disease but also improve health outcomes in older people, indicating the necessity of individualized nutritional advice in older people. Exploring the relationship between race and cardiovascular disease in elderly people shows that disparities are linked to dietary habits. Studies have found that older African Americans in general have elevated blood pressure levels compared to Whites, even when their utilization of anti-hypertensive medication is similar or higher (Ford et al., 2015). This disparity reflects the complex interplay between lifestyle, diet, and cardiovascular well-being. While nutritional interventions in general might hold promise, determination of specific community needs—e.g., culturally appropriate nutrition education—could maximize their effectiveness. By bridging dietary disparities, health care providers could more effectively promote heart-healthy practices among the elderly. Focusing on race-specific dietary interventions, maximizing the control of hypertension and minimizing cardiovascular risk factors among disenfranchised populations might be optimal. Patient-specific nutritional care profile development is of utmost importance in cardiovascular disease management, particularly among the elderly population. Some dietary patterns, such as the Mediterranean diet, have been noted to decrease the risk of cardiovascular disease by virtue of their anti-inflammatory components as well as by balancing lipid profiles. Taking them in conjunction with holistic support from the healthcare team could empower geriatric patients to have control over their health path and promote long-term self-care. Furthermore, the involvement of caregivers and family members in nutritional planning can offer a support system that reinforces healthy dietary habits (The Stern Center for Evidence-Based Policy, 2015). Besides promoting diet compliance through collaborative planning, it supports the provision of an environment that fosters long-term habit change. Application of nutrition, thus, goes beyond the mere formulation of diets; it is at the core of a holistic intervention for cardiovascular disease prevention and management in the elderly (Figure 15.6).

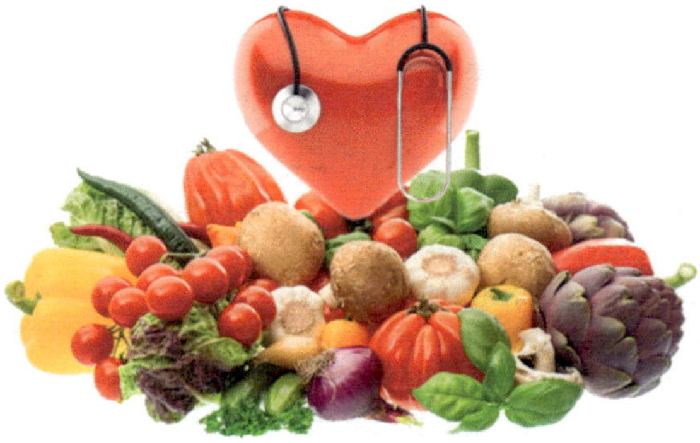

Figure 15.6. Men's health, heart disease and nutrition.

Source: https://gfnc.gov.gd/wp-content/uploads/2024/06/heart.jpg.

15.2.2. Nutrition's Influence on Diabetes Management

Nutrition is a significant factor in the control of diabetes, particularly among the geriatric population, where the interaction among aging, chronic disease, and dietary consumption becomes determinative. As elderly people are likely to experience issues such as compromised metabolism, diminished physical activity, and nutrient deficiencies, their diet can be a determining factor in glucose control and overall well-being. A properly planned diet, rich in unprocessed foods like fruits, vegetables, whole grains, and lean meats, can not only control blood sugar but also support weight management, an important component of diabetes care. To this end, one should acknowledge that tailored nutritional intervention, depending on a person's health status and individual taste, can improve the quality of life among elderly people with diabetes. Furthermore, research has determined that malnutrition and inadequate nutrient consumption are very prevalent among the elderly, particularly those suffering from chronic diseases like diabetes. Research has also determined that geriatric patients often do not consume the proper level of nutrition, exacerbating their existing medical condition and rendering diabetes more difficult to treat. For instance, the impact of malnutrition on diabetic complications recovery is tremendous, resulting in an elevated rate of hospitalization and increased mortality. Management of these issues with specific nutritional interventions forms a two-fold benefit: improving glycemic control along with solving the negative impacts of malnutrition that can hamper the healing and recovery process. This emphasizes the need to give priority to nutritional care and education among older diabetic patients via healthcare policy, as evidenced by results correlating specific dietary interventions with success in enhancing resilience and reducing health complications (The Stern Center for Evidence-Based Policy, 2015). Furthermore, effective diabetes management among older people extends beyond the physical effects of nutrition to encompass psychological and social factors as well. To a large extent, eating habits for the majority of the elderly are intertwined with cultural values and social interaction; hence, changing their diets is challenging. Blending a full diabetes care program involving nutritional education, community support, and involvement of family members can offer an ideal environment for better eating habits. The literature supports that multi-component plans that engage caregivers and physicians can help promote elderly people to control their food intake for autonomy and also promote compliance with dietary advice. Thus, the healthcare sector must recognize and integrates the intricate role of nutrition in diabetes care among elderly people to ultimately enhance their quality of life and health outcomes (Malafarina et al., 2017).

15.2.3. The Connection Between Nutrition and Osteoporosis

The nexus between nutrition and osteoporosis is an important area of study within geriatric health because nutrient consumption has a direct influence on bone mineral density and the overall health of bones. Vitamins such as vitamin D and minerals such as calcium are all essential in performing significant roles in bone metabolism to allow for healthy bone formation and upkeep. Calcium is tasked with functioning as a structural component of bone, while vitamin D facilitates adequate absorption of calcium in the digestive tract. Deficiency of both of these substances helps to enhance low bone density, thereby leading to increased vulnerability to osteoporosis among the elderly. Further, malnutrition itself worsens the problem since aging has a direct influence on gastrointestinal tract functional status, reducing the digestion and absorption of vital nutrients, thereby promoting a cycle of health worsening (Rémond et al., 2015). In addition to calcium and vitamin D, several other micronutrients have been proven to contribute to bone health, and this defines the complicated nature of osteoporosis. Vitamins K and D are particularly important, as newer evidence suggests that they have a synergistic effect on bone metabolism. Patients with impairments of the mind, such as those experiencing dementia, are usually deficient in these vitamins, making them even more susceptible to osteoporosis (Downey et al., 2017). The interplay between nutritional deficiencies and cognitive impairment can cause an increased risk of fractures from osteoporosis, a reason why holistic approaches to the elderly's nutrition are needed. Therefore, nutritional interventions targeting the promotion of these vitamins and calcium may be a critical component of preventing and controlling osteoporosis in the elderly. In addition to this, the socio-economic determinants of nutrition of the elderly cannot be overlooked. Most of the aged population is disadvantaged by issues such as low income, social isolation, and poor access to dense foods that are rich in nutrients, which can render them unable to enjoy proper nutrition. Such issues can render malnutrition common among them, a situation closely linked with many health complications, including osteoporosis. It is necessary to create and execute customized dietetic interventions and education programs targeting these barriers to optimize nutrient intake in older adults. By creating environments that place emphasis on healthy eating and convenient access to nutrient-rich foods, health care practitioners can play a critical role in osteoporosis prevention strategies, which will enhance the quality of life among older adults (Rémond et al., 2015) (Figure 15.7).

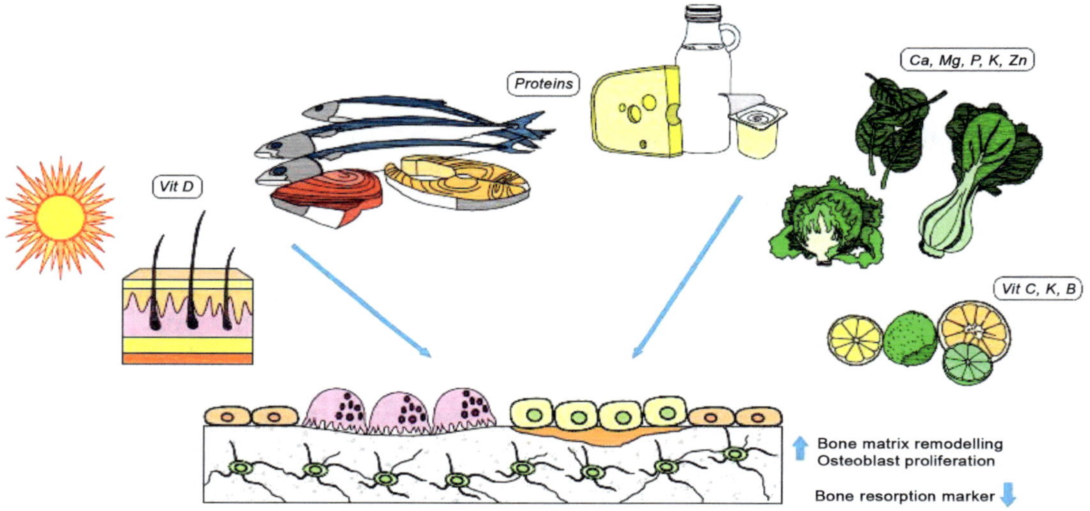

Figure 15.7. Nutrients and dietary patterns related to osteoporosis.

Source: https://www.mdpi.com/nutrients/nutrients-12-01986/article_deploy/html/images/nutrients-12-01986-g001.png.

15.3. Nutritional Strategies for Disease Prevention

Healthy preventive strategies for nutritional disease are crucial in the elderly, where food actually influences overall health and survival. Because older adults are more likely to develop chronic diseases such as cardiovascular disease, diabetes, and osteoporosis, an eating pattern rich in fruit, vegetables, whole grains, and lean protein becomes essential. These food groups provide critical vitamins, minerals, fiber, and antioxidants that are essential to immune function and to cellular repair. Individualized dietary therapies may not only enhance quality of life but also save healthcare dollars associated with chronic disease management. Emphasizing the importance of nutrient-dense foods avoids situations that are prevalent among the elderly individuals, ultimately leading to better health outcomes and increasing life expectancy in this vulnerable population (The Stern Center for Evidence-Based Policy, 2015). Moreover, understanding the relationship between food and mental health is essential for optimizing geriatric care. One large problem within the older population is undiagnosed depression, which may hinder nutritional education and compliance with dietary recommendations. It is estimated that up to 40% of older individuals with long-term illness have undiagnosed depression, which affects cognitive function and overall well-being (Wynn-Grundy, 2016). This connection highlights the significance of health care practitioners not just focusing on nutritional interventions but also exercising special care with mental health checks.

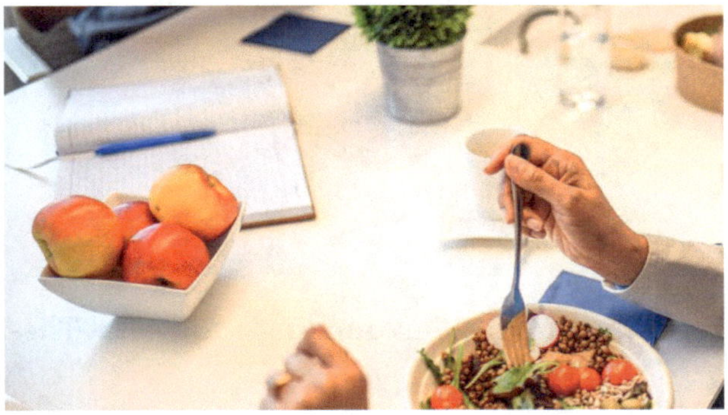

Figure 15.8. Nutritional strategies for disease prevention.

Source: https://media.licdn.com/dms/image/sync/v2/D4E27AQHz-zUYhKFu0A/articleshare-shrink_800/B4EZc1yF8DHIAI-/0/1749769662475?e=2147483647&v=beta&t=eX_IPzThErvfDaWzOtzwrP--SpogsXj--EXIL8lmhP8.

Combining psychological care with nutrition counseling can allow older people to adopt improved dietary behaviors, which may improve their mental health as well as increase the effectiveness of prevention strategies against chronic diseases. Lastly, embracing community-based nutritional interventions will bridge the knowledge-practice gap among older adults. These programs can potentially offer services such as cooking lessons, nutritional education sessions, and personalized meal planning based on the nutritional needs of older individuals. These programs can also promote social interaction and, therefore, attenuate social isolation, which is a factor leading to worse mental and physical well-being in old age. By emphasizing collaboration between healthcare professionals and community resources, these programs have the potential to create long-term models for promoting healthy diets. The harmony of community support with successful nutritional strategies is the secret to prevention of disease, ultimately yielding longitudinal care of geriatric individuals and placing in perspective the synergistic interface between nutrition, mental health, and community interaction (The Stern Center for Evidence-Based Policy, 2015) (Figure 15.8).

15.3.1. Importance of a Balanced Diet

The requirement of a balanced diet is even more evident when one takes into consideration the nutritional needs of the elderly. With advancing age, physiological alterations impair the digestive system's functioning, affecting the ingestion, digestion, and absorption of the nutritional needs. This loss can lead to malnutrition, which increases the susceptibility to various conditions such as cardiovascular disease, frailty, and immune dysfunction. These age-related changes can be offset by a properly balanced diet that includes all the essential vitamins, minerals, proteins, and good fats. Proper intake of nutrients assists older individuals in maintaining their immune systems, gaining muscle mass, and enhancing overall health outcomes. Therefore, nutrition interventions specific to the elderly's needs are needed to reverse the undesirable outcomes of malnutrition on their condition, as highlighted in the recent study on the aging impact on nutrient consumption (Rémond et al., 2015). As evidenced by studies, the diet and health interaction among the elderly cannot be overstated. Institutions of evidence-based dietary guidelines addressing the unique requirements of the elderly are imperative in preventing malnutrition. Aside from the macronutrients needed for energy and muscle preservation, the guidelines must encompass micronutrients essential for cognition as well as bone health. In addition, the incorporation of foods with minimal mechanical disintegration can overcome the reduced efficiency in digestion that is prevalent in this age group. Promoting healthy eating habits, with a focus on whole foods and nutrient-rich foods, can ease the disparity between dietary requirements that are specific to aging and food consumption.

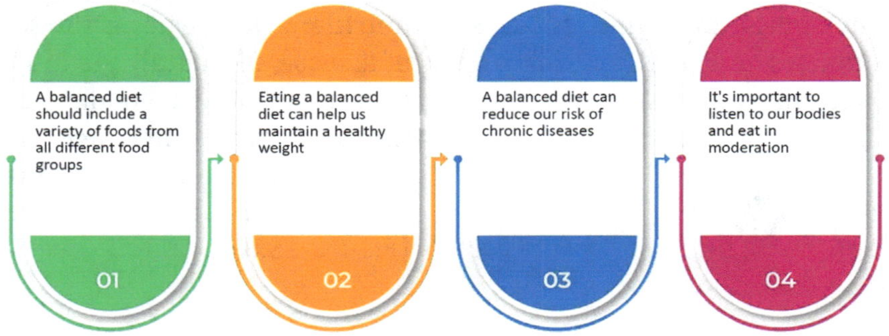

Figure 15.9. A balanced diet.

Source: https://fastercapital.co/i/Health-Caveats--Debunking-Myths-Surrounding-Fad-Diets--The-Importance-of-a-Balanced-Diet.webp.

The research findings presented in a systematic mapping of research into policy proposals also clearly establish why comprehensive dietary approaches are needed to improve health outcomes for elderly individuals (The Stern Center for Evidence-Based Policy, 2015). Besides, both the psychological and social facets of nutrition must be resolved in the creation of a well-settled diet among the elderly. The changing family role and caregiving are likely to have an influence on food intake and dietary wants. Social isolation is likely to reduce motivation for meal preparation, and therefore it is more susceptible to nutrient deficiencies. Thus, shared meal programs and interventions based on community level that encourage common meals or nutrition education have the potential to play a role in enforcing healthy eating in the elderly. Their inclusion in dietary recommendations further adds to the potential for interventions to be effective. By considering both physiological and psychosocial dimensions of nutrition, an international viewpoint emerges that emphasizes the critical function of balanced diets in preventing disease and enhancing longevity in older populations (Rémond et al., 2015; The Stern Center for Evidence-Based Policy, 2015) (Figure 15.9).

15.3.2. Role of Hydration in Health Maintenance

Hydration plays a very essential role when it comes to health maintenance, especially in the elderly, where the functions of the body in relation to fluid loss and replenishment are more impaired. Elderly individuals have a defective thirst mechanism, thus resulting in inadequate fluid intake and subsequently dehydration, which exacerbates health issues like urinary tract infection, kidney stones, and even dementia. As dehydration affects overall health and nutritional status as much as it does, nutrition care should have the highest priority to maintain sufficient, easily accessible fluid consumption unique to elderly patients. The characterization of hydration as a component of comprehensive health care is with evidence as results indicate that all older people should be routinely screened for low-intake dehydration, and there is a need to promote adequate fluid consumption as a routine health practice among older adults (Volkert et al., 2019). Secondly, aging adversely affects gastrointestinal function which can impair hydration among older people. Perturbations such as diminished gastric motility, decreased secretion of digestive enzymes, and alterations in the intestinal wall function inhibit the nutrient and fluid absorption process by the body. The three-dimensional deterioration of gastrointestinal strength not only undermines the consumption of nutrients but also increases the assimilative efficiency for hydration (Rémond et al., 2015). Ensuring proper hydration of older adults is a complex task involving nutritional intervention and individualized attention to fluid intake and its impact on health. Healthcare providers need to advocate for personalized hydration regimes meeting specified needs and monitoring fluid intake to prevent dehydration, with positive results for aging individuals. The effects of hydration are more than just physical health; they also play a significant role in the quality of life among older adults. It has been discovered through studies that hydration can improve mood, cognitive function, and total vigor, all necessary for a sustained active life as one ages. Hydration also contributes to various physiological processes, including thermoregulation and cell functions, thus optimizing body function and disease resistance typical in old populations. However, the proposal of proper hydration must go along with education about fluid choices, as not all fluids will equally enhance the state of hydration. For instance, added nutrient-rich fluids can provide hydration as well as provide essential vitamins and minerals that can complement the overall nutrition regimen (Volkert et al., 2019). Embracing optimal hydration habits in geriatric care not only aids in the sustenance of optimal health but also greatly promotes the overall quality of life, making it the main focus of disease prevention and management among the elderly.

15.3.3. Benefits of Dietary Supplements for Older Adults

As people age, they are more likely to develop adverse effects concerning nutrient absorption and consumption, thereby predisposing them to malnourishment. Dietary supplements are also a significant component in combating such deficiencies, thereby ensuring good health and well-being among elderly individuals. Elderly individuals mostly lack appetite or have changed tastes, and therefore, it is difficult for them to obtain the needed quantities of essential nutrients. Application of dietary supplements that include vitamins, minerals, and essential fatty acids can encourage the delivery of essential nutrients to ensure that elderly individuals enjoy good health. Also, these supplements can enhance immune function, which is crucial for this age group that experiences perpetual declines in immune function due to the aging process. Taking proper dietary supplements, elderly individuals can alleviate complications due to malnutrition and maintain overall body functions. Dietary supplements have also been found to facilitate recovery and minimize complications due to age-related conditions. For example, malnutrition among older adults with hip fractures is exceedingly common, as indicated by research that demonstrates clearly that nutritional intervention can drastically change outcomes and decrease mortality among this population. In particular, malnutrition's effect on recovery can be dramatic, in that poor nutrient intake has been found to contribute to higher hospitalization complications and reduced functional recovery rates. By consuming targeted dietary supplements during the recovery phase, the elderly can restore vital nutrients that are often lacking in their diet, ensuring a stronger healing process. This highlights the imperative role of nutrition in geriatric patient care and the quintessential role played by dietary supplements in building resilience and recovery. Besides, awareness of the alterations in the physiological gastrointestinal tract during aging is essential to inform oneself of the efficacy of dietary supplements in elderly people. With increasing age, the gastrointestinal tract may lose efficiency in food digestion and absorption of nutrients, leading to nutrient deficiencies in the long run. This reduction in gastrointestinal function can exacerbate malnutrition, making the person more prone to multi-organ system diseases. Dietary supplements may be able to overcome some of these barriers by providing bioavailable nutrients that are less difficult for the aging physiology to absorb. Through coordination between dietary intake and supplementation with the functional needs of aging physiology, health professionals can effectively avoid the pathological effects of malnutrition. Intermittent or regular nutritional supplementation also helps prevent malnutrition but is particularly important for improving the overall health status of older people and thus their quality of life (The Stern Center for Evidence-Based Policy, 2015) (Figure 15.10).

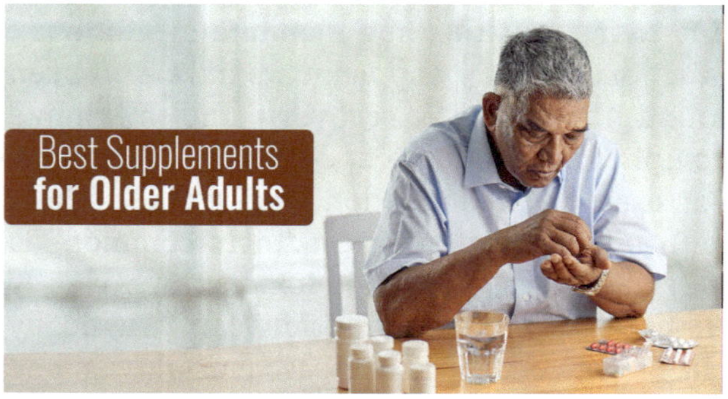

Figure 15.10. Best supplements for older adults.

Source: https://www.steadfastnutrition.in/cdn/shop/articles/best_supplement_for_olde_radults_46ba3c3d-94ff-4b6a-9a90-ef578a99f771.jpg?v=1741341999.

15.4. Challenges in Geriatric Nutrition

Geriatric nutrition problems are multifaceted and involve physiological, psychological, and social factors that adversely affect food intake and health among the elderly. The population growth of elderly individuals is matched with the prevalence of chronic illnesses that make nutritional needs more complicated. The elderly tend to lose their sense of taste and smell, resulting in reduced appetite and aversion to food. Besides that, mobility limitation will avoid shop visits, which lead to spoiled food choices. Further, the interaction between nutrient intake and management of chronic disease grows increasingly important. Addressing these challenges necessitates monitoring and intervention aimed at promoting proper nutritional behaviors in this vulnerable population, as deficiency can further exacerbate underlying medical conditions and increase healthcare costs, highlighting the need for geriatric nutritional care strategies (The Stern Center for Evidence-Based Policy, 2015). Psychological problems, particularly depression, are significant barriers to effective nutrition among the elderly. Evidence shows that depression that has not been diagnosed is common in older people, particularly those with long-term diseases, with as many as 40% estimated to go undiagnosed (Wynn-Grundy, 2016). Presenting symptoms of decreased concentration and decreased motivation severely compromise proper eating habits and will cause deficiency states. These elderly will struggle with understanding or remembering elementary health education and thus perpetuate the cycle of poor nutrition and further deteriorating health. Thus, depression screening in the elderly must become a mainstay of any nutritional intervention strategy to promote better health outcomes and reduce the risk of complications from inadequate nutrition intake. These programs emphasize the importance of adding mental health education to the geriatric nutrition overall plan. Lastly, social problems such as loneliness and economic deprivation have a huge impact on the nutritional status of elderly people. Elderly individuals reside alone, possess impaired mobility, or lack support systems necessary to encourage sound eating habits. Economic difficulties typically limit their ability to purchase foods rich in nutrients, and they are reliant on processed foods that typically contain fewer essential nutrients. Furthermore, access to community resources, such as meal delivery programs or nutrition education, can be unequal in rural or poor urban environments. Combating these issues of social isolation and economic difficulties needs to be done in order to improve the nutritional status of older adults. Effective responses may include enhancing social engagement initiatives and developing caring programs to ensure proper access to healthy food, thus enhancing overall health and well-being among the aging population (The Stern Center for Evidence-Based Policy, 2015).

15.4.1. Physical and Cognitive Barriers to Proper Nutrition

As one grows old, physical barriers significantly impair the ability of individuals to access appropriate nutrition. Restricted mobility, which is usually brought about by diseases such as arthritis or other musculoskeletal disorders, restricts the access of older people to supermarkets and fresh foods. Furthermore, sensory capabilities such as taste and smell can decline, decreasing the quality of food, hence leading to less food intake and micronutrient deficiencies. These constraints are reinforced by economic limitations; many elderly individuals live on fixed incomes, and therefore, it is challenging to obtain healthy foods. Correspondingly, the trial of mobility, sensory impairment, and economic constraints necessitates targeted interventions that can present pragmatic solutions to ensure the elderly receive adequate nutrition, thereby enhancing their health status and well-being (The Stern Center for Evidence-Based Policy, 2015). Cognitive impairment, particularly with mental conditions such as depression and dementia, adds a layer of complexity to eating habits among older individuals. There is evidence that undiagnosed depression in this group is as high as 40% and that this has a negative effect on their capacity to absorb and retain education about healthcare, such as about nutrition (Wynn-Grundy, 2016). The greater the cognitive impairment, the greater the decline in planning and preparing good, healthy meals, which typically results in the consumption of convenience meals that are potentially rich in empty calories but poor in nutrient requirements. Furthermore, memory impairment will make recall of nutritional advice impossible, so that older people cannot adhere to nutritionally indicated diets. Elimination of such cognitive obstacles is a necessary part of any comprehensive plan to improve geriatric nutrition and, hence, disease prevention and treatment. Successful intervention against the physical and mental obstacles to geriatric nutrition is a multi-component approach. These may involve community programs to access fresh foods, and nutrition education that is adjusted for cognitive capacity among older adults. For instance, workshops utilizing simple, visually based materials may help older adults to better understand the importance of good nutrition and how to achieve it. In addition, involving caregivers and relatives in education programs can reinforce support systems so that older individuals are given skilled support for food selection. Such programs not only enhance geriatric nutritional patterns but also minimize healthcare costs in the future for diseases caused by malnutrition, ultimately aligning with health policy goals for maximizing geriatric outcomes (The Stern Center for Evidence-Based Policy, 2015) (Figure 15.11).

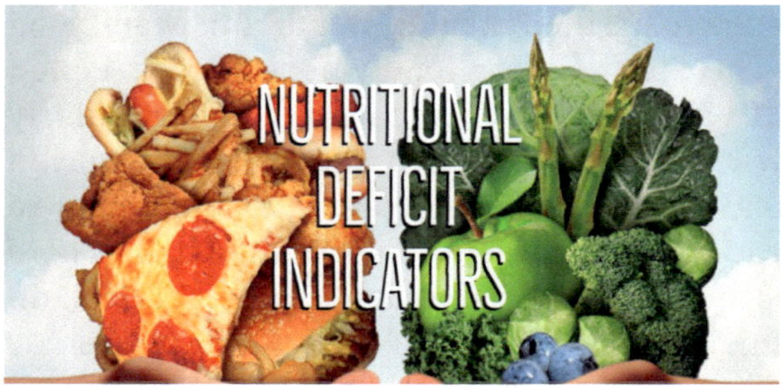

Figure 15.11. Nutritional deficit indicators.

Source: https://naturalfittherapy.com/wp-content/uploads/2018/03/nutri-deficit-indicators-1200x628.jpg.

15.4.2. Social, Psychological, Economic, and Cultural Factors Affecting Dietary Choices

The combination of social and psychological factors significantly affects the eating behavior of older people because they typically face special issues in their dieting behavior. The elderly often face social isolation, which can decrease their motivation to cook and consume nutritious food. The majority of geriatric individuals dine alone, thus without the social sharing typically derived from dining together. Such a lack of social sharing diminishes the pleasure of eating, usually augmented by common experience. Dining alone, thus, could lead to decreased food intake and reliance on convenience foods, which are typically less healthy. Treatment of these social factors is important in order to enhance the quality of life and health status among this group, since evidence reveals that social dining while eating can have a beneficial influence on food intake levels and overall nutritional status. Psychological factors also play an important role in determining the diet of the elderly. Depression, anxiety, and mental deterioration are issues that can have a dramatic influence on appetite and food craving. For instance, depressive symptoms may lead to decreased appetite for food, and therefore malnutrition and other illnesses. Mental impairment may hamper awareness of hunger feelings or the importance of consuming nutritious foods, and thereby it is increasingly difficult for older people to maintain diets in equilibrium. Personal backgrounds and culture can shape food attitudes and develop patterns that may be contradictory to dietary counseling. Accordingly, awareness of psychological dynamics is crucial in order to develop efficacious interventions to improve dietary behaviors and campaign for the elderly's nutritional needs. Furthermore, integration of social support systems might be helpful in countering the adverse impacts of social and psychological determinants on diets. Meals that are volunteer-supported have been found to significantly increase food intake in older people. By providing companionship and assistance while eating, volunteers can alleviate loneliness and promote healthier eating. Research has discovered that volunteer-assisted patients had a 15% increase in food intake, far higher than those who consumed meals alone. This illustrates how the building of social relationships enhances the eating experience, as well as resulting in better overall health outcomes. The quest for nutritional solutions for older individuals must therefore adopt an understanding of these social and psychological factors to design interventions that are holistic and person-centered in focus (Presley, 2014; Rémond et al., 2015). The lack of nutrition education can enhance poor diets that are not meeting the requirements for essential vitamins, putting individuals at risk for deficiencies of significant nutrients such as iron, folate, and vitamin B12. As these nutrients play significant roles in the prevention of malnutrition-related disease, these deficiencies have the potential to contribute to the negative impact on the health and quality of life in older adults. Socioeconomic determinants play a crucial role in shaping nutritional outcomes, particularly among geriatric patients. These aspects include a variety of factors, such as income level, educational attainment, and availability of health care, which all play significant roles in the selection of foods and overall nutritional status. Those who have lower socioeconomic status tend to be disadvantaged in purchasing healthy food, as fresh fruits and vegetables can be seen as out of reach. They may also not have the necessary educational information to decipher nutritional facts or prepare wholesome meals. Thus, the outcome of this disinformation can be a reliance on highly sugary and fatty processed foods that further lead to malnutrition among older adults. Addressing these socioeconomic challenges is an interdisciplinary endeavor with the participation of not only healthcare providers but also policymakers, who can provide support and programs towards increasing food access to the ageing population. Support systems from society, such as family ties and community services, are also key drivers in the diet of the ageing. Social support may also enable access to healthy food, with relatives participating in preparing and making purchases of food, thereby influencing food consumption. Social isolation leads to reliance on take-out or convenience food, which could be non-optimal in terms of diet. Training in healthy food and community programs for improving food security is important in addressing improved food choices among the elderly. Comprehending preventive interventions and care coordination, as presented in studies of health benefits for older people, can lead to long-term positive impacts on nutritional status and overall well-being. Finally, the intersection of socioeconomic status and environmental and cultural conditions also must be considered in the determination of food selection among older adults. Cultural constructs of food, concepts of health, and customary eating patterns significantly control what older individuals accept or prefer. Moreover, other environmental determinants, including local grocery stores and fresh produce markets, can ease or hinder food availability, ultimately deciding eating habits. Processes that include community participation and reinforce cultural dietary liking, in addition to promoting healthy eating, can have a beneficial effect on the geriatric diet. By intervening on such multifaceted socioeconomic determinants, healthcare practitioners and policymakers have the opportunity to utilize impactful interventions that, in addition to improving the nutritional status among older adults, also impact their overall quality of life and health outcomes, particularly in the area of managing chronic illness and comorbidities, as confirmed in previous research outcomes.

15.4.3. Cultural Influences on Food Preferences

Cultural determinants significantly affect older adults' food choices, dictating how people eat, what food people prefer to eat, and what they know and believe about nutrition. As an individual ages, their origins, including tradition, ethnicity, and social standards, play important roles in what is healthy or desirable food. Traditional culture often influences recipes, food preparation, and food consumption habits, and may have an impact on nutrient intake and the quality of the diet. In some diets, for instance, legumes, vegetables, and whole grains may be the choice, while others will select meat and processed foods. This variability mirrors the need for health promotion strategies modified to respect and include cultural choices to support food compliance and satisfaction in older adults. Recognition of cultural factors through appreciation can support more effective interventions in the management of geriatric nutrition, generating both health and respect for personal identities. Social context, such as family and community, constitutes another key element of diet preference among the geriatric population. Several food-related cultural activities involve communal meals, family customs, and communal feasts, which are advantageous for both nutrition and socialization. In the elderly, particularly those with social isolation, these communal elements have a huge influence on their choice of food and overall nutrition. Loneliness or lack of motivation to cook can lead to unhealthy eating habits, evidenced by studies that indicate older adults living alone find it difficult to prepare food for one person and consequently experience problems of food accessibility (Whitelock & Ensaff, 2018). Thus, socially addressing the issue of eating is critical in the preservation of quality of life among older adults because promoting communal eating environments can have the potential to enhance not only nutrition but also affective state. In addition, the intersection of cultural contexts and individual experiences, such as perceptions of health and aging-related changes, complicates dietary habits in late life. Older individuals may experience age-related physiological changes, e.g., decreased appetite or altered taste, which may be misinterpreted culturally (Matringe et al., 2007).

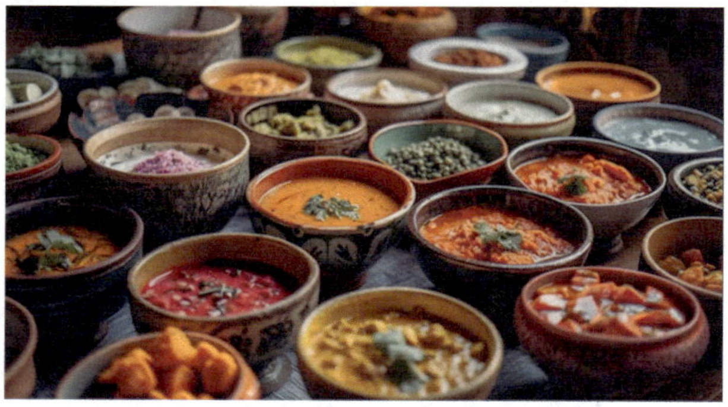

Figure 15.12. The cultural concept of food: influences and significance.

Source: https://i0.wp.com/calxylian.com/wp-content/uploads/2023/07/The-Cultural-Concept-of-Food.webp?fit=1200%2C675&ssl=1.

For instance, culturally established dietetic conceptions may lead individuals to avoid certain nutrient foods, thereby negatively impacting them. The identification of barriers and facilitators impacting older people's nutritional behaviors is critical. Such complication also underscores the necessity for healthcare providers and caregivers to seek input from older adults regarding background, taste, and unique nutritional needs. By doing so, providers are able to craft culturally relevant nutrition strategies that not only address health complications but also address older adults' living experience, improving diet compliance and overall well-being (Figure 15.12).

15.5. Nutrition Interventions in Clinical Settings

The increasing appreciation for the role of nutrition intervention within the clinical setting has been more and more apparent in the domain of geriatric care. Given that aging populations have distinct nutritional requirements, healthcare professionals are tasked with the strategic implementation of nutritional interventions appropriate to the individual needs of older adults. These interventions can have a pivotal role in both the prevention of, and the management and even reversal of, many chronic diseases common in the elderly. For instance, the implementation of customized meal plans that cater to the specific dietary requirements and limitations of geriatric patients can enhance their nutrition in general, hence reducing the threats of malnutrition and associated medical complications, such as cardiovascular disease and diabetes. These targeted nutrition strategies not only improve clinical outcomes but also instill a sense of independence and well-being in older adults, underscoring the central position that nutrition holds as a cornerstone of geriatric care. Nutritional education becomes an important component of successful interventions in elderly patients within the clinical setting. By the provision of comprehensive education regarding nutrition, health providers can empower older adults to make healthy dietary choices that have positive impacts on their health. However, the effectiveness of such training may be diminished by mental illness, such as depression, which remains undiagnosed in older age groups. Studies have established that undiagnosed depression compromises the capacity of older adults to hold onto relevant healthcare information, illustrating the need for combined interventions on nutritional and psychological aspects of care. As noted, unrecognized depression has consequences regarding the retention of learning content about nutrition and points to the need for multicomponent interventions in clinical practice focusing on mental health along with nutritional education, ultimately improving health outcomes among the at-risk population (Wynn-Grundy, 2016). Moving forward, health systems must continue to refine how they implement nutrition interventions as part of geriatric care. T

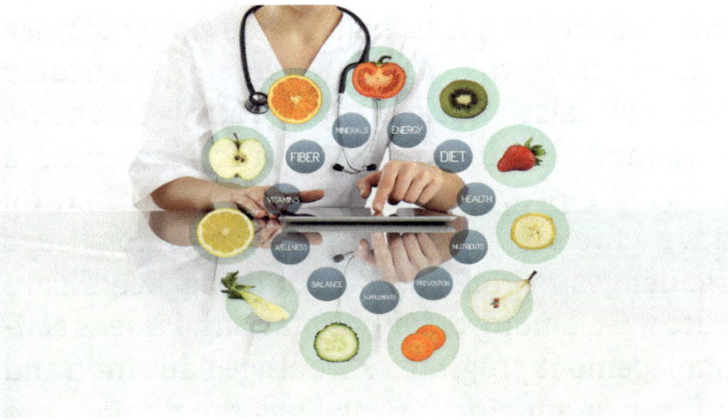

Figure 15.13. Comprehensive nutrition consultation.

Source: https://kajabi-storefronts-production.kajabi-cdn.com/kajabi-storefronts-production/themes/781684/settings_images/yfcSkjmURquyWLRrXZYM_file.jpg.

he inclusion of evidence-based policies to improve preventive care, such as food security programs and efficient care coordination, is significant for the advancement of nutrition among the elderly. Furthermore, studies show that most crucial areas, like patient self-management and palliative care, are under-studied despite having solid evidence (The Stern Center for Evidence-Based Policy, 2015). By shifting the emphasis more to these aspects in clinical interventions, health care professionals can significantly enhance the quality of life and well-being of older patients. In the end, an integrative approach to nutrition interventions—congruent with mental health care and evidence-informed—can contribute to enhanced health outcomes, reduced health care costs, and a healthier older population (Figure 15.13).

15.5.1. Role of Dietitians in Managing Elderly Nutrition

The role of dietitians in the management of elderly nutrition extends far beyond the provision of dietary information; it is an overall package specially prepared to address the unique demands of the older individual. As nutritional deficiency rises with age, particularly in institutional-aged care populations, dietitians play a key role in the recognition and rectification of these nutritional issues. There is evidence to demonstrate that nearly half of all residents in aged care facilities are malnourished due to multiple factors affecting appetite and nutrient absorption, and thus the need for specific nutrition interventions. Some of the interventions they provide comprise individualized meal planning and nutrient-dense foods that can benefit overall health outcomes among older adults and thus warrant the dietitians' important role in the interprofessional healthcare team as a chaperone for nutrition care among geriatric patients (Agarwal et al., 2016). In addition to direct nutritional management, dietitians have a key role in planning and implementing effective nutrition schemes in residential aged care facilities. They enable regular nutrition screenings and assessments, which are essential for the early detection of malnutrition and attendant health risks. In addition, dietitians work together with other healthcare providers to develop effective nutrition interventions that are tailored to an individual's dietary requirements and preferences. These interventions are specifically essential in light of the complex healthcare situation encountered by the elderly, such as comorbidities and functional impairments. By ensuring that such protocols are monitored and altered regularly, dietitians avert losses of nutritional status that can lead to severe complications, such as rising hospitalization rates and declining quality of life. Their training allows for an integrated solution in which not only clinical nutrition but also eating as a social and emotional activity is taken into consideration (The Stern Center for Evidence-Based Policy, 2015). They also contribute to the role of geriatric nutrition through participation in geriatric nutrition, lobbying for policy advocacy for healthy aging and optimal nutrition. Their input is significant in shaping best practice, which serves to give high priority to prevention and care coordination, both being key to the response of healthcare systems to population ageing.

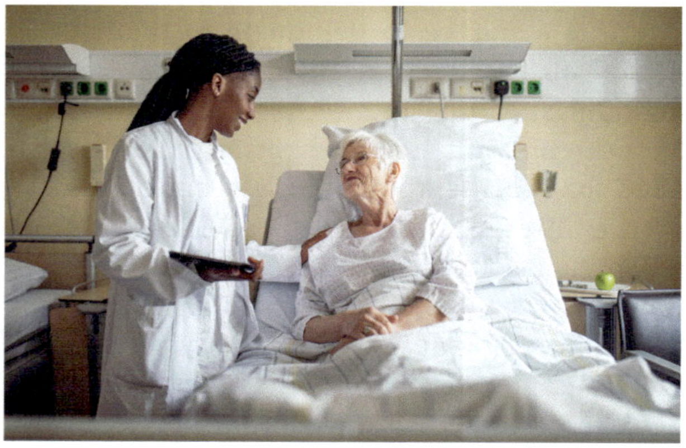

Figure 15.14. Role of dietitians in managing elderly nutrition.

Source: https://s3-us-west-2.amazonaws.com/utsw-patientcare-web-production/original_images/patient-hospital.jpg.

Through research and policy debate, dietitians are able to place the importance of patient self-management of nutritional health and the need for palliative considerations when providing dietary advice in front of the public. In doing so, the full breadth of dietetic practice in geriatrics is highlighted with clinical, teaching, and advocacy competencies being integrated. Lastly, continued engagement by dietitians in these disciplines is essential to improve health outcomes and the quality of life for elderly adults, with nutrition being key to the prevention and management of age-related diseases (The Stern Center for Evidence-Based Policy, 2015) (Figure 15.14).

15.5.2. Evidence-Based Dietary Interventions

The utilization of evidence-based dietary interventions is a significant component of promoting geriatric nutrition, particularly in averting the negative health effects attributed to aging. As the elderly are faced with unique nutritional issues, such as malnutrition and multi-morbidity, it is crucial to employ dietary interventions that not only remain practicable but are also backed by quality scientific evidence. Evidence-based practices with a focus on prevention and care coordination have shown promise to overcome these challenges, significantly enhancing healthcare outcomes among older populations. Patient self-management programs encourage education and a focus on nutrition, which has the potential to empower older adults to make knowledge-based food choices, leading to improved nutritional status and overall health. By being part of existing health systems, professionals can enact a more integrated geriatric care that is sustainable and effective (The Stern Center for Evidence-Based Policy, 2015). Malnutrition is an emergent situation in RAC facilities, where prevalence may be staggering. Evidence indicates, across the board, that nearly half of all residents in these types of facilities are malnourished, usually as a consequence of issues related to appetite, dietary intake, and nutrient absorption. Directly associated with all these numerous adverse health effects is the heightened risk of infection, falls, and pressure ulcers, which increase healthcare costs and lower the quality of life for elderly patients. These results indicate the need for formalized dietetic interventions that enhance food quality as well as integral nutritional programs. Employment of routine nutrition screening, precise assessments, and multidimensional dietetic interventions can significantly decrease the risk of malnutrition, enhancing the well-being of older people living in RACs (Agarwal et al., 2016). Besides, the effectiveness of dietary management relies on the contribution of a multidisciplinary team to give a balanced touch to geriatric nutrition. Under these collaborative efforts, multiple stakeholders enter the arena, including health caregivers, nutritionists, and caregivers at home, who are critical in recognizing and treating food and nutritional issues. Through ongoing monitoring and regular reevaluation of nutrition strategies, these multidisciplinary teams can efficiently tackle individual dietary needs. An evidence-driven model of geriatric nutrition not only outlines the applicability of individualized nutritional interventions but also highlights the need for ongoing education and communication between all parties involved in the care of an older adult. Interprofessional collaboration like this will ultimately lead to long-term health gains that benefit physical as well as emotional well-being in older adults navigating the complexities of their healthcare journey (The Stern Center for Evidence-Based Policy, 2015).

15.6. Community and Family Support in Nutrition

Family and community support in nutrition is significant to the overall well-being of the elderly, exerting a crucial impact on their quality of life and health condition. Families also serve as vital caregivers, often playing a central role in encouraging healthy dietary practices and adherence to dietary recommendations. Support from the community can also help older adults overcome the issues of nutrition, particularly when confronting long-term diseases. Family-based interventions draw on family involvement and tend to foster enhanced dietary compliance and facilitate a healthy environment that fosters enhanced habits. As rates of chronic diseases among the aged increase, structural community resources and family participation become a rising necessity, highlighting a dual process of social and individual support in effective nutrition interventions. Furthermore, community programs aimed at the elderly's nutritional care may significantly enhance their social relations and overall well-being. These programs may include meal delivery services, nutrition education, and garden programs, which provide not just food but also opportunities for sociability. Research suggests that social contact encourages active participation in eating habits, which may specifically help counteract issues like loneliness and depression. According to studies, the policy for patient self-management and care coordination in communities is a key driver in the improvement of the nutritional well-being of the elderly (The Stern Center for Evidence-Based Policy, 2015). Such interventions use common resources to establish a sustainable system of support within the elderly, thus highlighting the importance of community in nutritional well-being. Further, the relationship between diet and mental health among the elderly creates a compelling argument for comprehensive family and community support systems. Depression that goes undetected can impair older adults' capacity to make appropriate dietary choices and retain nutrition knowledge that they must have to remain healthy. Research indicates that a significant proportion of elderly people may be having challenges with undiagnosed depression, which affects their cognitive functions and consequently their food intake (Wynn-Grundy, 2016). Creating accommodating settings that are actively involved in working on mental issues can result in enhanced nutritional education and information absorption, creating a domino effect towards improving overall health outcomes. Through the establishment of a socially conscious community, nutrition and mental health can be influenced positively, providing an integrated approach to disease prevention and treatment in the elderly (Figure 15.15).

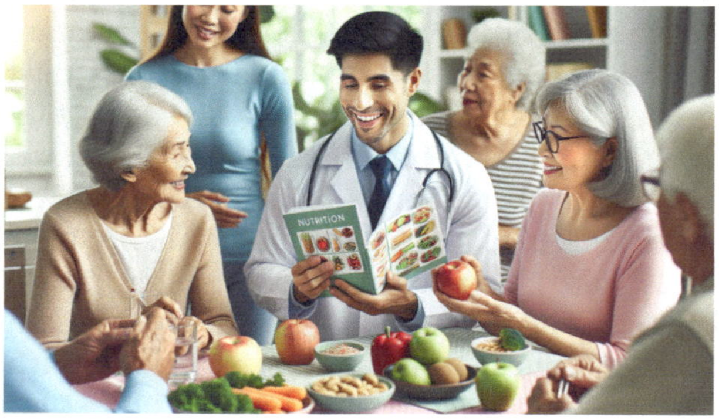

Figure 15.15. Community and family support in nutrition.

Source: https://cdn.growtha.dev/64f58746ad542d8781e2bab0/66307cb4ac39dfb386083853_1695575082593x234550197059517630-1714453233002x647831488737293800-dalle-LHILQ.png.

15.6.1. Importance of Social Support for Healthy Eating

Social support plays an important role in geriatric nutrition in determining healthy eating in the elderly. When people get older, they tend to have substantial life changes, for example, losing their loved ones, hence depression and feelings of loneliness. According to studies, social networks, for example, family, friends, and neighbors, help in promoting eating habits.

These support structures can assist in promoting healthy meal preparation and a social environment to facilitate eating well, ultimately influencing food intake and nutritional status among the aged. Curiously, people engaging in communal meals with friends or relatives tend to embrace a balanced diet and hence reduce the vulnerability to nutritional inadequacy as well as improve the general health status among the elderly (Wynn-Grundy, 2016). In addition, good eating and social support are inextricably linked with the mental well-being of older adults. Untreated depression could have a significant effect on an older adult's capacity to acquire health care information, such as diet. Greater symptoms of depression were correlated with diminished retention of diet education in one study among older adults, suggesting that peer emotional support can act as a buffer against these effects. By the creation of a health-conducive setting in which conversation about nutrition and health is encouraged, families and caregivers can enhance the effectiveness of health interventions among older people. It demonstrates how the encouragement of social integration not only maintains mental well-being but also enables the facilitation of enhanced understanding and adherence to dietary recommendations essential for the treatment of chronic diseases prevalent among older people (Wynn-Grundy, 2016). Moreover, social support also plays an important role in community-based initiatives that seek to enhance nutritional health among the elderly.

Empirical policy interventions, such as promoting community involvement, for instance, group meals and nutrition education, have been reported to enhance better dietary intake for the aged. Social support through meals can lead to greater fruit and vegetable intake and hence offset issues in dietary inadequacy. In addition, family caregivers also form a crucial part of these social support networks because they can coordinate meal provision and promote healthy dietary choices. Implications for future research and policymaking lie in how to weave in community resources with family-based support networks to create a better environment for the optimal promotion of healthy dietary habits among older people, thereby also improving their overall well-being and quality of life.

15.6.2. Community Programs Promoting Geriatric Nutrition

Effective community programs for the promotion of older people's nutrition are of critical importance to enhancing older persons' health. Such programs will usually tackle problems about having healthy foods available and dietary education on healthy eating habits, specifically for older people. The majority of community agencies, such as senior centers and local health departments, offer meal delivery programs and nutrition courses that provide older people with the ability to make nutritional decisions. These programs not only address the immediate nutritional needs of older individuals but also involve them socially, which is necessary for mental well-being. By encouraging participation in these programs, communities can significantly reduce the likelihood of malnutrition and associated health issues prevalent among seniors. This action works with the overall mission of public health by improving the quality and length of life for older individuals. Further, research has established that community nutrition programs have the potential to cause tangible improvements in the health of older individuals. The programs encourage emphasis on nutrient-rich diets, which can help prevent the occurrence of chronic ailments typical of older adults, such as diabetes and high blood pressure. Interaction between various stakeholders like caregivers, decision-makers, and community leaders helps to enhance the efficacy of such programs. For instance, evidence from research shows that evidence-based interventions such as exposure to healthy food and nutrition education have the capacity to influence the health trajectory of older adults (The Stern Center for Evidence-Based Policy, 2015). Through a systematic process of overcoming obstacles towards optimal nutrition, i.e., food deserts and mobility restrictions, community programs are capable of making choices that not only enhance dietary well-being but also offer a better aging approach in general. The development of such community-based programs points toward a shift toward more conceptualization of geriatric care with an increased emphasis on prevention as well as treatment. According to the Health Care Task Force, the activity participation of the elderly in nutrition-related activities can yield long-term returns like enhanced quality of life and reduced healthcare costs for preventable diseases. By an intergenerational approach to health and nutrition, these programs can facilitate the sharing of knowledge between generations, with healthy behaviors passed down and maintained. As communities recognize the importance of geriatric nutrition, continued investment in such programs will be needed in order to care for an expanding population of older people, vindicating the importance of nutrition as a key part of disease prevention and control programs in public health systems (Figure 15.16).

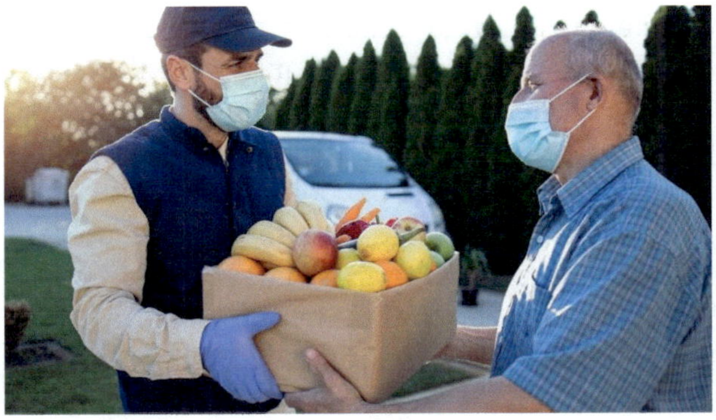

Figure 15.16. Community nutrition programs.

Source: https://eac-network.org/wp-content/uploads/2022/03/nutrition-programs-scalia-gallery-fullwidth.jpg.

15.6.3. Family Involvement in Meal Planning and Preparation

Family involvement in meal planning and preparation plays a unique role in older people in the sense that it has a direct impact on their nutritional status and overall health outcomes. The increasing occurrence of malnutrition among older individuals in various care settings has made familial involvement in eating habits very pertinent. These individuals can be assisted by their relatives, who can provide nutritionally adequate meals, with the requirements of older relatives properly catered for. This collaboration not only contributes to improved food quality but also to a sense of belonging and the emotional well-being of the elderly, factors that are crucial in countering health issues brought about by isolation and loneliness. By incorporating the dietary likes and limitations of older relatives, family members help deliver a more personalized diet plan that promotes higher dietary adherence and satisfaction, ultimately producing better health outcomes. Furthermore, family support can reduce some of the special challenges related to meal preparation for older individuals. As one becomes older, they can acquire physical impairments that affect their ability to prepare food for themselves, leading to nutritional deficiencies and adverse health effects. Mutual food preparation among family members not only provides functional assistance but also the chance for intergenerational bonding. It allows for the sharing of cooking techniques and nutritional knowledge, enhancing the dietary habits of the older and younger generations. Evidence shows that a healthy family unit, engaged in meal planning, can successfully reduce the malnutrition-associated risks, which are very prevalent in aged care facilities where elderly individuals have multi-morbidities and decreased appetite (Agarwal et al., 2016). This kind of collaboration ensures the nutritional needs of older individuals are fulfilled at all times, thus promoting their well-being and health. Furthermore, the requirement for family support in food planning grows with age groups of older adults, particularly in those regions where fast ageing populations are dominating, e.g., northern New England (Fox et al., 2015). With the number of older adults, particularly older-than-85-year-olds, steadily rising, the demand for efficient nutritional interventions grows more urgently. Members of the family can be primary stakeholders in calling for an assortment of nutrition interventions tailored for their relatives, which can include refining the sensory characteristics of food or adjusting meals according to specific conditions. Including family collaboration in programs of nutrition care not only addresses the physical needs of elderly individuals but also helps to aid them in their emotional and psychological welfare, thereby creating an all-around approach to geriatric nutrition that is vital in disease prevention and treatment among this vulnerable population.

SUMMARY

The contribution of geriatric nutrition in preventing and treating disease among the elderly cannot be emphasized enough. As the population of older people increases and a projected 20% population is anticipated by 2029, their unique nutritional needs constitute a vital public health concern. Malnutrition in this population is often the consequence of both physiological alterations and psychogenic influences, such as undiagnosed depression, that can cause severely compromised intakes and health status. Studies recognize that as many as 40% of older people with chronic disease may be suffering from hidden depression, thereby compromising their ability to retain key healthcare information related to nutrition (Wynn-Grundy, 2016). Understanding the matters, therefore, becomes critical for offering effective intervention measures for improving nutritional status and overall health in this vulnerable group. Moreover, the inclusion of careful assessments factoring in nutritional well-being as well as mental health is essential to optimizing the provision of healthcare to the older population. For instance, the application of geriatric assessments can provide useful insights into the specific needs of elderly patients so that healthcare givers can deliver the right treatment. Although geriatric assessments remain underutilized, their worth, particularly in morbidity and mortality forecasting in relation to nutritional and psychological well-being, cannot be overlooked (Lampugnane, 2017). As the health care systems undergo the shift to address the nuances of geriatric care, focusing on nutrition as a preventative and therapeutic intervention should take priority, considering the provisions provided to assure older persons' optimization of quality of life. Finally, interdisciplinary teamwork between healthcare professionals like dietitians, geriatricians, and mental health professionals is essential in maximizing the effectiveness of nutrition intervention among older people. With this kind of teamwork, it will be more manageable to have a more coordinated effort where nutritional teaching and screening of mental health are simultaneously done. Emphasizing the role of diet in the prevention as well as treatment of diseases will improve health outcomes among older people tremendously. As the discipline of geriatric medicine continues to evolve, it is essential that practitioners in the future possess the knowledge and training necessary to deal with the intricate interfaces between diet and health among the elderly population. Such integrative treatment will eventually translate to better handling of health conditions among the elderly and encourage healthier aging.

When the importance of nutrition in older people is considered, it becomes increasingly clear that impaired nutritional status is a key determinant in the onset of many diseases in the elderly. It is well argued that malnutrition in this age group not only accelerates existing conditions but also disrupts healing and general health. Particularly, the elderly with chronic diseases are prone to being undiagnosed with depression, thus also making them lose concentration and learn the required healthcare information. This relationship was demonstrated in a study where higher Geriatric Depression Scale scores were associated with poorer retention of nutrition education in older adults, and the desperate need for targeted interventions to address both mood and nutrition in the geriatric population (Wynn-Grundy, 2016). Prioritizing nutrition can thus be considered an umbrella approach in disease prevention and treatment in the elderly. Furthermore, geriatric nutrition is not only a matter of short-term nutritional problems but also encompasses broader systemic health interventions. Integrated healthy aging has been advocated by the International Longevity Centers Health Care Task Force. This vision subscribes to the view that better nutrition can have a direct influence on a range of health outcomes and thus stem healthcare costs while improving the well-being of older individuals. By demonstrating the intersection of nutrition with medical care, the Task Force raises the imperative for health care structural change aimed at prevention. Such effort can reverse the dual peril of illness and mental illness in the aging population and create conditions for resilience and longevity in this growing demographic. In general, the confluence of nutrition, mental health, and healthcare reform provides a compelling case for an integrated approach in the provision of geriatric care. Awareness of the multifaceted relationship between these aspects is critical in developing effective interventions to improve the health outcomes for the elderly. To deal with nutrition not only avoids disease but is also a vital component in mitigating the role of depression, as well as maximizing cognitive ability in the aged. Additional research needs to be focused on exploring these connections with an eye towards creating holistic health programs that encourage the provision of adequate nutritional care for older people and ensure their health and well-being through the difficulties of aging. The importance of such policies cannot be overstated, so that the ageing population can thrive in a health system devised to meet their individual needs.

A CLOSER LOOK

PREVENTION AND TREATMENT OF MALNUTRITION IN OLDER ADULTS

Prevention and malnutrition treatment in older adults are crucial components in effective ageing, as malnutrition has been found to result in frailty, impaired immunity, delayed wound healing, muscle wasting, and death. Preventive interventions begin with routine nutritional screening using standardized tools such as the Mini Nutritional Assessment (MNA) or the Malnutrition Universal Screening Tool (MUST), which allow for early identification of those at risk before actual clinical presentation. Identification in its initial stages is crucial, as malnutrition tends to present insidiously in the elderly because of factors like decreased appetite, oral problems, polypharmacy, depression, or intellectual impairment. Treatment methods involve individualized nutrition care plans according to the medical condition and individual needs of the elderly (Figure 15.17).

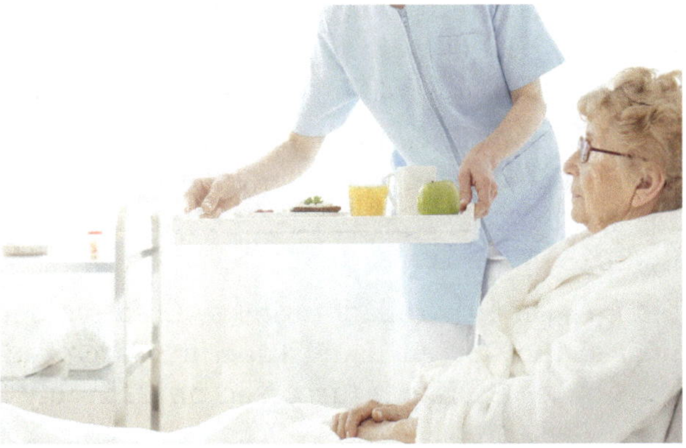

Figure 15.17. Malnutrition in hospitalized adults.

Source: https://effectivehealthcare.ahrq.gov/sites/default/files/styles/product_hero_desktop/public/images/ehc-assistant-meal.jpg?itok=wjxvmJ85.

Delivering adequate energy and protein intake is significant, with older individuals being more likely to need higher amounts of protein—1.0–1.5 grams per kilogram body weight per day—to favor muscle mass and prevent sarcopenia. Micronutrients such as calcium, vitamin D, vitamin B12, and zinc are also essential since deficiencies are common and can exacerbate illness. Nutrient-dense foods, oral nutritional supplements, and fortified foods are most generally used to enhance intake, particularly in patients with reduced appetite or difficulty eating. Social and environmental reasons, such as meal eating alone, poverty, or unavailability of quality food, also need to be addressed by supportive community schemes, home meal delivery programs, or caregiver assistance. Multidisciplinary team care with dietitians, physicians, and caregivers results in improved outcomes through ensuring continuous surveillance and optimization of nutritional interventions. In the institutional setting, restructuring the eating environment and offering food choices can improve intake and satisfaction. Ultimately, an active and multi-faceted approach to the prevention and treatment of malnutrition in older adults not only improves physical health and cognitive function but also preserves independence and quality of life.

REFERENCES

1. Agarwal, E., Isenring, E., Marshall, S., et al. (2016). Optimizing nutrition in residential aged care: A narrative review. https://core.ac.uk/download/196601588.pdf (accessed on 12th July 2025).
2. Ford, C. D., Sawyer, P., Parmelee, P., Clay, O. J., Crowther, M., & Allman, R. M. (2014). Race and Sex Differences in Correlates of Systolic Blood Pressure in Community-Dwelling Older Adults. *Journal of health disparities research and practice*, *7*(4), 32–50.(accessed on 12th July 2025).
3. Volkert, D., Beck, A. M., Cederholm, T., Cruz-Jentoft, A., Goisser, S., Hooper, L., Kiesswetter, E., Maggio, M., Raynaud-Simon, A., Sieber, C. C., Sobotka, L., van Asselt, D., Wirth, R., & Bischoff, S. C. (2019). ESPEN guideline on clinical nutrition and hydration in geriatrics. *Clinical nutrition (Edinburgh, Scotland)*, *38*(1), 10–47. https://doi.org/10.1016/j.clnu.2018.05.024(accessed on 12th July 2025).
4. Rémond, D., Shahar, D. R., Gille, D., Pinto, P., Kachal, J., Peyron, M. A., Dos Santos, C. N., Walther, B., Bordoni, A., Dupont, D., Tomás-Cobos, L., & Vergères, G. (2015). Understanding the gastrointestinal tract of the elderly to develop dietary solutions that prevent malnutrition. *Oncotarget*, *6*(16), 13858–13898. https://doi.org/10.18632/oncotarget.4030(accessed on 12th July 2025).
5. Downey, C. L., Young, A., Burton, E. F., Graham, S. M., Macfarlane, R. J., Tsapakis, E. M., & Tsiridis, E. (2017). Dementia and osteoporosis in a geriatric population: Is there a common link?. *World journal of orthopedics*, *8*(5), 412–423. https://doi.org/10.5312/wjo.v8.i5.412 (accessed on 12th July 2025).
6. Fox, S., Davie, L., & Rataj, A. (2016). Collaborating to Create Elder Friendly Communities in New Hampshire: A Scan of the Current Landscape. Research report completed for the NH Endowment for Health, Concord, NH..pdf (accessed on 12th July 2025).
7. Lampugnale, C. A. (2017). Surgical assessment of the geriatric oncology patient. *BU*. https://open.bu.edu/bitstream/2144/26707/5/Lampugnale_bu_0017N_13146.pdf (accessed on 12th July 2025).
8. Malafarina, V., Reginster, J. Y., Cabrerizo, S., et al. (2017). Nutritional status and nutritional treatment are related to outcomes and mortality in older adults with hip fractures. https://core.ac.uk/download/pdf/212756692.pdf (accessed on 12th July 2025).
9. The Stern Center for Evidence-Based Policy (2015). The Stern Center for Evidence-Based Policy, 2015. The Stern Center for Evidence-Based Policy ("Stern Center"), University of Pittsburgh's Health Policy Institute. (accessed on 12th July 2025).
10. Wynn-Grundy, N. J. (2016). Undiagnosed depression in the elderly and healthcare education. https://core.ac.uk/download/70426926.pdf (accessed on 12th July 2025).
11. Whitelock, E., & Ensaff, H. (2018). On Your Own: Older Adults' Food Choice and Dietary Habits. *Nutrients*, *10*(4), 413. https://doi.org/10.3390/nu10040413(accessed on 12th July 2025).

INDEX

C

F

G

H

I

J

K

L

M

N

O

P

W

Z